Medical Office Procedures

10TH Edition

Nenna L. Bayes, AAS, BBA, M.Ed., CPC
Professor, Program Coordinator of Office Systems
Administration and Medical Information Technology,
Retired Ashland Community and Technical College

Amy L. Blochowiak, MBA, RHIT, ACS, AIAA, AIRC, ARA, FLHC, FLMI, HCSA, HIA, HIPAA, MHP, PCS, SILA-F
Healthcare Business Professional Program Director
& Instructor
Northeast Wisconsin Technical College

McGraw Hill

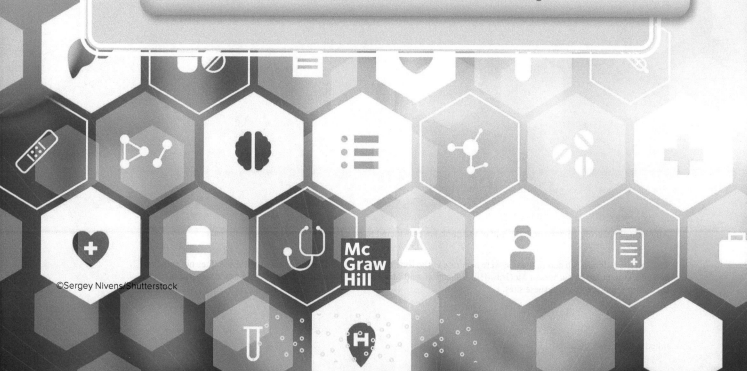

MEDICAL OFFICE PROCEDURES

Published by McGraw Hill LLC, 1325 Avenue of the Americas, New York, NY 10019. Copyright ©2022 by McGraw Hill LLC. All rights reserved. Printed in the United States of America. No part of this publication may be reproduced or distributed in any form or by any means, or stored in a database or retrieval system, without the prior written consent of McGraw Hill LLC, including, but not limited to, in any network or other electronic storage or transmission, or broadcast for distance learning.

Some ancillaries, including electronic and print components, may not be available to customers outside the United States.

This book is printed on acid-free paper.

2 3 4 5 6 7 8 9 CPI 24

ISBN 978-1-260-59792-9
MHID 1-260-59792-X

Cover Image: ©*Tyler Olson/Shutterstock*

mheducation.com/highered

Brief Contents

Table of Contents

About the Authors

Nenna L. Bayes, AAS, BBA, M.Ed., CPC, has coauthored and reviewed various titles within the medical administrative fields. She earned an associate of applied business degree, a bachelor of business administration degree, and a master of arts degree in education from Morehead State University. During her tenure, she has taught numerous courses within the administrative and medical administrative curriculum. She is a retired professor and program coordinator for the Office Systems Technology and Medical Information Technology programs at Ashland Community and Technology College in Ashland, Kentucky, and has received many teaching excellence awards. She is also a Certified Professional Coder (CPC). Prior to teaching, she worked in various medical office environments. Additionally, she is a member of the American Academy of Professional Coders (AAPC) and the American Health Information Management Association (AHIMA).

She lives in Flatwoods, Kentucky, with her husband and is blessed to have two children (a daughter and a son), a daughter-in-law, and three granddaughters. She is actively involved in music and enjoys camping in her leisure time.

Amy L. Blochowiak, MBA, RHIT, ACS, AIAA, AIRC, ARA, FLHC, FLMI, HCSA, HIA, HIPAA, MHP, PCS, SILA-F, has coauthored and reviewed various textbooks within the medical administrative and insurance fields. She earned associate degrees in medical office mid-management and health information technology from Northeast Wisconsin Technical College, bachelor's degrees in both business administration and marketing from Lakeland College, and a master's degree in business administration from Lakeland College. She is currently the program director and instructor for the Healthcare Business Professional program at Northeast Wisconsin Technical College, where she sits on many committees and shares her passion for student success. Prior to teaching, she worked in various insurance industry roles for over 16 years. She is a member of the American Health Information Management Association (AHIMA).

Preface

The medical profession is complex and demanding. The typical physician rarely has time to attend to the administrative responsibilities of the office. Successfully performing the work of an administrative medical assistant requires a foundation of procedural knowledge as well as continuing education to keep up to date with technology, including computer skills, new computer software, and legal guidelines. This tenth edition of *Medical Office Procedures (MOP)* provides the required background for the responsibilities of the administrative medical assistant. To prepare students for the ever-increasing use of technology in the medical office, this revision places continued importance on the computerization of routine tasks and of communications.

Job opportunities in the medical field often change with varying degrees of education and specialization required. This textbook allows for the integrated application of office procedures, skills, and knowledge in the classroom through the use of projects and simulations. Students learn to perform the duties of the administrative medical assistant under realistic conditions and with realistic pressures that require them to organize the work and set priorities.

HERE'S WHAT YOU AND YOUR STUDENTS CAN EXPECT FROM *MOP*:

McGraw-Hill's new electronic health record tool, EHRclinic, provides a practice environment, giving students the look and feel of a real EHR system. EHRclinic is fully integrated with Connect and autograded.

- Chapter projects, end-of-chapter material, and simulations are available online in Connect, making it even easier for you and your students to access all the necessary materials in one convenient place.
- Connect provides simulated EHRclinic exercises in select chapters. These exercises simulate the use of a practice management software system to complete various tasks.
- Each chapter has been matched up with updated ABHES and CAAHEP competencies, which are listed in the chapter opener.
- The end-of-chapter material—including the Using Terminology matching questions, Checking Your Understanding multiple-choice questions, and Thinking It Through critical-thinking questions—has been updated.
- The chapter projects have been updated and aligned with the organization of the book.
- The updated Working Papers are both at the back of the book and available electronically on the Instructor Resource site in Connect.
- Art and screenshots have been updated.

ORGANIZATION OF *MOP*

MOP is divided into four parts:

Part	Coverage
Part 1: The Administrative Medical Assistant's Career	Introduces the administrative medical assistant's career, defining the tasks, describing the work environments, and introducing medical ethics and medical law as they apply to the administrative medical assistant. Includes section on HIPAA as it relates to the role of the administrative medical assistant.
Part 2: Administrative Responsibilities	Introduces specific administrative responsibilities, including a chapter on managing health information with technology, and provides opportunities for practice.
Part 3: Practice Financials	Discusses procedures for preparing and organizing patients' charts and bills/insurance. Includes section on compliance and introduction to the new *ICD-10-CM* code set.
Part 4: Preparing for Employment	Prepares students for employment by covering all steps of the job-search process, from completing applications to interviews and follow-up.

NEW TO THE TENTH EDITION!

The following are the key changes in the tenth edition. Chapter updates include:

- new EHRclinic exercises available in Connect.
- CAAHEP and ABHES competencies aligned with that chapter.
- updated photos.
- updated key terms.
- updated professional organization information.
- new Breach Notification section.
- updated medical laws.
- end-of-chapter tabular summary correlated with the learning outcomes.
- end-of-chapter matching and multiple-choice review questions.
- updated Thinking It Through questions.
- updated EHRclinic screenshots.

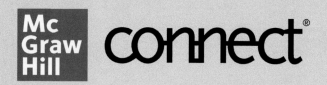

Instructors: Student Success Starts with You

Tools to enhance your unique voice

Want to build your own course? No problem. Prefer to use our turnkey, prebuilt course? Easy. Want to make changes throughout the semester? Sure. And you'll save time with Connect's auto-grading too.

65%
Less Time
Grading

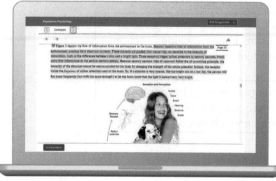

Laptop: McGraw Hill; Woman/dog: George Doyle/Getty Images

Study made personal

Incorporate adaptive study resources like SmartBook® 2.0 into your course and help your students be better prepared in less time. Learn more about the powerful personalized learning experience available in SmartBook 2.0 at **www.mheducation.com/highered/connect/smartbook**

Affordable solutions, added value

Make technology work for you with LMS integration for single sign-on access, mobile access to the digital textbook, and reports to quickly show you how each of your students is doing. And with our Inclusive Access program you can provide all these tools at a discount to your students. Ask your McGraw Hill representative for more information.

Padlock: Jobalou/Getty Images

Solutions for your challenges

A product isn't a solution. Real solutions are affordable, reliable, and come with training and ongoing support when you need it and how you want it. Visit **www. supportateverystep.com** for videos and resources both you and your students can use throughout the semester.

Checkmark: Jobalou/Getty Images

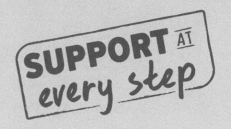

Students: Get Learning That Fits You

Effective tools for efficient studying

Connect is designed to make you more productive with simple, flexible, intuitive tools that maximize your study time and meet your individual learning needs. Get learning that works for you with Connect.

Study anytime, anywhere

Download the free ReadAnywhere app and access your online eBook or SmartBook 2.0 assignments when it's convenient, even if you're offline. And since the app automatically syncs with your eBook and SmartBook 2.0 assignments in Connect, all of your work is available every time you open it. Find out more at **www.mheducation.com/readanywhere**

> *"I really liked this app—it made it easy to study when you don't have your textbook in front of you."*
>
> - Jordan Cunningham,
>   Eastern Washington University

Calendar: owattaphotos/Getty Images

Everything you need in one place

Your Connect course has everything you need—whether reading on your digital eBook or completing assignments for class, Connect makes it easy to get your work done.

Learning for everyone

McGraw Hill works directly with Accessibility Services Departments and faculty to meet the learning needs of all students. Please contact your Accessibility Services Office and ask them to email accessibility@mheducation.com, or visit **www.mheducation.com/about/accessibility** for more information.

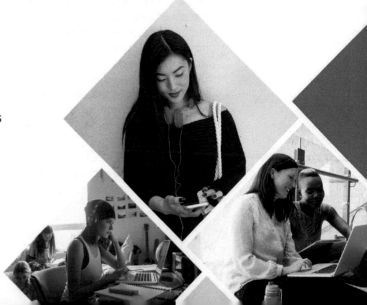

SIMULATIONS

We know that hands-on experience is an extremely valuable tool for your students. To provide that "real-life" experience, *Medical Office Procedures* features simulations that help students understand what it feels like to work in a medical practice. A 4-day simulation appears at the end of Chapters 5 and 9. The text provides instructions for the completion of the simulation. In each simulation, the student listens to the "Simulation Recordings" that accompany the program (available on Connect). The recordings contain conversations between Linda Schwartz (the doctor's administrative medical assistant, with whom the student will identify) and Dr. Karen Larsen, various patients, and other office callers. (*Note:* The student may use the simulation recordings individually, or the recordings may be assigned for use by the class as a whole. A complete transcript of the Simulation Recordings appears in the *Instructor's Manual* located within the Instructor Resources on Connect.)

Student Materials

In the "Working Papers" section at the back of the text, there are forms, medical histories, handwritten drafts, incoming correspondence, and other communications needed to complete the projects and the simulations that are provided. These Working Papers, as well as additional Project Resource Materials, are available on the Instructor Resource site in Connect.

EHRclinic Exercises ⏰EHRclinic

The tenth edition of *Medical Office Procedures* now includes McGraw-Hill's new electronic health records tool, EHRclinic. EHRclinic provides realistic experiences in online electronic health records, practice management applications, and interoperable physician-based functionality. Integrated within Connect, EHRclinic allows instructors to easily incorporate these exercises into their curriculum with assignments that are assignable and autograded. EHRclinic exercises are closely aligned with course content and include assessments that measure and map student performance, allowing instructors to save time while improving outcomes.

Chapter Projects

Chapter projects, which are a critical part of practice associated with *Medical Office Procedures,* give students the opportunity to get hands-on experience with medical office tasks. Completing on-the-job tasks, especially those related to practice management software, is an important aspect of an administrative medical assistant's work. *MOP* now offers these options for completing these tasks:

- Connect Simulated EHRclinic Exercises: Connect provides EHRclinic exercises that *simulate* the use of a practice management software system. The simulated exercises cover key practice management tasks to provide experience in working with patient, insurance, procedure, diagnosis, and transaction databases. Students will experience the look and feel of using live software, without actually having to download any software. Instructors can add them to their course by accessing them in "Assignments." Students can follow the instructions printed in the relevant chapter projects and simulations. More detailed instructor information can also be found in the Instructor Resources site in Connect.
- Hardcopy or manual work: As always, your students will also have the option of experiencing the manual version of these practice management exercises, using the various resources included in the Working Papers and Connect. See the chapter projects for specific instructions regarding the manual options.

Instructor Resources

You can rely on the following materials to help you and your students work through the exercises in the book. The following supplements can all be found with the Instructor Resources, located through the Library tab on Connect:

- Instructor's Manual with course overview; sample syllabi; project and simulation documents; answer keys for end-of-chapter questions; and correlations to competencies from several organizations, such as ABHES and CAAHEP.
- A PowerPoint slide presentation for each chapter, containing teaching notes correlated to learning outcomes. Each presentation seeks to reinforce key concepts and provide a visual for students. The slides are excellent for in-class lectures.
- Test bank for use in classroom assessment. The comprehensive test bank includes a variety of question types, with each question linked directly to its learning outcome, Bloom's Taxonomy, and difficulty level. The test bank is available in Connect, a Word version, and a computerized version (TestGen).
- Instructor Asset Map to help you find the teaching material you need. These online chapter tables are organized by learning outcomes and allow you to find instructor notes, PowerPoint slides, and even test bank suggestions with ease! The Asset Map is a completely integrated tool designed to help you plan and instruct your courses efficiently and comprehensively. It labels and organizes course material for use in a multitude of learning applications.
- Additional materials needed to complete chapter projects.

Knowing the importance of flexibility and digital learning, McGraw-Hill has created multiple assets to enhance the learning experience no matter what the class format—traditional, online, or hybrid. This product is designed to help instructors and students be successful, with digital solutions proven to drive student success.

To the Student

You have chosen a fascinating, challenging profession. The field of healthcare is growing at a rapid pace, providing many opportunities for the trained professional. Welcome to an educational resource designed to prepare you for immediate and long-range success as an administrative medical assistant. In this course, you will use *Medical Office Procedures (MOP)* not only as a source of practical information but also as an instrument for realistic practice in applying what you have learned. Throughout the chapters, you will be asked to apply your newly acquired knowledge—not simply to tell how or why you would use the information on the job. You will then repeatedly apply the information throughout the text.

As you complete the designated projects within the text, you will accumulate many of the medical records and correspondence needed in the simulations that occur after Chapters 5 and 9. You will be asked to assume the role of Linda Schwartz, an administrative medical assistant. During each simulation, you will handle various tasks assigned by the physician, the patients, and other office callers after listening carefully to recorded conversations. With some instructor guidance, you will perform your duties in an appropriate manner. You will be performing a variety of closely related administrative medical office tasks in the simulations: answering the telephone, scheduling appointments, taking messages, filing, preparing bills, and so on. You will gain proficiency in performing a wide range of administrative activities and in coping with a variety of problems and pressures in the medical office. All these activities will help you strive to organize work, set priorities, relate one task to another, and manage time. After completing these simulations, you will find that you are well prepared for the transition from classroom to office.

Starting with Part 2, you will be "working" for Dr. Karen Larsen, a family practitioner. As directed, ***save your work from the chapter projects.*** This work will form the basis for your "office files." In the simulations, you will use and add to these files. Essential patient data and forms are provided in the Working Papers section of the book, Connect, or your instructor's learning management system. You will also need the following supplies:

- File folder labels and 31 file folders
- A ring binder or a file folder to serve as your appointment book if you are not using Connect to complete exercises
- An expandable portfolio to serve as your file cabinet (all your office files can be stored in this portfolio)
- Paper for printing
- External storage device, such as a USB flash drive, to store the projects as directed
- Miscellaneous items—rubber bands, a notepad, pens, pencils, paper clips, and so on

Acknowledgments

Suggestions have been received from faculty and students throughout the country. This is vital feedback that is relied upon with each edition. Each person who has offered comments and suggestions has our thanks. The efforts of many people are needed to develop and improve a product. Among these people are the reviewers and consultants who point out areas of concern, cite areas of strength, and make recommendations for change. In this regard, the following instructors provided feedback that was enormously helpful in preparing the tenth, and previous editions, of *MOP*.

REVIEWERS FOR THE TENTH EDITION

Many instructors assisted in reviewing the ninth edition manuscript, helping us shape the content for this tenth edition, and we thank them for their feedback and insightful suggestions:

Beverly Bartholomew, M.Ed., CPC, CPC-I
Wake Tech Community College

Dr. Melba Bolling
Virginia Highlands Community College

Lisa Branham, MLIS, MEd
Greenville Technical College

Sharon Breeding, MAE
Bluegrass Community and Technology

Tanya Byrd-Johnson, BBA, MEd
West Georgia Technical College

Tammy A Davis, MHA, RHIA, CHTS-PW, CAHIMS
Southeast Community and Technical college

Mary Donahee-Rader, BBA, CMA(AAMA)
Schoolcraft College

Maya Fernandez, Ed.D., MBA
Cedar Valley College

Savanna Garrity, MPA, CPC
Madisonville Community College

Brandy V. Gustauvs, DHSc, MS, RHIA, CCA
St. John's River State College

Starra Herring, BSHA, BSAH, CMA(AAMA), AHI, MBA, MAHA
Stanly Community College

Coleen S. Jones, MSEd
Valencia College

Jackie Jones, MS, RHIA
Delgado Community College

Jane A. Jones, BS, MAT, COI, CMAA, CEHRS
Mountain Empire Community College

Bette Keeny, MS
Reading Area Community College

Sheryl Krey, MBA, CMPB, CHRS, CHIS
Washtenaw Community College

Kathleen Locke, MBA
Spartanburg Community College

Christine Malone, Ed.D, MBA, MHA,
CMPE, CPHRM, FACHE, EvCC
Everett Community College

Candice Milam, CMA (AAMA), MEd.
Danville Area Community College

Cheryl A Miller, MBA/HCM
Westmoreland County Community
College

Tiffinee Morgan, Professor, CMAA
West Kentucky Community and
Technical College

Julie L. Myhre, BA, CMT-R, RHIT
Century College

Rose Nelson, (MAAC), (BCSC),
(EHRC), (PHIC)
The Workforce Institutes City College

Barbara Parker, BSEd, CMA (AAMA),
CPC
Olympic College

Patricia A. Saccone, MA, RHIA, CDIP,
CCS-P, CPB
Waubonsee Community College
Aurora Illinois

Wendy Sammons, CMA, AAT, LPN
Lanier Technical college

Sonya L. Sample, MSHRD
Clemson University

Stephanie Vergne, MAED, RHIA, CPC
Hazard Community & Technical
College

ACKNOWLEDGMENTS FROM THE AUTHORS

To the students and instructors who use this book, your feedback and suggestions have made *MOP* a better learning tool for all.

I especially want to thank the editorial team at McGraw-Hill—Michelle Vogler, Marah Bellegarde, Erin DeHeck, and Ann Courtney—for their enthusiastic support and their willingness to go the extra mile to get this book revised.

And to my loving and supportive family: my husband, Bruce; my children, Jennifer and Andrew and his wife, Ashley; my three amazing granddaughters, Addison, Alianna, and Aubriella for their unending love and support. To my loving and supportive mom who lost her brief battle with pancreatic cancer during the final stage of MOP10 but remained a constant source of encouragement and to my dad, who passed away but continues to encourage me. To each of you—your constant encouragement keeps me moving forward. Thank you.

Nenna Bayes

Thank you to the students and instructors that use this textbook. Your suggestions and feedback helps us make improvements to ensure we put forth the best learning tool for everyone.

I also want to thank the editorial team at McGraw-Hill for their continued support.

To my family: my husband, Tom; my children, Brandon and his wife Maria, Bryanna and her significant other Ken, thanks for always encouraging me to try new things and providing support when I need it most.

Amy Blochowiak

PART 1

The Administrative Medical Assistant's Career

CHAPTER 1
The Administrative Medical Assistant

CHAPTER 2
Medical Ethics, Law, and Compliance

Welcome to *Medical Office Procedures*! This textbook has been written specifically to provide you with the skills and knowledge you will need to succeed as an administrative medical assistant. In Part 1, you will learn about the role of the administrative medical assistant, as well as legal and ethical aspects of the career.

CONSIDER THIS: Physicians' offices, hospitals, clinics, and other employers hire administrative medical assistants. *In what type of medical setting do you intend to pursue your career?*

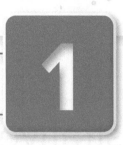

The Administrative Medical Assistant

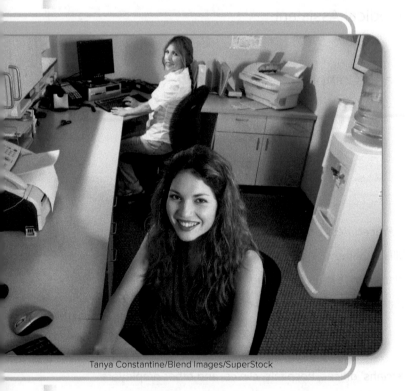

Tanya Constantine/Blend Images/SuperStock

LEARNING OUTCOMES

After studying this chapter, you will be able to

1.1 describe the tasks and skills required of an administrative medical assistant.

1.2 list and define at least three personal attributes essential for an administrative medical assistant.

1.3 describe the employment opportunities in various medical settings and specialties and nonmedical settings.

1.4 identify and define at least six positive work attitudes that contribute to the work ethic and professionalism of an administrative medical assistant.

1.5 list three advantages of professional affiliation and certification.

1.6 apply elements of good interpersonal communication to relationships with patients and others within the medical environment.

KEY TERMS

Study these important words, which are defined in this chapter, to build your professional vocabulary:

AAMA	certification	good judgment	punctuality
accuracy	confidentiality	honesty	self-motivation
administrative medical assistant (AMA)	dependability	IAAP	tact
	efficiency	initiative	team player
AHDI	empathy	maturity	thoroughness
AMT	ethnocentrism	problem-solving	work ethic
assertiveness	flexibility	professional image	

ABHES

1.a. Describe the current employment outlook for the medical assistant.

1.c. Describe and comprehend medical assistant credentialing requirements, the process to obtain the credential, and the importance of credentialing.

1.d. List the general responsibilities and skills of the medical assistant.

4.h. Demonstrate compliance with HIPAA guidelines, the ADA Amendments Act, and the Health Information Technology for Economic and Clinical Health (HITECH) Act.

5.a. Respond appropriately to patients with abnormal behavior patterns.

5.b.1. Use empathy when communicating with terminally ill patients.

5.c. Assist the patient in navigating issues and concerns that may arise (i.e., insurance policy information, medical bills, and physician/provider orders).

5.f. Demonstrate an understanding of the core competencies for Interprofessional Collaborative Practice (i.e., values/ethics; roles/responsibilities; interprofessional communication; teamwork).

5.h. Display effective interpersonal skills with patients and healthcare team members.

5.i. Demonstrate cultural awareness.

7.g. Display professionalism through written and verbal communications.

8.j. Make adaptations for patients with special needs (psychological or physical limitations).

10.b. Demonstrate professional behavior.

10.c. Explain what continuing education is and how it is acquired.

www.abhes.org/accreditationmanual

The ABHES standards appear with permission of The Accrediting Bureau of Health Education Schools

CAAHEP

V.C.3. Recognize barriers to communication.

V.C.4. Identify techniques for overcoming communication barriers.

V.C.18.a. Discuss examples of diversity—cultural.

V.C.18.b. Discuss examples of diversity—social.

V.C.18.c. Discuss examples of diversity—ethnic.

V.P.5.a. Coach patients appropriately considering cultural diversity.

V.P.5.c. Coach patients appropriately considering communication barriers.

V.A.1.a. Demonstrate empathy.

V.A.3.a Demonstrate respect for individual diversity, including gender.

V.A.3.b. Demonstrate respect for individual diversity, including race.

V.A.3.c. Demonstrate respect for individual diversity, including religion.

V.A.3.d. Demonstrate respect for individual diversity, including age.

V.A.3.e. Demonstrate respect for individual diversity, including economic status.

V.A.3.f. Demonstrate respect for individual diversity, including appearance.

X.A.1. Demonstrate sensitivity to patient rights.

X.C.5. Discuss licensure and certification as they apply to healthcare providers.

XI.C.1.a. Define *ethics*.

XI.C.1.b Define *morals*.

XI.C.2. Differentiate between personal and professional ethics.

XI.C.3. Identify the effect of personal morals on professional performance.

2015 Standards and Guidelines for the Accreditation of Educational Programs in Medical Assisting, Appendix B, Core Curriculum for Medical Assistants, Medical Assisting Education Review Board (MAERB), 2015.

INTRODUCTION

As the population ages, new healthcare reforms are implemented, and newer technologies, medicine, and treatments are introduced into the healthcare industry, the opportunities for rewarding careers in medical environments increase. These changes also pose new challenges for healthcare professionals. Legal and ethical issues abound. Following procedures that comply with government regulations concerning patients' privacy and security is also critical.

Because of rapid changes and the increasing complexity of the healthcare industry, continuing education is necessary to succeed in performing the role of an administrative medical assistant. Equally important is exhibiting the personal attributes and work ethic that contribute to the smooth and efficient operation of the medical practice team.

1.1 TASKS AND SKILLS

The healthcare industry focuses on preventing, diagnosing, treating, and managing diseases. Delivery of healthcare services is provided by trained professionals such as doctors, nurses, dietitians, physical and occupational therapists, nurses, and medical assistants in a variety of settings. Medical assistants are medical office professionals who capably perform a number of tasks in a wide variety of settings. Administrative tasks are those procedures used to keep the offices in medical practices running efficiently. Clinical tasks are those procedures the medical assistant may perform to aid the physician in the medical treatment of a patient. General tasks are skills and knowledge that enable the medical assistant to function within the office and patient environment. The American Association of Medical Assistants' Role Delineation Chart outlines the areas of competence you must master as an entry-level medical assistant. It provides the basis for medical assisting and evaluation. Students in an accredited medical assisting program are required to master the three areas of competence: clinical, administrative, and general. The AAMA Role Delineation Chart is also a good reference source that identifies the skills, duties, and procedures that medical assistants (administrative, clinical, and general) are educated to perform. For more information on the AAMA, please visit www.aama-ntl.org. Students in an administrative medical assistant program need to master the administrative and general competencies.

This textbook concentrates on administrative responsibilities, which involve the technical skills and personal traits required in most medical office careers. Throughout the text, the administrative medical assistant is often referred to as the "assistant" or as the "AMA" rather than by the full title. Other occupational titles for the administrative medical assistant are "medical receptionist" and "front office specialist."

Administrative Medical Assisting Tasks

The **administrative medical assistant (AMA)** is a professional office worker dedicated to assisting in the care of patients. To effectively perform all the required tasks, an assistant must be proficient in a number of skills. Hard skills, which are teachable, measurable skills, are used by the administrative medical assistant to perform many of the required office tasks.

The following are the major categories of tasks performed by an administrative medical assistant:

- Front desk procedures
- Scheduling
- Records management
- Administrative duties
- Financial

Front Desk. The administrative medical assistant greets patients and other visitors, such as family members and pharmaceutical representatives. The assistant also verifies and updates personal and demographic data about patients, explains the fees that will be charged for services, collects payments, and guides patients through their medical office encounters. The area should be kept clean and well-organized. All information should be maintained in a manner that protects the confidentiality of all patients. This is discussed in more detail later in this chapter and in a later chapter.

Scheduling. The administrative medical assistant answers the telephone; schedules future office appointments either by phone, electronically, or in person; schedules out-of-office encounters, such as hospital admissions, laboratory testing, and referrals to specialists; and forwards telephone calls and/or takes messages according to office procedures.

Records Management. The administrative medical assistant creates and maintains patient medical records (referred to as charts, electronic medical records, and/or electronic health records); stores and retrieves the records for use during encounters with physicians; and files other kinds of documents. The assistant begins the electronic chart by inputting patient demographic and financial information into the electronic database. As offices continue the process of converting to electronic health records, the assistant may assume the responsibility for scanning hardcopy charts into the electronic database.

Administrative Duties. The administrative medical assistant opens and sorts incoming mail, prepares outgoing mail, and composes routine correspondence. The assistant also maintains physicians' schedules, which involves keeping track of the time required for office encounters with patients, meetings, and conferences, as well as coordinating patients' hospital admissions and surgical procedures.

Financial. The administrative medical assistant codes or verifies codes for diagnoses and procedures; processes and tracks insurance claims; posts payments and prepares patients' bills; assists with banking duties; guides patients to available financial arrangements for payment; and maintains financial records.

Administrative Medical Assisting Skills

The work of an administrative medical assistant, which requires many technical and personal skills, is interesting and varied. Customer service to patients and other medical office team members is also provided by the administrative medical assistant. The role of the administrative medical assistant differs from that of the clinical medical assistant in that the clinical portion deals exclusively with the performance of medical tasks, such as taking blood samples and preparing a patient for a medical procedure. Administrative medical assistants focus on administrative tasks ("front office skills"), such as those listed in subsequent sections.

Communication Skills. The assistant must understand and use impeccable English grammar, style, punctuation, and spelling in both writing and speaking. These skills enable the assistant to handle correspondence, to maintain medical records, and to interact professionally with staff members, patients, and other medical personnel.

Electronic communication is the most common and efficient mode of communication for many messages. Even though this method of communication is fast, it requires proper grammar, punctuation, and structure. Taking the time to proofread all documents prior to transmission is extremely important. Errors lead to misinformation, which can lead to mistreatment.

In the communication cycle, our nonverbal communication style is as important as—if not more important than—our verbal message. Body posture, voice tonality, and facial expressions are just a few examples of our nonverbal communication techniques. We will discuss communication skills in more depth in a future chapter.

Communicating with other medical personnel requires the knowledge, correct spelling, and proper use of anatomy, physiology, and medical terminology, including nationally recognized medical abbreviations. Both correct pronunciation and written usage of the medical language are essential communication skills within the medical environment.

Mathematics Skills. The assistant must have accurate math skills to be able to maintain correct financial records, bill insurance carriers and patients, and order and arrange payment for office supplies. Many questions asked of the medical office assistant involve a patient's financial responsibility—for example, what will be the patient's balance after insurance has paid its portion. Addition, subtraction, and percentage calculations are three math skills the assistant needs. Extracting payment information from insurance data and correctly posting to patient accounts are areas of responsibility for the administrative medical assistant.

COMPLIANCE *TIP*

The administrative medical assistant plays an important role in ensuring that the medical office's procedures comply with government regulations concerning patients' records. These rules include keeping patient information private and following guidelines for release of this information. The Medical Ethics, Law, and Compliance chapter presents information on how to stay in compliance.

Organizational Skills. Controlling the usually hectic pace of the medical environment requires the assistant to have the skills of managing time and setting priorities. Systematic work habits, the willingness to take care of details, and the ability to handle several tasks at the same time (multitasking) are essential. Scheduling, updating and maintaining records, and keeping an orderly office require strong organizational skills. The most organized individual may still encounter many days when established priorities must be rearranged. When those days happen, the administrative medical assistant must be flexible and willing to reorganize and/or reprioritize.

Data Entry Skills. Accuracy in keying data and proficiency in proofreading are vital skills in the medical office. Patient personal and financial information is keyed into the electronic database and assimilated with the medical data to produce health claim forms and patient billings, as well as many other types of integrated reports. Errors in keyed information can have drastic effects on financial and medical information. As an example, a physician prescribes 0.025 mg of a medication, and the information is keyed erroneously as 0.25 mg. The patient may suffer serious or fatal complications, and the practice could incur legal consequences. Another example would be the patient's first name being keyed in as Bill when it is listed as William on his insurance card. This error would result in the insurance claim being denied, causing a delay in payment until the claim is corrected and resubmitted.

AMAs must possess strong keyboarding and word processing skills, including mastery of the alpha, numeric, and symbol keys and functions, such as mail merge, in order to effectively process administrative medical data. Producing professional letters, manuscripts, envelopes, and reports sends a nonverbal message about the professionalism of the office. Templates for chart notes and other commonly used formats save time and provide fewer opportunities for errors.

Computer and Equipment Skills. A basic understanding of a variety of technologies and the ability to use computers with mastery are essential workplace skills. Computers are used in every kind of healthcare setting for many different tasks. Computer programs handle electronic health records, word processing, financial spreadsheets, databases, and charts and visuals for speeches and presentations. With practice management programs, the assistant may handle patient and insurance billing and tracking, scheduling, account updating, records management, integrated reports (such as aging reports for patients and payers), and other tasks. Electronic scheduling is a popular feature because of its ease of searching and time-saving convenience.

Wireless technologies allow healthcare professionals who are away from their offices or facilities to contact staff members and computers from any location. They also have constant accessibility to patient records through interconnected electronic health records programs. Voice-recognition technology enables the physician to dictate notes using voice commands. The use of e-mail and text messaging to communicate is as widespread as telephone communication, both within the medical practice and among medical practices, hospitals, and insurance companies.

To assist effectively in patient care, the medical assistant must be able to use a computer to:

- process claims and bills and perform other routine financial tasks.
- maintain the office schedule.
- edit, revise, and generate documents.
- scan and send documents to other locations.
- communicate electronically within and outside the workplace.
- research and obtain information from electronic sources, such as the Internet.

Knowing how to use basic technologies, such as copiers, fax machines, scanners, and calculators has long been a requirement for every office professional. Multiple-line telephone systems are also standard office equipment. Records must be kept on service agreements, in addition to warranties, repair records, and instructional materials for each piece of equipment. Knowing where and whom to call when equipment malfunctions is critical to the efficient flow of the office environment. Continuing to develop computer skills and learning new technological applications are crucial to the effectiveness and career advancement of administrative medical assistants.

Interpersonal Skills. Excellent interpersonal skills often come from a genuine desire to work with people. This desire and these interpersonal skills are essential for the administrative medical assistant, who is usually the patient's first contact with the medical office. That contact sets the tone for the patient's visit and influences the patient's opinion of the physician and the practice.

Many patients need someone to assist them with understanding the medical jargon sent to them from parties such as insurance carriers. The medical office assistant serves as a liaison or advocate for the patient to help translate the insurance language into everyday language and explain other medical office information.

The assistant skilled in positive communication with patients is warm, open, and friendly. Patients appreciate attention and concern—for their schedules and their comfort. Effective interpersonal skills involve looking directly at the person being spoken to, speaking slowly and clearly, listening carefully, and checking for understanding of the communicated message. Communication is discussed in a future chapter.

Respect for and openness to the other person are often shown by a pleasant facial expression and a genuine, natural smile. At the heart of interpersonal skills is sensitivity to the feelings and situations of other people.

1.2 PERSONAL ATTRIBUTES

In addition to essential office hard skills, the success of the administrative medical assistant depends on a variety of soft skills. Soft skills are less tangible, more subjective attributes of an individual. A positive attitude toward work and a cheerful personality are examples of soft skills. *Personality* has been defined as the outward evidence of a person's character. Many aspects of personality are important in dealing with patients and other medical professionals.

Because patients entering a healthcare setting may be anxious, fearful, or unwell, most of them value a friendly, pleasant personality as the most important attribute of a medical assistant. The qualities discussed here are components of a pleasant personality and are useful professional and personal skills.

Genuine Liking for People

A genuine enjoyment of people and a desire to help them are keys to success in a medical assisting career. These qualities are expressed in the way you communicate with people through speech and body language.

Because patients may worry that they will be viewed only as numbers and notes on their patient charts, it is important that they feel recognized as individuals. In communicating with patients, your warmth and attentiveness help reassure patients and signal your desire to help. Looking directly at the patient and listening with attention communicate acceptance of the person. A pleasant facial expression, a natural smile, and a relaxed rather than rigid body posture are all body language signs that express openness and acceptance.

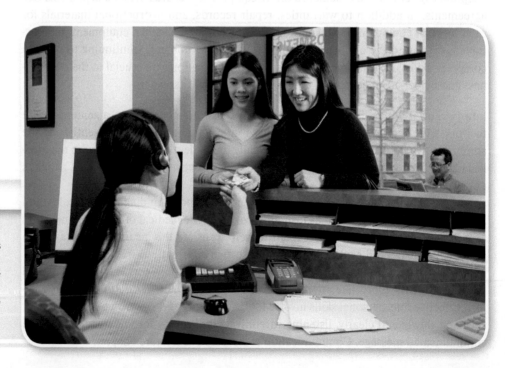

Figure 1.1

The administrative medical assistant enjoys working with people. *How do assistants show their care and concern for patients?* Fuse/Corbis/Getty Images

Viewing yourself and colleagues as integral medical office team members creates an atmosphere of cooperation and respect for individual differences. At times, personalities may seem to be in conflict; however, the individual who has a genuine liking of people will be able to respect differences within the team environment and accentuate the positiveness of cooperation through differences. Individuals change or lose positions more frequently due to the inability to get along with others than they do for lack of skills. Never underestimate the value of an open mind and of "playing nicely."

Cheerfulness

The ability to be pleasant and friendly is an asset in any career. Lifting patients' spirits helps build goodwill between them and the physician. A pleasant assistant can frequently head off difficulties that occur when patients become worried, anxious, confused, or irritable.

EXAMPLE: CHEERFULNESS TOWARD A FRUSTRATED PATIENT

It is five o'clock, normal closing time for the office. The doctor is behind schedule because of several difficult cases, and there are two patients yet to be seen in the waiting room. One of the patients approaches the assistant.

Patient: I've been waiting a long time to see the doctor. How much longer will I have to wait?

Despite feeling tired at the end of the day and ready to go home, the assistant remains cheerful and explains the situation without frustration.

Assistant: Dr. Larsen has had several difficult cases today that have caused this delay. She will see you next, but it may be another 20 to 30 minutes. Would you like to wait or would you prefer to reschedule your appointment?

In this example, the patient may be feeling forgotten or ignored. Frequently, delays do occur. Patients should be kept apprised of delays and given the opportunity to choose to continue to wait or to reschedule their appointment.

Empathy

Many of the personal traits needed to be a successful medical assistant spring from **empathy,** a sensitivity to the feelings and situations of other people. Empathy enables you to understand how a patient feels because you can mentally put yourself in the patient's situation. Empathetic phrases such as "Insurance forms can be confusing" or "You seem confused; may I help?" may be used to show the patient you are concerned about his or her situation. Phrases that emphasize yourself or give false impressions, such as "I completely understand how you feel," should be avoided. Everyone has had some personal experience with an illness or with not feeling well. Reminding yourself of how you felt and of how you wanted to be treated in that situation will help you treat patients with kindness.

EXAMPLE: EMPATHY TOWARD A PATIENT

Assistant: Mr. Patient, I realize you are not feeling well after your surgery yesterday. Would you feel more comfortable lying down while you wait?

Understand that nervous patients may not be listening clearly to your instructions. Offering to repeat them and answering questions are other examples of empathy.

The U.S. Department of Labor projects this field will grow much faster than the average, ranking medical assistants among the fastest-growing occupations for the 2016–2026 decade. In 2016, the Department of Labor *Occupational Outlook Handbook* reported 634,400 persons employed as medical assistants, with a projected 818,400 employed in 2026, a 29 percent increase. Fueling the rapid growth are advances in technologies, an aging population, and healthcare reform. Job opportunities are predicted to be excellent, especially for those applicants with formal training, experience, and/or certification.

The employment forecast for administrative medical assistants (formerly called medical secretaries) is projected to increase faster than the average for other occupations. This field is projected to increase by 15 percent or higher from 2016 to 2026. The number of people employed as administrative medical assistants in 2016 was estimated to be 574,000 with a projected increase to 654,800 by 2026. Administrative medical assistants have opportunities to advance into management positions, such as office manager or compliance officer. There are many organizations, institutions, and companies that operate in areas within or closely related to healthcare. Workers familiar with the healthcare environment are of value and in demand.

A thorough training in technical skills, the development of good interpersonal skills, and ongoing professional development help ensure a successful career for administrative medical assistants. Because the healthcare industry is booming, a well-trained medical assistant has a wide variety of opportunities in many different settings.

Physician Practice

The most common place of employment for the administrative medical assistant is in a physician practice. Many physicians are associated with a group practice—in which space, staff, and physical resources, such as equipment and laboratory facilities, are shared. A group practice may consist of physicians who are all generalists or who all have the same specialty, or it may be a combination of generalists and specialists.

There are many advantages to both doctors and patients in these larger practices. Doctors may better control spiraling overhead costs of operating an office. Such practices also give new physicians the opportunity to join an established practice and to acquire new patients to add to their clientele. Because of the large volume of patients, the administrative medical assistant may specialize in a task area, such as patient scheduling, or may perform a variety of duties.

Some administrative medical assistants work in a small office where one or two physicians practice. The assistant acts as the doctor's right hand, taking care of all administrative tasks. Working in a small office gives the assistant a great deal of responsibility, variety in the tasks to be completed, and an opportunity to develop close ties with patients and the physician.

There are job opportunities for assistants in a wide range of practices. Many such medical specialties are listed and defined in Table 1.1. In addition to these specialties, the American Medical Association (AMA) lists many other medical specialities and subspecialties. Many of the specialties on this expanded list are surgical practices related to the specialties shown in Table 1.1. However, there are also specialties that deal with new areas, such as undersea and aerospace medicine. Other specialties reflect the increased use of new technologies to treat illness. Interventional radiology is an example of such a specialty; it uses tools guided by radiologic imaging to perform procedures that are less invasive than those required with surgery.

Table 1.1 Examples of Medical Specialties and Subspecialties

Addiction Medicine: An addiction medicine specialist is a physician who diagnoses and treats the complications of substance abuse addiction, including the physical and psychological complications.

Allergy and Immunology: An allergist/immunologist diagnoses and manages disorders of the immune system.

Anesthesiology: An anesthesiologist maintains pain relief and stable body functions of patients during surgical, obstetric, and diagnostic procedures.

Bariatric: A bariatric physician specializes in the causes, treatment, and prevention of obesity.

Chiropractic: A chiropractor studies the disease process as a result of deviations/changes to the normal workings of the neuromuscular system. Common treatment options include body manipulation and other forms of therapy.

Dentistry: A dentist is concerned with the care and treatment of teeth and gums, especially prevention, diagnosis, and treatment of deformities, diseases, and traumatic injuries. Subspecialties include the following:

An **endodontist** specializes in root canal work.

A **forensic dentist** applies dental facts to legal issues.

An **oral surgeon** specializes in jaw surgery and extractions.

An **orthodontist** straightens teeth.

A **pedodontist** provides dental care for children.

A **periodontist** specializes in gum disease.

A **prosthodontist** specializes in dentures and artificial teeth.

Dermatology: A dermatologist diagnoses and treats diseases of the skin and related tissues.

Emergency Medicine: A physician who provides immediate decision making and necessary action to prevent further injury or death.

Family Practice: A family practice physician provides total healthcare for the individual and for the family.

Geriatrics: A geriatric specialist diagnoses and treats conditions and diseases that are specific to the older population.

Gynecology: A gynecologist is concerned with the diseases of the female genital tract, as well as female endocrinology and reproductive physiology.

Hospice: This field of medicine renders interdisciplinary care to individuals with life-threatening conditions. Physical (pain management), psychological, and spiritual services are given to the patient and the family. The primary focus of hospice care is quality of life.

Internal Medicine: An internist diagnoses a wide range of nonsurgical illnesses. Subspecialties include the following:

Cardiovascular Medicine: A cardiologist diagnoses and treats diseases of the heart, blood vessels, and lungs.

Endocrinology: An endocrinologist diagnoses and treats endocrine gland diseases.

Gastroenterology: A gastroenterologist diagnoses and treats diseases of the digestive tract and related organs.

Gerontology: A gerontologist treats the process and problems of aging.

Hematology: A hematologist diagnoses and treats diseases of the blood.

Immunology: An immunologist diagnoses and treats symptoms of immunity, induced sensitivity, and allergies.

Infectious Disease: A specialist in infectious disease diagnoses and treats all types of infectious diseases.

Nephrology: A nephrologist diagnoses and treats disorders of the kidneys and related functions.

Oncology: An oncologist diagnoses and treats cancer.

Pulmonary Disease: A pulmonologist diagnoses and treats lung disorders.

Rheumatology: A rheumatologist is concerned with the study, diagnosis, and treatment of rheumatic conditions.

Neurology: A neurologist diagnoses and treats disorders of the nervous system.

Obstetrics: An obstetrician provides care during pregnancy and childbirth.

Occupational Medicine: A specialist in occupational medicine works with companies to prevent and manage occupational and environmental injury, illness, and disability and to promote health and productivity of workers and their families and communities.

Ophthalmology: An ophthalmologist cares for the eyes and vision system.

Osteopathology: This field of medicine specializes in the diagnosis and treatment of the neuromusculoskeletal system.

Orthopedics: An orthopedic surgeon or orthopedist provides treatment of the musculoskeletal system.

Otorhinolaryngology: A physician in otorhinolaryngology specializes in the diagnosis and treatment of illnesses of the ears, nose, and throat (ENT).

Pathology: A pathologist investigates the causes of disease using biological, chemical, and scientific laboratory techniques.

Pediatrics: A pediatrician specializes in the comprehensive treatment of children. There are many pediatric subspecialties.

Physical Medicine/Rehabilitation: A physiatrist evaluates and treats all types of disease through physical means, such as heat, cold, massage, traction, therapeutic exercise, stimulation, and medications.

Plastic Surgery: A plastic surgeon repairs, replaces, and reconstructs physical defects through surgical means.

Psychiatry: A psychiatrist diagnoses and treats mental, emotional, and addictive disorders.

Radiology and Nuclear Medicine: A radiologist uses radioactive materials to diagnose and treat disease.

Thoracic Surgery: A thoracic surgeon uses surgery to diagnose or treat diseases of the chest.

Urology: A urologist diagnoses and treats diseases of the urinary tract and the adrenal glands.

Clinics

The administrative medical assistant may be employed by a clinic. A clinic may specialize in the diagnosis and treatment of a specific disorder—back pain, headache, mental health, or wound treatment, for example—and is considered an outpatient setting. Many clinics have a number of specialties within one building. The specialties may be related, so that the patient moves from department to department for extensive examination and specialty consultations.

Hospitals and Medical Centers

Hospitals and the large physical complexes that make up medical centers employ many administrative support personnel, particularly those skilled in specific medical office management tasks. Assistants may work in the admissions department in several areas of a hospital or medical center—the main admitting office, where patients are received for a stay in the hospital; admissions to the emergency room; or admissions for patients in same-day surgery clinics. Departments such as patient education, insurance, billing, social services, and medical records also need skilled and knowledgeable assistants. Career opportunities for assistants in these facilities will continue to grow along with the technological advances in diagnosis and treatment and the size of the aging population.

Care Facilities

Many facilities specialize in the short-term care of patients recovering after hospital stays. There are also patients who enter rehabilitation centers to improve the functioning of their back, arms, legs, hips, or hands. Other facilities provide long-term care for patients with chronic mental or physical illnesses. All of these facilities rely on skilled personnel who understand patients and their care.

Insurance Companies

The healthcare industry is subject to great pressure because of high health costs and the reality that people are living longer and often require greater care as they age. Insurance companies and government health insurance programs must ensure that claims from healthcare providers are "clean claims"—in other words, the claim forms are correct and complete. They employ administrative medical assistants who are skilled in handling medical documents and understand medical procedures. Other professionals who may be utilized by the insurance industry are Certified Medical Coders, Certified Medical Billers, and Certified Reimbursement Specialists. Assistants may work for the following:

- Large insurance companies specializing in healthcare, such as Anthem, Humana, Centene, WellCare Health, UnitedHealth Group, Aetna, and Cigna
- Government-sponsored programs, such as Medicare, Medicaid, Children's Health Insurance Program (CHIP), and Tricare
- Other insurers, some of which are sponsored by clubs, unions, and employee associations
- Managed care organizations and accountable care organizations

All areas of employment have complex needs and require the handling of tasks such as completing and checking reports received from doctors, coding diagnoses and procedures, adjusting claims, sending payments of claims, and renewing contracts.

Positive personality traits are developed into habits and skills that help the administrative medical assistant deal effectively with tasks and people. These habits and skills, which form a **work ethic,** greatly enhance employees' value in any medical work setting. Both hard skills and soft skills help develop a positive work ethic and professional display of work conduct.

Work Ethic

Employers responding to research surveys about employees rank certain habits and skills the highest. These habits and skills make the employee valuable to the practice. They are also often predictors of success in a medical office setting.

For centuries, work ethic, the outward display of an employee's values and standards, has been one of the foundation stones of business. Businesses have either been successful or failed as a direct result of employees' work ethics. We will discuss several areas in which employees outwardly display work ethic.

Accuracy. Because even a minor error may have major consequences for a patient's health, physicians rank **accuracy** as the most important employee trait. Although physicians may give exact instructions, they may not oversee tasks to completion. The physician counts on the assistant to perform tasks with complete correctness, including constant attention to detail.

Thoroughness. The careful and complete attention to detail required for accuracy is known as **thoroughness.** The thorough assistant produces work that is neat, accurate, and complete. This trait involves

- listening attentively.
- taking ample notes.
- paying attention to details, such as who, what, when, why, where, and how.
- verifying information.
- following through on details without having to be reminded.

The physician and other team members should be able to depend on the assistant to accomplish any task in a complete, accurate, and timely manner.

Dependability. The administrative medical assistant who finishes work on schedule, does required tasks without complaint (even when they are unpleasant), and

HIPAA *TIPS*

Patient confidentiality is an important part of Health Insurance Portability and Accountability Act (HIPAA) compliancy. Never discuss confidential patient information when using a speakerphone feature. Unauthorized parties may be able to overhear the conversation. It is important and courteous to advise speakers that they are being broadcast and to advise them of all other listeners in the room. If there is a possibility of being overheard by patients or visitors, the speakerphone should not be used. The voice should be kept sufficiently low even when not using a speakerphone.

You are responsible for making patient callbacks prior to leaving for the afternoon. The other medical office professional is absent, so you are also responsible for prepping charts for the next day's appointments. Using the speaker option on the telephone means that you can do other things at the same time, such as charting in patients' files. If you decide to use this option, what would you say to the patient on the phone to advise him or her that you are on speakerphone?

always communicates willingness to help is said to be a dependable employee. **Dependability** is closely related to accuracy and thoroughness. The dependable assistant

- asks questions and repeats instructions to avoid mistakes.
- asks for assistance with unfamiliar tasks.
- enters all data, such as insurance claim information and lab values, carefully.
- takes clear and complete messages.

Others can depend on the assistant to accomplish tasks effectively and as efficiently as possible. When an emergency situation occurs and the administrative medical assistant must miss work, contact the designated staff member, such as the office manager, immediately so tasks and responsibilities can be completed on time.

Efficiency. Effective individuals accomplish tasks, but efficiency has higher value in the work environment than effectiveness alone. Using time and other resources to avoid waste and unnecessary effort when completing tasks is the defining mark of **efficiency.** An example of an efficient administrative medical assistant is one who plans the day's work in advance, makes a schedule for completion, and assembles the materials and resources necessary to complete the tasks. Efficiency also includes the organizational ability to divide large, complex tasks into smaller, more manageable components. Rearranging resources to complete tasks efficiently may require change. Flexibility is a key component when working within a medical office environment.

Flexibility. The ability to adapt, to change gears quickly, and to respond to changing situations, interruptions, and delays is **flexibility.** The flexible assistant is able to respond calmly to last-minute assignments, to meet deadlines under pressure, and to handle several tasks at once. The ability to grasp new situations and new concepts quickly is an important aspect of flexibility. Being able to implement new ideas and good suggestions with self-confidence is a mark of flexibility.

The medical setting is very fluid. Advances in computer technology, new medical coding systems, and updates to the Health Insurance Portability and Accountability Act (HIPAA) and other healthcare laws pose frequent challenges to members of the

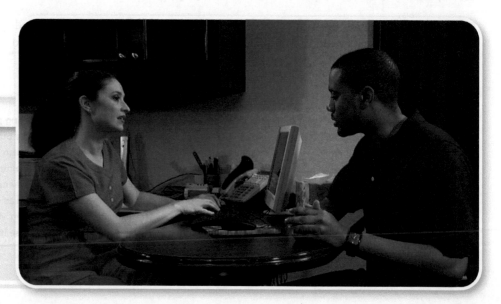

Figure 1.2

The administrative medical assistant shown here is entering insurance information for a new patient. *How can assistants ensure accuracy in their work?* Take One Digital Media/ McGraw-Hill

healthcare team. Flexibility and good judgment are key contributors to a smooth transition when changes occur in the medical office environment.

Good Judgment. The quality of **good judgment** involves the ability to use knowledge, experience, and logic to assess all the aspects of a situation in order to reach a sound decision. Frequently, good judgment is expressed by the administrative medical assistant who knows when to make a statement and when to withhold one. For example, choosing the right time and right words when making a suggestion to an employer or to other staff members shows good judgment. It may also be good judgment to decide that the suggestion should not be made because, based on your objective and honest evaluation of past experience, the suggestion will not be accepted.

Honesty. Telling the truth is **honesty.** It is expressed in words and actions. It is the quality that enables the physician to trust the administrative medical assistant at all times. The trustworthy assistant understands the serious nature of the physician's work and the confidential nature of the patient's dealings with the physician. The assistant can be trusted not to reveal any of a patient's data, any conversations, or any details, which must always remain confidential. Honesty is central to the integrity that allows the assistant to effectively represent the profession. Finally, the honest assistant demonstrates initiative by quickly reporting mistakes without attempting to cover them up or blame others.

Initiative. To take action independently is to show **initiative.** The administrative medical assistant works with certain routine administrative activities every day. Dealing with these often requires the assistant to take action without receiving specific instructions from the physician. The assistant's ability to move work forward and to resolve issues by using initiative is a valuable skill in a busy office.

Initiative also involves making unsolicited offers of help that mark a valued employee, one who goes beyond the job's regular responsibilities. For example, offering to stay late to help the physician or coworkers finish extra work is always appreciated. To give patients additional help, you may offer to call for a taxi after an appointment, obtain a wheelchair when needed, write out instructions, or open a door for a struggling patient. Medical office assistants who demonstrate initiative also have critical-thinking skills and problem-solving abilities.

Problem-Solving Ability. **Problem-solving** involves logically planning the steps needed to accomplish a task. Asking for advice when appropriate and acting wisely also demonstrate the ability to solve problems effectively. The administrative medical assistant who is adept at solving problems also has a basic understanding of the goals and requirements of the work environment. Critical-thinking skills and problem-solving skills work together to establish steps and reach solutions. Just as problem-solving involves logically planning steps, the assistant who uses critical-thinking skills looks at all possible resources to build the steps. Critical thinkers use past experiences and present resources and knowledge to form future solutions. In other words, they think "in and outside their box." Brainstorming, listing all possible ideas, with others allows the assistant to gather information that otherwise may not have been considered. Being able to produce solutions in a timely manner should be one of the goals of a problem-solving team.

Problem-solving is best accomplished when these steps are followed:

Step 1 Identify the problem.

Step 2 Set a goal (resolution of the problem).

Step 3 Gather information.

Step 4 Brainstorm possible solutions.

Step 5 Select and implement a solution.

Step 6 Evaluate the result(s).

Step 7 If the desired results did not meet the established goal, begin again with Step 1.

Punctuality. Being on time—**punctuality**—is important for the administrative medical assistant because of the physician's schedule and the need to complete routine duties before patients arrive. A medical office is often open for the staff a half hour before patient appointments. This is not a time for employees to use in getting from home to work. It is a time for planning the day's work, organizing tasks, and greeting patients who arrive before the start of business hours. It is common for an answering service to continue answering calls during this time to allow the assistant and other team members time to prepare. Given enough time, the self-motivated employee may prepare the next day's tasks prior to leaving at the end of the work shift.

Self-Motivation. The quality of **self-motivation** is expressed by a willingness to learn new duties or procedures without a requirement to do so. The administrative medical assistant who helps with work that needs to be done and learns new aspects of job responsibilities is self-motivated. Alertness is an aspect of self-motivation. This alertness enables the assistant to see and undertake jobs that need to be done and to anticipate the patients' and the physician's needs. A mix of self-motivation and tact should be used when seeking areas to assist fellow team members.

Tact. The ability to speak and act considerately, especially in difficult situations, is known as **tact.** Working with people in ways that show you are sensitive to their possible reactions helps you achieve the purpose at hand smoothly and without giving offense. Tactful manners and speech create goodwill with patients and other members of the medical office team.

Being a Member of the Team. Those who have the positive attitude of a **team player** are generous with their time, helping other staff members when necessary. A good team player observes stated office policies and quickly learns the unwritten rules of office life, such as

- when it is acceptable to sit at another employee's desk.
- whether it is acceptable to eat or drink at your workstation.
- how to time a break and determine how long it should be.
- when and in what manner it is acceptable to converse with coworkers.

Being a good team player also involves the simple courtesies: avoiding personal activities, phone calls, text messaging, and other social media; knocking before entering an office, even if the door is open; being careful about sharing details of your personal life in ordinary polite conversation; and avoiding the use of profanity and coarse language. Team players, moreover, are always careful to observe confidentiality by not discussing patients or commenting in any way about them or any other staff members.

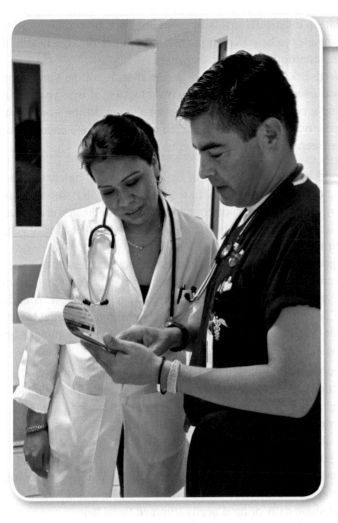

Working outside the traditional office environment, such as processing medical insurance claims from home, still requires the staff member to work as part of and consider the needs of the medical office team. Missing a deadline or keeping materials longer than anticipated can cause a ripple effect. Aggressive behavior within a team promotes ill feelings and a lack of cooperation; however, professionally assertive behavior among those working together as a team can promote positive attitudes toward daily responsibilities and a willingness to cooperate to accomplish goals.

Assertiveness. **Assertiveness** is the ability to step forward to make a point in a confident, positive manner. In some ways, assertiveness is the result of having acquired many of the habits, attitudes, and skills discussed here. Administrative medical assistants who are accurate, dependable, and honest and who understand and perform tasks with intelligence and good judgment are confident employees. They are able to step forward and contribute to a more efficient, more cordial work environment. Assertiveness is always a positive force. It is unlike aggressiveness, which is a hostile and overbearing attitude. Assertiveness assumes that the assistant not only is competent but also has established cordial and cooperative working relationships.

Professional Image

Few professions are as highly respected as the medical profession, which has an image of health, cleanliness, and wholesomeness. If you choose to work in a healthcare setting, your appearance and bearing must reflect this image. Patients expect your positive personality and pleasing manner to be reflected in your appearance through healthful habits, good grooming, and appropriate dress.

Being in style, as advertisements and magazines define style, is not the same thing as projecting a **professional image.** Style reflects a personal vision of who you are in the way you act, dress, and groom, such as hairstyle and nail care. In the workplace, however, you reflect not your own personal vision but the employer's preferences about how the practice should be seen by patients and the community.

Physical Attributes. Good health is the result of eating a properly balanced diet, getting sufficient rest, and exercising regularly. These good health habits show in the energy of your body when you move, walk, or communicate; in the healthful appearance of your skin; in the alertness and clarity of your eyes; and even in the shine of your hair and the health of your nails.

Habits that promote good health are essential to maintaining a professional image. These good health habits are complemented by good grooming habits. Although cleanliness is the basis of good grooming, grooming means more than cleanliness. A daily bath or shower, the use of deodorant, regular dental care along with daily dental brushing and flossing, and a neat overall appearance are all elements of good grooming. Also included in good grooming habits are the following:

- Nails should be manicured, so that the hands look well maintained. Employees should avoid bright or unusual nail polish colors and stenciled nails. Nails should not be so long that they pose a threat to others or interfere with working at the keyboard. Office policy on artificial nails should be followed.
- Hair requires frequent shampooing and should be arranged in a style that will not require a great deal of attention during working hours.
- The patient and the assistant should be able to look at each other eye to eye; therefore, hair should not cover the eyes or interfere with sight.
- Male employees should shave daily or have neatly trimmed facial hair.
- Perfumes or colognes should be avoided in the office. Staff members and patients may be irritated by fragrances, especially those with a floral base. Lotions should also be unscented.
- Makeup should be used moderately and should complement the assistant's skin type and color.
- Clothes must always be freshly laundered and wrinkle free. If you are required to wear a white uniform, it must be kept *snow* white and should never be worn over dark undergarments. If business casual clothes are worn in the office, they should be simple and should fit well. Tight or revealing clothes are not appropriate.
- Shoes should be closed toe, comfortable, and in good repair.
- Jewelry and hair ornaments are not good accompaniments to uniforms. Jewelry that is worn with street clothes in the office should be small and unobtrusive. Large bangles and bracelets with dangling parts are often noisy and interfere with completion of tasks.
- Most professional work environments have a stated policy concerning the amount and type of jewelry that may be worn—for example, one ring per hand (engagement ring/wedding band is considered one). Piercings and tattoos are common in today's society, and office policy will state what may be worn and/or shown. Common policies state that no more than two earrings per ear are permitted and that no other piercings may have jewelry, such as tongue, nose, eyebrow, or lip. Tattoos should be covered.

Maturity. Many administrative and personal skills contribute to the achievement of **maturity.** And maturity *is* an achievement. It takes great determination to acquire and practice the attitudes, habits, and skills that contribute to maturity.

Emotional and psychological maturity is not dependent on age. It is made up of many aspects of personality and of many skills. The mature person is able to work with supervisors and under pressure, even in unpleasant or frustrating conditions. The mature person sees a job through and gives more than is asked. Maturity enables a person to gather and use information to make good decisions. It is reflected by independence of judgment as well as by ambition and determination. As maturity becomes evident in the administrative medical assistant, it inspires the confidence of managers, patients, and coworkers.

Professionalism. Patients and society have an expectation of the medical care team to use technical skills and knowledge, communication, image, behavior, attitude, and respect to benefit patients, and, ultimately, society. In healthcare, all aspects from applying proper personal hygiene to using protective equipment are considered evidence of healthcare professionalism. Perception of healthcare quality is often determined by how the medical team demonstrates professionalism. Patients who experience high-quality, professional healthcare are more likely to return for future medical needs. Demonstrated positive professionalism

- earns patients' trust.
- creates a positive public perception of the practice.
- encourages a positive work environment.
- increases patient satisfaction.

Professional organizations emphasize professionalism within their individual codes of ethics, which will be presented in a later chapter.

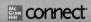 **GO TO PROJECT 1.1 AT THE END OF THIS CHAPTER**

1.5 PROFESSIONAL GROWTH AND CERTIFICATION

When an employee stops being willing to learn, he or she stops growing professionally and becomes less valuable to his or her employers and other colleagues. Learning and growing in the field allow the administrative medical assistant to become more successful and to enjoy an enviable professional status. Once assistants have completed specific requirements, they are eligible to join several national associations. By passing examinations, medical assistants and medical administrative assistants may become certified. **Certification** is the indication given by certain associations that a person has met high standards and has achieved competency in the knowledge and tasks required. Through continuing education, seminars, conferences, and meetings with other professionals in the field, these organizations provide opportunities to grow as office professionals and to advance in a chosen career.

The medical field is constantly changing; completing continuing education through providers, educational institutions, and/or professional organizations is a must for an individual to remain current in his or her chosen medical area of expertise.

American Association of Medical Assistants
20 North Wacker Drive, Suite 1575
Chicago, IL 60606
Phone: 800-228-2262
Website: www.aama-ntl.org
E-mail: membership@aama-ntl.org

American Medical Technologists
10700 West Higgins, Suite 150
Rosemont, IL 60018
Phone: 847-823-5169
Website: www.americanmedtech.org
E-mail: mail@americanmedtech.org

Association for Healthcare Documentation Integrity
4120 Dale Road, Suite J8-233
Modesto, CA 95356
Phone: 800-982-2182
Website: www.ahdionline.org
E-mail: ahdi@ahdionline.org

AAMA. The American Association of Medical Assistants **(AAMA)** is a major nationwide organization. The AAMA recommends to the Commission on Accreditation of Allied Health Education Programs (CAAHEP) those formal education programs that have met AAMA curriculum standards. Further, the AAMA sponsors the national certification examination for medical assistants in three areas: general, administrative, and clinical. As stated earlier in the chapter, specifics within each of the three areas are outlined at the AAMA website (www.aama-ntl.org). Those who pass the examination are certified and receive the designation of Certified Medical Assistant (CMA).

The AAMA requires CMAs to be recertified, either by exam or by submission of qualifying points, every 5 years. This practice ensures that medical assistants keep up with developments in the field. There are hundreds of continuing education courses sponsored by the AAMA to help assistants keep current and become recertified.

Although medical assistants need not be certified to be employed as assistants, certification improves the chances of career advancement and provides motivation for continued professional growth.

AMT. The American Medical Technologists **(AMT)** is another nationwide organization offering certifications for medical assistants. AMT offers several national examinations of which two directly relate to medical assistants and administrative medical assistants. Successful completion of the one examination earns the credential of Registered Medical Assistant (RMA). Another certification exam to become a Certified Medical Administrative Specialist (CMAS) is offered through AMT.

Certified members must maintain active member status and comply with the Certification Continuation Program (CCP) requirements. To maintain the RMA and CMAS certification, a member must earn 30 points over a 3-year period for each credential held. AMT will evaluate the submitted points for any points that can be used in both recertification areas.

AHDI. The Association for Healthcare Documentation Integrity **(AHDI),** formerly known as the American Association of Medical Transcription (AAMT), is a nationwide organization that promotes professional standards of practice related to the field of healthcare documentation. AHDI works to ensure the highest level of quality, privacy, and security as it relates to patient and other healthcare information.

AHDI offers credentialing examinations related to healthcare documentation: Registered Healthcare Documentation Specialist (RHDS) and Certified Healthcare Documentation Specialist (CHDS). The former credential, Certified Medical Transcriptionist (CMT), is no longer offered by AHDI; however, both the RHDS and the CHDS have transcription components. The RHDS examination is designed for recent graduates of a healthcare documentation/medical transcription curriculum. Individuals who have already earned the RHDS credential *and* have a minimum of 2 years' experience in an acute-specialty or multispecialty transcription setting may take the CHDS certification exam. If an individual meets the qualifications to take both the RHDS and the CHDS exams, a third exam, Combined RHDS/CHDS Credential Qualifying Exam (CQE), is available.

Recertification for both the RHDS and the CHDS must be completed every 3 years. RHDS recertification candidates must take and successfully pass a recertification course. A minimum score of 75 percent on each section and as a final score is required. CHDS recertification candidates must submit 30 continuing education credits (CECs) with at least 24 CECs in four core areas.

Until electronic health records are fully implemented in the medical field, transcriptionists may still be utilized. The transcriptionist's skill in English usage, grammar, and style ensures the competent editing and correction of materials. Taking advantage of certification and opportunities for continued study in this field, as in medical assisting, helps in career advancement.

IAAP. The International Association of Administrative Professionals **(IAAP),** previously known as Professional Secretaries International (PSI), is a worldwide nonprofit organization working with career-minded office and administrative professionals to promote opportunities for their membership to connect, to lead, to learn, and to excel. Core values of IAAP include authenticity, community, passion, relevance, and resilience.

This organization sponsors a comprehensive examination—the Certified Administrative Professional (CAP). Individuals successfully completing the CAP examination demonstrate competence in six areas:

1. Communications, organizational
2. Documentation production and business writing
3. Records and office management
4. Distribution of information and technology
5. Project and event management
6. Operational functions

Two speciality exams are offered by IAAP as add-on certifications once an individual has achieved the CAP credential: Organizational Management (OA) and Technology Applications (TA).

The organization, which maintains chapters all over the United States, makes professional contacts easy. The IAAP provides study materials and information about available review courses.

There are companies that offer salary incentives to those who become Certified Administrative Professionals. In this area, as in all other areas of most professions, certification improves the chances for advancement.

AAPC and AHIMA. The American Academy of Professional Coders (AAPC) and the American Health Information Management Association (AHIMA) offer certifications in areas related to coding and health information management.

AAPC offers five medical coding credentials reflecting the various locations, such as outpatient and inpatient, and aspects of medical coding. Individuals may demonstrate knowledge in medical coding through the following exams:

1. Certified Professional Coder (CPC)
2. Certified Outpatient Coder (COC)
3. Certified Inpatient Coder (CIC)
4. Certified Professional Coder–Payer (CPC-P)
5. Certified Risk Adjustment Coder (CRC)

Credential exams are also available in many specialty areas, such as dermatology and family practice. Also offered by AAPC are credentials that allow individuals to demonstrate knowledge of the revenue cycle, compliance regulations, auditing, and medical practice management:

1. Certified Professional Biller (CPB)
2. Certified Professional Compliance Officer (CPCO)
3. Certified Professional Medical Auditor (CPMA)
4. Certified Physician Practice Manager (CPPM)
5. Certified Documentation Expert-Outpatient

Recertification must be completed every 2 years by submitting continuing education units (CEUs). The number of CEUs to submit is based on the number of credentials to be renewed. One credential requires 36 CEUs up through five credentials, which require 52 CEUs.

International Association of Administrative Professionals
10502 N. Ambassador Drive,
Suite 100
Kansas City, MO 64153
Phone: 816-891-6600
Website: www.iaap-hq.org

American Academy of Professional Coders
2233 S. Presidents Drive, Suite F
Salt Lake City, UT 84120
Phone: 800-626-CODE (2633)
Website: www.aapc.com
E-mail: info@aapc.com

American Health Information Management Association
233 N. Michigan Avenue, 21st Floor
Chicago, IL 60601-5809
Phone: 312-233-1101 or
800-335-5535
Website: www.ahima.org
E-mail: info@ahima.org

National Healthcareer Association
11161 Overbrook Road
Leawood, KS 66211
Phone: 800-499-9092
Website: www.nhanow.com
E-mail: info@nhanow.com

AHIMA offers three certifying exams in coding—Certified Coding Associate (CCA), Certified Coding Specialist (CCS), and Certified Coding Specialist–Physician Based (CCS-P). Six exams are offered to allow individuals to demonstrate their competency in areas dealing with health information and medical records, including electronic medical records:

1. Registered Health Information Technician (RHIT)
2. Registered Health Information Administrator (RHIA)
3. Certified Health Data Analyst (CHDA)
4. Certified in Healthcare Privacy and Security (CHPS)
5. Certified Documentation Improvement Practitioner (CDIP)
6. Certified Healthcare Technology Specialist (CHTS)

Knowledge of medical, administrative, ethical, and legal requirements as they pertain to medical record information is required. Applicants will also be asked to demonstrate their competence in computer information systems.

Recertification is required every 2 years by submission of qualified CEUs. The number of CEUs required depends on the credential. For each additional credential to be recertified, an additional 10 CEUs is required, up to a maximum of 50 CEUs.

NHA. Another organization that works to improve competency within the area of healthcare is the National Healthcareer Association (NHA). Through education and certification exams, the NHA strives to provide the healthcare field with confident and prepared employees.

Several certifications are offered through the NHA. Four of them are listed here:

1. Certified Medical Administrative Assistant (CMAA)
2. Certified Electronic Health Records Specialist (CEHRS)
3. Certified Billing and Coding Specialist (CBCS)
4. Certified Clinical Medical Assistant (CCMA)

Individuals who have successfully completed a training program through an accredited or state-recognized program or provider may qualify to take a certification exam. Additionally, individuals who have successfully completed formal medical services training through the military are also qualified to take an NHA certification exam. Another option for qualifying to take an NHA certification exam is work experience. To qualify, an exam applicant must have completed a minimum of 1 year's work experience within a health field covered by an NHA exam within the last 3 years. Study materials for each certification exam are offered though the National Healthcareer Association.

Every 2 years, individuals possessing certifications through NHA must renew the credential. An applicant for renewal must submit evidence of successfully completing 10 continuing education credits within the past 2 years. Continuing education credits may be completed through the NHA or through an organization recognized by NHA for providing NHA-recognized continuing education credits.

Mc Graw Hill connect GO TO PROJECT 1.2 AT THE END OF THIS CHAPTER

1.6 INTERPERSONAL RELATIONSHIPS

The administrative medical assistant is usually the first person the patient comes into contact with when making an appointment or going to the doctor's office. The way in which the assistant receives and welcomes the patient, whether by phone or physically in the office, establishes the tone of the visit, the professionalism of the office, and the patient's expectations about the doctor and the treatment.

The responsibility to make patients feel that they are important and that enough time is available to them for treatment is of major concern for the medical assistant. Although the office may be busy and both the doctor and the patients may want to speak to the assistant at the same time, the assistant must remain calm, reassuring, and pleasant to everyone.

Taking Care of Patients

Greeting a patient by name, if possible, contributes to making that patient feel important. If you are away from the desk when a patient arrives, acknowledge the patient with a smile and a greeting as soon as you return.

Every person is to be shown the same degree of respect and concern without regard to race, age, gender, or socioeconomic situation. Every doctor's office accepts patients who receive care for a nominal fee or even completely free. The physician's aim in all cases is the same: to make the person well in the shortest possible time. The assistant's aim in all cases is to treat all patients with the same amount of empathy, concern, and attention.

Familiarity

A physician may choose to establish a less formal tone in the office in order to make patients feel more comfortable. Even when this is the case, the office is still a professional setting. Certain ways of expressing familiarity, either with the physician or with the patients, are not appropriate.

The doctor should always be referred to and spoken to by title and last name: "Dr. Larsen will see you now." This courtesy is observed even if the physician and administrative medical assistant are relatives or have a personal relationship. Conversation in front of patients should never indicate anything other than a professional relationship.

Patients may have preferences about the way they are addressed. It shows respect to address the patient by the appropriate title and last name: "Mr./Mrs./Ms./Miss/ Reverend Lopez." If a patient wishes to be addressed in some other way, such as by a first name or nickname, that patient will invite you to do so. The assistant should make a notation of the preference for future use. Names that are difficult for the assistant should have the pronunciation noted. It is acceptable to call children by their given name.

EXAMPLE: ADDRESSING A PATIENT

Assistant: Mrs. Patient, Dr. Larsen is ready to see you now.

Patient: Thank you, Linda, but please call me Margaret. I'm not used to being called Mrs. Patient.

Social Relationships

In many offices, the policy discourages, or may even forbid, a social relationship between a patient and a staff member. Such a policy reflects the physician's belief that these relationships are not consistent with a professional atmosphere and may interfere with the proper medical management of the patient's case. Under no circumstances should you make a social engagement with a patient without first checking office policy and discussing the situation with your employer.

Conversation with Patients

If the administrative medical assistant has to spend considerable time with a patient, the patient is the one who decides whether or not to start a conversation. If the patient wishes to talk, the patient should also choose the subject. The assistant should listen and respond courteously. General subjects, such as the weather, sports, hobbies, or local events, may be ideal topics. Try to avoid controversial subjects, such as politics or religion. Keeping the conversation to general topics should also ensure that you are not in a situation in which you argue with a patient or try to persuade a patient that a certain view is correct. If possible, try to use the patient's name at least one time during the conversation.

Because the patient identifies the administrative medical assistant with the doctor, the patient also believes that the assistant carries the doctor's authority. For this reason, the assistant should not offer a patient medical advice or comment on the patient's treatment. Very few patients have a substantial knowledge of medicine, anatomy, or physiology. They may easily misunderstand a remark made by the assistant, especially if the remark contains a technical term. If the patient seeks advice or asks a question related to treatment, the medical assistant should respond tactfully: "That is a question the doctor should answer for you. Be sure to ask about that during your examination."

Difficult Patients. The best test of interpersonal skills may be the successful handling of difficult, unreasonable, or unpleasant patients. The patient's self-control may be undermined by the pain and worry that accompany the illness. Dealing with short-tempered or irritable patients requires the medical assistant to show patience, understanding, and restraint. Calmly repeating instructions to an uncooperative patient may be difficult, but it may prevent having to ask a patient to redo a procedure or task or having to repeat the instructions later.

EXAMPLE: PROVIDING INSTRUCTIONS TO A DIFFICULT PATIENT

Assistant: Mr. Public, here are the instructions for the x-ray you are going to have on Monday, October 3, at Riverview Clinic. Let me go over them with you again to see whether you have any remaining questions.

Patient: You do not need to repeat the instructions to me again. I understand!

Assistant: OK, Mr. Public. If you think of any questions at a later time, you may call me. I have written my name and telephone number at the bottom of the instructions. I will be happy to help answer any questions you may have.

A patient who has had to wait a long time to see the doctor may become restless or impatient. In such instances, the medical assistant should make some gesture of attention. Introduce a general topic of conversation or reassure the patient that you are aware of the lateness of the schedule and thank the person for understanding.

There are times when patients become angry. A mistake in an insurance payment, a long wait to see the doctor, or even the patient's physical pain or discomfort may trigger an outburst of bad temper. The medical assistant must remain calm and courteous. A gentle tone and soothing voice sometimes help calm a patient. Separate facts from feelings and do not argue. Politely offer to help correct a situation in any way you can. The offer by itself may help reduce or even eliminate the patient's anger.

EXAMPLE: CLARIFYING A BILL TO AN UPSET PATIENT

Patient: My insurance company sent me this form that says you have been paid for my last office visit and I do not owe you any money. So, why did you send me this bill?

Assistant: Mr. Patient A, may I please see the form so that I can compare your form with the form sent to us by your insurance company?

You are correct, you do not owe any more money for your last office visit. The bill you received is for the strep test you had during your last visit. The insurance paid its portion and the bill you received is for your remaining portion. *[Assistant points to the correct places on the insurance form.]* This is the insurance payment for the office visit, this is its payment portion of the strep test, and this is your portion of the strep test, which is the same amount as on your bill. Does this help clarify why you received a bill?

Every patient should leave the doctor's office with a feeling of goodwill. Frequently, the medical assistant will have an opportunity to talk to the patient as the patient prepares to leave the office. Calling the patient by name, if possible, and extending a pleasant goodbye will have beneficial results. A patient who leaves the office on a positive note may tell others about a good experience with the staff. Likewise, patients will also share a bad experience.

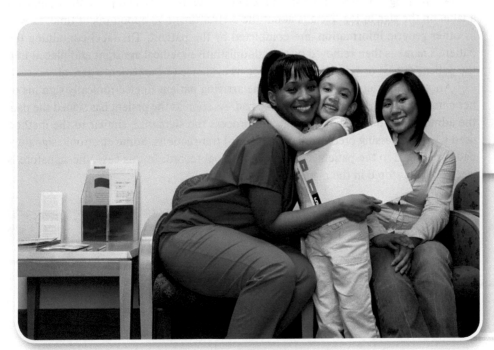

Figure 1.4

The administrative medical assistant ensures that patients leave the office with a feeling of goodwill. *What actions and attitudes cause patients to feel positive about their office visits?* XiXinXing/Shutterstock

Terminally Ill Patients. If you know a patient is terminally ill and he or she engages you in conversation, be sensitive to the situation by avoiding certain questions that you would ordinarily ask, such as "How are you?" Try to keep the conversation short and general. Patients who are terminally ill usually are willing and eager to discuss topics such as pets, children and/or grandchildren, spouses/partners, or other individuals of whom they are proud. Many patients have hobbies, such as gardening or music, about which they are excited to share. Select topics that are short-term instead of long-term in nature, such as plans for the next New Year's celebration. The bottom line is to be empathetic to the patient's condition and emotional state.

Confidentiality

Maintaining the **confidentiality,** or privacy, of patients' medical information is a legal requirement. A doctor who gives information about a patient without a patient's permission, except to another doctor who is involved with the patient's care, can be prosecuted under the law, and the doctor's license may be revoked. Similar legal requirements and penalties apply to employees in the doctor's office.

Patient Sign-In Log. Documentation of a patient's visit, in his or her own handwriting, is provided when the patient signs in on the log. The patient's privacy is to be protected at all times, which includes when he or she is in the check-in and waiting area.

Traditionally, a patient arrives at the office and signs his or her name and other pertinent information, such as arrival time, appointment time, and doctor to be seen, on a check-in log. Leaving this information available to be viewed by others or asking for nonpertinent personal health information, such as reason for the visit or insurance information, on the check-in log is a violation of HIPAA (which will be covered in a later chapter). Many offices still use this format; however, as soon as the patient arrives, the name is marked through with a broad, dark marker. This method of concealing patient check-in information complies with current medical law as long as the patient information is nonreadable. The problem with this method is that the written documentation of the patient's visit in his or her own handwriting has been eliminated.

Another sign-in method is a label method. Patients arrive and place their name on a label on the sign-in log. Details about the arrival time and appointment time, as well as other generic information, are completed by the patient. The label containing the patient's name is then removed by the administrative medical assistant and placed into the patient's chart or on a daily patient log as evidence of the patient's arrival.

Another popular method is to ask the arriving patient to electronically sign his or her name using a stylus and an electronic pad. As soon as the patient has signed the pad, the administrative medical assistant will process the signature, similar to the method used when processing credit card or debit card transactions. Some electronic signature pads are linked to the patient's electronic medical record. In this case, the signature is electronically stored in the medical record.

COMPLIANCE *TIP*

The responsibility for confidentiality extends beyond the office environment. Neither a patient's name nor any other information should ever be mentioned outside the office. A patient may not wish to tell family members or business associates that medical care is needed. The doctor's specialty may be an indication of the disease for which the patient is being treated, and the patient may not wish this to be known.

Assigning numbers to patients on their arrival is another method of protecting patient confidentiality. Their numbers, instead of their names, are used when addressing them in the waiting area.

Sometimes patients will verbally check in on their arrival. The administrative medical assistant should ask the patient to sign in/register and will make a notation of his or her arrival on the daily schedule.

During times when extreme circumstances exist, such as COVID19, patients may be asked upon arrival to remain in their vehicles and call or send a text message to a stated phone number in order to check in to the medical facility. The patient will receive a call, text message, or other form of communication when it is time to enter the medical facility.

Medical Histories. Medical histories of patients contain a great deal of confidential information, not only about the patients but also about their families and perhaps other contacts, such as friends. Employees may not disclose any information about a patient's illness, personal history, or matters relating to family or others without a written release from the patient. The written release-of-information form and the exceptions to the release will be discussed in a later chapter.

Confidentiality about medical records is also to be observed in any conversations the administrative medical assistant has with the patient. It is not the administrative medical assistant's place to share with the patient the doctor's diagnosis or prognosis. The doctor is the sole judge of what information is to be given to, or withheld from, the patient. The assistant must refuse to discuss the patient's case and should refer the patient to the doctor for information.

Many people other than the patients themselves may ask the medical assistant for information about a patient's case. There are some patients who are curious about other patients whom they may know or may have seen in the doctor's office during their own visits. There are some curious patients who may try to obtain personal information about the doctor, staff, or other patients. Friends or relatives of a patient may inquire about the doctor's opinion, the method of treatment, or the duration of the illness. A courteous but firm refusal, such as "I'm sorry, but that information is confidential," should prevent further attempts to get information.

Record Security. The administrative medical assistant must be aware of the location of the front desk and of various work areas in relation to public spaces, such as the lobby or waiting room. Location is important in safeguarding the confidentiality of records because they may be read if left where other patients, staff members, or visitors can see them. Because patient records, schedules, and billing information are now often computerized, the locations of computer screens at the front desk and in work areas are also important. Sensitive information should not remain on the screen when you need to be away from the desk. Screen savers should be used when away from the computer area, and access to computer data should be password-protected. Screens should not be viewable by patients, either on their arrival or on their departure. Monitor protectors that allow data to be viewed only from the front may also prevent accidental disclosure of medical information. Mobile computers should never be left in a room with a patient. When exiting a patient examination room, take the mobile device with you.

Hardcopy medical charts are often placed outside the exam room for the physician to review prior to entering the room. As other patients pass this area, they can see the name on the chart. This is illegal disclosure of protected medical information and a violation of HIPAA Privacy and Security Rules. These rules will be discussed in another chapter. A very simple solution is to turn the chart around, so that the name and any other medical information are not exposed.

In areas close to the waiting room or lobby, caution should also be exercised in conversations, whether over the phone or face to face. Conversations between a patient and the assistant or among employees may easily be overheard. Unless soundproof glass is being used, simply sliding the glass window closed does not prevent information from being heard.

In general, nothing that happens in the office should be repeated at home or to friends. A patient can sometimes be identified by the circumstances of the case or by some other detail, even when the patient's name is not mentioned.

There is wisdom in the adage "What you see here, what you hear here, must remain here when you leave."

Cultural Diversity

People's beliefs, value systems, and language, as well as their understanding of the world, grow out of the culture into which they were born and in which they were raised. It is important to understand that, just as the elements of your culture are formative for you, so the cultures of others are formative for them. Be aware that people from cultures different than yours may express themselves and present themselves in a different way from what your own culture has taught you to expect. **Ethnocentrism** is the tendency to believe that one's own race or ethnic group is the most important and that some or all aspects of its culture are superior to those of other groups. This, in and of itself, can be a barrier within the office team environment and in interactions with patients. Be respectful of people of all cultures and backgrounds. This does not mean that you accept the beliefs and customs of the culture as your own but that you are considerate of each individual's right to express individualism within cultural practices, such as dress. Never assign patients to stereotypes that are racial, ethnic, or religious.

Language Barriers. Although most aspects of other cultures do not present barriers, a cultural barrier may occur when the patient and staff do not speak the same language. Diversification of patient populations is increasingly common. When communicating through language barriers, maintaining the privacy and confidentiality of patients' medical health information is essential.

Medical environments should look at the community's and the medical office's cultural mix and identify patients within the medical practice who are Limited English Proficient (LEP) and the frequency of LEP patients' visits. LEP patients do not speak, read, or write using English as their primary language of communication. Under the Health and Human Services (HHS) LEP Guidelines, medical settings that receive money from federally funded programs must develop and implement steps to provide LEP patients with meaningful, accurate, and timely medical services. Medical settings which receive only Medicare Part B payments are exempt from the HHS guidelines; however, the number of exempted settings is very small. Office personnel then determine their patients' primary communication language(s) and if there is a need for an on-site or a qualified medical interpreter. If the patient prefers an interpreter, the interpreter should be trained and familiar with medical terminology and medical language. Patients may not be charged a fee for the interpreter's services. Use of friends and family members as medical interpreters should be discouraged in the medical environment due to issues such as confidentiality, competency, conflict of interest, and privacy. However, friends and family members can provide cultural definition for the patient. For example, through a medical interpreter, the physician tells the patient to remove her shoe so that the foot can be examined. In her culture, this is a violation of her religious norm. In this case, a friend or family member who speaks both languages and knows the patient's culture could explain the medical need to remove the shoe.

Other communication modes may be used to effectively communicate with LEP patients. Telephonic services, videoconferencing using a medical interpreter, and bilingual staff members can be effective methods of communicating through language barriers. Using voice-activated translation software may also assist in communications with LEP patients. Forms and other office materials may be printed in different languages relevant to the patient population. Reference materials with frequently used terms and phrases can be a helpful tool when communicating with LEP patients. Another consideration is the type of services being rendered to the LEP patient(s)—administrative medical services, routine medical services, or emergency services.

Not having appropriate cultural resources to meet the needs of the day's patients can create a disruption in the schedule, just as not having the appropriate medical instruments can stop the day's schedule. Following are additional guidelines for communicating with LEP patients either directly or through other communicative methods:

- Speak slowly and clearly.
- Do not raise your voice above an ordinary conversational tone. Speaking loudly does not improve understanding.
- Use simple words, not technical terms.
- Be brief.
- Have key phrases, such as "your next appointment is" or "thank you," translated into languages used by patients within the practice. Staff members should practice the phrases and be ready to use them when needed.

Another form of language barrier may occur in the office when the assistant needs to effectively communicate with patients who are deaf. Effective communication ensures that these patients have obtained the same results and benefits as hearing patients. Following are tips for communicating successfully with deaf or hard-of-hearing (HOH) patients:

- Determine the patient's preferred form of communication: signing, writing, or speech/lipreading. Make note in the patient's chart, and be prepared when the patient arrives. If the patient relies on American Sign Language (ASL), prior to the medical visit ask the patient if an interpreter will be accompanying him or her to the visit. If not, make arrangements to have a medical sign language interpreter present. According to the Americans with Disabilities Act, the provider may not bill the deaf or HOH patient for the interpreter's fee.
- Establish the type of service that is to be rendered to the patient. If the patient will be receiving new medications, having a procedure, or giving medical consent, a medical sign language interpreter should be used.
- Head nodding by the patient does not necessarily mean understanding. The patient may be relying on another individual to explain the details.
- Larger, quicker, more forceful motions by the patient may be an expression of heightened emotions.
- Body language, especially facial expressions, of the administrative assistant are keenly observed by the patient.
- Key phrases, such as "good morning" or "your copayment today is," should be learned and practiced by the staff member.
- "Positive" and "good" are closely linked in ASL. Positive test results may be interpreted as good test results. A patient may be confused by the statement "Your test results for MRSA were positive" as meaning "Your test results for MRSA were good."

Follow these suggestions when the communication mode is lipreading:

- Make sure you have the patient's complete attention prior to beginning the communication process. A simple statement such as "Are you ready to begin?" will ensure that both parties are ready to communicate.

- Maintain direct face-to-face contact with the patient at all times during the communication process.
- Clear your mouth and mouth area of all items that may be intrusive to communication, such as gum or candy.
- Provide adequate lighting in the area, and ensure that no shadows will interfere with lipreading. This should be checked with another office member prior to communication with the patient.

If the patient's mode of communication is writing, provide writing tools, such as a whiteboard and marker or pen and paper. Written communications, when possible, should be free of medical language. For many deaf and hard-of-hearing (HOH) individuals, ASL is their primary means of communication, and English is a second language. Written communication containing standard medical language may be challenging for the patient to understand. All written communication should be maintained in the patient's medical record.

Many patients, both deaf and hearing, communicate faster with electronic devices. A small computer may be used to communicate between the administrative assistant and the patient. Examples of other methods or devices that may be used to communicate with deaf, hard-of-hearing (HOH), and/or nonverbal patients are (1) a qualified notetaker, (2) real-time captioning, (3) written materials, and (4) amplifiers. Whether the preferred mode of communication is signing, writing, or speech/lipreading, the privacy and confidentiality of the patient's medical information must be protected.

Patients who are blind or who have vision loss should be provided the same effective medical/administrative communication as sighted patients. Accommodations for blind or loss-of-vision patients may include

1. a medically "qualified" reader—a person trained in effective, impartial, and accurate reading of medical information.
2. information printed in braille or large print.
3. a computer screen-reading program.

If the patient uses a mobility device, such as a cane or a sight dog, clear the walking path for the patient.

The bottom line is, do not make assumptions about LEP patients or those with other communicative disabilities. Ask the patient his or her preferred method of receiving effective medical care and communication, and be guided by his or her choices.

Nonpatients

All visitors to the doctor's office should be treated courteously. Often, a patient's friend or relative may accompany the patient.

Visitors on business, such as pharmaceutical company sales representatives, call on the office frequently. The doctor may not wish to take time away from the patient schedule and may ask the administrative medical assistant to get information on the product, obtain samples, and keep the business cards on file. Some offices schedule a specific time each week and/or month for pharmaceutical representatives. This gives the representative an opportunity to present materials to the physician and allows the physician to devote time exclusively to the representative.

There may be other visitors who take up the doctor's time unnecessarily, and most doctors appreciate an assistant who screens and tells the visitor that the doctor is seeing patients, is out of the office, or so on. Be truthful when deterring nonpatients who request the physician's time without an appointment. Even one unscheduled visitor can disrupt the daily appointment schedule. Request that the physician provide names (or positions) of individuals who should not be seen during office hours.

 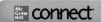 **GO TO PROJECT 1.3 AT THE END OF THIS CHAPTER**

1.1 Describe the tasks and skills required of an administrative medical assistant.	• The administrative medical assistant has task responsibilities in the following areas: — Front office procedures — Scheduling — Records management — Administrative duties — Financial • These tasks require skills in the following areas: — Communication — Mathematics — Organization — Computers — Interpersonal relationships
1.2 List and define at least three personal attributes essential for an administrative medical assistant.	• Personal attributes needed for the successful administrative medical assistant are equally as important as required tasks and skills. Among the personal attributes needed are the following: — Genuine liking for people: enjoying people and having a desire to help them — Cheerfulness: the ability to be pleasant and friendly — Empathy: sensitivity to the feelings and situations of other people
1.3 Describe the employment opportunities in various medical settings and specialties and nonmedical settings.	• Employment opportunities for administrative medical assistants are increasing in physician practices (single and multiphysician practices), clinics, hospitals and medical centers, care facilities, and insurance companies. Other opportunities are increasing in the field of education and accounting firms.
1.4 Identify and define at least six positive work attitudes that contribute to the work ethic and professionalism of an administrative medical assistant.	• Habits and skills that make up the work ethic of an administrative medical assistant include — accuracy: the ability to be correct, clear, and thorough. — thoroughness: the ability to apply careful and complete attention to detail. — dependability: the ability to be relied upon to fulfill instructions and to complete tasks on time.

- efficiency: the ability to use time and other resources in such a way as to avoid wasted efforts.
- flexibility: the ability to respond quickly to changed situations, last-minute assignments, and delays; the willingness to accept and implement new ideas.
- good judgment: the ability to use knowledge, experience, and logic to assess all the aspects of a situation in order to reach a sound decision.
- honesty: the ability to always tell the truth and to quickly assume responsibility for mistakes.
- initiative: the ability to take action independently.
- problem-solving: the ability to use logic to plan needed steps to accomplish a goal.
- punctuality: the ability to be on time.
- self-motivation: the ability to express a willingness to learn new duties and/or procedures without a requirement to do so.
- tact: the ability to speak and act considerately, especially in difficult situations.
- team membership: the ability to work positively with others, to be generous with his or her time, to assist others, to be courteous, and to observe rules of confidentiality.
- assertiveness: the ability to step forward to make a point in a confident, positive manner.
- a professional image: that of a friendly, capable professional who inspires confidence. From the assistant's manner, speech, posture, and appearance, patients and others have the impression of someone who is mature and dedicated to competent service.

1.5 List three advantages of professional affiliation and certification.	• Certification
	   — often favorably influences an employer's opinion.
	   — contributes to career advancement.
	   — fosters professional growth by the need to be recertified, continuing education programs, seminars, webinars, conferences, and the opportunity to network with others in the same profession.

1.6 Apply elements of good interpersonal communication to relationships with patients and others within the medical environment.	• Administrative medical assistants should treat patients, physicians, colleagues, and others with courtesy, always maintaining a calm, pleasant, reassuring manner. • They should refrain from revealing confidential information, and they have a professional relationship with the physician(s), colleagues, patients, and visitors in the office. • Medical team members need to create an atmosphere of interest in others by using positive nonverbal communications—body language, facial expressions, eye contact, and so on. • Patients are to be provided medical services in a meaningful, accurate, and timely manner using their preferred mode of communication.

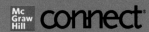

Project 1.1 **(LO 1.4) Professionalism in the Medical Office Environment**

List six examples, three hard skills and three soft skills, of an administrative medical assistant's professionalism in the medical environment. State how the examples are beneficial to the patient.

Project 1.2 **(LO 1.5) Internet Research: Professional Organizations**

Using the Internet, research the websites of three professional organizations listed in Chapter 1. Write down the student membership requirements of each and the advantages of belonging to each.

Project 1.3 **(LO 1.2, LO 1.4, and LO 1.6) Personal Attributes, Work Ethic and Professionalism, and Interpersonal Relationships**

 On Working Paper 1 (WP 1) in an end section of this book, match each of the terms in Column 2 with its definition in Column 1.

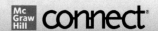

Self-Awareness (LO 1.2)

Do you ever find time to think about who you are, your strengths and weaknesses, or your personality? What about your habits and values? Many people are not inclined to spend much time on self-reflection; consequently, many of us have a low level of self-awareness. Self-awareness can improve, and it can help us identify opportunities for professional development and personal growth. **Describe your level of self-awareness. What do you think needs to be changed in your life to improve your self-awareness?**

Self-Confidence (LO 1.2)

Self-confidence is extremely important in almost every aspect of our lives. People who lack self-confidence can find it difficult to become successful. Self-confident people have qualities that others admire, and they inspire confidence in both their personal and professional lives. Gaining the confidence of others is one way in which a self-confident person finds success. The good news is that self-confidence can be learned, practiced, and expanded. **How can you work to build up your level of self-confidence? Why is self-confidence so important to success?**

Multicultural Sensitivity (LO 1.6)

Multicultural sensitivity includes learning about others and celebrating similarities while accepting differences. Race and ethnicity are difficult subjects to discuss, but cultural similarities and differences can be discussed and embraced. **How can you promote multicultural sensitivity?**

USING TERMINOLOGY

Match the term or phrase on the left with the correct answer on the right.

_____ **1.** [LO 1.2] Empathy

_____ **2.** [LO 1.6] Ethnocentrism

_____ **3.** [LO 1.4] Thoroughness

_____ **4.** [LO 1.5] AHDI

_____ **5.** [LO 1.5] Certification

_____ **6.** [LO 1.4] Accuracy

_____ **7.** [LO 1.4] Problem-solving

_____ **8.** [LO 1.4] Initiative

_____ **9.** [LO 1.4] Dependability

_____ **10.** [LO 1.4] Tact

a. Completing tasks with correctness and attention to detail

b. A trait that results in complete, neat, and correct tasks

c. Sensitivity to other people's feelings and situations

d. A trait characterized by working independently and offering to help others

e. Recognition given by associations that an individual has met high standards and has demonstrated competency in given knowledge and tasks

f. Provides certification opportunities for healthcare documentation specialists

g. Believing that one's own race, ethnic group, and/or culture is superior to all other groups

h. The ability to speak and act considerately in various situations

i. Logically and systematically planning steps to accomplish a task

j. Finishing tasks on schedule, without complaining, and offering to assist others

CHECKING YOUR UNDERSTANDING

Select the most correct answer.

1. [LO 1.1] Nenna worked as an administrative medical assistant but was dismissed from her AMA position after numerous patients complained about how they were greeted. Nenna claims she always used an appropriate verbal greeting with each patient. Which of the following might have contributed to the miscommunication between Nenna and the patients?

   a. Lack of professional certification
   b. Not enough reading material in the waiting area
   c. Nonverbal facial expressions and tone of voice
   d. An unclean uniform

2. [LO 1.4] During his first 6 months at a local medical clinic, Aaron completed and submitted insurance claims to various carriers. He used a software program to check and process his claims prior to submitting them for payment. This demonstrated that he accurately completed claims using very few resources. Which of the following was he demonstrating?

   a. Tact
   b. Ethnocentrism
   c. Assertiveness
   d. Efficiency

3. [LO 1.5] While searching online for a medical coding position, Maria noticed that several opportunities required CCS-P, CPC, or other current coding credentials. Which of the following key words or phrases could she use to search for their meaning on the Internet?

   a. Certification
   b. Interpersonal relationship skills
   c. Computer skills
   d. Records management skills

4. [LO 1.3] Addison would like to work in a medical-related administrative field but is not interested in a medical office setting. Which of the following may offer the best choice of a career for Addison?

   a. Food management
   b. Teacher's aide
   c. Home health sales
   d. Both teacher's aide and home health sales

5. [LO 1.1] During her interview, Ashley stated she has worked within the physical medical office setting and from the home setting using electronic health records and insurance claim processing programs. Her records show she received high evaluations and was frequently given more administrative authority. She had demonstrated competence in

   a. communication skills within the team environment.
   b. organizational skills.
   c. computer skills.
   d. All of these.

6. [LO 1.2] After he finishes his shift at the Flatwoods Medical Clinic for Burned Children, Andrew volunteers his time with the local equestrian program for physically challenged children. Which of the following personal attributes is Andrew demonstrating most clearly?

   a. Dependability
   b. True and genuine liking of other individuals
   c. Resourcefulness
   d. Cheerfulness

7. [LO 1.4] An AMA should always be aware of the impression and professional image given by his or her actions and presentation because

   a. the physician and practice are represented through the AMA.
   b. it is part of the job description.
   c. it may lead to an increase in salary or wages.
   d. None of these.

8. [LO 1.6] A lipreading patient needs to have a fasting glucose tolerance test completed at the local hospital. Prior to communicating directions for the test, the administrative medical assistant should

   a. look directly at the patient when conveying instructions.
   b. remove breath mints from his/her mouth.
   c. confirm the patient is ready to receive the instructions.
   d. All of these.

9. [LO 1.6] When verbally communicating with a patient who speaks a different language than the dominant language used in the medical office, the administrative medical assistant should

    a. speak loudly.

    b. use medical jargon.

    c. be brief.

    d. speak for a minimum of 5 minutes.

10. [LO 1.5] To maintain certification, a CMA must successfully meet requirements for recertification every

    a. 5 years.

    b. 10 years.

    c. 1 year.

    d. 2 years.

THINKING IT THROUGH

These questions cover important points in this chapter. Using your critical-thinking skills, play the role of an administrative medical assistant as you answer each question. Be prepared to discuss your responses.

1. [LO 1.1, 1.2] What qualities and skills are needed by the assistant who is responsible for the front desk? Why are these critical skills?

2. [LO 1.2] How can imagining yourself in someone else's situation help you develop empathy for patients?

3. [LO 1.1, 1.3] Why do you think that assistants working in various medical settings have similar types of assignments? Why would some employers assign assistants a single task or related task, such as processing insurance claims, while in other settings the assistant is likely to perform a variety of tasks? Provide examples to support your answers.

4. [LO 1.4] Why is it important to be a team player in the office?

5. [LO 1.4] What qualities project a professional image in an administrative medical assistant?

6. [LO 1.5] An assistant is asked by another team member why he/she decided to meet the requirements to become certified. What might the assistant answer?

7. [LO 1.6] How should an assistant communicate with LEP patients and with patients who are visually and/or hearing impaired?

Medical Ethics, Law, and Compliance

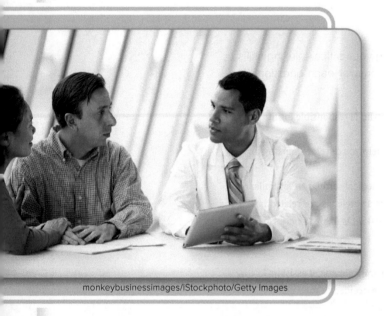

monkeybusinessimages/iStockphoto/Getty Images

LEARNING OUTCOMES

After studying this chapter, you will be able to

2.1 define *medical ethics, bioethics,* and *etiquette.*

2.2 discuss medical law, statutes, and legal documents, such as advance directives, and give three examples.

2.3 identify and discuss several key components of the HIPAA Administrative Simplification Act.

2.4 state the purpose of a medical Compliance Plan and explain compliant methods the assistant can use to safeguard against litigation.

KEY TERMS

Study these important words, which are defined in this chapter, to build your professional vocabulary:

advance directives	durable power of attorney	implied consent	POLST
arbitration	emancipated minor	informed consent	registration
assault	ethics	liability	release of information (ROI)
authorization	etiquette	licensure	respondeat superior
battery	express consent	litigation	settlement
bioethics	fraud	living will	statute of limitations
compliance	Good Samaritan Act	malpractice	subpoena
contributory negligence	Health Insurance Portability and Accountability Act (HIPAA)	mature minor	subpoena duces tecum
defensive medicine		medical abandonment	summons
deposition		medical practice acts	

ABHES

4.a. Follow documentation guidelines.

4.b.1. Institute federal and state guidelines when releasing medical records or information.

4.b.2. Institute federal and state guidelines when entering orders in and utilizing electronic health records.

4.c. Follow established policies when initiating or terminating medical treatment.

4.d. Distinguish between employer and personal liability coverage.

4.e. Perform risk management procedures.

4.f. Comply with federal, state, and local health laws and regulations as they relate to healthcare settings.

4.g. Display compliance with code of ethics of the profession.

4.h. Demonstrate compliance with HIPAA guidelines, the ADA Amendments Act, and the Health Information Technology for Economic and Clinical Health (HITECH) Act.

5.f. Demonstrate an understanding of the core competencies for Interprofessional Collaborative Practice (i.e., values/ethics; roles/responsibilities; interprofessional communication; teamwork).

7.a. Gather and process documents.

7.g. Display professionalism through written and verbal communications.

10.b. Demonstrate professional behavior.

www.abhes.org/accreditationmanual

The ABHES standards appear with permission of The Accrediting Bureau of Health Education Schools

CAAHEP

V.C.8. Discuss applications of electronic technology in professional communications.

VIII.C.5. Differentiate between fraud and abuse.

X.C.1. Differentiate between scope of practice and standards of care for medical assistants.

X.C.3. Describe components of the Health Information Portability and Accountability Act (HIPAA).

X.C.4. Summarize the Patient's Bill of Rights.

X.C.5. Discuss licensure and certification as they apply to healthcare providers.

X.C.7.a. Define *negligence*.

X.C.7.b. Define *malpractice*.

X.C.7.c. Define *statute of limitations*.

X.C.7.d. Define *Good Samaritan Act(s)*.

X.C.7.f. Define *living will/advanced directives*.

X.C.7.g. Define *medical durable power of attorney*.

X.C.7.l. Define *risk management*.

X.C.12.a. Describe compliance with public health statutes: communicable disease.

X.C.12.b. Demonstrate compliance with public health statutes: abuse, neglect, and exploitation.

X.C.12.c. Describe compliance with public health statutes: wounds of violence.

X.C.13.a. Define the medical legal term *informed consent*.

X.C.13.b. Define the medical legal term *implied consent*.

X.C.13.c. Define the medical legal term *expressed consent*.

X.C.13.e. Define the medical legal term *emancipated minor*.

X.C.13.f. Define the medical legal term *mature minor*.

X.C.13.g. Define the medical legal term *subpoena duces tecum*.

X.C.13.h. Define the medical legal term *respondeat superior*.

X.C.13.k. Define the medical legal term *defendant-plaintiff*.

X.C.13.l. Define the medical legal term *deposition*.

X.C.13.m. Define the medical legal term *arbitration-mediation*.

X.C.13.n. Define the medical legal term *Good Samaritan laws*.

X.P.2.a. Apply HIPAA rules in regard to privacy.

X.P.2.b. Apply HIPAA rules in regard to release of information.

X.P.4.a. Apply the Patient's Bill of Rights as it relates to choice of treatment.

X.P.4.b. Apply the Patient's Bill of Rights as it relates to consent for treatment.

X.P.4.c. Apply the Patient's Bill of Rights as it relates to refusal of treatment.

X.A.2. Protect the integrity of the medical record.

XI.C.1.a. Define *ethics*.

XI.C.1.b. Define *morals*.

XI.C.2. Differentiate between personal and professional ethics.

XI.C.3. Identify the effect of personal morals on professional performance.

XI.P.1. Develop a plan for separation of personal and professional skills.

XI.P.2. Demonstrate appropriate response(s) to ethical issues.

XI.A.1. Recognize the impact that personal ethics and morals have on the delivery of healthcare.

2015 Standards and Guidelines for the Accreditation of Educational Programs in Medical Assisting, Appendix B, Core Curriculum for Medical Assistants, Medical Assisting Education Review Board (MAERB), 2015.

INTRODUCTION

Daily news headlines reflect legal and ethical questions: Should life support be ended for a patient when there are no signs of brain function? How should scarce healthcare resources be divided? When may a healthcare provider refuse to treat a patient? Consumers of healthcare services are interested in these legal and ethical healthcare issues. As healthcare professionals, administrative medical assistants have an even greater interest in such issues. Understanding the legal and ethical aspects of healthcare helps them act according to the highest professional standards. Such knowledge also helps assistants resolve issues of confidentiality and patients' rights.

2.1 MEDICAL ETHICS

All professions, as well as people's lives, are governed by standards of conduct. The standards of conduct that grow out of one's understanding of right and wrong are known as **ethics.** Medical ethics that govern the healthcare professions are usually found in written policies or codes for each profession. These standards are not laws. A person acting within the law may nevertheless do something that is not ethical. A person may also do something right, or ethical, while breaking the law. Ethics are statements of right and wrong behaviors that hold members of the profession to a high degree of behavior.

Principles of Medical Ethics

Hippocrates, a Greek physician who lived during the fourth and fifth centuries BCE, is called "the father of medicine." He made the first statement of principles governing the conduct of physicians. This statement, known as the Hippocratic oath, is the foundation of modern medical ethics. In part, the oath requires the physician to pledge the following:

> I will follow that method of treatment which, according to my ability and judgment, I consider for the benefit of my patients, and abstain from whatever is deleterious [harmful] and mischievous. . . . Whatever, in connection with my professional practice or not in connection with it, I may see or hear in the lives of men which ought not to be spoken abroad, I will not divulge, as reckoning that all such should be kept secret.

Today, physicians follow the Principles of Medical Ethics developed by the American Medical Association (AMA) and based on the Hippocratic oath. The code requires physicians, among other rules, to practice high standards of patient care, to respect patients' rights, to treat patients with compassion, and to safeguard patient confidences. Additionally, physicians are to continue advancing and improving their medical skills and knowledge, contribute to the welfare of the community, and maintain patient care as the most important aspect of healthcare.

The Medical Assistant's Ethical Responsibility

Most other associations that regulate healthcare professions also have codes of ethics to set levels of competence and patient care. The American Association of Medical Assistants (AAMA) has developed the Code of Ethics and Creed, which outlines moral and ethical behaviors for the medical assistant in relation to the medical profession and specifically to the career field of medical assisting. Because the administrative medical assistant is considered an agent of the physician while performing tasks related to employment, the AAMA code is based on AMA standards.

Medical assistants and administrative medical assistants, in their roles and within the boundaries of their job responsibilities, are required to (1) treat all patients with respect, (2) maintain confidentiality of patients' protected health information, (3) conduct professional activities in a manner that honors the profession, (4) improve knowledge and skills, and (5) contribute to the community. As an example, many medical offices organize teams to walk or run in community charity events to raise money for medical research. Attending continuing education workshops, seminars, and conferences that update skills and knowledge within the AMA field is another way to uphold the AMA code of ethics. In addition, assistants should endeavor to merit the respect of the public and of the medical profession. The creed emphasizes the qualities of effectiveness, loyalty, compassion, courage, and faith.

Medical coders can find their respective code of ethics at either the website for the American Academy of Professional Coders (aapc.com) or the website for the American Health Information and Management Association (ahima.org).

Bioethics

The area of **bioethics** deals with the ethics of medical treatment and technologies, processes, and scarcity of resources. Advances in the sciences, rapid developments in technology, and new kinds of treatment have dramatically increased the number of bioethical issues and questions. However, monetary resources—of both the patient and the medical provider—and medical availability impact decisions relating to the use of scarce medical advances. Professional guidelines in these areas are, in some cases, being legislated by federal and state laws and others may still need to be established. These issues are associated with abortion, the definition of *death,* patients' rights, and types of medical care. The response to bioethical issues may require a restatement or a new application of existing ethical guidelines.

Issues. Because physicians have always faced life-and-death situations, they have also faced difficult decisions. Today, their ethical responses have been made even more difficult by the increased power of technology and scientific knowledge. Consider the ethical aspects of these questions:

- What rights are involved with using a human fetus?
- Should genetic engineering—the altering of cells to produce physical traits or to eliminate disease—be encouraged? Suppose one of the outcomes is the cloning of a human being.
- How should scarce usable body organs be fairly allocated?
- When is it acceptable to remove a patient from life support? Who makes that decision?
- Should the physician be criminally responsible for assisting a terminally ill patient in his or her own suicide?
- Do individuals have the right to produce a child for the sole purpose of providing cells for another individual?
- Should providers have the right to refuse healthcare to morbidly obese patients?
- Should allocation of healthcare be based on the anticipated life-expectancy contribution of the patient, such as withholding life-sustaining care from the aged or chronically ill?

The ability to create, sustain, or end life is a major concern for individuals and for society. Many people who fear that their lives may be sustained without their consent have made living wills. In a **living will,** a person may clearly state the intent to refuse certain life-sustaining measures and specifies the length and methods of these measures. Examples of life-sustaining measures include

- receiving artificial hydration.
- receiving artificial nutrition.

- being revived using cardiopulmonary resuscitation (a Do Not Resuscitate [DNR] form must be completed by the patient and on file with the medical provider).
- being intubated.

The patient's wishes may also be stated in regard to organ donation.

Should the patient become unable to make medical decisions, another person may be appointed to carry out the requirements of the living will or make decisions regarding medical issues not covered in the living will. The medical durable power of attorney is discussed later in this chapter. The living will, which is valid in most states, is one response to a bioethical issue.

Moral Values. The link between moral values, or concepts of what is good, and professional behavior is shown in ethics by the use of words such as *compassion, honesty, honorable,* and *responsibility.* The primary ethical obligation of the physician is to put the benefit of the patient first. Moral values may dictate that physicians take certain actions and refrain from others. For example, considering the patient's well-being, the physician may agree to perform an abortion. However, every physician also has the right, based on his or her moral views, to refuse to perform abortions. Physicians also make moral choices about treatment based on how the treatment will benefit the patient. Some patients may request a particular treatment for their illness. A physician may ethically refuse to use the requested treatment if it does not meet the recognized standard of acceptable care.

Many times, physicians find moral values contained within the laws of the state where they practice; these laws must be obeyed. For example, violence against children must be reported in many states. However, even if the law does not require this notification, the physician must respond ethically by reporting such cases. The physician's own belief system, good judgment, and decision-making skill all contribute to the ethical practice of the profession.

Etiquette

Etiquette is defined as those behaviors and customs that are standards for what is considered good manners. While codes of ethics specify standards for capable patient care, *etiquette* is a broad term for behaviors that mark courteous treatment of others.

Proper office etiquette should be used by the administrative medical assistant at all times—including when upholding the respective code of ethics. Consider the following scenario and the application of etiquette.

SCENARIO

Patient A comes into the office and presents medical coverage through a state assistance program. Patient B checks in and presents a Blue Cross Blue Shield (BCBS) card for medical coverage. The administrative medical assistant addresses the BCBS patient with a friendly, warm tone and a smile. Patient A is not acknowledged with a verbal greeting, and the administrative medical assistant uses hand sanitizer while looking at Patient A.

The administrative medical assistant exhibited poor etiquette by treating Patient A as a lesser patient by refusing to offer a warm, friendly greeting and by the implied behavior that Patient A is unclean. The AMA and the AAMA codes of ethics say patients will be treated with human dignity. The administrative medical assistant did not uphold the code of ethics.

Frequently, an employer's rules of etiquette are found in the policy and procedures manual of the medical practice. Examples of good manners and proper etiquette in the office include

- dressing appropriately to show respect for others and for the profession.
- using proper forms of address for both the physician and patients.
- extending a cheerful greeting to all who visit the office.
- using proper telephone techniques.
- observing the use of polite everyday phrases: "Please," "Thank you," "Excuse me."

Etiquette forms the basis of effective communication and fosters satisfying interactions in all cultures and settings. Using good manners and following those aspects of etiquette that may be unique to the workplace help create a pleasant environment in an efficient office.

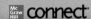 **GO TO PROJECT 2.1 AT THE END OF THIS CHAPTER**

2.2 MEDICAL LAW

Law is a set of rules made and enforced by a recognized authority. For example, federal, state, and city laws require some actions and forbid others. Law protects citizens and helps society work smoothly. Physicians and other healthcare professionals may be affected by the law—both criminal and civil statutes. The law, then, as it applies to standards of acceptable care, is known as *medical jurisprudence,* or *medical law.*

Law and the Right to Practice

Medical law regulates the right to practice and the granting of various licenses and certifications. Each state governs the practice of medicine within its borders through laws known as **medical practice acts.** These acts

- define *medical practice.*
- explain who must be licensed to give healthcare.
- set rules for obtaining a license and renewal of a license.
- state the duties imposed by the license.
- cover the grounds on which the license may be revoked.
- list the statutory reports that must be sent to the government.

State medical practice acts also protect users of healthcare services. To do this, the acts set forth the penalties for practicing medicine without a valid license. The acts also define *misconduct,* including conviction of a felony, such as insurance fraud; unprofessional conduct, such as sexual behavior with a patient; personal or professional incapacity, such as mental illness; and inappropriate use, or overprescribing, of drugs. The penalty for such acts may be the suspension or revocation of a license.

Licensing. The license to practice medicine, called **licensure,** is granted by a state medical board established in each state. Licenses are issued to applicants once they have completed the educational requirements and have successfully passed an examination. Licenses may also be issued as a result of reciprocity, the recognition by one state of another state's requirements for licensure. Those who have passed the examination given by the National Board of Medical Examiners receive licenses from the state through what is called *endorsement.*

Relicensure is required either annually or every other year. Those who hold licenses may be relicensed by paying a fee and providing proof, such as certificates of course completion, that they have met continuing education requirements, commonly referred to as CEUs (continuing education units). As an example, for a medical coder holding the CPC credential through AAPC to renew certification, membership must be maintained and at least 36 approved CEUs must be completed every 2 years. To renew the RHIT credential through AHIMA, 20 CEUs must be completed every 2 years.

Certified Specialization. The American Board of Specialties determines the competency of, and then certifies, those doctors who intend to practice within a medical specialty. The board requires additional academic in-hospital training in which the medical student, known as a *resident,* concentrates on a specialty and takes a comprehensive examination. Fulfilling the requirements, the candidate becomes *board-certified.* This certification is an essential minimum standard of competence in a particular medical specialty.

Narcotics Registration. A physician in clinical practice who will have occasion to prescribe or dispense drugs must register for a permit. This **registration** (permit), issued by the registration branch of the Drug Enforcement Administration (DEA), must be renewed every 3 years.

The Physician's Practice

In today's complex healthcare environment, the physician's practice has many elements of both a health service and a business, such as providing good patient care, scheduling, performing billing and insurance procedures, hiring and training staff, and maintaining the physical resources of the office, such as office premises and equipment. Every part of the practice is affected by legal and ethical considerations.

Because the physician's primary responsibility is to practice an acceptable standard of patient care, the laws, responsibilities, and ethical considerations that surround the physician-patient relationship are of great importance.

Contracts. The relationship between the physician and the patient starts when the patient goes to the physician for care. This initial contract is implied; it is not expressed in either words or writing. The physician does not say, "I am here to offer you care." The patient does not say, "I am requesting care." The patient usually has a medical need, and the physician treats it. The physician's behavior, in having a practice open to patients, and the patient's behavior, in going to the physician's office, together establish an implied contract. At times a written, or expressed, contract is provided, and both physician and patient sign a document. For example, the physician may provide a standard written contract to allow a patient to pay for services over an extended period of time, or the patient is to receive an injection that has stated risks.

Once the physician-patient relationship is established, the physician is legally required to

- possess the ordinary skill and learning commonly held by a reputable physician in a similar locality. The patient has the right to believe that the physician is so qualified. Accordingly, the physician's license should be displayed in the office.
- use his or her learning, skill, and best judgment for the benefit of the patient.
- preserve confidentiality.
- act in good faith.
- perform to the best of his or her ability.
- advise against needless or unwise treatment.
- inform and advise the patient when the physician knows a condition is beyond his or her scope of competency.

The physician is not legally required to

- accept as patients all those who seek his or her services.
- restore a patient to the same condition that existed before illness occurred.
- obtain recovery for every patient.
- guarantee successful results from an operation or a treatment.
- be familiar with all possible reactions of patients to various medicines.
- be free from errors in complex cases.
- possess the maximum amount of education possible.
- continue care after a patient discharges himself or herself from a hospital, even if harm could come to the patient.

In the physician-patient relationship, the patient also has certain responsibilities. The patient must give the information necessary for the physician to make a correct diagnosis; follow the physician's instructions and any orders for treatment, provided that these are within the bounds of similar standards of care for physicians who practice in that area of medicine; be, in general, cooperative; and pay for all services rendered.

Consent. When a patient goes to a physician's office for treatment, that patient's consent to treatment, like the contract itself, is not stated outright. This **implied consent** applies to routine treatment only. For more complicated procedures, especially surgery, diagnostic tests, and x-ray treatments, it is important to have **expressed consent.** The patient may express consent either in writing or orally. It is standard practice for the patient to give expressed consent by signing a special consent form before any special procedure is performed. An exception to this practice is the patient who is incapable of giving consent when an emergency requires immediate action. Express written consent is important to avoid later lawsuits or, even more seriously, criminal accusations.

When oral consent is acceptable, it may be given in a phone conversation, provided that the call is a three-way conversation involving the patient and two office personnel. Both office employees then must sign as witnesses to the conversation in which the patient expressed consent.

There is another aspect of patient consent, whether implied or express. The patient must give **informed consent,** meaning that the patient has had the illness or problem explained by the physician in simple, understandable language. The patient has also been given options for treatment and for the refusal of treatment, with the individual benefits and risks of each, along with the physician's prognosis. Also, the medical team personnel must give the patient an opportunity to ask questions and provide time, if needed, for the patient to discuss the plan with his or her family or advisors. Patients also have the right during informed consent to have their questions answered to their satisfaction—not necessarily to their liking, but to their satisfaction. Also, a check on the patient's comprehension should be conducted. The physician will know what he or she intended the patient to understand, but the physician must check to be sure the patient actually received and processed the information as intended. Also addressed during informed consent are the likelihood of success, treatment alternatives, and the potential outcome without treatment. In other words, the patient has been given enough information to make a knowledgeable decision. The final part of informed consent is the patient's consent to have the procedure or treatment performed. A sample consent form is shown in Figure 2.1.

Adults who are *legally competent* are able to give informed consent. The law requires that, in order to be competent, a person must have attained legal age of *majority* (adult age as defined by law) and must be of sound mind. When a patient is not able to give consent, that consent must be given by the next of kin, the legal guardian, or a court-appointed guardian, such as a court-appointed surrogate or proxy. A **durable**

Figure 2.1

Informed Consent Form

CONSENT FOR INFLUENZA (FLU) VACCINE
Office of Karen Larsen, MD

Purpose of the Influenza Vaccine

Influenza is a highly contagious respiratory tract infection. Symptoms may include chills, fever, headache, cough, sore throat, and muscle aches. Generally, the illness lasts several days to a week or more. The flu may be severe or even life-threatening for some people.

Each year the influenza vaccine is updated because viruses that cause the flu often change.

Influenza Vaccine

The flu vaccine contains inactive (dead) influenza viruses selected by the U.S. Food and Drug Administration. Because it is an inactive virus vaccine, the vaccine will not give you the flu.

Protection from the flu vaccine develops within 2 weeks after receiving the vaccine and may last up to a year.

Risks and Side Effects

The risk of the flu vaccine causing serious problems is very small. Mild side effects may include soreness, redness, and swelling of the injection site; fever; and muscle aches. If any side effects occur, they may begin upon receiving the vaccine injection and last 1 to 2 days.

NOTE: People who have an allergy to eggs, chicken, or chicken feathers should not receive the influenza vaccine. Also people who currently have an active infection should not receive the vaccine.

If you have any questions or concerns, please check with your physician before receiving the flu vaccine.

Freedom of Consent

The influenza vaccine is a voluntary injection. You are free to deny this consent.

Patient's Consent

I have read this form. I understand the purpose of the influenza vaccine and the risks and benefits of the vaccine. I have expressed any questions or concerns about the flu vaccine to my physician.

_____   _____
Patient receiving the vaccine (Please print)   Date of birth

_____   _____
Signature of patient or guardian   Date

Figure 2.1

Informed Consent Form

power of attorney might have been executed by the patient. A durable power of attorney (DPA) gives someone else, of the patient's choosing, the right to make decisions for the patient. Specifically, a medical durable power of attorney gives another individual the legal right to make decisions relating to a patient's medical issues such as long-term care. Copies of all legal documents must be on file in the patient's record prior to granting permission for another to give informed medical consent.

An **emancipated minor** is a minor who has gained independence (emancipation) either by situation or by court order from parents or legal guardians prior to adulthood, which in many states is 16 or 18 years of age. If the minor is emancipated through a court order, a copy of the order should be obtained and placed into the emancipated minor's medical record. State laws may vary in legal requirements for emancipated minors. A medical administrative assistant should consult both federal and state requirements for emancipated minors. In many states, minors may be emancipated and give consent in the following cases:

- By court order
- A minor who is in the military service

- A minor who is living away from his or her parents and is managing his or her own financial day-to-day affairs
- A college student who is living away from home
- A minor who is married or divorced

An emancipated minor may decide for himself or herself what medical treatment will be received, from whom it will be obtained, and how often the treatment will be received. An emancipated minor may also refuse treatment. Following are the kinds of medical care that minors may usually consent to:

- Pregnancy tests and/or prevention of pregnancy
- Prenatal care
- Diagnosis and treatment of a sexually transmitted disease
- Diagnosis and treatment of alcohol or drug abuse
- Diagnosis and treatment of rape, incest, or child abuse
- HIV testing
- Mental health treatment, counseling, or residential shelter (The minor must demonstrate to the healthcare provider that he or she has the maturity level to participate in healthcare decisions in an intelligent manner. Also, the minor must be deemed a danger to herself or himself or to others if treatment is not rendered.)
- Treatment as an alleged victim of incest or child abuse

Records for emancipated minors must be kept confidential and not accessible to parents or legal guardians unless consent is given by the patient for disclosure of information.

Some states have placed into law the **mature minor** doctrine, and state laws vary on the requirements for a minor to be legally declared "mature." However, not all states have adopted the common-law mature minor doctrine. Therefore, state law should be consulted prior to rendering medical services to a minor who states he or she is mature enough to make medical decisions for him/herself. A mature minor is a minor who has demonstrated that he or she possesses the maturity to make decisions about his or her own medical care. An example would be that a mature minor may either accept or refuse a blood transfusion based on religious beliefs. Medical decisions made by the mature minor can be made with or without the input of parents or guardians. Several factors, which vary from state to state, are evaluated during the decision-making process of evaluating a minor as "mature":

- Age of the minor
- Ability to comprehend the nature, risk, and consequences of the medical treatment
- Exhibition of the minor's degree of maturity (conduct and demeanor of the minor)
- Education and/or training of the minor
- Circumstances of each individual case

Again, state laws vary regarding minors (unemancipated, emancipated, and mature) and medical care, so state law should be consulted before treating a minor without parental consent.

For medical and legal purposes, written or electronic verification of informed consent should be maintained for each treatment option discussed with a patient, whether emancipated or adult by law. Topics, questions, and answers (discussed earlier in the chapter) are recorded on a consent form. Although there is no one consent form required by law, the informed consent that the patient signs should usually contain the following:

- The name of the patient and the date
- The name of the procedure to be performed

- The name of the physician performing the procedure
- An explanation of the procedure
- A statement of risks and benefits
- A statement that the patient signs to signify understanding of the procedure and the information given in the form
- The patient's signature
- The signature of a witness (optional) testifying to the patient's signature
- Alternative(s) to treatment and risks and benefits of the alternative(s)

In addition to written, informed consent for procedures, there are other reasons for obtaining patient consent. For example, if a physician wishes to videotape a patient visit or procedure for training purposes, the physician must obtain the patient's written consent. An example of this type of consent form is shown in Figure 2.2.

COMPLIANCE *TIP*

The assistant should always bring to the physician's attention any confusion noticed in a patient about directions or any lack of understanding. If the patient has questions, the assistant should inform the physician. Alertness on the part of the assistant will help ensure informed consent.

In addition to consent forms, the medical chart for a patient should contain all legal documents that may be used for the care of the patient. **Advance directives** are legal documents stating the patient's wishes for medical care, should he or she not be able to make these decisions. Living wills (discussed earlier in this chapter) should be maintained in the patient's medical record. When a patient does not want to be resuscitated, a DNR (Do Not Resuscitate) should be executed and on file with the medical office.

Figure 2.2

Consent for Videotaping Form

CONSENT FOR VIDEOTAPING

I, _____Any Patient_____ , give my consent for the videotaping of my appointment with Karen Larsen, MD, including medical history and examination on this date.

I understand that I have a right to private, confidential medical consultation and treatment, and I voluntarily waive that right so that the videotape may be used for teaching purposes at the University Medical School.

I am in agreement that my medical history, which is related to the taped examination, may be disclosed during the described use of the videotape for
_____teaching purposes_____.

I further understand that at any future time I may request in writing that certain parts or the entire recording be deleted and not used.

Signature _____Any Patient_____   Date _____7/10/20-_____

Witness _____Any Witness_____   Date _____7/10/20-_____

Copies of a durable power of attorney, medical and/or financial, should also be filed in the patient's record. When a patient is admitted to the hospital, each of these documents should also be forwarded to the hospital if they are not available through the patient's electronic health record.

Most states have adopted a newer method to help patients who are not able to express desired life-sustaining interventions. The Physician Orders for Life-Sustaining Treatment (**POLST**) is a multisection medical order form that allows the patient to choose the level of life-sustaining services in areas such as cardiopulmonary resuscitation, medical interventions, antibiotics, and artificially administered nutrition. The difference between this type of form and other healthcare advance directives is that it is signed by both the patient and the physician, making it a set of medical orders. Also, the POLST moves with the patient and is part of his or her medical record. However, it is not meant to replace advance directives but is used as a medical order to render services in various medical situations.

SCENARIO

A terminally ill cancer patient completes and signs a POLST, and the physician also signs the form. If the patient becomes ill and must be taken to the hospital by ambulance, the form (which the patient has in his or her possession) is given to the emergency medical technicians (EMTs). The EMTs now have a signed physician order for advanced life-sustaining services or nonservices. When the patient reaches the hospital, the POLST travels with the patient and becomes part of the hospital record. When the patient is discharged, the POLST is returned to the patient. It is a "traveling" form. As electronic patient charts are becoming more accessible between medical providers, the POLST will be viewable by multiple providers.

Administrative medical assistants will recognize the form by its bright color—many states use bright, lime green forms—and by its name. The program name may differ by state. In addition to POLST, state program names include MOLST (Medical Orders for Life-Sustaining Treatment), MOST (Medical Orders for Scope of Treatment), and POST (Physician Orders for Scope of Treatment).

 connect **GO TO PROJECT 2.2 AT THE END OF THIS CHAPTER**

Medical Liability and Communications

Liability means legal responsibility. In many areas of life, people are liable, or legally responsible, for actions (or nonactions) and their consequences. The owner of a home may be liable for an injury caused to a guest in the home.

Physicians have liability in their roles as providers of healthcare and as owners of a medical practice. Under the legal doctrine of **respondeat superior,** an employer is liable for employees' actions when employees are acting within the scope of their employment. Therefore, physicians are responsible for the actions of their staff. If the medical coder releases information on a healthcare claim that is not directly related to the services rendered on the claim, the physician is ultimately responsible for the breach of confidentiality. In general, physicians are responsible not only for the quality of the care they give to patients but also for

- *the safety of employees.* An office policy and procedures manual will often contain regulations that relate to observing state laws for safety, including the handling of discarded waste and hazardous materials.
- *the safety of the premises.* Rules that help ensure protection from injury, theft, and fire need to be specified. This is important not only for patients and employees but also for the safety of records.

Physicians wishing to protect themselves from lawsuits brought by patients sometimes practice **defensive medicine.** This means that physicians order tests and/or additional tests and follow-up visits to confirm a diagnosis or treatment result. The physician's liability as it relates to patient care is discussed in the following sections.

Malpractice. **Malpractice** is the improper care or treatment of a patient by a physician, hospital, or other provider of healthcare as a result of carelessness, neglect, lack of professional skill, or disregard for the established rules or procedures. In spite of vigilance on the part of the physician and the office staff, accidents may occur during treatment. Some patients may be dissatisfied with the care they have received. In cases such as these, a patient may file a malpractice suit against the physician. A patient who files a suit is required to prove that there is an injury, as the law defines *injury,* and that the physician's inadequate care was the direct cause of the injury.

Termination. As discussed earlier, the contractual agreement between the patient and the physician calls for the physician to furnish care to the patient for a particular illness as long as care is required. At times, a physician may choose to terminate, or end, the physician-patient relationship because a patient does not follow treatment instructions or because the patient has stated (either orally or in writing) an intent to seek care from another physician. If a patient is unreasonably demanding or has threatened the provider and/or any member of the medical team, it may be necessary to discontinue providing medical care to the patient. Other reasons may be due simply to patient relocation, retirement of the physician, or nonpayment of charges by the patient.

The physician is required to notify the patient of the decision to terminate the patient-physician relationship and to allow the patient a reasonable amount of time to obtain another physician. The AMA (American Medical Association) recommends using the following steps to appropriately terminate the patient-physician relationship:

1. Provide written notice to the patient of the termination. Certified mail, Return Receipt requested, is recommended. In the letter, provide a brief explanation for the termination of the relationship—for instance, noncompliance with medical advice or consistent failure to keep appointments.
2. Provide medical treatment for a reasonable amount of time, such as 30 to 45 days for minor conditions or 2 to 3 months for more complex cases, allowing the patient

time to secure medical care from another provider. It is appropriate to provide the patient with resources and recommendations to help the patient locate another physician of the same or closely related specialty.

3. Offer to transfer the patient's records to the new physician. Secure a signed and dated authorization from the patient before transferring records.

After a withdrawal letter has been sent, the physician should provide the patient's name to the administrative medical assistant who schedules appointments. If the patient calls and requests an appointment, the call should be transferred to the physician, who will explain to the patient what needs to be done to reestablish care.

Abandonment. Unless the patient is discharged in an appropriate way, either because the treatment was completed or because the physician followed the procedure for termination, the patient may sue the physician for abandonment. **Medical abandonment** is when the physician-patient relationship is terminated at an unreasonable time and without providing the patient an opportunity to locate another physician of the same or similar specialty. When a patient claims to have been medically abandoned, he or she must prove that the physician ended the relationship at a critical stage of the patient's care without a justifiable reason or sufficient notification and that, as a result of the abandonment, the patient sustained an injury. Good documentation is essential to proving that the physician did not abandon the patient.

EXAMPLE: PATIENT'S APPOINTMENT HISTORY TO AVOID MEDICAL ABANDONMENT

Notations in patient medical record:

4/6/20-	Patient canceled appointment. Rescheduled for 4/13/20-.
4/13/20-	Patient did not show up for follow-up appointment.
4/13/20-	Patient was sent a letter requesting her to reschedule her 4/13/20- missed appointment.
4/16/20-	Patient reschedules missed 4/13/20- appointment. Rescheduled for 4/20/20-.
4/20/20-	Patient did not show up for rescheduled follow-up appointment.

As a precaution, patients should be notified of any physician absences from the office for vacation, conferences, or emergencies. The name and telephone number of the substituting or covering physician should be made available to patients. The assistant may post a notice of the physician's absence or mail a notice to patients. The notice or letter should be kept on file. As electronic health records are implemented in the medical field, notices of absence and coverage during the absence should also be posted at the website or other social media sites for the physician.

The following example could constitute medical abandonment.

EXAMPLE: MEDICAL ABANDONMENT

Patient A had a surgical procedure scheduled with Dr. Public on Tuesday. The patient arrived at the hospital and registered. After several hours, the surgical unit phoned the physician's office and received a recorded message that Dr. Public was out of town and would not return for 3 weeks. Information for coverage was not given. No patients were notified of his absence. Dr. Public has also missed scheduled patient appointments in the past.

Assault and Battery. The clear threat of injury to another is called **assault.** Any bodily contact without permission is called **battery.** In medical law, *battery* is interpreted to include surgical and medical procedures performed without the patient's consent or procedures that go beyond the degree of consent that was given.

> EXAMPLE: MEDICAL BATTERY
>
> A badly damaged uterus is removed during exploratory surgery, even though the patient had not signed a consent for the removal.

In this example, even though the procedure may have been in the best interest of the patient, the physician may be sued for battery. Unless a physician acts in a grave emergency, he or she may well lose a lawsuit in court as a result of not having proper patient consent.

Fraud. An intentionally dishonest practice that deprives others of their rights is called **fraud.** Fraud is often committed by medical professionals to gain monetary payment or other benefits to which they would otherwise not be entitled. Depending on the laws of the state where the physician practices, the penalty may range from reprimand to the revoking of a license.

A wide range of activities is included under the definition of *fraud.* Examples include

- making false statements to a patient about the benefits of a particular drug or treatment.
- falsifying diplomas or licenses.
- submitting false or duplicate claims for payment to the federal government or an insurance company.

All members of the medical office team should be cautious about making fraudulent claims (verbal or written) or claims that may be interpreted as fraudulent. Physicians who are convicted of medical fraud may face fines, imprisonment, and possible loss of the right to practice medicine.

Litigation. The bringing of lawsuits, or **litigation,** against the physician is not uncommon. Many lawsuits arise out of civil law. Civil law deals with crimes against persons committed by other persons or institutions, such as the government or a business. While criminal law handles the actual commission of a crime, civil law gives a person the right to sue. For example, a physician may be convicted of battery in a criminal court and then may be sued by the patient in civil court for injuries resulting from the battery. The civil court may decide to award the patient a certain amount of money for the injuries.

One common type of civil suit that patients may bring is for malpractice. However, the law also covers many other aspects of the physician's practice, such as the hiring process, drug testing of employees, equal opportunity, sexual harassment, fair labor laws, and workers' compensation.

If called to court, follow the directions and advice of the practice's attorney. It is not advisable to go to court without legal representation. If the practice does not have an attorney on retainer, contact other practices that do and retain his or her services. Additionally, medical office personnel may purchase liability insurance.

Steps in Litigation

Once a lawsuit is begun, there are several steps involved in resolving it:

- *Summons.* A written notice—the **summons**—is sent to the person being sued (the *defendant*), ordering the defendant to answer the charges made. The summons is sent by the court along with a copy of the complaint filed by the other party (the *plaintiff*).
- *Subpoena.* A **subpoena** is a legal document in which the court orders an individual to appear in court. It can also order that certain documents relevant to the case be delivered to the court. A **subpoena duces tecum** requires a person who has information related to the case to appear in court *and* to bring documents or other tangible legal evidence related to the case.
- *Deposition.* A sworn statement to the court before any trial begins, and usually made outside of court, is called a **deposition.**

The Physician's Response to Litigation

Complete, accurate documentation is critical in physician-patient disputes. The documentation may provide the physician with evidence of **contributory negligence.** A patient's refusal to have tests, x-rays, or vaccinations or a patient's failure to follow the physician's instructions may be considered contributory negligence. The physician's notations in the patient record, made at the time of the patient's actions, would protect the physician against a later claim that reasonable precautions had not been taken. Any contact by telephone, letter, electronic communication, or face-to-face encounter regarding, for example, the patient's refusal to have laboratory or x-ray reports, should also be indicated.

EXAMPLE: CONTRIBUTORY NEGLIGENCE

Notation in patient's medical record:

3/12/20-   Patient refused to have chest x-ray. Patient did accept medication.

Alternatives to Trial

The complaint may be heard in court at a trial. However, the case may also be resolved through settlement or arbitration. In a **settlement,** the plaintiff and the physician's insurance company reach an agreement and the case does not go to court. In **arbitration,** through a process fair to both sides, an *arbitrator* (an unbiased third party) is chosen. This person, rather than a judge, hears evidence and helps both sides resolve the dispute or makes a decision if the two sides cannot agree. Because the defendant and the plaintiff agree beforehand to abide by the arbitrator's decision, the arbitration also ends the case before it reaches court.

Statute of Limitations

A law that sets a time limit for initiating litigation is called a **statute of limitations.** This time limit varies from state to state, and federal statutes establish the time limits for federal cases. The time span during which a lawsuit for malpractice may be brought may begin when the claimed negligence first occurred, when the claimed negligence was first discovered, or when the physician-patient relationship ended. In pediatric cases, the time span may begin after the patient reaches the state's legal age of majority. When children are treated, physicians should retain records long enough to cover this span of time. Information about particular state laws is available from state offices and their websites.

Good Samaritan Act

When someone voluntarily renders aid in an emergency situation to an injured individual, that person is legally referred to as a *good samaritan*. When rendering aid to someone, a good samaritan should be reasonably careful not to cause further injury. The **Good Samaritan Act** is designed to protect individuals who render care to an injured person from liability for civil damages that may arise as a result of providing emergency care. If first aid is part of a good samaritan's job description, then he or she is obligated by law to render first aid.

There are many variations of the Good Samaritan Act from state to state. In some states, it is considered an act of negligence if a person fails to at least call for help. Other states offer immunity to good samaritans when an unintentional injury is sustained by the injured party. However, when the injury is the result of negligent care or reckless treatment, the good samaritan may not receive immunity. States that offer immunity under Good Samaritan laws will not hold a good samaritan liable for damages when the following two conditions are met:

1. Aid must be rendered at the scene of an emergency.
2. Motive was strictly to render aid, without expecting to receive any type of payment for services.

Because of the minor variations from state to state, the medical assistant's role in emergency situations is defined by the state in which the assistant is employed.

False Claims Act

The original False Claims Act was passed by Congress in 1863. Since that time, it has been updated and amended and is currently a major legislative weapon in the fight against fraud. Areas such as nursing facilities, physicians' offices, and hospitals are governed by the False Claims Act. Other areas, including federal weapons and defense contracts, are also required to be compliant.

Under the False Claims Act, whistleblowers—individuals who have evidence of fraud involving federal funding, such as Medicare dollars, were given increased protection against retaliation. Additionally, the financial reward to whistleblowers in successfully prosecuted cases was increased. When a whistleblower has evidence of misuse of federal funds, a claim is filed under the False Claims Act and is referred to as a "qui tam" action. In a qui tam action, a suit is brought by a whistleblower on behalf of the federal government. Whistleblowers typically include healthcare administrators, nurses, patients, and doctors. Private individuals and companies may file an action only through an attorney. A few examples of fraud under the False Claims Act are

- billing for services, pharmaceuticals, and tests that were never rendered to the patient.
- billing for services at a higher level than the actual rendered service.
- accepting healthier patients, as opposed to sicker patients who will require more medical services, in order to receive a higher reimbursement from medical plans that pay on a set reimbursement amount for each patient or condition.

Stark Law/Anti-Kickback Laws

Under the Stark Law, physicians are not permitted to make patient referrals to an entity that provides designated health services (DHS) and receives payment from a federal health program *if* the physician or an immediate family member has a financial relationship with the provider(s). A financial relationship, as defined by the Stark Law, exists when the referring physician has a direct or indirect investment or ownership in the rendering entity or will receive payment or compensation from the rendering entity for the referral. Services defined as DHS include

- clinical laboratory services.
- physical and occupational therapy.
- outpatient speech-language pathology services.
- radiology and other imaging services.
- DME (durable medical equipment).
- parenteral and enteral nutrients, equipment, and supplies.
- prosthetics and orthotics.
- prosthetic devices and related supplies.
- outpatient prescription drug treatment.
- home health services.
- inpatient hospital services.
- outpatient hospital services.
- nuclear medicine.
- a financial relationship.

Physicians may apply for an exception to the Stark Law. Currently, there are approximately 35 exceptions under which a physician may refer a patient for DHS in which he or she has a vested interest. These can be found at the OIG and other legal websites. Penalties for violation of the Stark Law include (1) repayment of all claims paid by Medicare and Medicaid that proved to be in violation of the Stark Law, (2) civil penalties of up to $100,000, (3) exclusion from both Medicare and Medicaid, (4) criminal fines ranging from $25,000 to $100,000, and (5) maximum jail incarceration of up to 10 years.

Stark laws and Anti-Kickback laws have similar features and intents. However, there are a few differences.

1. Anti-Kickback laws prohibit a provider from receiving, paying, offering, or soliciting *anything of value* in order to receive referrals. Stark laws prohibit the provider from referring to a DHS entity in which he or she or a family member has a *vested interest.*
2. Anti-Kickback laws prohibit referrals from *anyone* in order to receive an incentive. Stark laws prohibit referral from *physicians* to a DHS entity.
3. Anti-Kickback laws cover *any items or services* received as a kickback for referrals. Stark laws cover *designated health services (DHS).*
4. Anti-Kickback laws apply to payments from *all* federal healthcare programs. Stark laws are specific to payments received from *Medicare and Medicaid.*
5. Anti-Kickback law violations include both *criminal and civil penalties.* Stark Law violations include *civil* penalties.

A newer Anti-Kickback law, the Eliminating Kickbacks and Recovery Act of 2018 (EKRA), was passed. This legislation was passed to address the problem of a third party (physician, clinic, etc.) enrolling an addicted patient into an insurance plan and then arranging for the patient to be admitted into a treatment facility, sometimes called a *sober home*. In exchange for placing the patient in the treatment facility, the third party (admitting provider) would receive a kickback payment from the treatment facility. The treatment facility would then bill the insurance plan for services. EKRA refers to this action as "patient brokering." Because Stark laws and other Anti-Kickback laws target only healthcare benefit programs or providers that receive federal payments (Medicare, Medicaid, etc.), entities receiving payment from private pay insurers could not be prosecuted under those laws. Therefore, a gap in Anti-Kickback laws existed.

EKRA states that *whoever* receives a kickback in exchange for brokering a patient to a treatment facility/sober home or certain clinical labs will be fined up to $200,000, be imprisoned for no more than 10 years, or both.

There are exceptions to EKRA, and since the legislation is new and its scope is still being defined as of the writing of this text, medical providers should consult EKRA regulations when referring patients to treatment facilities/sober homes, recovery homes, and some clinical laboratories.

Patient's Bill of Rights

In 1997, the original version of the Patient's Bill of Rights was passed by Congress. Its main goals were to increase and strengthen consumers' confidence in the healthcare system, to establish a stronger foundation on which to build physician-patient relationships, to emphasize a patient's right to receive quality care, and to make patients more responsible by stipulating that the patient must take an active role in the management of his or her own healthcare. Specifically, eight patient rights were stated in the original version:

1. Patient's right to an accurate and easy-to-understand health plan, provider, and facility information in the patient's preferred mode of communication
2. Patient's right to choose high-quality healthcare providers
3. Patient's right to emergency services, without waiting for authorization or incurring a financial penalty, *if* the patient feels his or her life is in imminent danger from severe pain, illness, or sudden injury
4. Patient's right to know his or her treatment options—explained in understandable, lay terms—and to participate in or refuse treatment
5. Patient's right to considerate and respectful healthcare
6. Patient's right to confidentiality of protected healthcare; to read and be provided a copy of his or her medical record, and the right to ask for corrections to the medical record if the record is incomplete or inaccurate
7. Patient's right to a fair and fast review process on a complaint as it relates to aspects of the patient's healthcare; areas included—but not limited to: actions of personnel, wait times, and facility inadequacies
8. Patient's right to take an active part in the management of his or her own healthcare

In 2010, additional patient rights federal regulations were provided to protect patients and place them in a more dominant role regarding their own healthcare. The new regulations placed bans on long-standing insurance practices. Basically, the regulations banned insurance companies from

1. dropping patient coverage due to an unintentional error on an insurance application form.
2. imposing lifetime coverage limits.
3. deciding which provider a patient must see (patients can choose their own provider from within the health plan's network).
4. charging more for using an out-of-network emergency center.
5. denying the patient's right to appeal a coverage/payment decision to a third party.
6. denying full coverage (no out-of-pocket expense) for recommended preventive services.
7. denying coverage for young adults up through their 26th birthday, unless coverage is provided to a young adult by an employer.

Medical Communications—Access to Information. All information a patient gives a physician is confidential. Administrative medical assistants who process physicians' correspondence and work with patients' records are authorized to read this information. However, no patient information may be conveyed to anyone outside of the practice without permission from the patient. Under the federal law known as the *Final Privacy Rule,* patients must provide a general consent to the sharing of information for the purpose of carrying out treatment or submitting insurance claims. They must also provide written **authorization** for specific items that are not covered by the general consent.

Patients have the right to see their medical records. Preferably, this is to be done with the physician's participation so that information can be interpreted for the patient in a meaningful way. The physician must always be notified when patients request to review their records.

Release of Information

It is often necessary to release information from patients' medical records to insurance companies, other medical facilities, or other physicians. These releases are connected to patient care, proper treatment, and accurate billing and may be released under HIPAA without written patient consent. HIPAA will be discussed later in this chapter. The strictest confidentiality must be maintained while providing requested data. The medical office follows a procedure to make sure that the party asking for the information has the right to receive it, that proper authorization to release the information has been granted, and that appropriate methods and security precautions are used to transmit the data.

The administrative medical assistant can ensure the proper transfer of information by carefully following the office's procedure and double-checking the source and validity of the request. If patient information is being requested for purposes other than patient treatment by another physician or facility, collection of insurance payment, or maintenance of workflow in the medical office, the patient must give permission in writing to release the information. For example, information about alcohol and drug abuse may not be released without a specific authorization form from the patient. "Use" of medical information refers to the entity's internal sharing of medical data, such as the medical coder asking a question of the physician in regard to a patient's diagnosis. Use of medical information does not require a written authorization from a patient. "Disclosure" of information refers to the entity's external sharing of medical data, such as sending medical treatment and diagnostic information on a claim form to a healthcare plan. Depending on the purpose of the disclosure, it may or may not require a written release. We will discuss this at a different time in this chapter. Written permission is in the form of an authorization for **release of information (ROI),** sometimes simply called a *release*. The authorization for release of information must meet several legal requirements in order to be valid. A sample authorization form is shown in Figure 2.3.

The release must be in plain English or in the patient's preferred mode of communication/language and include the following information:

- A description of the information to be used or disclosed
- The patient's full name and date of birth
- The name or other specific identification of the person(s) or entity authorized to receive the information
- A description of the purpose of each requested use or disclosure
- An expiration date
- The signature of the individual (or authorized representative)
- The date the form was signed
- A statement that the patient may revoke the release of information

COMPLIANCE *TIP*

The physician's office may only forward information about a patient that is part of the patient's care in that office. Information about patients that comes from hospital or clinic records cannot be forwarded by the physician's office. Such information must be requested from the source that generated it.

Figure 2.3

Authorization for Release-of-Information Form

AUTHORIZATION TO RELEASE MEDICAL INFORMATION

Original Authorization MUST be attached to the patient's permanent medical record.
A copy of this Authorization should be attached to the forwarded medical record.

DATE: _____

TO: Karen Larsen, MD
      2235 South Ridgeway Avenue
      Chicago, IL 60623-2240
      312-555-6022, 312-555-0025 fax

RE: Patient name _____
      Patient street address _____
      Patient city, state, ZIP _____
      Patient telephone _____
      Patient date of birth _____

The undersigned hereby requests and authorizes Karen Larsen, MD, to release to (INSERT NAME OF RECIPIENT OF PATIENT RECORDS) or any of his/her/their assigned representatives, copies of any and all records and documents regarding the undersigned's past and current medical treatment, medical condition(s), and medical expenses. The information to be released includes any and all medical and hospital records currently within your possession, including, but not limited to, any and all x-ray films, pathology slides, laboratory reports, medical histories, consultation reports, prescriptions, medical correspondence, consent forms, employment information, and billing information.

In addition to authorizing the release of the above stated medical records and documents, the undersigned expressly authorizes Karen Larsen, MD, to release the following information to the designated individual or entity: (Please initial the items below for release, if appropriate)

____ Psychiatric information ____ Drug/Alcohol information ____ HIV-related information

The physician is instructed to comply with this request by providing copies of my records only, with the understanding that my original medical record will be maintained within the possession of Karen Larsen, MD.

A copy of this authorization **shall not** be used in lieu of an originally signed authorization.

This authorization may be revoked by the undersigned at any time by a written notice to the physician except to the extent that action has already been taken.

This authorization will expire sixty (60) days from the date of this request OR _____ (specify other date) and will be null and void thereafter.

_____   _____
Signature of patient   Date

Patient is a minor, or patient is legally unable to sign because _____

_____   _____
Signature of authorized person   Date

_____   _____
Print name of authorized person   Relationship to patient

Disclosure statement: This information is being disclosed to you from records whose confidentiality is protected by federal and state law. Federal and state law prohibit you from making any further disclosure of this information without the specific written authorization of the person to whom it pertains, or as otherwise permitted by law.

Helping Ensure Confidentiality

The administrative medical assistant can help protect confidentiality by

- avoiding any conversation, either in person or on the telephone, with a patient or others, about any aspect of treatment, patient records, or financial arrangements; when speaking on the phone, avoiding using the caller's name or the name of any patient.

- being careful when calling patients about test results, which includes never leaving a message on the answering machine or with any other person except to request a return call from the patient.
- keeping documents shielded from view in areas where fax machines, copy machines, and printers are located.
- removing documents from these areas and shredding them, rather than putting materials in the trash.
- protecting computerized records and other information, which includes not leaving information showing on any unattended screen and being careful of access to the network if the computer shares programs and data files.

Exceptions to Confidentiality. Under some circumstances, the physician is required to file reports containing confidential information to state departments of health or social services. These are called *statutory reports*. The government needs this information to protect the health of the whole community. Each state has its own requirements for statutory reports. Each state is responsible for making and enforcing the laws related to the reports it needs. The following are examples of circumstances requiring statutory reports:

- Births
- Deaths
- Abuse of a child, a vulnerable or elderly adult, or a battered person (State law requires teachers, physicians, and other licensed healthcare workers to report cases of suspected abuse; and any private citizen may, at any time, file a complaint with a protective agency.)
- Injuries resulting from violence, such as gunshot or stab wounds, or any other evidence of criminal violence
- Occupational illnesses, such as chemical poisoning
- Communicable diseases, including acquired immune deficiency syndrome (AIDS), hepatitis, neonatal herpes, Lyme disease, rabies, and sexually transmitted diseases
- Cases of food poisoning

Another exception to the requirement for a release of information is a court-ordered release of patient information. As discussed earlier in this chapter, a subpoena may be issued for patient information. A subpoena duces tecum may also be issued requiring the stated individual, such as the physician, to appear in court and to also bring stated patient records.

COMPLIANCE *TIP*

To comply with the HIPAA Privacy Rule, medical offices must give each patient a copy of their Notice of Privacy Practices (NPP) at the patient's first encounter. The written notice explains how patients' information may be used (internally) or disclosed (externally) and describes their privacy rights. Patients must then sign and date an acknowledgment showing that they have read and understand the document.

Transmission of Information Electronically. In today's medical practice, it is very common to transmit information electronically. To ensure that health information is protected from misuse, a federal law, the **Health Insurance Portability and Accountability**

Act (HIPAA) (pronounced hip-uh), regulates how electronic patient information is stored and shared. The administrative medical assistant must be conscientious about the following:

- If information is faxed, the assistant should carefully check the fax number and then call to confirm receipt.
- The assistant should use a cover page for the fax, requesting the return of the information if it has reached the wrong person.
- The assistant should not send confidential information by e-mail. Most e-mail networks are not secure.

The following section (Section 2.3) discusses HIPAA in detail.

  GO TO PROJECT 2.3 AT THE END OF THIS CHAPTER

2.3 HIPAA

HIPAA (the Health Insurance Portability and Accountability Act of 1996) became Public Law 104-191 in 1996. A major provision of HIPAA, known as Administrative Simplification, affects medical practices as well as hospitals, health plans, and healthcare clearinghouses. Its rules have gradually been passed and then implemented in the healthcare industry.

Implementing HIPAA has changed administrative, financial, and case management policies and procedures. There are now strict requirements for the uniform transfer of electronic healthcare data, such as for billing and payment; new patient rights regarding personal health information, including the right to access this information and to limit its disclosure; and broad new security rules that healthcare organizations must put in place to safeguard the confidentiality of patients' medical information.

There are three parts to HIPAA's Administrative Simplification provisions:

1. **HIPAA Electronic Transaction and Code Set Standards Requirements**
   National standards for electronic formats and data content are the foundation of this requirement. HIPAA requires every provider who does business electronically to use the same healthcare transactions, code sets, and identifiers.
2. **HIPAA Privacy Requirements**
   The privacy requirements limit the release of patient-protected health information without the patient's knowledge and consent beyond that required for patient care.
3. **HIPAA Security Requirements**
   The security regulations outline the maximum administrative, technical, and physical safeguards required to prevent unauthorized access to protected healthcare information. The security standards help safeguard confidential health information during the electronic interchange of healthcare transactions.

Who Must Comply?

Covered Entities. There are three categories of what are termed *covered entities (CEs)*—healthcare providers, health plans, and healthcare clearinghouses—that must comply with HIPAA. The Department of Health and Human Services has established standards for transmitting healthcare information. If a healthcare provider, health plan, and/or healthcare clearinghouse electronically transmits healthcare information for which the HHS has established standards of transmission through HIPAA, that entity by legal definition is considered a covered entity.

- *Healthcare providers.* "Healthcare provider" includes any person or organization that furnishes, bills, or is paid for healthcare in the normal course of business. Providers include, among many others, physicians, hospitals, pharmacies, nursing homes, durable medical equipment suppliers, dentists, optometrists, and chiropractors. A healthcare provider is a covered entity under the HIPAA Privacy Rule only if it conducts any HIPAA standard transactions electronically or if another person or entity conducts the HIPAA standard transactions electronically on its behalf (such as a billing service company and a hospital billing department).
- *Health plans.* A health plan is an individual or a group plan that provides or pays for the cost of medical care. Health plans include employee welfare benefit plans as defined under the Employee Retirement Income Security Act of 1974 (ERISA), including insured and self-insured plans, except plans with fewer than 50 participants that are self-administered by the employer.
- *Healthcare clearinghouses.* Healthcare clearinghouses are companies that "translate" or "facilitate" translation of electronic transactions between the providers of healthcare and the healthcare plans. In other words, they are a "go-between," electronically formatting the provider's claim and billing information in the HIPAA-approved electronic standards needed by the healthcare plan and transmitting the information to the healthcare plans.
- *Business associates (BA).* HIPAA also affects many others in the healthcare field. For instance, software billing vendors and third-party billing services that are not clearinghouses may need to make changes in order to be able to continue to do business with someone who is a covered entity. Under the *original* HIPAA business associates (BA) requirement, business associates were required to apply only "reasonable and appropriate" security practices. Through business associate agreements, healthcare providers are responsible for making sure that associated business partners (BAs) are fully HIPAA compliant. Examples of businesses associated as covered entities are software vendors, lawyers, third-party billers used to process claims, accounting firms, ambulance transport services, and so on. Each BA must be able to produce HIPAA-compliant transactions.

  Under *updates* to HIPAA, business associates (BAs) must be compliant with all HIPAA rules essentially classifying business associates as a covered entity. Additionally, BAs must now comply with the breach notification requirements under HIPAA updates. They are mandated to investigate all breaches of patient data, to conduct risk assessments for possible breaches, and to make reports to their covered entities.

Almost all physician practices are included under the HIPAA standards. A practice is *not* a covered entity only if it does not send any claims (or any other HIPAA transaction) electronically *and* does not employ someone else, such as a billing agency or clearinghouse, to send electronic claims or other electronic transactions to payers or health plans on its behalf. Because the Centers for Medicare & Medicaid Services (CMS) refuses to pay any Medicare claims that are not filed electronically from all but the smallest groups (those that have fewer than 10 full-time employees or the equivalent of 10 full-time employees), noncompliance is not practical for physician practices.

Additionally, a patient's medical information may become "unprotected," as defined by HIPAA, if the information is released from a covered entity to an uncovered entity. As an example, a patient may request a work excuse from the physician to validate missed work while seeing the physician for an appointment. Once the work excuse is given to the employer (a noncovered entity under HIPAA), the privacy of the employee's medical information may be unprotected. However, other federal or state laws may govern the use of the information by the employer. As a general rule of thumb, once protected medical information leaves a covered entity and is transmitted or given to a noncovered entity, the medical information is generally then outside the HIPAA scope of legal protection.

HIPAA Transaction and Code Set Standards

The HIPAA Transaction and Code Set Standards require standardization in healthcare e-commerce. These standards enable any provider to fill out a claim for a patient— regardless of the payer—and submit that claim electronically in the same format. Every payer must accept the standard format and standard codes and send electronic messages back to the provider, also in standard formats, advising the provider of claim status, remittance, and other key information necessary for payment to proceed.

Standard Transactions. The HIPAA transactions standards apply to exchanges for the most common business communications between providers and payers, greatly expanding the amount of health information that is exchanged electronically, as well as the types of patient information involved in electronic communications.

Technically described as *X12 transactions,* HIPAA standards for electronic transactions have been adopted. If a covered entity conducts an electronic transaction that has a HIPAA-approved standard for transmitting the medical data, that electronic transmission standard must be used. Examples of HIPAA-approved standards for electronically transmitting protected medical data include the following:

- Claims or encounters: X12 837P, version 5010 for physicians, and X12 847I, version 5010A2 for hospitals (equivalent to the paper CMS-1500, UB-04, and ADA dental claim forms)
- Claim status inquiry and response: X12 276, X12 277, respectively
- Eligibility inquiry and response: X12 270, X12 271, respectively
- Enrollment and disenrollment in a health plan: X12 834
- Referral Certification and Authorization: X12 278
- Payment and remittance advice: X12 835
- Health plan premium payments: X12 820
- Coordination of Benefits (COB): X12 837; uses the same number as the healthcare claim because it sends a claim to both the primary and secondary healthcare plans
- Healthcare claim attachment (Patient Information Transaction): X12 275 (currently waiting adoption into the Transaction Code Set)
- First Report of Injury: X12 148 (currently waiting adoption into the Transaction Code Set)

Standard Code Sets. Under HIPAA, a code set is any group of codes used for encoding data elements, such as tables of terms, medical concepts, medical diagnosis codes, or medical procedure codes. Medical data code sets used in the healthcare industry include coding systems for diseases, impairments, other health-related problems, and their manifestations; actions taken to diagnose, treat, or manage diseases, injuries, and impairments; and any substances, equipment, supplies, or other items used to perform these actions.

Code sets for medical data are required for data elements in the administrative and financial healthcare transaction standards adopted under HIPAA for diagnoses, procedures, and drugs. The following are the HIPAA standard code sets:

- For diseases, injuries, impairments, and other health-related problems: *International Classification of Diseases, 10th edition, Clinical Modification (ICD-10-CM)*

- For procedures or other actions taken to prevent, diagnose, treat, or manage diseases, injuries, and impairments:
  - Inpatient hospital services: *International Classification of Diseases, 10th edition, Procedure Coding System (ICD-10-PCS)*
  - Dental services: *Code on Dental Procedures and Nomenclature (CDT)*
  - Physicians' services: *Current Procedural Terminology (CPT)*
- Other hospital-related services: *Healthcare Common Procedure Coding System (HCPCS)*
- Drug code: *National Drug Code (NDC) Directory*

HIPAA Privacy Rule

The HIPAA Privacy Rule provides the first comprehensive federal protection for the privacy of health information. It is designed to provide strong privacy protections that do not interfere with patient access to or the quality of healthcare delivery. It creates for the first time national standards to protect individuals' medical records and other personal health information. The Privacy Rule is intended to

- give patients more control over their health information.
- set boundaries on the use and release of health records.
- establish appropriate safeguards that healthcare providers and others must achieve to protect the privacy of health information.
- hold violators accountable, with civil and criminal penalties that can be imposed if they violate patients' privacy rights.
- strike a balance when public responsibility supports disclosure of some forms of data—for example, to protect public health.

Before the HIPAA Privacy Rule, the personal information that moved across hospitals, doctors' offices, insurers or third-party payers, and state lines fell under a patchwork of federal and state laws. This information could be distributed—without either notice or authorization—for reasons that had nothing to do with a patient's medical treatment or healthcare reimbursement. For example, unless otherwise forbidden by state or local law, without the Privacy Rule, patient information held by a health plan could, without the patient's permission, be passed on to a lender, who could then deny the patient's application for a home mortgage or a credit card, or to an employer, who could use it in personnel decisions. The Privacy Rule establishes a federal floor of safeguards to protect the confidentiality of medical information. State laws that provide stronger privacy protections will continue to apply over and above the federal privacy standards.

Protected Health Information (PHI). The core of the HIPAA Privacy Rule is the protection, use, and disclosure of protected health information (PHI). Health information (HI) means any information, whether oral or recorded in any form or medium, that is created or received by a healthcare provider, a health plan, a public health authority, an employer, a life insurer, a school or university, or a healthcare clearinghouse and that relates to the past, present, or future physical or mental health or condition of an individual; the provision of healthcare to an individual; or the past, present, or future payment for the provision of healthcare to an individual.

Protected health information means individually identifiable health information that is transmitted or maintained by electronic (or other) media. The Privacy Rule protects all PHI held or transmitted by a covered entity, in any form or media, whether electronic, paper, or oral, including verbal communications among staff members, patients, and/or other providers. Under this definition, a report of the number of people who have diabetes and have been treated by a physician is not PHI, but the names of the patients are protected. PHI includes many facts about people, such as names; addresses; dates (birthdates/admission/discharge/death); certificates or license numbers; telephone numbers; Social Security, medical record, or account numbers; bioidentifiers (such as a fingerprint or voiceprint); photos; and health plan beneficiary numbers—any of which could be used to identify the patient. The following are also identified as protected health information:

- Web: Internet Protocol (IP) address, uniform resource locator (URL), and e-mail address
- Fax numbers
- Vehicle identification number (VIN) and license plate numbers
- Instrument or device identifier and number
- Any other unique identifying characteristic, number, or code

Provider Responsibilities. The HIPAA Privacy Rule recognizes that medical offices and payers must be able to exchange PHI in the normal course of business. The Rule says there are three everyday situations in which PHI can be released *without* the patient's permission: treatment, payment, and healthcare operations (TPO).

- *Treatment* means providing and coordinating the patient's medical care. Physicians and other medical staff members can discuss patients' cases in the office and with other physicians. Laboratory or x-ray technicians may call to clarify requests they cannot process because of the missing data. This information can be provided by the physician or another medical staff member.
- *Payment* refers to the exchange of information with health plans. Medical office staff members can take the required information from patients' records and prepare healthcare claims that are transmitted to health plans.
- *Healthcare operations* are the general business management functions needed to run the office.

For the average healthcare provider or health plan, the Privacy Rule requires activities such as

1. notifying patients about their privacy rights and how their information can be used.
2. adopting and implementing privacy procedures for its practice, hospital, or plan.
3. training employees and documenting the training, so that they understand the privacy procedures.
4. designating an individual to be responsible for seeing that the privacy procedures are adopted and followed.
5. securing patient records containing individually identifiable health information, so that they are not readily available to those who do not need them.

Medical office staff should be careful not to discuss patients' cases with anyone outside the office, including family and friends. Avoid talking about cases, too, in the practice's reception areas, where other patients may overhear comments. Close charts on desks when they are not being worked on. When leaving a chart outside the examination room for the physician to review, place the patient's chart so that the name or number is not visible to other patients who are passing by that room. Simply stated, place the chart backward. A computer screen displaying a patient's records should be positioned so that only the person working with the file can view it. Using a filter over the monitor will provide more protection from unauthorized disclosure of information. Files should be closed when the computer is not in use.

A covered entity must disclose protected health information in only two situations: (1) to individuals (or their personal representatives) specifically when they request access to, or an accounting of disclosures of, their protected health information; and (2) to HHS when it is undertaking a compliance investigation or review or enforcement action.

The Privacy Rule must be followed by all covered entities—health plans, healthcare clearinghouses, healthcare providers, and contracted business associates (BAs).

Acknowledgment of Receipt of Notice of Privacy Practices. To comply with the HIPAA Privacy Rule, medical offices, as well as other providers and health plans, must give each patient an explanation of privacy practices at the patient's first contact or encounter. To satisfy this requirement, medical offices give patients a copy of their Notice of Privacy Practices (NPP) and/or display a copy of the NPP in the waiting area. It must be visible for patients to view. The notice explains

1. how the covered entity will use and disclose PHI.
2. how the covered entity will protect PHI.
3. privacy rights of the patient, including the patient's right to file a complaint with the covered entity and with HHS.
4. how the patient can contact the covered entity to make a complaint.

The office must also ask patients to review this notice and sign an Acknowledgment of Receipt of Notice of Privacy Practices, showing that they have read and understand the document. This is usually completed on the patient's first visit, unless care is given in an emergency situation. If care is given in an emergency situation, the provider must give the patient a copy of the Acknowledgment as soon as possible after the emergency. If a patient refuses to sign the Acknowledgment, the provider must keep a record of the attempt to gain the patient's signature. Refusing to sign the Acknowledgment will not prevent the medical practice from using and disclosing PHI as stated by the Privacy Rule.

Unless changes have been made to the NPP after the patient originally signed the Acknowledgment, an annual signature is not required. If changes have been made to the Notice of Privacy Practices, a new Acknowledgment of Receipt of Notice of Privacy Practices should be given to the patient and a new signature obtained.

If a patient requests a copy of the Notice of Privacy Practices, provide a copy. If the practice has a website or other electronic presence, the NPP should be available through the electronic venue. Another option is to post a copy of the NPP in a clear and easily accessible location within the waiting area. Health plans are required to send a copy of the NPP to the subscriber upon enrollment, then to send a reminder at least once every 3 years that the subscriber can request a copy of the NPP from the health plan.

Minimum Necessary. When using or disclosing protected health information, a provider must make reasonable efforts to limit the use or disclosure to the minimum amount of PHI necessary to accomplish the intended purpose. "Minimum necessary" means taking reasonable safeguards to protect a person's health information from incidental disclosure. State laws may impose more stringent requirements regarding the protection of patient information.

These minimum necessary policies and procedures also reasonably must limit who within the entity has access to protected health information and under what conditions, based on job responsibilities and the nature of the business. The minimum necessary standard does not apply to disclosures, including oral disclosures, among healthcare providers for treatment purposes. For example, a physician is not required to apply the minimum necessary standard when discussing a patient's medical chart information with a specialist at another hospital.

Treatment, Payment, and Healthcare Operations. Patients' medical care information can be shared (used and disclosed) by providers—without a written release of information from the patient—to treat the patient, to obtain payment for services, and to conduct the healthcare operation of the medical provider, such as transmitting daily information to the entity's Certified Public Accountant (CPA). Use and disclosure of PHI without the requirement for the patient's written authorization falls under TPO (treatment, payment, and healthcare operations) as previously explained. Examples of use and/or disclosure of PHI without written authorization include:

- *Treatment:* forwarding patient's PHI to a specialist who will continue care of the patient (continuity of care); clarifying information to a pharmacist concerning a patient's new prescription
- *Payment:* supplying requested information to a healthcare plan in order to obtain payment for services
- *Healthcare operations:* submitting statutory reports; supporting compliance programs and fraud/abuse detection

Patient Rights. Under HIPAA, patients have an increased awareness of their health information privacy rights, including the following:

- The right to access, copy, and inspect their health information
- The right to request an amendment to their healthcare information
- The right to obtain an accounting of certain disclosures of their health information
- The right to alternative means of receiving communications from providers
- The right to complain about alleged violations of the regulations and the provider's own information policies

For the healthcare provider, these rights apply to the patient's designated record set (DRS), which includes medical and billing records maintained for the patient. However, mental health information, psychotherapy notes, and genetics information are not included in the designated record set. For the healthcare plan, the DRS includes items such as enrollment, claim decisions (such as denials and payments), and the medical management system of the healthcare plan.

A patient's request for a copy of medical records cannot be denied due to nonpayment of the bill. Also, the records must be sent in the patient's preferred format: paper, electronic, or e-mail. If a fee is allowed by state regulations for the cost of supplies and postage, the patient must be notified of the amount when the request is made. Some states mandate one copy of medical records at no cost. Requests for medical records under HIPAA must be completed within 30 calendar days of the request.

For use or disclosure of PHI other than for treatment, payment, or healthcare operations (TPO), the patient must sign an authorization to release the information.

Patients who observe privacy problems in their providers' offices can complain either to the designated privacy officer at the medical office or to the Department of Health and Human Services (HHS). Complaints must be put in writing, on paper or electronically, and sent to the Office of Civil Rights (OCR), which is part of HHS, usually within 180 days. The office must cooperate with an HHS investigation and give HHS access to its facilities, books, records, and systems, including relevant protected health information.

Exceptions to the Privacy Rule. In addition to TPO, there are a number of exceptions to the Privacy Rule. All these types of disclosures must also be logged, and the release information must be available to the patient who requests it.

- *Release under court order.* If the patient's PHI is required as evidence by a court of law, the provider may release it without the patient's approval upon judicial order. In the case of a lawsuit, a court sometimes decides that a physician or medical practice staff member must provide testimony. The court issues a subpoena, an order of the court directing a party to appear and testify. If the court requires the witness to bring certain evidence, such as a patient's medical record, it issues a subpoena duces tecum, which directs the party to appear, to testify, and to bring specified documents or items.

- *Workers' compensation cases.* State laws may provide for release of records to employers in workers' compensation cases. The law may also authorize release to the state workers' compensation administration board and to the insurance company that handles these claims for the state.

- *Statutory reports.* Some specific types of information are required by state law to be released to state health or social services departments. For example, physicians must make such statutory reports for patients' births and deaths and for cases of abuse. Because of the danger of harm to patients or others, communicable diseases (such as tuberculosis, hepatitis, and rabies) must usually be reported.

- *HIV and AIDS.* A special category of communicable disease control is applied to patients with diagnoses of human immunodeficiency virus (HIV) infection and acquired immune deficiency syndrome (AIDS). Every state requires AIDS cases to be reported. Most states also require reporting of the HIV infection that causes the syndrome. However, state laws vary concerning whether only the fact of a case is to be reported or if the patient's name must also be reported. The medical office's guidelines will reflect the state laws and must be strictly observed, as all these regulations should be, to protect patients' privacy and to comply with the regulations.

- *Public Employees.* Performing within the scope of their duties, PHI may be disclosed to coroners, medical examiners, and organ procurement agencies. In a limited capacity, law enforcement may also receive PHI.

- *Research data.* PHI may be made available to researchers approved by the practice. For example, if a physician is conducting clinical research on a type of diabetes, the practice may share information from appropriate records for analysis. When the researcher issues reports or studies based on the information, specific patients' names should not be identified.

- *De-identified health information.* There are no restrictions on the use or disclosure of "de-identified" health information, which does not identify an individual.

HIPAA Security Rule

The regulations of the HIPAA Security Rule work in concert with the final privacy standards and require that covered entities establish administrative, physical, and technical safeguards to protect the confidentiality, integrity, and availability of health information covered by HIPAA. The Security Rule covers electronic PHI (e-PHI) that is either produced, saved, transferred, received, and/or maintained by the covered entity. It specifies how a covered entity must secure such protected health information (e-PHI) on computer networks, the Internet, disks and magnetic tape, external hard drives, removable storage devices, smart devices and PDAs, and extranets. Basically, the Security Rule provides the guidelines for the physical "how-to-protect" PHI as stated in the Privacy Rule.

Security Rule Standards. National standards have been federally mandated, which allows the medical workforce to use more technological methods, such as EMRs and CPOE (Computerized Physician Order Entry), which, in turn, means greater mobility and efficiency when providing patient care. While the Security Rule guidelines are standardized, there is flexibility within the Rule that allows covered entities (CEs) to establish their own security policies and procedures. The CEs demonstrate that they have developed security policies and procedures based on the CEs' needs and size, available technologies, cost of implementation, and the likelihood and potential impact of a breech of e-PHI to the CEs.

Each covered entity must demonstrate policies and procedures that

- protect the confidentiality and integrity of all maintained e-PHI.
- provide availability of e-PHI to the patient and to authorized entities or individuals.
- verify compliance by all individuals within the workforce.
- identify and protect against reasonable and anticipated illegal use and disclosure of e-PHI.

Covered entities are to use three general areas of safeguards to protect e-PHI: administrative, technical, and physical.

Administrative Safeguards. Covered entities are required to implement the following administrative safeguards:

- A security official must be assigned responsibility for the entity's security.
- All staff, including management, must receive security awareness training. The training should be documented, and a sanction policy and procedure must be stated for security violations.
- Covered entities must conduct risk analyses to determine information security risks and vulnerabilities.
- Covered entities must establish policies and procedures that allow access to electronic PHI on a need-to-know basis.
- Administrative policies and procedures must periodically be evaluated to assess their effectiveness in meeting HIPAA Security Rule standards.

Technical Safeguards. Technical safeguards involve protecting e-PHI through electronic methods. Covered entities must

- implement audit controls that record and examine workers who have logged into information systems that contain PHI.
- employ technical measures to deter unauthorized use of e-PHI. The use of an encryption program is encouraged.
- implement policies and procedures to protect the integrity of e-PHI and to document that e-PHI has not been improperly destroyed or altered in any way.
- employ technological methods that guard against the illegal or improper transmission of e-PHI.

Physical Safeguards. Covered entities must use physical safeguards policies and procedures to protect ePHI, and the buildings and equipment containing ePHI, from hazards, both natural and environmental. They must

- limit physical access to areas that contain electronic PHI while allowing access to authorized individuals.
- implement policies and procedures for the proper use of workspace and electronic media.
- implement policies and procedures that protect e-PHI throughout the phases of transfer, removal, reuse, and disposal.

Physical safeguards are often easy to implement but can be more easily overlooked. Following are examples of HIPAA violations.

1. Allowing a friend or relative to enter the work area with patient information visible on the computer screen

    Violation: ePHI is visible on the screen.

    Compliance: *(1) Do not allow anyone, other than authorized team members, in the work area. (2) Always remove e-PHI from the computer screen when there is a possibility of illegal disclosure. Minimize data and/or use a screen saver.*

2. Posting a picture on social media of office team members dressed in Halloween costumes and a patient exiting an exam in the background

    Violation: Patient is seen in the photo and can be identified.

    Compliance: *Do not post photos of the medical environment on social media. If pictures are posted, there must be no evidence of patients or e-PHI.*

3. Asking a patient to state his or her address and birthdate at the patient reception area

    Violation: Others in the reception area can hear the patient's e-PHI.

    Compliance: *If possible, verify patient's e-PHI in a confidential, private area.*

4. Disposing in the office trash (not in the shredding container) of a patient's list of scheduled appointments

    Violation: Patient's e-PHI (it was created and maintained on the computer) can be retrieved and used illegally.

    Compliance: *Shred all patient e-PHI.*

HIPAA Breach Notification Rule

Since the implementation of the HIPAA Privacy Rule and Security Rule, health information has gained increased protection. However, breaches of PHI can still occur. In broad terms, a breach occurs when there is an unauthorized or impermissible use and/or disclosure of information which compromises the security of patients' PHI.

Under the HIPAA Breach Notification Rule, covered entities are required to notify affected individuals when a breach of PHI has occurred. In cases of more than 500 affected patients, the covered entity must also notify HHS of the breach and also notify local media that serve areas in which affected individuals live. Notifications must be made within 60 calendar days following discovery of the breach. A breach affecting fewer than 500 individuals may be reported annually to HHS. If a breach occurs at or by a business associate, the BA must notify the covered entity of the breach.

Once a breach has been discovered, a severity risk assessment of the improper use and/or disclosure of the PHI must be made. The following four factors are part of the severity risk assessment:

1. *PHI involved.* Determine the nature and extent of the affected PHI. The types of PHI identifiers should be evaluated and the likelihood that the breached PHI may be re-identified.

2. *Who received the PHI.* Analyze who actually used the breached PHI and to whom the information was given
3. *What happened to the PHI.* Evaluate if the breached PHI was actually acquired or if it was viewed.
4. *What has been done since the breach was discovered.* Demonstrate that risk to the PHI has been lessened or eliminated.

HIPAA National Identifiers

The HIPAA law requires identifiers for the following:

- Providers
- Employers
- Health plans
- Patients

The Centers for Medicaid & Medicare Services has issued identifier rules for three of the four: the employer, the national provider, and the health plan.

Employer Identifier. HIPAA requires employers to use national, standardized identifiers in business transactions, such as submitting a medical insurance claim form to obtain payment for services to a patient. The Employer Identification Number (EIN) issued by the federal government (IRS) was chosen by HIPAA as the national employer identifier.

National Provider Identifier. The National Provider Identifier (NPI) Rule provides a unique provider identifier for each provider. It is a 10-position numeric identifier with a check digit in the last position to help detect keying errors. In May 2008, the NPI officially replaced all other identifying numbers for providers, such as the previously used UPIN numbers from providers. Claim forms have been modified to accommodate the NPI numbers.

Health Plan Identifiers. The Final Rule was published by HHS in 2012. Most health plans, with the exception of very small plans, will be required to obtain a federally issued Health Plan Identifier (HPID). Covered entities must use HPIDs in all standard electronic transactions. The Final Rule also establishes an Other Entity Identifier (OEID) for entities that are not classified as health plans, healthcare providers, or individuals but still need to be identified in HIPAA standard transactions. Examples include third-party administrators (TPAs) and transaction vendors. Although the Final Rule does not mandate that other entities obtain and use an OEID, they may obtain and use one if they need to be identified in health plan transactions.

On October 31, 2014, the Centers for Medicare & Medicaid Services announced the indefinite delay and implementation of the mandatory HPID/OEID requirement. Health plans and other entities that had already obtained their HPID/OEID numbers should maintain a record of the HPID/OEID numbers for future use.

Patient Identifiers Not Issued. Due to the public concern over privacy, a patient identifier standard has not yet been adopted. CMS has not proposed such an identifier, and it is no longer being pursued.

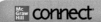 **GO TO PROJECT 2.4 AT THE END OF THIS CHAPTER**

MEDICAL COMPLIANCE PLANS AND SAFEGUARDS AGAINST LITIGATION

Medical practices must take steps to reduce the risk of accusations of fraud and abuse when submitting claims to insurance companies and federal agencies, such as Medicare. The processes involved in coding and billing are complicated, and there is much room for error. Although many errors are not intentional, medical practices are required to show their resolve to behave with **compliance,** or adherence to rules and regulations.

To assist in this process of ensuring that procedures are in compliance, the Office of the Inspector General (OIG), an agency of the U.S. Department of Health and Human Services (HHS), has issued *Compliance Program Guidance for Individual and Small Group Physician Practices.* This voluntary plan is a positive step toward helping physicians protect themselves and their practices from violations related to claims and reimbursements. Using the guidance provided by the OIG, physicians can develop an effective Compliance Plan for their practices.

There are specific risk areas in practices that a medical Compliance Plan addresses:

- *Coding and billing.* The risks include billing for services not rendered; submitting claims for equipment or medical supplies that are not reasonable; and double billing, which results in duplicate payment.
- *Reasonable and necessary services.* The practice must offer the patient only necessary procedures and treatments that meet Medicare's definitions and may not offer more complex and more expensive methods when simpler, less expensive alternatives exist.
- *Documentation.* Great care is to be taken in entering data and maintaining and retaining all information related to treatment, claims, and reimbursements. Proper documentation forms, such as consent forms and advance directives, should be maintained within the medical record.
- *Improper inducements, kickbacks, and self-referrals.* Neither the physician nor anyone on staff may accept payment for awarding contracts or for purchasing anything *(inducements).* Nor may anyone knowingly offer, pay, solicit, or receive bribes to influence getting business that is reimbursable by federal government programs *(kickbacks).* The physician may not refer a patient to any health service with which the physician or any member of the physician's immediate family has a financial relationship *(self-referral).*
- *HIPAA compliance.* Medical office team members should comply with HIPAA's Administrative Simplification Act and its three parts: Privacy, Security, and Transaction Code Set.

The Medical Compliance Plan

The major purpose for creating and implementing a Compliance Plan, sometimes referred to as Incident Management, within the practice is to prevent, discover, and correct noncompliant behaviors, including the submission of erroneous claims or unlawful conduct involving the federal healthcare programs. Even though it may seem negative, if there are no noncompliant behaviors discovered and corrective actions taken, the Compliance Plan may be noneffective.

The OIG's *Compliance Program Guidance* suggests seven basic elements for any Compliance Plan set up within the practice:

- *Written policies and procedures.* There should be written policies (what is to be accomplished) and procedures (how it is to be accomplished) for patient care, billing and coding, documentation, and payer relationships. These should be written in user-friendly language and should be up-to-date.

- *Designation of a chief compliance officer.* The officer may be an office manager or a biller. The officer's duties include monitoring the plan, conducting audits periodically, keeping the policies and procedures updated, and investigating reports or allegations of fraud.

- *Training and education programs.* Education is an essential component because the physician relies on staff members to follow procedures that reduce the practice's vulnerability to fraud. Topics such as fraud, waste, and abuse should be covered on a continuing basis. Documentation of all training (i.e., topics, participants, dates, length of training) should be placed in the Compliance Manual. All employees should receive training on how to perform their jobs according to the standards and regulations of the practice. Employees should also understand through their training programs that compliance is a condition of their continued employment.

- *Effective line of communication.* The practice should create an environment where there is an open-door policy of communication and employees feel encouraged to report mistakes promptly and to report any potential problems without fear of retribution. Additionally, a method for anonymously submitting thoughts and concerns should be encouraged.

- *Auditing and monitoring.* An internal audit should be conducted at least once a year by a designated staff member or an outside consultant. The audit includes areas such as checking for data entry errors, billing and/or coding errors, medical documentation errors, contract compliance, and other areas that are specific to the business of the practice and to the field of speciality.

- *Well-publicized disciplinary directives.* Every staff member should understand the policies/procedures for compliance and the penalties for noncompliance. Disciplinary guidelines should include the circumstances under which someone would receive any one of a range of penalties, from a verbal warning to dismissal to referral for criminal prosecution.

- *Prompt corrective action for detected offenses.* Corrective action should be taken within 60 days from the date on which the problem is identified. Problems must be investigated at once and corrective action taken. A review of policies/procedures should be conducted for clarity and possible modifications.

The Administrative Medical Assistant's Role in Compliance

The potential for accusations of fraud is always present in the complex areas of patient care, billing and coding, and documentation. If fraud is detected and not reported or corrected, the reputation and legal standing of the practice are put at grave risk. The administrative medical assistant has job responsibilities related to all of these areas and plays a central role in helping to ensure that the practice is in compliance.

The administrative medical assistant who is working efficiently and effectively is key to the success of a Compliance Plan. In the following areas of responsibility, the assistant helps the practice stay in compliance:

- *Accurate data entry.* Accurate work speeds the correct payment of claims and lessens the chances of federal audit.

- *Accurate documentation.* Good documentation reduces the chances for mistakes and provides an excellent trail if proof of corrective action is required. In addition to protecting the practice, accurate documentation contributes to improved patient care.

- *Timely filing and storing of electronic and hardcopy records.* Keeping records in good order and for an appropriate length of time can show the physician's good faith efforts to apply the principles of compliance.
- *Prompt reporting of errors or instances of fraudulent conduct.* The assistant has the ethical and professional responsibility to help the physician correct mistakes and investigate instances of unlawful behavior.

Safeguards Against Litigation

The administrative medical assistant needs to be aware that liability for negligence is recognized by law to include not only the physician's actions but also the actions of the physician's employees. An assistant who is performing tasks within the job description and as a proper assignment is considered to be the agent of the physician. It is the physician's responsibility to define the assistant's job properly, to state and regulate office policies, to assist in teaching the policies, and to see that policies and procedures are implemented. It is the assistant's responsibility to understand thoroughly his or her job description and the office policies/procedures. The assistant, then, must act responsibly within the scope of his or her job and according to office policies/procedures.

It is easier to prevent a malpractice claim than to defend one. Administrative medical assistants who maintain good interpersonal relationships with patients and other staff members help reduce the likelihood of litigation. In particular, the following guidelines are useful:

- Keep everything that you hear, see, and read about patients completely confidential.
- Never criticize a physician to a patient.
- Do not discuss a patient's condition, diagnosis, or treatment with the patient, with other patients, or with staff members. What the physician tells the assistant about a patient is to be kept confidential, even from the patient.
- Refrain from discussing patient information in hallways or outside patient rooms.
- Do not diagnose or prescribe, even though you feel sure you know what the physician would prescribe. There are often circumstances of which you are unaware. Prescribing constitutes the practice of medicine and is unlawful unless you are licensed.
- Notify the physician if you learn that a patient is under treatment by another physician for the same condition.
- Inform the physician of all information given by the patient, such as when the patient has questions, appears confused, or seems not to understand directions or instructions given.
- Inform the physician about any unpleasant incident that may have occurred between the patient and any staff member. In this case, the assistant writes a notation to the physician, which does not become part of the patient's record.
- Notify the physician if the patient mentions that he or she has no intention of returning to the office or complying with the treatment plan.
- Be available to assist the patient and the physician.
- Obtain proper authorizations for release of information and consents. Maintain these with the patient's records.
- Keep complete and accurate records, including notations about a patient's failure to keep an appointment, cancellation of an appointment, or failure to follow treatment instructions.
- Be selective in giving information over the telephone. Many practices accept requests for information only when they are written.

- Observe the confidentiality of computerized records by shielding computer screens from the view of patients or other staff members, protecting passwords, and following practice security guidelines when using e-mail to transmit information.
- Keep prescription pads (if hardcopy prescription pads are being used by the physician) and medications in a secure place.
- Be safety conscious. See that all equipment is in safe working condition, and be alert to potential safety hazards.

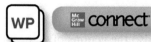 **GO TO PROJECT 2.5 AT THE END OF THIS CHAPTER**

2.1 Define *medical ethics, bioethics,* and *etiquette.*	• Ethics are the standards of conduct that grow out of one's understanding of right and wrong. Medical ethics require physicians to practice high standards of patient care, respect patients' rights, treat patients with compassion, and safeguard the privacy of patients' communications. • Bioethics deals with the ethical issues involved with medical treatments, procedures, and technology. • Etiquette involves following medical manners and customs, such as using the proper form of address for the physician, greeting cheerfully all visitors to the office, and using proper telephone techniques.
2.2 Discuss medical law, statutes, and legal documents, such as advance directives, and give three examples.	• Advance directives are legal documents prepared in advance by the patient, stating the patient's wishes for receiving or not receiving certain medical care, should the patient be unable to make decisions at that time. Advance directives give the medical team specific directions as to the type of care to render. • Advance directives include DNRs (Do Not Resuscitate), living wills, and durable power of attorney.
2.3 Identify and discuss several key components of the HIPAA Administrative Simplification Act.	• HIPAA defines three categories of covered entities: — Healthcare providers: individuals or entities that render services — Healthcare plans: entities that provide payment for healthcare services — Clearinghouses: entities that electronically process health claim information from providers and transmit data to plans • Both health information and protected health information contain health information and health payment information about a patient's past, present, and possible future. Both can be used by covered entities and business associates to conduct business. • Health information is any information used by a covered entity; protected health information could be the same information, but it would contain information that would allow the individual to whom the health information refers to be identified. • The purpose of an Acknowledgment of Receipt of Notice of Privacy Practices is to — inform the patient of how his or her protected health information may be used and/or disclosed by the covered entity.

	— describe the patient's rights concerning his or her protected health information.
	• The following are exceptions to the Privacy Rule as it relates to the patient's protected health information: — Court-ordered release of information — Workers' compensation cases — Statutory reports — HIV and AIDS reports — Public employees within the scope of their duties — Research data submission — De-identified health information
	• Another provision of the HIPAA Administrative Simplification Act describes how protected health information is to be protected through security guidelines. Administrative, physical, and technical policies and procedures are implemented to protect the confidentiality, integrity, and availability of protected health information. Six of the safeguards the covered entities are to implement are — assigning an officer to oversee the security measures. — training all personnel on the policies and procedures for PHI security. — auditing controls to document who has accessed PHI. — limiting physical access to facilities containing PHI. — conducting risk analyses to identify areas of risk and vulnerability. — establishing written policies and implementing procedures that limit access to and protect PHI.
	• Under the Breach of Notification Act, covered entities are required to report unauthorized or impermissible use and/or disclosure of patients' PHI. A risk assessment containing four primary factors must be conducted by the covered entity. The four factors are — PHI involved. — who received the PHI. — what happened to the PHI. — what has been done since the breach was discovered.
2.4 State the purpose of a medical Compliance Plan and explain compliant methods the assistant can use to safeguard against litigation.	• The purpose of the implementation of policies and procedures stated in a Compliance Plan is to prevent the submission of erroneous claims or unlawful conduct involving federal programs and laws.

- The administrative medical assistant can contribute to compliance in several ways:
  - Entering data accurately and documenting thoroughly
  - Maintaining the flow of records, especially if the provider is using hardcopy patient records
  - Reporting errors or instances of fraudulent/abusive situations promptly
- It is easier to prevent a malpractice suit and litigation than to defend one. Some of the ways all members of the medical team can help prevent litigation are to
  - keep all patient PHI confidential and all information to yourself.
  - refer all medical questions to the clinical personnel.
  - keep any critical thoughts of others, including the physician, away from patients.
  - notify the physician if you learn of a patient who is seeking treatment for the same condition from another source.
  - forward information to the physician when a patient seems confused or has not understood the physician's instructions.
  - inform the physician of any unpleasant situations between the patient and a medical team member.
  - notify the physician if the patient states he or she has no intention of returning or of following the treatment plan. This should be documented in the patient's record.
  - be available to patients and to others in the medical team.
  - obtain and document all needed forms and authorizations, such as releases of information and advance directives.
  - keep thorough and updated documentation in all patient records. Remember, if it is not documented, it was not done.
  - attempt to get all requests for PHI in writing and keep a list of all disclosures of PHI.
  - implement security safeguards to protect confidentiality.
  - keep prescription pads and medications secured.
  - maintain a safe work/patient environment.

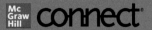
Project 2.1   (LO 2.1) Internet Research: Bioethical Topics

Using the Internet, research articles on two different bioethical issues of interest to yourself, referencing at least two difference sources for each issue. Read the articles on each issue. Upon completion of your research, submit a written document regarding what you have learned.

Project 2.2   (LO 2.2) Physician's Obligations and Medical Law

Working Paper 2 (WP 2) in an end section of this book contains statements that refer to the obligations of the physician and/or medical law. Mark each statement with either "T" for *true* or "F" for *false*. For each *false* answer, document what makes the statement *false*.

Project 2.3   (LO 2.2) Medical Liability and Communications

Working Paper 3 (WP 3) contains statements that refer to the obligations of the physician and/or medical law. Mark each statement with either "T" for *true* or "F" for *false*. For each *false* answer, document what makes the statement *false*.

Project 2.4   (LO 2.3) Protecting Patients' PHI

Read the following case scenarios and decide whether the patient's PHI is being protected or is a possible breach of PHI. Submit a written document stating your decision and your justification(s) for that decision.

Scenario 1
Alianna, a medical biller, missed 2 days of work due to illness. Upon returning, she asked to take home an office laptop to get caught up on her work.

Scenario 2
A patient is moving to another area and has requested to bring an external storage device to the office to have medical records copied.

Scenario 3
The physician assistant has a patient on hold and needs to access the patient's electronic PHI. The PA asks to borrow your password.

Scenario 4
While taking a patient's history, the medical assistant was called out of the examination room to answer a question. The laptop was left in the examination room and the medical assistant was logged into the computer.

Scenario 5
Over the past few years, your area has seen a change in the weather pattern. More severe storms, tornadoes, and floods have occurred. Electronic data are safe because a backup copy is made each night and is locked in the physician office.

Project 2.5   (LO 2.1, LO 2.2, LO 2.4) Legal Terms

Using Working Paper 4 (WP 4), match each legal term in Column 2 with the correct definition in Column 1.

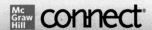
Problem-Solving (LO 2.1, LO 2.2, LO 2.4)

Problems are something that we all have in common. Not one person can avoid problems, whether professional or personal. Murphy's law states: If something can go wrong, it will. Our ability to overcome challenges is what allows us to achieve goals. When you encounter a problem, take a step back and spend time thinking about the cause of the problem. No matter what, when you are dealing with any challenge, becoming frustrated or emotional will not help you succeed. You need time to rationalize and figure out all of the details of the problem in order to come up with an effective solution. **Reflect on a time that you were faced with a problem. Describe the situation as it happened and what you could have done to change the way you handled the problem.**

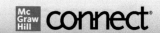
USING TERMINOLOGY

Match the term or phrase on the left with the correct answer on the right.

_____ 1. [LO 2.2] Assault

_____ 2. [LO 2.2] Battery

_____ 3. [LO 2.3] Release of information

_____ 4. [LO 2.2] Subpoena

_____ 5. [LO 2.2] Liability

_____ 6. [LO 2.3] Summons

_____ 7. [LO 2.3] HIPAA

_____ 8. [LO 2.4] Compliance

_____ 9. [LO 2.1] Ethics

_____ 10. [LO 2.2] Licensure

a. Standards of conduct that result from one's concept of right and wrong

b. Being legally responsible for actions and consequences

c. A clear threat of injury to an individual

d. Bodily contact without permission

e. A written notice by a court for the defendant to answer all charges

f. A legal document ordering all related documents and/or persons with knowledge of the case to appear in court

g. A legal document that must be on file from the patient before transferring medical information

h. A legal statute that covers the electronic transmission of patient medical information

i. Adhering to legal rules/regulations as well as high standards through practices and procedures

j. The written, legal right granted by a state or an organization to practice, after education and training, within a field by meeting the practice requirements of the specified discipline

CHECKING YOUR UNDERSTANDING

Select the most correct answer.

1. [LO 2.2] At the physician's office, blood must be drawn from a patient to check cholesterol levels and possible reasons for consistently elevated blood pressure. The patient arrives and blood is drawn. Which of the following has the patient given?

   a. Expressed consent
   b. Implied consent
   c. No consent
   d. Written consent

2. [LO 2.2] When the results of the blood work in Question 1 were returned, the physician decided to schedule the patient for a heart catheterization. Other courses of treatment had been tried, unsuccessfully, to lower the blood pressure and cholesterol levels. Which of the following must the patient give prior to the procedure?

   a. Expressed consent
   b. Implied consent
   c. Informed consent
   d. Implied and informed consent

3. [LO 2.1] During a recent political campaign, the candidates stated varying positions on stem cell research. Under which category does this topic fall?

   a. Ethics
   b. Etiquette
   c. Compliance
   d. Bioethics

4. [LO 2.2] When Bruce was diagnosed with Alzheimer's disease, he decided he might need another individual to make informed medical decisions if he was not able to make them for himself. Which document would he need to complete?

   a. Medical durable power of attorney
   b. Expressed consent form
   c. Certificate of deposit
   d. Deposition

5. [LO 2.3] Of the following, which is *not* a covered entity?

   a. Clearinghouse
   b. Healthcare providers
   c. Office supply delivery service
   d. Healthcare plans

6. [LO 2.3] The following information was displayed on the computer screen containing electronic health information data: Sandy Smith, insurance ID number B4059962, DOB 07-07-1959. Upon checkout, Sandy's neighbor saw the data on the screen and later called Sandy to ask why she was seeing an OB/GYN. This is a breech of confidentiality because

   a. protected health information was disclosed without permission.
   b. health information was disclosed.
   c. the phone number was incorrect.
   d. the blood type was not listed.

7. [LO 2.3] How an office will contact a patient to remind him or her of an appointment should be stated within the

   a. informed consent.
   b. disclosure log.
   c. release of information.
   d. Notice of Privacy Practices.

8. [LO 2.4] Jennifer is asked to develop and implement policies and procedures to protect medical data. Before beginning, which of the following would most likely be the first step?

   a. Assign a security officer.
   b. Assign passwords to individuals who need access.
   c. Identify areas of vulnerability.
   d. Conduct staff training.

9. [LO 2.4] Upon checkout, Francisco seemed upset and stated he would not be returning to the physician for treatment and was not going to take the prescribed medication. Which of the following courses of action would be appropriate for the AMA?

   a. Make a notation of the patient's statement in his medical record and notify the physician.
   b. Wait to see if Francisco comes to his next appointment.
   c. Follow the patient and attempt to change his mind.
   d. Make a notation of his comments in his medical record.

10. [LO 2.2] When does the contract between the patient and the physician begin?

   a. When the first procedure is performed
   b. After the patient leaves the office
   c. Before the physician leaves the exam area
   d. When the patient seeks the services of the physician

THINKING IT THROUGH

These questions cover important points in this chapter. Using your critical-thinking skills, play the role of an administrative medical assistant as you answer each question. Be prepared to discuss your responses.

1. [LO 2.1] What are the major standards, as set forth in the AMA code of ethics, that doctors are expected to adhere to in their practices? What qualities does the AAMA creed emphasize for administrative medical assistants?

2. [LO 2.2] You hear Mr. Washington enter the office. He has come to keep a 3 P.M. appointment with the doctor. You are busily trying to rearrange the afternoon appointments to accommodate an emergency that occurred in the morning. You do not feel that you can raise your eyes from the complicated list of appointments before you. You simply say, in response to Mr. Washington's greeting, "Please have a seat." Have you violated any principles of office etiquette? Please give reasons for your answer.

3. [LO 2.2] In what ways would patients be in danger if it were not for medical practice acts?

4. [LO 2.2, LO 2.4] In a casual conversation, a patient boasts that he has made his stomach pains disappear without taking any of the medicine prescribed by the doctor. He also says that, although he had had these pains far longer than he admitted to the doctor, his home cure worked. He then informs you, quite seriously, that he does not expect to receive a bill for services from the physician. How do you respond to the patient? What is wrong with the way this patient thinks about the doctor-patient relationship?

5. [LO 2.3] On what basis would you decide whether an individual's request for access to a patient's record should be fulfilled?

6. [LO 2.3] A request for a patient's medical record is sent by fax to your office. The fax cover sheet contains the letterhead of a nearby medical facility. You do not recognize the name of the physician, fax number, or telephone number stated for the physician's office. How do you respond to the request?

7. [LO 2.4] Payment from an insurance company has just arrived at the office. In processing the paperwork, you notice that an error has been made in coding the procedure. The error has resulted in an overpayment to the practice. The error is only the latest mistake in a growing number of errors, all made by the same staff member. What are your responsibilities in this situation?

8. [LO 2.2] In a dispute between a patient and the doctor, both parties have agreed to an alternative to trial. What happens in an arbitration? What advantages may arbitration have over a court trial?

9. [LO 2.4] What are the aspects of an administrative medical assistant's behavior and attention to procedure that help the practice avoid litigation?

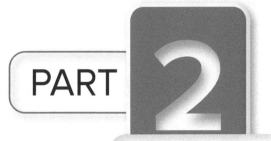

PART 2

Administrative Responsibilities

Part 2 discusses the important duties of the administrative medical assistant concerning oral and written communications. It also presents the tasks involved with scheduling the physician's appointments and handling mail. Aspects of office management include how to manage the physical environment and one's personal stress.

CONSIDER THIS: Communication skills are at the heart of successful relations with the medical staff, patients, and others in the physician's practice. *What steps can you take to improve your effectiveness in speaking and writing?*

Office Communications: An Overview of Verbal and Written Communication

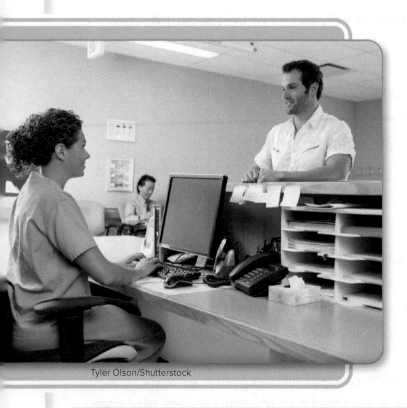

Tyler Olson/Shutterstock

LEARNING OUTCOMES

After studying this chapter, you will be able to

3.1 list the steps of the communication cycle and give an example of a barrier to each step.

3.2 explain how the verbal message is affected by nonverbal communication.

3.3 apply effective written communication techniques to compose written medical office correspondence.

KEY TERMS

Study these important words, which are defined in this chapter, to build your professional vocabulary:

bibliography	encoding	message	noise
block-style letter	endnotes	modified-block-style	open punctuation
channel	feedback	letter	proofreading
decoding	first draft	mixed/standard	title page
editing	footnotes	punctuation	

ABHES

4.a. Follow documentation guidelines.

5.h. Display effective interpersonal skills with patients and healthcare team members.

7.a. Gather and process documents.

7.g. Display professionalism through written and verbal communications.

7.h. Perform basic computer skills.

10.b. Demonstrate professional behavior.

www.abhes.org/accreditationmanual

The ABHES standards appear with permission of The Accrediting Bureau of Health Education Schools

CAAHEP

V.C.1. Identify styles and types of verbal communication.

V.C.2. Identify types of nonverbal communication.

V.C.3. Recognize barriers to communication.

V.C.4. Identify techniques for overcoming communication barriers.

V.C.5. Recognize the elements of oral communication using a sender-receiver process.

V.C.7. Recognize elements of fundamental writing skills.

V.C.8. Discuss applications of electronic technology in professional communication.

V.P.1.b Use feedback techniques to obtain patient information, including restatement.

V.P.1.c. Use feedback techniques to obtain patient information, including clarification.

V.P.2. Respond to nonverbal communication.

V.P.3. Use medical terminology correctly and pronounce accurately to communicate information to providers and patients.

V.P.8. Compose professional correspondence utilizing electronic technology.

V.P.11. Report relevant information concisely and accurately.

V.A.1.a. Demonstrate empathy.

V.A.1.b. Demonstrate active listening.

V.A.1.c. Demonstrate nonverbal communication.

V.A.2. Demonstrate the principles of self-boundaries.

XI.A.1. Recognize the impact personal ethics and morals have on the delivery of healthcare.

2015 Standards and Guidelines for the Accreditation of Educational Programs in Medical Assisting, Appendix B, Core Curriculum for Medical Assistants, Medical Assisting Education Review Board (MAERB), 2015

INTRODUCTION

In the healthcare profession, an important part of the administrative medical assistant's job is interacting with patients, building relationships with co-workers, and representing the physician and the quality of the practice. These are all good reasons to develop outstanding positive communication skills.

It is not only in interpersonal relationships but also in letters, memos, reports, and e-mail that the assistant represents the practice. Successful communication as an administrative medical assistant is due as much to oral and written communication skills as to technical skills.

3.1 | THE VERBAL COMMUNICATION CYCLE

Have you ever played the game of telling one person something, and the message is passed on to others until finally the last person says what he or she heard, and it is nothing like the original message? Communication between individuals or groups is what creates the web of our lives. Everything we do is interactive, even if we are interactive with only ourselves, and our communications have a ripple effect on others, which alters the context in which we live. Understanding this interactivity is crucial to healthy communication. How efficiently we use the communication cycle and how well we identify barriers to effective communication will contribute to the effectiveness of our communications.

The Circular Communication Cycle

For communications to be sent, received, and understood as intended, each step of the communication cycle must be completed effectively. If not, misunderstanding and conflict can create a nonproductive atmosphere in the work environment and in our personal lives. Time will be lost and productivity will decrease when the cycle breaks down. Each step is interconnected with the other steps.

Origination of Message by the Sender. At the beginning of the communication cycle, the sender must organize the message. The communicator should ask questions such as those that follow:

- What and why do I want to communicate? The sender will formulate ideas he or she wants to communicate. These ideas, known as the **message,** can be influenced by the sender's background, physical well-being, and beliefs, as well as the context in which the message is formulated.
- Who is my receiver or audience? The audience may be one person or a group of individuals. When preparing the message, the sender must consider the background of those who will be receiving the message. The educational level, professional field, and cultural background of the receiver are just a few of the items to consider when composing a message.
- What is the best method to communicate the message? Some messages are best delivered verbally; some can be effectively communicated through written methods. The chosen method for transmitting the message is called the **channel.**
- When should I communicate the message? The timing of the delivery is critical to the effectiveness of the communication. The receiver's perception of the message can be greatly influenced, positively or negatively, by the time at which the message is delivered and received. One example is giving a patient pre-surgery instructions when the patient is giving you the medical chart and charge sheet from the visit. The patient is not ready to receive the information.

Encoding of the Message by the Sender. Expressing ideas through words and gestures is known as **encoding.** Words and gestures have different meanings to individuals in different cultures. Concrete words should be used in place of relative terms. A patient may need to arrive 30 minutes prior to the scheduled procedure time. If the assistant tells the patient to arrive early for the procedure, the patient's perception of *early* may be only 5 minutes.

Other items to consider when encoding a message are the receiver's background knowledge of the message, physiological considerations (such as hearing loss), and language barriers.

Transmitting the Message Through a Channel. It is vital to transmit clearly what you want to say, to properly time your message, and to select the appropriate method, or channel, to communicate your message. Consider the following before transmitting a message:

- Are there any barriers that will disrupt the communication process? Anything that can break down the communication transmission process is known as **noise.** Noise can come from external sources, such as cell phone static, others talking, equipment running, or even typographical errors in a message. Internal noise, such as other thoughts or illness, can disrupt the cycle as well.
- Is the receiver ready to accept the message? If the patient is looking away or is talking or texting on a phone, he or she is distracted and is not ready to listen to the message. As discussed previously, timing of the message can help or hinder the receiver's interpretation of the message.
- Does the nature of the message lend itself to a particular channel of communication? Messages that are general in nature, such as providing an appointment, are effectively transmitted through verbal or written channels. Messages of a more sensitive nature should be evaluated for the most effective channel. Disciplinary actions or warnings should be delivered using a face-to-face channel, not by phone or e-mail. Examples of current channels of communication include written (such as reports and letters), visual (photos), electronic (including fax, e-mail, text), and telephone. Selecting the channel to match the nature of the communication helps to ensure the intended message is received.

Receiving and Decoding the Message by the Receiver. A person's perception is a person's reality, and the way a message is received and perceived is the meaning of the message for the receiver. Factors such as different backgrounds, noise, and knowledge base often make successful communication difficult. **Decoding** is the receiver's application of meaning to the transmitted message. A patient may be greeted with "Good morning," but the voice tone is angry and short. The words transmitted are verbally correct, but the accompanying nonverbal cues may cause the patient to decode the message as "Good morning, but leave me alone."

Checking for Understanding Through Feedback. **Feedback,** the receiver's responses, helps the sender determine if successful communication has occurred. Responses include both verbal and nonverbal reactions. A slightly tilted head or a perplexed look may indicate the receiver is confused. A receiver should ask questions for clarification. As the sender, ask the patient to repeat information. You may also restate information or question the patient to check for understanding. Figure 3.1 shows an example of the complete flow of communication between the administrative medical assistant and a patient.

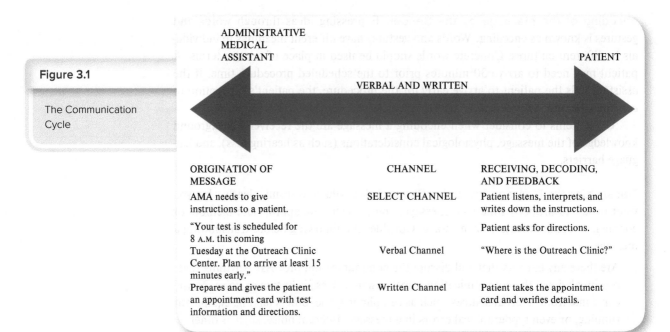

Figure 3.1

The Communication Cycle

ADMINISTRATIVE MEDICAL ASSISTANT		PATIENT
VERBAL AND WRITTEN		
ORIGINATION OF MESSAGE	CHANNEL	RECEIVING, DECODING, AND FEEDBACK
AMA needs to give instructions to a patient.	SELECT CHANNEL	Patient listens, interprets, and writes down the instructions.
"Your test is scheduled for 8 A.M. this coming Tuesday at the Outreach Clinic Center. Plan to arrive at least 15 minutes early."	Verbal Channel	Patient asks for directions. "Where is the Outreach Clinic?"
Prepares and gives the patient an appointment card with test information and directions.	Written Channel	Patient takes the appointment card and verifies details.

Barriers to the Communication Cycle

Many factors can create a barrier within and to the communication cycle. The best-planned message may not be received properly if barriers have not been considered. Each message sent and received must pass through a cultural, personal, and ethical bias base. This filtering process can hinder the intended message from being received.

Physical barriers can make it difficult to send and/or receive an intended message. Noisy surroundings, poor acoustics, and dim lighting can negatively affect the message. Physiological barriers can also affect the intended sent and/or received message. Hearing loss, fatigue, pain, hunger, anger, mental capacity, anxiety, and illness are all examples of physical status or needs that could affect how a message is sent or how it is received.

EXAMPLE: BARRIERS TO COMMUNICATION

Mr. and Mrs. Patient Public brought their 6-year-old daughter to the office today with symptoms of a high fever, congestion, fatigue, and blood in her urine. The patient's father and mother had both recently lost their jobs due to company closure. After the PA's evaluation, it was decided that the child needed to be admitted to the hospital for more testing and evaluation.

Upon checkout, the administrative medical assistant gave admission information to the parents. The parents were overwhelmed with the information. Their thoughts were on how to pay for today's office visit, the testing, and then the hospital admission. Their daughter was crying.

There are two hospitals in the local service area. The parents took their daughter to the wrong hospital.

The parents' anxiety, concern for their daughter's health, their daughter's distress, and their worry about how to pay the bill, as well as the administrative medical assistant's lack of checking for feedback, all contributed to the parents going to the wrong hospital.

Selecting the proper wording can enhance the meaning and interpretation of the message. Using words that are unfamiliar to the receiver, such as medical insurance jargon, can destroy the intended message. Use words that create a receptive environment for the message. It is important to remember that most individuals think much faster than they speak—up to three times faster. As you verbally send a message, concentrate on the current message and words and refrain from thinking ahead. This can cause receivers to become bored with the message, allowing their minds to wander.

Another barrier to effective communication is inactive listening. As a sender and receiver, we become involved in the cycle. The fast pace of society has conditioned many individuals to fake attention to messages and simply wait for the sender to stop talking so that they can begin talking! This can cause miscommunication and failure to hear all the facts.

The first step to becoming an active listener is to stop talking and begin listening when someone else is speaking (sending a message), even if we don't agree with the message. Try to listen objectively and patiently before responding. Judging a message based on the sender's appearance is another contributor to inactive listening. If you must judge, judge the message, not the sender's appearance.

3.2 NONVERBAL COMMUNICATION

We have all heard the old saying "Actions speak louder than words," and nowhere is that more true than in communication. Since communication is interactive and contributes largely to the web of life in which we live, we must be very aware of not only our verbal messages but also the nonverbal communication we send with them. It has been estimated by many body language experts that up to 93 percent of all human communication is nonverbal. Our verbal message may have all the right elements, which we discussed earlier in this chapter, but our nonverbal message may say something different.

Facial expression, tone of voice, eye contact, body movement and posture, our use of space, and appearance all contribute to our unspoken message. When our verbal message says one thing but our body language communicates another, we confuse our audience and lose credibility. When a listener must choose between the spoken message and the nonverbal one, the nonverbal message wins!

Facial Expression

The face is one of the most visible and expressive parts of the body. It is capable of many expressions, which reflect our thoughts and emotions. Few people have a true "poker face," which doesn't display their emotions. Most individuals have a wide variety of facial expressions, which they use many times during a conversation. A smile, a frown, pressed lips, and a wrinkled brow are just a few of the ways people can express emotions. It is common for a medical office to employ individuals with varying cultural backgrounds. Gestures may have different meanings to individuals, even within a small grouping. In American culture, a smile is considered a gesture of approval, satisfaction, or happiness. However, other cultures perceive a smile as an expression of nervousness or embarrassment.

Tone of Voice

Tone of voice may, on the surface, seem to be a verbal communication barrier. However, when the words of a message give one meaning but the sender's tone of voice gives another, the tone of voice becomes a nonverbal communication cue. Feelings can be hurt by the tone of voice used by another. For example, you discover an error in a patient's account and realize it was your error. Right away, you go to the office manager and inform him of the error and your intent to correct it. The office manager says, "That's fine," but the tone of voice is very sharp and loud. Do you believe it is fine and the office manager is not upset? The tone of voice used says the office manager is upset, and that is the conveyed message.

Eye Contact

Confidence and interest are expressed nonverbally by making and keeping eye contact with an audience. Whether the audience is an individual or a group, maintaining eye contact allows the sender and the receiver to be attentive and show respect for the other. When direct eye contact is maintained, a level of trust may be established. These characteristics are true of the American culture. However, in other cultures, direct eye contact can be offensive and make the communicators uncomfortable.

Body Movement and Posture

Gestures, or movements we make with our body, attach meaning to a message. The ways in which we sit, talk, and stand tell their own tale. Leaning toward a person conveys interest in the message, while stepping away conveys a perception of distrust or offense. Leaning back in a chair can convey the message of being relaxed, while tapping a finger or pencil signifies that the conversation should end. Standing tall and straight is associated with high position, but slumping of the shoulders and lowering of the head make us appear shy or lacking in self-confidence. Our posture should support our verbal message and can be a powerful nonverbal cue.

Each culture has its own values associated with body movement. As an administrative medical assistant, you should know the different cultures represented among your patients and colleagues and use body movement and posture accordingly.

Space

Just how close should you stand to another person while communicating? Have you ever invaded someone's space? The spaces, or zones, around us have meaning and serve as social areas for interaction with others. The public zone (12 feet or more from your audience) is used for most public speaking events. A social zone is used for communications within 4 to 12 feet of our audience. Many individuals begin to feel uncomfortable when others enter their personal zone, which is 1.5 to 4 feet away, and become extremely uncomfortable with people in their intimate zone (1 to 1.5 feet). Too close, and our message will take second place to the discomfort the listener is feeling from our invasion of their zone. Too far away, and we send the message of being aloof and cold. In some cultures, however, it is considered rude not to stand extremely close (within the American intimate zone) when talking with an individual.

ROLE-PLAYING EXERCISE:

Ask a fellow student if he or she can tell you what the last assignment was for class. Listen intently and then pretend you did not hear. Move into the student's personal zone and ask the question again.

Notice any changes in the other individual, such as moving away from you or changing his or her tone of voice.

Appearance

Clothing and grooming send their own message about the communicator. Professional clothing in the medical office environment helps create a positive atmosphere for patients and colleagues. Scrubs should be clean and wrinkle-free. Underlying clothing should not be visible through the scrubs. If scrubs are not worn, casual office or professional office clothing should be worn. No holes or tears should be visible in clothing. Even on "dress-down" or "casual" days, clothing should be professionally presentable.

Hygiene and grooming also convey a nonverbal message. Nails should be clean and kept to a minimal length; hair should be washed and neat; and most individuals need to shower every day. Cleanliness, or lack thereof, affects our ability to be taken seriously. It is true that "we never get a second chance to make a first impression." The Administrative Medical Assistant chapter provides more details on professional appearance.

3.3 WRITTEN COMMUNICATION

Writing and speaking effectively have these points in common:

- The communication has an appropriate tone—a way of phrasing ideas, announcements, directions, and requests that is pleasant, positive, and reassuring.
- The communication has a clear purpose, aim, or goal.
- The message is directed to a person, or "listener," who is to receive it.
- Correct English is used—including acceptable grammar, spelling, and punctuation.
- Complete information is given in a direct, concise, and courteous way.

This section focuses on preparing written communications and the office procedures that deal with receiving and sending correspondence. However, the qualities of positive tone, clear purpose, a sense of the intended audience, good use of the English language, and a direct and courteous delivery of complete information are necessary whether you are speaking or writing.

Reasons for Written Rather Than Oral Communication

Because there are so many issues of law, ethics, and confidentiality in medical offices, written communication may often be preferable to a conversation or phone call. Written communication may be required for many reasons, including the following:

- *Giving complex directions or instructions.* Patients who are anxious or distracted may need to read information at a time when they are calm. Repeating the physician's instructions or other information in writing may be more effective than oral communication.
- *Being efficient.* Writing a brief message may not require the time and effort of a phone call or face-to-face conversation.
- *Documenting an event or a fact.* The written documentation of aspects of patient care and practice management helps protect the practice from legal problems.
- *Providing for confidentiality.* It may be difficult or improper to use the telephone for certain communications with a patient.

COMPLIANCE *TIP*

Test results, arrangements for a surgical procedure, and messages about a patient's condition may be better protected in written messages. These messages should always be placed in envelopes marked "Confidential" or "Private."

Formatting

Before dealing with the content of correspondence, it is necessary to consider the appearance of the letter on the page. When a letter from your office is received, it should be pleasing to the eye and invite the reader's attention.

The arrangement, or format, of the letter on the page may be one that your employer has selected and is shown in the office procedures manual. For example, the preferred office-style letter for a physician may be to place the subject line above the greeting, rather than below the greeting; or a double space may be used between the reference initials, enclosure notation, and copy notation. If this is not the case, you will need to choose one of the accepted formats for correspondence. There are two frequently used letter formats that give the letter a well-balanced and attractive appearance—block and modified-block style. In addition to the two letter styles, two formatting styles are now being used—those prepared in a contemporary style using a word processing software, such as the most current version of Microsoft Word or a similar word processor, and those prepared in a traditional format. Documents prepared in the newer formatting style are the preferred layout, and examples in this chapter have been prepared using this format.

Block Style. All lines in a block-style letter are flush with the left margin. The major rules for a **block-style letter** prepared in the new format are described here and shown in Figure 3.2a:

- Place the dateline at 2 inches, or place the dateline at least 0.5 inch below the letterhead. If preferred, center a one-page letter vertically, from top to bottom, on the page.
- Press Enter twice beneath the date, and key in the letter address. Single-space the letter address by removing the 1.5 spacing from the address.
- Press Enter once, key in the salutation, and then press Enter once after the salutation to begin the body of the letter.

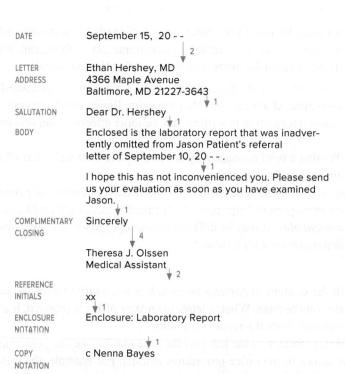

Figure 3.2a

Block-Style Letter with Open Punctuation

- Use either 1 or 1.5 spacing for the body of the letter. Some consider the extra 0.5 line spacing excessive and change the default line spacing from Normal to No Spacing. Press Enter twice between paragraphs.
- Place the complimentary closing one Enter below the body of the letter, and capitalize only the first word of the closing (e.g., *Very truly yours*).
- Press Enter twice, and key in the writer's name and title.
- Key reference initials, lowercase, one Enter below the writer's name if you are not the author of the document.
- Press Enter once to key in Enclosure or Enclosures. To list and align enclosures, tab to 1.0 inch.
- Place a copy (c) notation one Enter below enclosures. If multiple names are listed, align the names using the Tab key.

Modified-Block Style. The major rules for a **modified-block-style letter,** shown in Figure 3.2b, are similar to those for a block letter, but with these two exceptions:

- Position the dateline, complimentary closing, and signature line at a tab stop at center of the horizontal line length; for example, if the line length is 6.5 inches, place the tab at 3.25 inches.
- Begin all other lines at the left margin, or if you wish, indent new paragraphs 0.5 inch.

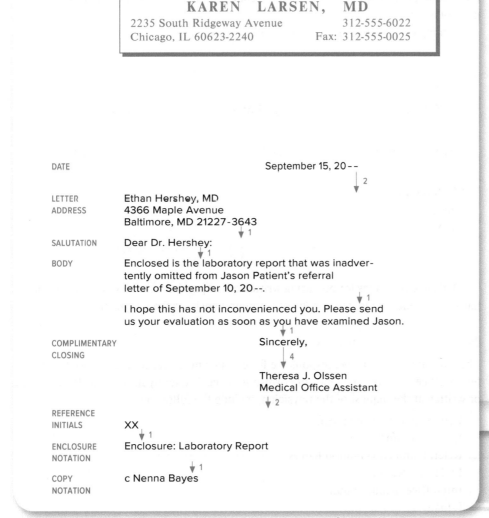

Figure 3.2b

Modified-Block-Style Letter with Mixed Punctuation

Punctuation

There are two styles of punctuation used in business letters:

- **Mixed/standard punctuation.** Place a colon after the salutation and a comma after the complimentary closing. This is also referred to as *closed punctuation*.
- **Open punctuation.** Do not use *any* punctuation after the salutation or complimentary closing. Open punctuation should be used when it is the preferred business letter punctuation style of the medical office.
- **Spacing after punctuation marks.** After punctuation marks, such as periods, commas, etc., insert either one or two spaces. More contemporary letter styles use one space after punctuation marks.

Continuation Pages

In business writing, it is commonly preferred to keep written correspondence to a one-page document. However, there are times when all necessary information cannot be placed on a single page. When a letter has more than one page, always use blank stationery of the same quality as that of the first page for the continuing pages. Do not use stationery with a letterhead, even when the first page has a letterhead. Use a top margin of 1 inch on pages after the first page, and add an appropriate heading, which includes the name of the recipient, page number, and date. Formatting of the second-page heading should match the formatting of the first page of the letter, and the second-page heading identifies the second and any subsequent pages with the first page of a letter.

Examples of second-page headings are shown here.

EXAMPLES: SECOND-PAGE HEADINGS

Ms. Susie Patient	Page 2 of 3	October 23, 20--
Ms. Susie Patient	2 of 3	October 23, 20--

Ms. Susie Patient
Page 2 of 3
October 23, 20--

Valuable resources for preparing written correspondence include a good dictionary, hardcopy or electronic, and a copy of a comprehensive reference manual.

Types of Correspondence

The assistant is, or may be, responsible for composing correspondence about many different office matters. The kinds of correspondence frequently initiated by the assistant, or written at the request of the physician, include the following:

- Letters of acknowledgment
- Letters of information
- Referral and consultation letters
- Follow-up letters
- Interoffice memorandums
- E-mail

Letters of Acknowledgment. The receipt of certain letters, materials, gifts, or requests for information requires a letter of acknowledgment. Such a letter may be written and signed by the administrative medical assistant or written by the assistant for the physician to sign. The letter of acknowledgment should include the date on which the item or request was received and a description of what was received. If the letter is a request for a response or decision, the assistant should acknowledge the inquiry but make no promises in the name of the physician about the exact date or nature of the response unless information was obtained from the physician.

The main purpose of a letter of acknowledgment is to let the sender know as soon as possible that a request is being handled. In the case of a gift, the letter states that the gift has been received and is appreciated. Because writing letters of acknowledgment is a frequent task, a form letter may be used. Such form letters are easy to create with the templates found in word processing programs.

Letters of Information. Letters of information must have clear and complete information. A concise statement of the information is also appreciated by the recipient. If the information contains instructions related to treatment, the letter usually has the physician's signature, although the physician may ask the assistant to compose the letter. Letters of Medical Necessity are sent to insurance providers to justify the use of a particular medication, procedure, or other treatment. Typical information in a Letter of Medical Necessity includes patient name, date of birth, insurance ID number, name of medication/procedure/treatment, and medical necessity justification and argument for the medication/procedure/treatment. Insurance providers may require the letter to be placed on the medical facility/provider's letterhead. Patient documentation may also need to be submitted with the letter to support the necessity. Before preparing a Letter of Medical Necessity, the administrative medical assistant should check with the insurance provider to be certain all information is included in the letter.

Referral and Consultation Letters. Referral letters are used when a physician transfers part or all of a patient's care to another physician. For example, a general practitioner may refer a patient with a heart condition to a cardiologist for an extended period of treatment. A request for a consultation happens when the physician asks another physician to examine a patient and report back findings on a specific question. For example, a general practitioner may ask a gastroenterologist to perform a colonoscopy and report the results of that examination as part of a patient's comprehensive physical examination.

Some practices send a brief letter thanking the physician who sent the patient when a patient is referred. The note is usually sent once the patient has been seen, so that a brief medical report can be included. Figure 3.3 is an example of this type of letter and may be used as a guide in drafting a letter of thanks for a referral. If a referred patient does not make or keep an appointment, a letter should be sent to the referring physician, explaining that the patient did not appear, after a reasonable period of time has passed.

Many medical insurance plans require patients to see a general practitioner before they can see a specialist. In these plans, the patient receives a referral letter or form from the general practitioner and takes it to the specialist's office. The referral contains an authorization number, which the assistant records as part of the patient's information. This type of referral may be handled differently by the medical office and generally does not require a thank-you note. The administrative medical assistant must learn the policies of the office for these situations.

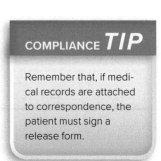

COMPLIANCE *TIP*

Remember that, if medical records are attached to correspondence, the patient must sign a release form.

Figure 3.3

Letter Thanking a
Physician for the Referral
of a Patient

KAREN LARSEN, MD
2235 South Ridgeway Avenue
Chicago, IL 60623-2240

312-555-6022
Fax: 312-555-0025

August 14, 20--

Hugh Arnold, MD
Suite 440
2785 South Ridgeway Avenue
Chicago, IL 60647-2700

Dear Dr. Arnold:

RE: FRANZ PATIENT   **DOB: 08/05/----**

Thank you for referring Franz Patient to me. I have
just completed his examination. Mr. Patient was first
examind by me on June 4. His diagnosis at that
time was otitis externa, bilaterally; defective
hearing, mixed type, bilaterally. The results of
the audiogram are enclosed.

In July, Mr. Patient had another audiogram (results
are also enclosed). At that time, a considerable
loss of high tones indicated a beginning degeneration of the auditory nerve, associated with
severe tinnitus.

Thank you for referring this patient to me.

Sincerely,

Karen Larsen, MD

nb

Enclosures: June Audiogram
             July Audiogram

To make a referral or ask for a consultation, the physician who is sending the patient usually writes or phones the other physician, giving the reason for the request and a summary of the results of the pertinent tests or treatments the patient has had. If the referral is discussed on the phone, a letter confirming the conversation is sent. The other physician then knows that a patient is expected and has a brief history of the patient's problem. The referring office may also schedule an appointment for the patient with the other physician. Figure 3.4 is an example of this type of letter and may be used as a guide in drafting a referral letter.

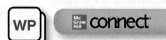

GO TO PROJECT 3.1 AT THE END OF THIS CHAPTER

Follow-Up Letters. Sometimes it is necessary to follow up on a request or a letter that has not received a response. In writing such a letter, be courteous, give the recipient the details of the original request and include a duplicate of the original request, and be clear about what action you wish the recipient to take.

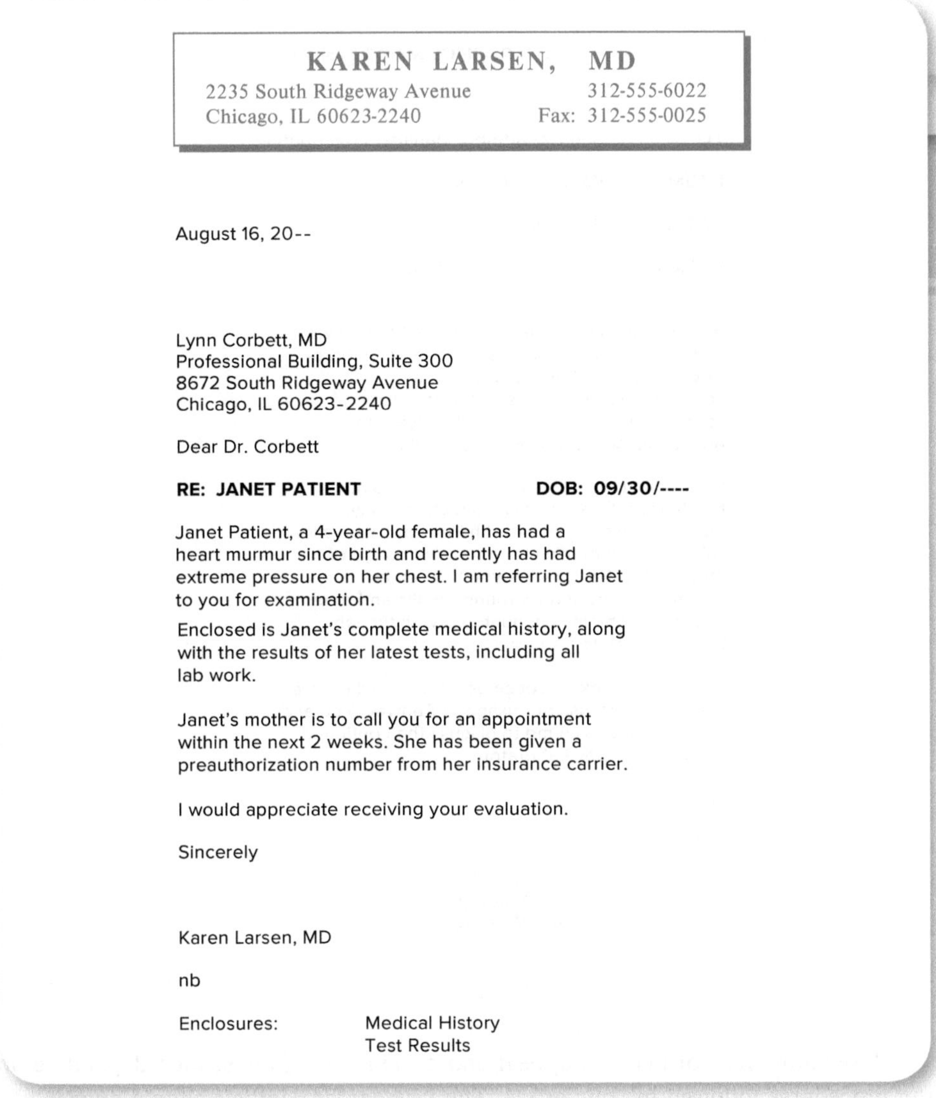

Figure 3.4

Letter Informing a
Physician of the Referral
of a Patient

KAREN LARSEN, MD
2235 South Ridgeway Avenue   312-555-6022
Chicago, IL 60623-2240   Fax: 312-555-0025

August 16, 20--

Lynn Corbett, MD
Professional Building, Suite 300
8672 South Ridgeway Avenue
Chicago, IL 60623-2240

Dear Dr. Corbett

RE: JANET PATIENT   **DOB: 09/30/----**

Janet Patient, a 4-year-old female, has had a
heart murmur since birth and recently has had
extreme pressure on her chest. I am referring Janet
to you for examination.

Enclosed is Janet's complete medical history, along
with the results of her latest tests, including all
lab work.

Janet's mother is to call you for an appointment
within the next 2 weeks. She has been given a
preauthorization number from her insurance carrier.

I would appreciate receiving your evaluation.

Sincerely

Karen Larsen, MD

nb

Enclosures: Medical History
                     Test Results

Interoffice Memorandums. Informal messages exchanged within an organization may be written as interoffice memorandums, usually referred to as "memos." Memos are written on stationery that may have a preprinted heading, such as *Interoffice Memorandum* or the name and logo of the practice.

There may be preprinted guide words near the top of the page, such as *TO:*, *FROM:*, *DATE:*, and *SUBJECT:*. If you require more guide words, such as *DEPARTMENT:* or *EXTENSION:*, you may use two columns, so that the memo heading does not take too much space.

If the memo is being sent to a number of people, after the guide word *TO:*, you may wish to key the words *See Distribution*. On the second line below the writer's initials at the end of the memo, key the word *Distribution* followed by a colon. Leave one line blank, and then type the names of those to whom the memo is to be sent, arranging the names either by rank or in alphabetic order.

Memos do not usually contain an inside address or complimentary closing, as a letter does. When memos are announcements to a number of people, there is no salutation. However, if the memo concerns only one individual, a salutation followed by a colon may be used, such as *Dear Tom:* or the name *Tom:* alone. If a salutation is used, a complimentary closing should also be used, such as *Sincerely,*.

Figure 3.5

Interoffice Memorandum

INTEROFFICE MEMORANDUM

TO: See Department Managers Distribution

FROM: Karen Larsen, MD

DATE: September 15, 20--

SUBJECT: Outside Laboratory Usage

After careful study, I have decided that Penway Laboratory will be our outside resource laboratory for the next 3 months. They have contracted to provide us with fast, reliable service. They are certified by Medicare to provide all necessary lab test results.

Our contact person at Penway will be Gina McPherson. She will bill us directly for any outside services we use with Penway. Also, she will send us monthly reports on our usage of their facility. Gary, I want you to keep an accurate report of turnaround results and other possible problems encountered with the lab tests we send to Penway.

During the week of December 20, we will have a meeting to discuss our usage of Penway. You and Gina will meet with me to discuss the continued usage of Penway Laboratory.

nb

Distribution:

Gary Libinski
Susan Solosky
Nancy Westing

A signature may or may not appear above the name of the sender, depending on the procedures followed in your office. The keyboarder's initials should appear two lines below the writer's name or initials or two lines below the body of the message. An example of an interoffice memo is shown in Figure 3.5.

Most, if not all, offices use computer-prepared or -stored documents to send communications. Templates can be prepared for routine correspondence, and each time a new correspondence is prepared using a stored template, the letter/e-mail has a clean, freshly prepared appearance. A template can be prepared using standardized wording and fill-in blanks to personalize the letter. Templates may also be referred to as *form letters*. If several copies, which are to be used at a later date, are made of form letters, each copied form letter (template) should be clean, legible, and have a freshly prepared appearance. The following section provides more information on electronic communication.

E-Mail and Other Electronic Communication Technologies. The most common and efficient form of interoffice communication is electronic mail (e-mail). It provides an immediate delivery of correspondence to one or many individuals. Preparing an e-mail is similar to preparing an interoffice memorandum. An e-mail address is keyed into the *TO:* field. Since a *FROM:* field is not included in the heading, many professionals include their names after the body of the message or compose a closing to be attached to each outgoing e-mail. Dates and time are automatically included with the e-mail.

A *SUBJECT:* line should be included. Mixed case may be used (capitalize the first letter of all words except prepositions and conjunctions), or the line may be keyed in all caps. Whichever format is used, the *SUBJECT:* line should be concise, enticing, and contain an active verb. Your e-mail is competing with other media for the reader's attention.

EXAMPLES: SUBJECT LINES

Outside Cardiology Services

Using Outside Cardiology Services Is Cost-Effective

The second example gives more detail of the message—it contains both a noun and a verb. If a subject line is not used, the recipient may perceive the e-mail as unimportant and not open it.

When composing the body of an e-mail, the standard protocol is to address only one topic and keep the e-mail to one page. Many writers include the recipient's name as a salutation or use the name in the first line of the body. If you use a salutation, such as Dear Nancy, also include the writer's name in the closing.

Engage your reader(s) by making your content empathetic to the reader. Tell the reader (1) what you are writing, (2) why it is important to them, (3) where action (or nonaction) is needed, and (4) how it will affect them. If action is required by a certain date, supply the required action and the date by which it is required. The following is a summary of the content of an effective e-mail:

1. Use a grabbing subject line.
2. Supply the what, when, where, why, and how of letter writing.
3. Give the reader information to support your purpose.
4. Provide a brief summary of the important facts.

Even though e-mail communication may be considered less formal than letters, it is still important to present a professional written image. Correct grammar, punctuation, and structure should be used. Always proofread an e-mail prior to hitting SEND. It is a good practice not to send anything through e-mail you do not want made public. Imagine your message being posted on the front page of your local paper or read on the evening news. Because of their ease, e-mails are often composed when the writer is angry or frustrated. If this is the case, go ahead and compose the e-mail but minimize it and allow yourself a cool-down period before hitting SEND. After you have allowed yourself this cool-down period, you may want to delete the e-mail or revise it before sending it to the recipient.

Always ask permission from the sender prior to forwarding an e-mail. Messages received may be intended only for the recipient. The sender may want to send a second e-mail with alternative wording, send an e-mail directly, or simply make a phone call.

Electronic technologies also allow medical team members to communicate with each other and with patients. It also establishes a Web presence and platform for the medical office through which patients and medical office team members can give and receive information. Following are some of these technologies:

- *VoIP (Voice over Internet Protocol):* allows switching from traditional telephone service to an Internet voice protocol. Broadband is used, allowing callers to communicate through the Internet instead of through long-distance calling. Depending on long-distance phone charges, VoIP can be a low-cost method of communication.

- *Blog:* journal-type entries made at a website. Usually, one person begins the blog and others may respond. Medical offices may use blogs to convey information, such as pros and cons of the shingles vaccine.
- *Podcasts:* files that can be listened to or viewed on a computer or mobile device. Podcasts can be informational, such as posting a podcast to update employees on new privacy regulations.
- *Wiki:* a website that allows employees and/or individuals to collectively create, contribute, and edit information. A wiki can be beneficial when collecting others' views and opinions. Information from a wiki source should be validated prior to use.
- *Voice conferencing (also known as conference calling):* allows two or more individuals from any location to participate in the same phone call. For example, a primary physician, cardiologist, and physical therapist may collaborate on a conference call to establish rehabilitation protocol for a patient after triple-bypass surgery.
- *Web conferencing:* Internet service that allows individuals to attend virtual meetings using a mobile device. Meetings are in real time and can be interactive. Slides and desktop screenshots can be used during the meeting. Attendees may view other attendees' computer screens. Chats can take place between attendees. A medical coder could use Web conferencing to gain training on *ICD-10-CM* coding procedures.
- *Video conferencing:* permits individuals to meet in a specially equipped area and conference with other individuals at a different location. Both sites are equipped with cameras and screens that allow attendees to see and interact with each other. A statewide meeting for nurse practitioners could be attended by many NPs without incurring large travel expenses.
- *Livestreaming:* allows individuals to send and receive information in a real-time electronic environment. A device, such as a smartphone, is used to convey or stream video and audio to an audience. Audience members can respond in real time. A monthly office meeting could be livestreamed and also recorded for medical office members who could not attend the live meeting to view at a later time.

McGraw Hill **connect**   GO TO PROJECT 3.2 AT THE END OF THIS CHAPTER

Preparing Professional Reports

Many physicians are involved in writing articles, books, or reports on the results of research. They may also need to prepare speeches or presentations. Helping prepare reports is often a duty of the administrative medical assistant.

Preparing Draft Manuscript. The manuscript that will eventually be submitted to a publisher starts out as a draft. Some writers begin with an outline, jotting down headings and subheadings. The rough draft may then be filled in with notes added to the outline. Other writers make many notes, ask the assistant to key the notes, and write from these.

The **first draft** is the first complete keying of the manuscript. All text should be spaced to allow ample room for corrections and additions. The manuscript may go through many drafts before it is final. Each draft should be identified by number—*Draft 1, Draft 2,* and so on. Before saving a draft to the computer file, be sure that you have labeled it with its correct draft number or used the word processor's automatic draft-numbering feature.

After each round of corrections, additions, and deletions, the physician will ask you to key the changes and to proofread and edit the draft. Suggestions for proofreading and editing are given later in this chapter.

Preparing Final Manuscript. The purpose of the writing determines the final format selected. The purpose of some reports is to share information; these reports may be meant for distribution only within the organization. Such reports may have an informal format and may even be prepared as a letter or memo. There are several templates for formats provided in word processing applications. If the procedures manual in your office does not dictate a format, you may want to choose one of these templates.

Formal reports, usually more complex and longer than informal reports, are often written for readers outside the organization. Documents meant as professional reports or manuscripts for publication often have special features, such as a table of contents, list of illustrations, summary, and list of sources consulted by the writer. The publisher of a journal article can give rules for format and style to help the assistant prepare the manuscript. A manuscript may be rejected by the publisher if the appropriate format, such as MLA (Modern Language Association) style, *AMA (American Medical Association) Manual of Style,* or APA (American Psychological Association) style, is not used. For other kinds of formal reports, the specifications for both a traditionally prepared report and a report prepared with Microsoft Word are given here.

- *Title page*

    Traditional: On the first manuscript page, called the **title page,** key the title of the report in all-capital letters. Key the subtitle, if there is one, in capital and small letters, double-spaced below the title. Boldface should be used for the title and subtitle. Key *Prepared by* 12 lines below the subtitle. Then double-space to key the writer's name and credentials; writer's title, if appropriate; and writer's affiliation on separate lines. Key the date of the report 12 lines below the affiliation. Center all the text horizontally and vertically on the page.

    Contemporary format: Within the word processing software, select to insert a cover page and select the desired cover page style. Key the requested information in the provided fields, such as "Key in the document title." Figure 3.6a shows the title page of a formal report prepared with Microsoft Word.

- *Text*

    Traditional: The text of the report should be double-spaced, with the first line of each paragraph indented 0.5 inch. There should be 1-inch margins on all sides.

    Contemporary format: Accept the preset default selection, usually 1.5, for spacing and the default font.

    The purpose of the report will determine which font is to be used. An acceptable font is 12-point Times New Roman. When a formal report is prepared, such as a manuscript to be submitted for publication, the font used will be determined by the organization that is publishing the document.

- *Numbering*

    Traditional and contemporary format: The title page should not be numbered; all other pages should be numbered in the upper right-hand corner. Pages are numbered consecutively, starting with the number 1, from the beginning to the end of the manuscript.

- *Headings*

    Traditional format: Section headings, such as *SUMMARY, INTRODUCTION,* and *CHAPTER 1,* should be keyed in all-capital letters in boldface type. Each section should start on a new page, with a 2-inch top margin, and there should be two blank lines below the section heading. Main text headings, which alert readers to new subjects within a section, should be keyed in all-capital letters and placed flush with the left margin on a separate line. Text subheadings should be keyed in capital and small letters, indented 0.5 inch, and followed by a period; text should follow right after the subheading on the same line.

Figure 3.6a

Title Page of a Formal Report

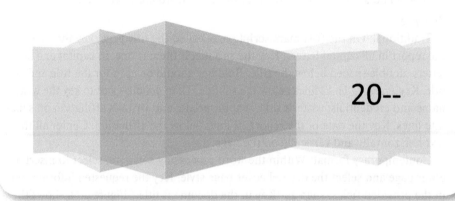

University Hospital

CHICKENPOX (VARICELLA)

An Overview

Karen Larsen, MD

20--

Boldface should be used for text headings, and there should be one blank line above headings.

Contemporary format: Side headings should be keyed at the left margin with the first letter of all main words capitalized. Select a heading style, such as Heading 1, and key in the heading. After the heading, press Enter one time.

- *Italics and underscoring:* Words within the text that are to be emphasized may be underscored or italicized. Although foreign words should also be italicized or underscored, medical terms that are foreign words but are in common use should not be either italicized or underscored.
- *Quotations:* If quotations are brief, they may be set in quotation marks and appear as part of the text. Longer quotations (four or more lines) should be single-spaced for traditional format or default normal spacing for current format and indented 0.5 inch from the left and right margins.
- *Notes:* Writers use notes in a report to (1) add parenthetical comments or (2) provide the sources for information or quotations. A raised number appears in the text at the point of reference for the note; the note itself is also numbered. Notes that are positioned at the bottom of the page on which the reference appears are called **footnotes.** Notes that are grouped together at the end of the report are called **endnotes.** Most word processing programs have a notes feature that enables the keyboarder to create footnotes and endnotes.
- *Illustrations:* If a manuscript that is to be sent to a publisher or printer contains photographs, tables, charts, or graphs, these illustrations may be submitted as digital computer files or as reproduction copy. If digital files are needed, a

Figure 3.6b

First Page of an Informal
Professional Report

CHICKENPOX (VARICELLA)

By Karen Larsen, MD,
University Hospital

January 25, 20--

DEFINITION

Chickenpox is a highly contagious, acute infection causing pruritic
rash, slight fever, malaise, and anorexia.

ETIOLOGY

Herpes virus varicella-zoster causes chickenpox. It is transmitted by
direct contact (respiratory secretions more prominently than skin lesions)
and by indirect contact (air waves). The highest communicable period is
the early stages of skin lesion eruption. Incubation period ranges from
13 to 17 days.

CLINICAL SYMPTOMS

The prodrome of chickenpox generally begins with slight fever, malaise,
and anorexia. The pruritic rash begins within 24 hours as erythematous
macules, then progresses to papules, and then to clear vesicles. The vesicles turn cloudy and break. Scabs then form. The rash begins on the trunk
and scalp. After the vesicles become cloudy and break, the rash spreads to
the face but rarely spreads to the extremities.

TREATMENT

The patient should remain in isolation for at least 1 week after the
onset of the rash. Local or systemic antipruritics, calamine lotion, cool
soda baths, and antihistamines should be used for relief of symptoms.
If a bacterial infection develops, an antibiotic should be prescribed.
Varicella-zoster immune globulin (passive immunity) can be given to
susceptible patients within 72 hours of exposure to varicella.

scanner can be used to create a computer file of the illustration. The file name should describe the illustration. If reproduction copy is to be submitted, each illustration should be mounted on a separate sheet of blank, letter-size paper and identified by a title, caption, or brief description written on the sheet of paper. The manuscript page number containing the reference to the illustration should also be noted on the paper. Every photograph submitted should be a glossy print. Care should be taken not to write on either the front or the back of the photograph.

- *Bibliography:* All the works consulted by the writer, including items given in notes, are listed, alphabetically by author, in a **bibliography** at the end of the report. The publisher or an appropriate reference manual should be consulted for the format and style required. The University of Chicago's *Chicago Manual of Style;* the *Publication Manual of the American Psychological Association;* the American Medical Association's *Manual of Style;* and *Scientific Style and Format: The CSE Manual for Authors, Editors, and Publishers,* published by the Council of Science Editors, are manuals that the writer may wish to consult for detailed descriptions of how to style and format notes and bibliographies.

An example of the first page of an informal report prepared with Microsoft Word is shown in Figure 3.6b.

Mc Graw Hill connect   GO TO PROJECT 3.3 AT THE END OF THIS CHAPTER

Proofreading and Editing

High quality in written communications is necessary because correspondence—both internal and external—represents your employer and the practice. The professional image of the practice depends in part on the impressions others form through the correspondence they receive. Incorrect, careless, or unclear communications may be damaging.

Two processes used to ensure accuracy and clarity are proofreading and editing. **Proofreading** is the careful reading and examination of a document for the sole purpose of finding and correcting errors. **Editing** is the assessment of a document to determine its clarity, consistency, and overall effectiveness. The good proofreader asks, Is this document entirely correct? Are sentence structure and punctuation used correctly? The good editor asks, Does this document say exactly what the writer intended in the best way possible? Are there any areas in the document that may confuse the reader?

EXAMPLE: PROOFREADING VERSUS EDITING

Proofreading:

"The prodrome of chickenpox begins with sight fever, malaise, and anorexia."

The proofreader would mark the error and/or change "sight" to "slight."

Editing:

"The incubation period varies."

The editor would mark the word "varies"—it is a relative term and can imply different meanings. A concrete or definite incubation period should be used, such as "The incubation period ranges from 13 to 17 days."

Proofreading Methods. Frequently, only one person reads a document for accuracy, comparing it to the original document. A single proofreader is all that is required for most routine correspondence and reports. For complex documents or highly technical materials, two proofreaders may work as partners. One person reads the original document aloud, including all punctuation and significant style and format elements; the other person examines the new copy carefully and makes the required corrections.

If you are the writer of the original document, proofreading is more difficult because there is no document against which to check for accuracy. For this task, an excellent working knowledge of English grammar, word usage, punctuation rules, and spelling is required. In cases where someone else has written the document, both the proofreader and the author should proofread the document.

Proofreading on the Computer Screen

Proofreading documents on the computer screen is an essential skill. You may want to use a piece of paper held against the screen to show only one line, so that you concentrate line by line on the text. Once you have examined the document line by line for errors and have corrected these, proofread your corrections carefully. Now you are ready to print and/or send a correct document.

Using Spell and Grammar Checkers

It is all too easy when you are proofreading on the screen to believe that the spell-check and grammar features in the word processing program have found all the errors for you. However helpful these features are, they simply cannot find many types of errors.

Spell-checkers have a dictionary of a certain number of words. Specialized words that are used frequently can be added to the spell-checker's dictionary. The software will highlight or underscore a word it does not recognize. You will then need to decide whether the word is correct. Specialized dictionaries, such as an electronic medical dictionary, are frequently installed to help minimize the number of errors recognized by the word processor. For example, without the installation of a medical dictionary, the word *hyperglycemia* would be noted as a misspelled word in most spell-checkers. The abbreviation *EHR* is frequently changed to *HER* in word processing programs without a medical dictionary. When words are manually added to a spell-checker, proofread the word to be sure it is spelled correctly. If words are added to the electronic dictionary and they are misspelled, the spell-checker will not catch the misspelling.

The spell-checker may not alert you to a word that is spelled correctly but misused. In some word processing programs, ordinary mistakes of this kind are underscored by the grammar checker. For example, using *their* where *there* should be used will be underscored by the software. However, certain other words that are frequently misused are not underscored. In the following examples, the mistakes may not be underscored by the software: "There are *too* of them (using *too* instead of *two*)"; "He did not *except* the gift (using *except* instead of *accept*)." The spell-check and grammar features are not adequate substitutes for a knowledgeable, alert reader.

Proofreading Symbols. Proofreaders and editors use standard symbols to indicate specific corrections to documents. If the document is to be published, the symbols will guide those who print the document. When corrections are made on the computer, these symbols on the paper copy guide the person keying the corrections. These proofreaders' marks, shown in Figure 3.7, should always be used when making corrections. Some physicians, however, may choose to use correction marks and symbols on hard-copy documents (e.g., transcribed reports) they have composed themselves.

Proofreading Techniques. It is always necessary to read every document several times. There are many elements in any written document and therefore many opportunities for error. Each time you read a document, you are concentrating on a different element:

1. Read for content. Does the document agree *exactly* with the original? Have any words been omitted? Have any words been repeated, especially at the ends of lines?
2. Read for correct grammar, spelling, usage (both words and numbers), and keyboarding errors. In addition to reading, use the spelling and grammar checkers but do not totally rely on them. Keep a good dictionary, medical dictionary, and English Reference manual close at hand.
3. Check the format. Has everything been keyed with correct spacing, margins, headings, centering, and page numbers? Is the format consistent throughout the document?
4. When you are reading for consistency, check that the writer always uses the same style for phone numbers and dates—for example, either *(212) 555-7952* or *212-555-7952*, and either *10/19/2025 or 10-19-2025.*

Figure 3.7

Proofreaders' Marks

Mark	Meaning	Example
∧	Insert word or letter	add it (*so*)
⌿	Omit word	and so it
····	No, don't omit	and so it
＼	Omit stroke	and sod it
/	Make letter lowercase	And so it
≡	Make a capital	if he is
☰	Make all capitals	I hope so
⌐	Move as indicated	and so
=	Line up horizontally	TO: John
‖	Line up vertically	‖ If he is
ss⌐	Use single spacing	and so it (ss)
∪	Transpose	(had it so)
ds⌐	Use double spacing	and so it (ds)
=/	Insert a hyphen	white hot
s⌐	Indent — spaces	s⌐ If he is
∼	Bold	He is not
∧#	Insert a space	add so it (#)
{	Insert a space	and so it
⊂	Omit the space	10 a.m.
—⊂	Underscore this	It may be
⟲	Move as shown	it is not
⌣	Join to word	the port (re)
word	Change word	and if he (so)
∘	Make into period	to him
◯	Don't abbreviate	Dr. Judd
○	Spell it out	1 or 2 if
¶	New paragraph	¶ If he is
∨	Raise above line	Hale says
+#↑	More space here	It may be
-#↑	Less space here	If she is
2#	2 line spaces here	It may be
—	Italicize	It may be

5. When proofreading for clarity, be sure that the most appropriate and concise words are used to communicate the idea. For example, do not use *demonstrate* for *show* or *utilize* for *use*.

6. In a separate step, proofread all numbers once again. Be sure that the number of digits in items such as addresses and ZIP Codes is correct. Be sure there are no transposed numbers.

7. Carefully check and confirm important data, such as the correct spelling of names, addresses, all numbers, and the use of titles, such as *Dr.* or *Rev.*

8. Read the document again after you have made all the corrections. Be sure that, in making required corrections, you have not introduced any new errors. It is helpful to read the document out loud.

Common Errors. The following is a list of common errors you may find when you proofread documents:

• Keyboarding mistakes, such as the omission or repetition of words and other typographical errors; misstrokes of keys—for example, keying *slepp* instead of *sleep*

• Errors of transposition in both letters and numbers—for example, keying *flies* instead of *files* or *appointment on October 13* instead of *appointment on October 31*

• Spacing errors, including not spacing correctly between words, such as keying *patientdoes* instead of *patient does;* incorrect spacing within a word, such as keying *the re* instead of *there;* too much spacing between lines

Editing Techniques. If you are the person who originates the document, you may find it difficult to assess your own work. However, you do have a thorough understanding of your purpose. When you are editing a document created by someone else, you need to be careful that you understand the writer and the situation well enough that you do not make inappropriate changes.

When you edit a document, you are judging clarity, organization, quality, flow, and consistency of format and style. In editing, you also use your proofreading skills. You have the overall objective of making the document as effective as possible. Use the following list to assess the document:

1. Read the whole document first to get a sense of its organization and purpose.
2. Look at sentence and paragraph structure to determine that it is correct. Look at sentences to be sure that they are not awkwardly constructed.
3. Assess the correctness of spelling, grammar, punctuation, and English usage.
4. Look for problems in the tone of the document. Is the tone appropriate for the intent of the document and for the intended audience (the reader)?
5. Determine that the content is complete and clear. If you have any questions, be sure to get clarification from the writer.
6. Look for any wording or content that may be confusing to the reader.

 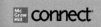

GO TO PROJECTS 3.4 AND 3.5 AT THE END OF THIS CHAPTER

3.1 List the steps of the communication cycle and give an example of a barrier to each step.	• The communication cycle has five steps: — Origination of the message by the sender. In this step, the sender analyzes the receiver and formulates the message. Barriers to consider are the knowledge base of the receiver and the physical environment. — Encoding of the message by the sender. In this step, the sender attaches words and gestures to the message. A barrier to consider would be a language barrier. — Transmission of the message. The sender determines the best channel for the message and sends the message to the receiver. A barrier to consider would be noise that disrupts the channel and the message. — Receiving and decoding of the message by the receiver. In this step, the receiver interprets the message. A barrier to consider is the inactive listening by the receiver. — Checking for understanding through feedback. In the last step, the sender verifies the receiver has interpreted the message as intended using techniques such as questioning and asking the receiver to paraphrase. A barrier to this step would be a judgmental assumption by the sender.
3.2 Explain how the verbal message is affected by nonverbal communication.	• Nonverbal communication has a greater impact on the receiver of a message than the verbal message. Most of our communication is through nonverbal channels. When the verbal message sends a communication but the nonverbal message, such as facial expression or body language, says something different, the nonverbal message is the one received.
3.3 Apply effective written communication techniques to compose written medical office correspondence.	• Written correspondences are a reflection of the medical practice and its employees. Documents should be prepared with proper grammar and word usage, sentence structure, and format. Prior to sending out any document, it should be carefully proofread and edited using personal knowledge and electronic methods, such as spelling and grammar checkers.

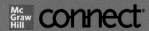

Project 3.1 (LO 3.3) Composing a Referral Letter

 Working Paper 5 (WP 5) contains a list of Dr. Larsen's Outside Services. Create a folder and label it SUPPLIES. Place Dr. Larsen's Outside Services listing in this folder, and refer to it when necessary. Add any new contact in the space provided.

Dr. Larsen has asked you to compose a referral letter for her signature. The purpose of the letter is to refer Florence Sherman to an ophthalmologist, Richard Diangelis, MD. Summarize the key points from the October 5 chart note, found in Working Paper 6 (WP 6). This referral letter confirms a conversation between the two physicians on October 8. Date the letter you write October 10. Address an envelope. Create a folder and label it SHERMAN, FLORENCE. Place a copy of the referral letter and October 5 chart note in Ms. Sherman's chart. Submit the letter, envelope, and chart note to your instructor.

NOTE: In a future project, you will be asked to prepare a folder/chart for each of Dr. Larsen's patients. Since a folder/chart has been created for Florence Sherman in this project, do not prepare a duplicate folder for Florence Sherman in Project 5.3.

Project 3.2 (LO 3.3) Composing an E-Mail

Dr. Larsen has asked you to prepare an e-mail *from her* to be sent throughout the medical center informing the staff of the following information. Compose the e-mail using your own wording, and do not directly copy the following information.

Wanda Norberg, MD, will start working part-time in January while Dr. Larsen takes a 2-month sabbatical to update the University Hospital Resident Program Guidelines (publication date is April 1). Dr. Norberg currently has an office at 2901 West Fifth Avenue, Suite 425, Chicago, IL 60612-9002. Her current phone number is 312-555-4525. Her hours will be 9 A.M. to 12 noon, Monday through Thursday, and Tuesday and Thursday evenings from 6 P.M. to 9 P.M. Employees are needed to work during these hours. If interested, contact Linda at extension 6022.

Remember to add Dr. Norberg's information to the Outside Services list (WP 5). Create a folder and label it MISCELLANEOUS. File a copy of the e-mail in this folder. Send the e-mail to your instructor.

Project 3.3 (LO 3.3) Internet Research: Journal Citations

Using your favorite Web browser, locate the American Medical Association's website. Visit the *Journal of the American Medical Association (JAMA),* and research author instructions. What are some of the criteria for acceptance of manuscripts? Can manuscripts be submitted electronically? Be prepared to discuss your findings.

Project 3.4 (LO 3.3) Editing and Proofreading Reports

 Dr. Larsen has asked you to proofread and edit two reports that she will use for her classroom teaching. The reports are on Connect, labeled Project 3.4a and Project 3.4b. The physician has marked the changes to be made on Working Papers 7 and 8 (WP 7 and WP 8). The reports also contain unmarked errors. First save the reports on your own storage device as Project 3.4 reports. Then proofread and edit the reports. Remember to save your work.

Project 3.5 (LO 3.3) Communications Terms

 On Working Paper 9 (WP 9), match the communications term in Column 2 with its definition in Column 1.

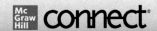

Communication (LO 3.2)

The act of communicating involves verbal and nonverbal components. The verbal component refers to the content of our message, that is, the choice and arrangement of our words. The nonverbal component refers to the message we send through body language and how we say what we say: the tone, pacing, and volume of our voice. Meaningful and effective communication is one of the most important of the soft skills, and its significance is growing due to the advancement of technology. **How can nonverbal communication interfere with the patient and healthcare provider interaction? Use role-playing to demonstrate the effects of nonverbal communication in the medical environment.**

Chapter 3 Review Questions

USING TERMINOLOGY

Match the term or phrase on the left with the correct answer on the right.

_____ 1. [LO 3.1] Barriers to communications

_____ 2. [LO 3.3] Block-style letter

_____ 3. [LO 3.1] Channel

_____ 4. [LO 3.1] Decoding

_____ 5. [LO 3.2] Noise

_____ 6. [LO 3.1] Encoding

_____ 7. [LO 3.3] Proofreading symbols

_____ 8. [LO 3.3] Bibliography

_____ 9. [LO 3.3] E-mail

_____ 10. [LO 3.1] Feedback

a. Standardized notations used to indicate corrections or changes to a document

b. Most common form of interoffice communication

c. Internal and external interferences with the communication cycle

d. Chosen method of transmitting a message

e. Applying meaning to a received message

f. An alphabetic listing of works used by a writer

g. Letter style in which all text is left-aligned

h. Applying gestures and words to a message or an idea

i. How a recipient responds to a message

j. Loud music, fatigue, and illness

CHECKING YOUR UNDERSTANDING

Select the most correct answer.

1. [LO 3.2] When Dr. Cary's AMA stepped toward a patient to explain the hospital preadmission procedure, the patient abruptly took a step backward. Which of the following is the most likely reason for the patient's movement during the communication process?

   a. The AMA had bad breath.
   b. The patient's cell phone was ringing.
   c. The patient needed to sit down.
   d. The AMA had intruded into the patient's personal space.

2. [LO 3.2] Aubriella felt she was being treated rudely by the medical office receptionist. When Aubriella arrived for her appointment, the receptionist greeted Aubriella, quickly shut the glass window, and began pointing her finger toward her. The receptionist was discussing a newly discovered crack in the wall with the office manager. Aubriella felt unwelcomed because

   a. the receptionist's verbal message did not match her nonverbal message.
   b. the receptionist's verbal and nonverbal message were the same.
   c. the crack on the wall was offensive to Aubriella.
   d. the receptionist did not offer Aubriella coffee or water.

3. [LO 3.3] A copy notation in a letter is placed

   a. immediately after the date.
   b. one Enter stroke below the complimentary closing.
   c. below the reference initials and any enclosure notation.
   d. one Enter stroke below the inside address.

4. [LO 3.1] The medical office team was confused by an e-mail Dr. Larsen sent. It said, "Employees must arrive early to work for the next few weeks." Employees did not know why or how early they must arrive. Which of the following is an encoding error used in Dr. Larsen's communication?

   a. Barriers to communication

   b. Using relative terms in place of concrete terms

   c. Sending the message through e-mail

   d. None of these

5. [LO 3.1] Which of the following is an example of concrete wording?

   a. The medical coder will be 15 minutes late today.

   b. Our lab will close early on Fridays.

   c. Dr. Larsen will be out of the office sometime next month.

   d. Your lab results will arrive next week.

6. [LO 3.2] Dr. Larsen asked Ali to refrain from wearing stained scrubs and provided Ali with a voucher to buy new ones. Why did Dr. Larsen ask Ali not to wear stained scrubs?

   a. Dr. Larsen did not like the color of Ali's scrubs.

   b. Ali was arriving 20 minutes late to work each day.

   c. The scrubs did not match scrubs worn by other medical staff.

   d. Stained scrubs may give a nonverbal impression to patients that the office is not concerned with cleanliness.

7. [LO 3.3] A second-page letter heading should contain the following:

   a. Inside address

   b. Complimentary closing and signature

   c. Reference initials and enclosure notation

   d. Recipient, page number, and date of the correspondence

8. [LO 3.3] Dr. Larsen is presenting a paper on gastroparesis. She asked a gastroenterologist to read the draft paper and check it for accuracy of the medical information. She has asked the gastroenterologist to

   a. edit the draft paper.

   b. proofread the draft paper.

   c. edit and proofread the draft paper.

   d. violate copyright laws.

9. [LO 3.3] Which of the following is a proofreading symbol?

   a. ¶

   b. $

   c. ☺

   d. ☆

10. [LO 3.3] Within a manuscript, a quotation of six lines should be formatted

   a. as all other lines of text in the manuscript.

   b. as a 0.5-inch indention from the left margin.

   c. as a 0.5-inch indention from the right margin.

   d. as a 0.5-inch indention from both the left and right margins.

THINKING IT THROUGH

These questions cover important points in this chapter. Using your critical-thinking skills, play the role of an administrative medical assistant as you answer each question. Be prepared to discuss your responses.

1. [LO 3.1] Mrs. Jenage was seen by the physician and needs to be admitted to the hospital. She is legally deaf but does read lips. How will you communicate hospital admission instructions to Mrs. Jenage and check to be sure the instructions were received correctly?

2. [LO 3.3] In a job interview, you are asked to describe the quality of your written communication skills and state why these skills are important. How do you respond?

3. [LO 3.3] Mrs. Court, who has a history of missed appointments, has just missed her latest one. The doctor asks that you contact her about the missed appointment, to mention politely that this has happened before, and ask her to reschedule as soon as possible. Why would you choose to write a letter rather than call the patient?

4. [LO 3.3] Prepare a draft of the body of the letter to Mrs. Court. Keep in mind the doctor's directions about the content and tone.

5. [LO 3.3] A colleague sends you this e-mail: "Please help! I need to prepare final manuscript for an article Dr. Trelando is submitting." You decide to e-mail the directions for preparing the title page and text pages for final manuscript. What does your e-mail say?

6. [LO 3.3] You receive a call from an assistant at Dr. Janis's office about a referral from your office. The referral is scheduled for today, but Dr. Janis cannot locate the referral letter sent by your office. How can e-mail help in this situation?

Chapter 4

Office Communications: Phone, Scheduling, and Mail

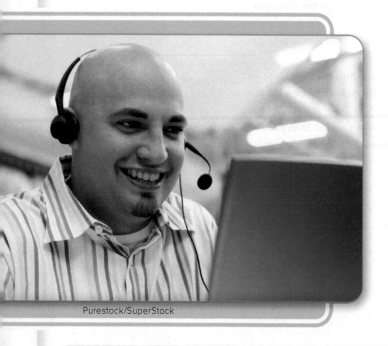

Purestock/SuperStock

LEARNING OUTCOMES

After studying this chapter, you will be able to

4.1 explain how proper screening and triage of patients during a phone conversation can assist the office environment.

4.2 recall and explain two different types of scheduling options and provide examples of practices that would be most suited to each of the schedules.

4.3 recall the steps in processing incoming and outgoing mail and discuss related safety recommendations.

KEY TERMS

Study these important words, which are defined in this chapter, to build your professional vocabulary:

annotate	established patient (EP)	POSTNET	Signature Confirmation
Certificate of Mailing	first-class mail	Priority Express Mail	Special Handling
Certified Mail	fixed office hours	Priority Mail	telephone etiquette
chief complaint (CC)	Insured Mail	Registered Mail	triage
cluster scheduling	new patient (NP)	Restricted Delivery	urgent
Collect on Delivery (COD)	no-show	Retail Ground	wave scheduling
Delivery Confirmation	open and fixed office hours	Return Receipt	ZIP
double-booking appointments	open office hours	screening calls	ZIP+4
emergency	optical character reader (OCR)	shared medical appointments	

ABHES

4.a. Follow documentation guidelines.

4.e. Perform risk management procedures.

5.h. Display effective interpersonal skills with patients and healthcare team members.

7.a. Gather and process documents.

7.e. Apply scheduling principles.

7.g. Display professionalism through written and verbal communications.

7.h. Perform basic computer skills.

8.g. Recognize and respond to medical office emergencies.

10.b. Display professional behavior.

www.abhes.org/accreditationmanual

The ABHES standards appear with permission of The Accrediting Bureau of Health Education Schools

CAAHEP

V.A.1.a. Demonstrate empathy.

V.A.1.b. Demonstrate active listening.

V.A.1.c. Demonstrate nonverbal communication.

V.C.7. Recognize elements of fundamental writing skills.

V.C.8. Discuss application of electronic technology in professional communication.

V.P.4.a. Coach patients regarding office policies.

V.P.6. Demonstrate professional telephone techniques.

V.P.7. Document telephone messages accurately.

V.P.8. Compose professional correspondence utilizing electronic technology.

V.P.11. Report relevant information concisely and accurately.

VI.C.1. Identify different types of appointment scheduling methods.

VI.C.2.a. Identify advantages and disadvantages of the following appointment systems: manual.

VI.C.2.b. Identify advantages and disadvantages of the following appointment systems: electronic.

VI.C.3. Identify critical information required for scheduling patient procedures.

VI.C.4. Define types of information contained in the patient's medical record.

VI.P.1. Manage appointment schedule using established policies.

VI.P.2. Schedule a patient procedure.

VI.A.1. Display sensitivity when managing appointments.

XII.C.8. Identify critical elements of an emergency plan for response to a natural disaster or other emergency.

2015 Standards and Guidelines for the Accreditation of Educational Programs in Medical Assisting, Appendix B, Core Curriculum for Medical Assistants, Medical Assisting Education Review Board (MAERB), 2015.

INTRODUCTION

Communication with patients and others who conduct business with the medical office must be documented in complete and accurate detail. Knowing how to access a patient's request for a medical visit and properly schedule the visit are critical to the smooth flow and operations of the medical environment. Different methods of scheduling appointments are used to accommodate various specialties and locations. Other forms of communications are received and sent through the United States Postal Service. Each of these will be discussed in this chapter.

4.1 TELEPHONE SKILLS

The traditional channel of communication between the patient and physician is the telephone. Most patients make their first contact with the physician's medical office by phone. Urgent and emergency cases are also reported by phone. The assistant must learn to recognize the situation in each type of call and handle it correctly. Often, the physician is engaged with another patient's care, and the assistant must be able to reassure the caller without interrupting the physician.

Attitudes are contagious. Patients judge the care they receive by the attitude of medical office personnel (reflected by the speaker's tone of voice and choice of words in telephone situations) as well as by the actual medical service provided by the physician. The caller should be paid the same attention given a person in a face-to-face conversation.

Telephone calls may be incoming, outgoing, or interoffice. Since administrative medical assistants typically handle all incoming calls to medical offices, they should use each call as an opportunity to present a positive image for the physician and the practice. An administrative medical assistant (AMA) must

- follow proper **telephone etiquette** (conduct).
- screen calls according to the office's policy.
- take complete and accurate messages.

Telephone Etiquette

When answering the telephone, try to visualize the person with whom you are talking. Think about who the caller is, what the caller is asking, how the caller feels, and whether he or she is a patient. If you do this, your voice will sound alert, interested, and concerned during the conversation.

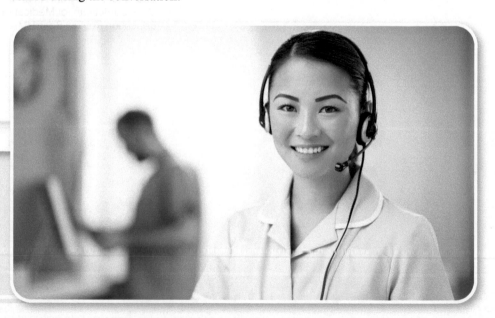

Figure 4.1

When answering the phone, the administrative medical assistant presents an image of the physician and the office. *How can the assistant present a positive image to callers?* Sturti/E+/Getty Images

Use a pleasant tone that conveys self-assurance, along with a genuine desire to be understanding and helpful. This is what is meant by the phrase *"using a voice with a smile."*

Use variations in pitch and phrasing to avoid sounding monotonous, and never indicate impatience or annoyance through the sound of your voice. Hold the mouthpiece of the phone about an inch from your mouth to avoid distortion or faintness of voice. When using a headset, follow the manufacturer's instruction for placement of the headset microphone. Speak clearly and distinctly; do not run words together or mumble. Even if you answer the phone with the same greeting many times a day, say the words slowly enough for the caller to understand. Always speak at a moderate pace throughout the conversation, giving the caller time to think about and understand what you have said.

When concluding a conversation, say "Goodbye," and use the caller's name. Refrain from using the phrase "bye-bye," which does not demonstrate professionalism. Thank the caller for calling by name. Remember, the caller had a choice of whom to call! This will leave the caller with a pleasant impression. Allow the caller to hang up first. Finally, replace the receiver gently when you hang up.

Promptness. Courtesy begins with promptness in answering the call. The ideal time to answer a call is on the second ring. This allows the caller a moment of preparation time to begin the conversation (the caller will expect to hear at least one ring before there is an answer). If you must place the caller on hold, always ask permission and briefly say why you must place him or her on hold.

EXAMPLES: PLACING A CALLER ON HOLD

Assistant: Dr. Larsen's office. I have another incoming call. May I place you on hold?

Assistant: Dr. Larsen's office. I am on another call. May I place you on hold?

Again, always ask permission prior to placing a caller on hold, wait for the patient to respond, and thank the person for holding when you return. If you must keep the individual on hold for more than 30 to 45 seconds, go back on the line and ask if the caller wants to continue holding or if you may take the caller's number and promptly return the call. Give the caller a time frame in which you will return the call. For example, say, "Mr. Patient, I need to talk with the nurse concerning your medication question. May I call you back within the next 30 minutes?" Then, call the patient back within the next 30 minutes. In other words, follow through with what you say you are going to do!

If the call is long distance, attempt to have another office team member respond to the call and not keep the caller waiting. If this is not possible, explain to the caller your need to complete another previous call and ask the person if he or she wishes to continue holding or call back. However, if you have phone service that includes a large number of long-distance calls or unlimited long-distance calling or VoIP, offer to return the phone call yourself.

Greeting and Identifying. There are many ways to answer the phone, but the preferred method is to answer with the name of the physician or clinic followed by the assistant's name. Using "Hello" as a greeting in an office environment is considered too casual and nonprofessional. Answering with "Good morning" or "Good afternoon" adds a personal touch but may be inefficient in a busy office. It is important to take time to say the name of the office slowly and distinctly. If the physician has a common surname, the physician's full name may be used to avoid confusion.

EXAMPLE: TELEPHONE GREETING

Assistant: Dr. Karen Larsen's office, Linda speaking. How may I help you?

In large clinics with multiple medical offices, the person who is operating a switchboard or multiline phone system may answer the call by identifying the name of the clinic and asking how the call should be directed. After a call has been transferred, employees in individual departments will then identify themselves.

EXAMPLE: TELEPHONE GREETING AND TRANSFER

Assistant: Northeast Clinic. How may I direct your call?

Patient: I'd like to make an appointment with Dr. Nasser.

Assistant: I can transfer you to Sharon at the appointment desk. She schedules Dr. Nasser's appointments. In case we are disconnected, her extension is 5555. Would you like for me to transfer your call to Sharon?

Patient: Yes, please.

Second assistant: Appointment desk. This is Sharon. How may I help you?

Following are some other tips to remember as part of proper telephone etiquette:

- Identify the nature of the call so that it can be properly handled. For example, calls may be categorized as routine versus emergency.
- Use courteous phrases, such as "please," "thank you," and "you are welcome."
- Actively listen to the caller. Engage yourself in the communication process by totally concentrating on the call and asking questions and/or repeating information back to the caller. Set your own thoughts aside while in the conversation. Listen objectively without judging the caller. By nature, when we hear something to which we object, we tend to miss information. Active listening is not a natural tendency—it needs to be practiced.
- Use words appropriate to the situation, but avoid using technical words.
- Offer assistance as necessary but, as an administrative medical assistant, do not offer medical advice.
- Avoid unnecessarily long conversations.
- Avoid using colloquial or slang expressions, such as *you know, ain't, like,* and *uh-huh.* Dialects are different and the "rule of thumb" is to respect local dialect but speak proper English.
- If necessary, repeat information at the close of the call.
- Speak at a moderate speed.
- Avoid overly personal conversations, even if initiated by the patient.

Screening Calls

Most incoming calls concern matters that can be handled by an administrative medical assistant guided by the preferences of the physician. Some physicians prefer to speak to patients, no matter what the circumstances. However, this routine is likely to be inefficient because it can cause interruptions to the patients who are being seen at the time by the physician. Also, medical records may not be available for the physician's reference at the time of the call. In some offices, a nurse is available to answer patients' questions. Other offices have a policy that nonemergency calls are returned by the physician or nursing staff during preset hours, such as after 4 P.M.

Screening calls, or evaluating calls to decide on the appropriate action, is often a difficult problem for the beginner, who may be afraid to assume the responsibility of making decisions. It is important to discuss this aspect of the job with the physician and/or office manager at the very beginning and to ascertain to what extent the administrative medical assistant will handle calls alone, what information should be given out, when messages should be taken, and when the patient should be told that the physician or nurse will return the call. A call-screening sheet, such as the one shown in Figure 4.2, can help you screen and transfer calls.

CALL-SCREENING SHEET

Purpose of Incoming Call	Doctor	Nurse	Message	Other
CLINICAL				
Emergency: Dr. in				Come in. In case of life-threatening emergency, call 911 and send medical emergency personnel to the caller's location.
Emergency: Dr. out of office				Send to ER
Seriously ill		✓		
Test results from lab			✓	
Information; advice; test results			✓	
Rx renewal			✓	
Doctor	✓			
Hospital: ER, ICU	✓			
Other				
ADMINISTRATIVE				
Appointment				Appt. desk
Medical records				Mesalina
Insurance				Tina
Billing/charges				Tina
Personnel				Gary

Figure 4.2

Call-Screening Sheet

The administrative medical assistant must be guided by the physician in deciding whether to handle a call or to transfer it to the physician. The first priority is to determine the name of the caller and nature of the call. You will then have a good idea of how to handle it.

Sometimes it may be hard to find out who is calling or what the call concerns. Phrases such as "May I please tell Dr. Larsen who is calling?" and "May I tell the nurse what you are calling about, please?" help you ascertain the information you need to complete or transfer the call. More on this topic is discussed later in this chapter.

Message-Taking Situations. Many calls can be handled by taking a message. The following are some examples:

- An ill new patient wants to talk with the physician about treatment.
- A patient already under treatment wants to talk with the physician.
- A patient's relative requests information about the patient.
- A personal friend or relative of the physician calls for the physician.
- Attorneys, financial planners, hospital personnel, and so on call about business.
- A patient calls with a satisfactory or unsatisfactory progress report (for example, a patient was told at the time of an appointment to call back with how a medication or treatment is working).
- Lab or x-ray results are called in.
- Prescription refills are requested.

The following calls are usually put through to the physician:

- Calls from other physicians.
- Emergency calls—for example, calls from the intensive care unit or the emergency room of the hospital.
- Calls from patients the physician has already identified (for example, out-of-town patients, the family of a seriously ill patient calling to check on the patient's condition, or a patient in labor).
- Calls from a patient with an acute illness, such as a severe reaction to a medication.

If there is a nurse in the office, many of these calls can be routed to the nurse, who will then decide whether or not to interrupt the physician in an examination room.

Some examples of various screening situations follow.

EXAMPLE: CALL TO SCHEDULE AN APPOINTMENT

Assistant: Dr. Karen Larsen's office, Linda speaking. How may I help you?

Caller: I would like to speak to Dr. Larsen.

Assistant: Dr. Larsen is with a patient. May I help you?

Caller: Well, I need to make an appointment for next week.

Assistant: Mary, at the appointment desk, will be able to help you. Would you like me to transfer your call to her?

or

I can schedule an appointment for you. Are you a patient of Dr. Larsen's?

The assistant can then proceed to schedule an appointment for the patient.

EXAMPLE: CALL TO DISCUSS A MEDICAL QUESTION

Assistant: Dr. Larsen's office, Linda speaking. How may I help you?

Caller: I need to talk to Dr. Larsen.

Assistant: Dr. Larsen is with a patient. May I help you?

Caller: I'm a patient of Dr. Larsen's, and I have some questions about my medications.

Assistant: May I ask who is calling?

Caller: This is Patient Chen.

Assistant: I will transfer you to the nurse, Ms. Chen. She should be able to help you.

or

The nurse should be able to help you with those questions, but she will need to access your medical records. May I take a message and ask her to return your call?

Transferring Calls. Telephone systems are provided with buttons for transferring a call to another line within the office. When calls are transferred, the system automatically puts the outside caller on hold. This means that the two people within the office can speak privately if necessary before one of them returns to the outside caller. For example, the administrative medical assistant can ask a question and relay the answer to the caller without having the physician or nurse speak to the patient, or the assistant can ask the physician or nurse to pick up the call and speak with the caller directly.

If a call must be transferred to another individual or department, be considerate of the caller. Explain that the call can best be handled by someone else, give the caller the name and extension (if available) of the party to which the call will be transferred, and offer to transfer the call. To be sure the call was transferred correctly, wait for the individual to whom the call is being transferred to answer the call and announce the caller. However, if the individual is not available, inform the caller and ask if he or she would like to leave a message on the individual's voice mail.

Emergency Calls. An emergency call may come at any time. The caller will probably be upset, and people who are excited often forget to give the most important information. It is imperative that the assistant remain calm and handle the call efficiently. The importance of obtaining the name, address, and phone number of the patient cannot be emphasized too strongly. The more information you can obtain, the better.

A physician or one of the other clinical personnel who are in the office when an emergency call comes through will normally speak with the patient. However, the administrative medical assistant answering the phone should screen the call, within the scope of his or her training, to determine if it is an emergency. In other words, do not offer medical advice—this would be outside the scope of training for the administrative medical assistant. Great tact and excellent judgment are needed to do this. These qualities are developed through training by the physician or office manager in what is a medical emergency as the practice defines it and how to handle the calls.

Prior to consulting the physician or other clinical personnel, the administrative medical assistant should obtain the following minimum information:

- Name and age of the patient
- Nature of the problem
- Duration (how long) the problem has existed
- Severity of the problem, using a rating scale such as 1 through 10, with 1 being least severe and 10 being most severe
- Patient's medical chart, if hardcopy patient charts are used

Many practices will assist nonclinical medical team members by providing a list of questions to ask the caller when determining needed action. Also, a "script" may be used to assist in making the correct determination. The list of questions and/or scripts should be developed by clinical medical team members and training provided to nonclinical team members on how to use these tools.

If the call is determined to be an emergency (i.e., sudden, sharp chest pain or headache with slurred speech), the caller should be instructed to hang up and go to the emergency department. The administrative medical assistant should immediately notify the physician and make a notation of the actions in the patient's medical record.

To assist in the decision-making process, the AMA must know the difference between an emergency situation and an urgent situation. The **Centers for Medicare & Medicaid Services** (CMS) defines an **emergency** medical condition as one that manifests itself by acute symptoms of sufficient severity, which includes severe pain, and that a layperson possessing an average knowledge of health and medicine could reasonably expect the absence of immediate medical attention to result in any of the following:

- Serious jeopardy to the health of the individual
- Serious jeopardy to the health of a pregnant woman or her unborn child
- Serious impairment to bodily functions, such as the ability to breathe
- Serious dysfunction of any bodily organ or part, such as the loss of an arm

CMS also defines **urgent** medical conditions as those for which treatments are medically necessary and immediately required as a result of an unforeseen illness, injury, or condition. This includes behavioral conditions. An urgent condition, left untreated, could result in an emergency condition.

Telephone calls from emergency departments are normally routed straight to the physician. In most offices, it is professional protocol to also directly route other physicians' calls straight to the physician.

Nonmedical Screening Situations. One of the most difficult situations to handle over the telephone is when a person refuses to state the purpose of the call, saying that it is a "personal call" or a "personal matter." A personal friend may not hesitate to state that fact. Similarly, a caller who is a patient will normally give a name and state the reason for the call. When the caller refuses to give his or her name, emphasize to the caller the importance of having complete information and that by supplying this information you can better assist him or her. The administrative medical assistant may explain, for example, that the physician will not return the call unless the nature of the call is known, if the physician has given such instructions, or that the call can be transferred to the office manager.

Caller: I need to talk to Dr. Larsen.

Assistant: May I ask who is calling?

Caller: It's personal. I'd rather not say.

Assistant: If you will please tell me your name, I can better assist you.

Caller: I'd rather not say.

Assistant: Without a name, office policy prevents me from transferring the call to Dr. Larsen. If you need immediate medical attention, call 911 or go to the nearest emergency department. Or, I can make an appointment for you with Dr. Larsen.

or

Assistant: Without a name, I will need to transfer your call to our office manager, Mr. Sanchez, at extension 3321. May I transfer your call?

If the caller absolutely refuses to give information, it is permissible to suggest that a letter be written and marked "Personal," so that the physician can become acquainted with the matter and give a response. A confident, pleasant voice will help you make the physician's position clear while avoiding needless disputes. When such situations occur, always keep the physician informed of the call and the attempted resolution.

Taking Messages

Because most calls cannot be taken immediately by a medical staff member, the assistant must take clear and accurate messages, so that the calls can be returned later.

Remember the following procedures for taking efficient, informative telephone messages:

- Always have pen and message pad on hand or have the electronic message center on the computer screen.
- Make notes as information is being given.
- Ask politely to have important information repeated.
- Verify information such as names, spellings, numbers, and dates for accuracy. You may ask, "Would you spell that prescription's name, please?" or "Let me repeat that to be sure I have noted it correctly."
- Make inquiries tactfully. A tactful question may be, "Will Gary know what this is about?" or "Could I tell Sue what this is about?" or "Is this a medical matter? If so, the physician will need your medical record."
- Use medical office abbreviations such as CC (chief complaint) or CHF (congestive heart failure) to save time when recording a message.
- Include the complete phone number, including the area code. Within the medical practice, patients may have numerous and varied area codes.
- Note all dates using month, day, year format. When using an electronic message board for telephone messages, the complete date may be automatically placed on the message. If not, or if using a handwritten message, the complete date will help to provide thorough documentation.

The more information you include in the message, the better. Be brief yet thorough.

COMPLIANCE *TIP*

Correctly maintaining patients' medical records, hardcopy and/or electronic, requires all communications from patients, including phone calls, to be properly documented. Correct documentation is legible, signed, and dated.

Figure 4.3

Telephone Message Slip

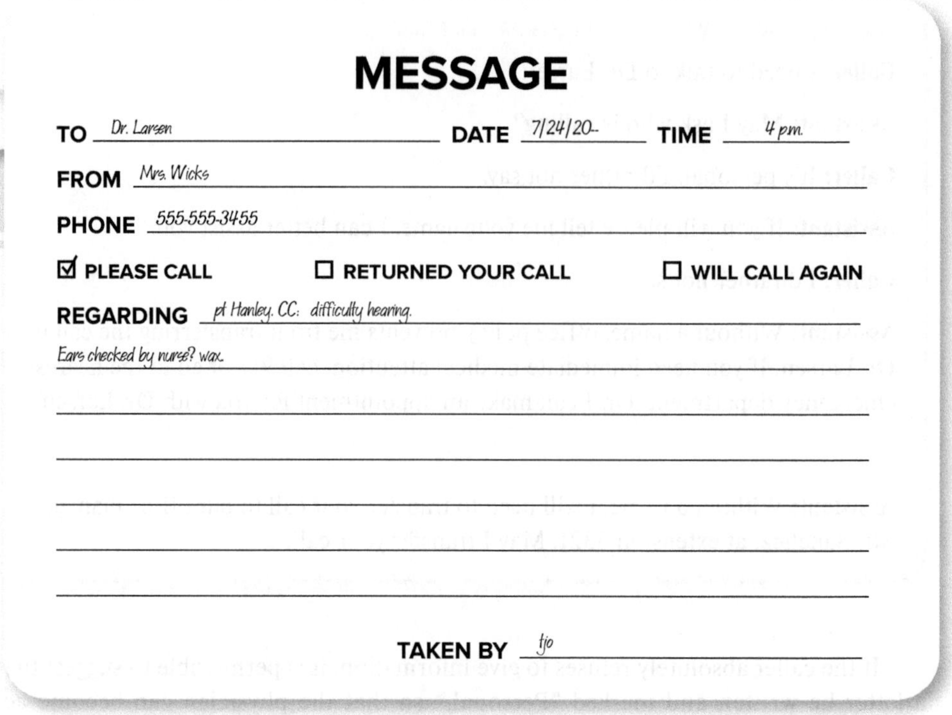

MESSAGE

TO _Dr. Larsen_   DATE _7/24/20-_   TIME _4 pm._

FROM _Mrs. Wicks_

PHONE _555-555-3455_

☑ **PLEASE CALL**   ☐ **RETURNED YOUR CALL**   ☐ **WILL CALL AGAIN**

REGARDING _pt Hanley. CC: difficulty hearing._

Ears checked by nurse? wax.

TAKEN BY _tjo_

When taking a phone message, do not say, "I will have the physician call you." This makes a commitment on behalf of the physician. It is better to say, "I will forward your message to the physician," or "I will ask the physician to call you."

If hardcopy records are being used, after taking a message regarding a patient's care, the assistant should obtain the patient's chart. The phone message should be attached to the chart with a paper clip and placed in the message center for the nurse or the physician. The message slip, or a transcription of it, as well as the physician's or nurse's actions, will be permanently documented in the patient's medical record.

Message Slips. Printed phone message slips are available from stationers for writing down messages efficiently and fully. See Figure 4.3 for an example of such a slip. Telephone message slips have blanks for noting basic information about the phone call, such as the date, time, to and from information, subject of the call, and requested actions. Message slip pads that make a copy of the written message should be used. In some offices, the computer system is used to enter and send messages to team members within the office.

Some physicians design their own telephone message slips and have them printed. A message slip customized for a physician's office will list the standard symptoms related to a given physician's specialty or field of practice. When a patient calls, the administrative medical assistant can take a message by checking off the symptoms that pertain to the patient. Figure 4.4 shows an example of a telephone message slip customized for a physician's office.

Verifying Information. When you are taking messages, it is a good idea to repeat important details, such as the date and time of an appointment or a telephone number. Verifying information reassures both parties of the call. If you are not sure of the correct spelling of a name, say, "I'm sorry. Will you spell your name again, please?" or "I want to record your name correctly. Will you please repeat that?" Sometimes questions about a message need to be asked or information needs to be clarified. Each message,

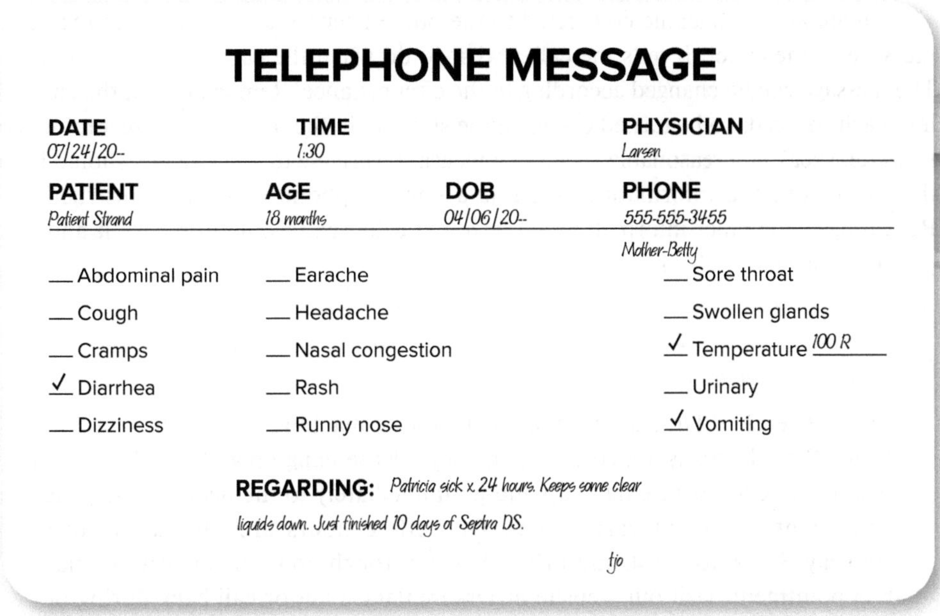

TELEPHONE MESSAGE

DATE	TIME		PHYSICIAN
07/24/20--	1:30		Larsen

PATIENT	AGE	DOB	PHONE
Patient Strand	18 months	04/06/20--	555-555-3455
			Mother-Betty

___ Abdominal pain   ___ Earache   ___ Sore throat

___ Cough   ___ Headache   ___ Swollen glands

___ Cramps   ___ Nasal congestion   ✓ Temperature _100 R_

✓ Diarrhea   ___ Rash   ___ Urinary

___ Dizziness   ___ Runny nose   ✓ Vomiting

REGARDING: Patricia sick x 24 hours. Keeps some clear liquids down. Just finished 10 days of Septra DS.

tjo

Figure 4.4

Customized Telephone Message Slip

whether electronic or handwritten, should include the initials or name of the individual taking the message. Taking ownership of the message demonstrates professionalism and confidence in your abilities.

Using Speakerphones. As a basic rule, calls to and from patients and medical professionals should not be placed on speakerphones. Speakerphones provide the assistant hands-free communication with the caller. However, unless precautions are taken, the conversation does not remain confidential. While the speakerphone has many advantages, it does have limitations.

In an office with a noisy environment, speakerphones are not the best choice for receiving and placing calls. Also, in a medical office, protected health information (as presented in the Office Communications chapter) is discussed during phone conversations. Using a speakerphone can allow a breach of confidentiality and the unintentional disclosure of PHI.

If a speakerphone must be used, there are a few things to remember:

- Always ask the caller's permission prior to conversing over a speakerphone or let the person know he or she is on a speakerphone.
- Ask the caller if the conversation reception is clear.
- Refrain from creating noise, such as moving papers or rolling chairs.
- Inform the caller if someone else is in the area and can hear the conversation.

Because of the possibility of breaching patient confidentiality by using a speakerphone, administrative medical assistants and others who answer phone calls in the medical environment use phone headsets. This allows hands-free communication by the medical office individual with the patient.

Answering Services. Many physicians' offices use commercial answering services or answering machines for phone coverage when the office is closed. Commercial answering services can answer the office's calls from a remote location. All unanswered calls are forwarded to an operator during nonoffice hours. This operator takes messages for routine calls or contacts the physician, covering physician, or appointed nurse if the call is an emergency. The physician or administrative medical assistant checks in with the answering service for any messages after returning to the office.

An answering machine connected to the office telephone line plays a prerecorded message to the caller. It tells the caller what to do when the call is urgent or routine. The message can be changed according to the circumstance. Remember that the answering machine needs to be turned off when the staff are in the office. When recording the message, speak at a reasonable speed in a pleasant, variable tone. Listeners should have time to record the information, such as a contact phone number or instructions. Repeating the contact information will give the caller extra time to record it and will provide an accuracy check.

> **EXAMPLE: ANSWERING MACHINE MESSAGE**
> You have reached Dr. Karen Larsen's answering machine. We are currently out of the office. If this is a medical emergency, please hang up and dial 911. If you need urgent care, please hang up and go immediately to the nearest emergency department or urgent care center. Our office hours are Monday through Thursday, 8 A.M. to 5 P.M. and Friday 8 A.M. through noon. If you want to make an appointment, visit our website at Drkarenlarsen.net or call back during our regular office hours. For insurance and billing questions, please call back during regular office hours. Thank you for your call.

 Mc Graw Hill connect   **GO TO PROJECT 4.1 AT THE END OF THIS CHAPTER**

Outgoing Calls

In addition to answering calls, administrative medical assistants place outgoing calls for the medical practice to patients, hospitals, clinics, and laboratories, as well as to insurance companies, suppliers, banks, and other businesses.

Planning the Call. Plan the conversation before making a call by gathering important documents (such as the patient's medical record), obtaining necessary information, and outlining questions to ask. Know the specifics of the call before you dial. Ask yourself who, what, when, where, and why, and make appropriate notations. Be aware of the following:

- Whom to call and ask for once the phone is answered
- What information to give or obtain/questions to ask/possible situations that may arise during the call (what-if situations)
- When to call
- Where to physically place the call so that PHI is not unintentionally divulged
- Why the call is being made (Can the information be gathered by other means, such as calling the patient's insurance carrier? Is the call being made for an emergency situation or for a referral to another physician?)

> **EXAMPLE: REQUEST FOR OUTGOING PHONE CALL**
> **Dr. Larsen:** Linda, please call Dr. Martin and ask him to see Patient Lucy.

To complete the call requested in the preceding example, Linda will need to confirm the following with Dr. Larsen:

- Who: Call Dr. Martin.
- What: Referral for Lucy; Lucy's diagnosis (if applicable). What are the contingency plans (what-ifs)? For example, what is the alternative if Lucy must be seen today but Dr. Martin is not in the office today?
- When: Call today to schedule an appointment date and time for Lucy to be seen by Dr. Martin.
- Where: Make the call in an area where others cannot hear Lucy's PHI.
- Why: The call must be made directly to Dr. Martin's office to schedule the appointment.

Always obtain the necessary information and have it on hand before scheduling services (such as referrals, laboratory and x-ray procedures, surgery, and hospital admissions). Insurance information should also be given to the provider. Under HIPAA's TPO provision, release of information from the patient is not needed when scheduling an appointment for continuity of the patient's care. Some medical providers will, however, still ask for the release.

Using Resources. Numerous resources are available to help the assistant place calls and manage the flow of calls in a medical office.

Telephone Directories

An alphabetic directory, or white pages, lists telephone customers by name in alphabetic order. The white pages usually contain other information as well, such as directory-assistance numbers, billing information, international long-distance calling procedures, and area code maps. Information concerning government agencies, including phone numbers, is often listed in the blue pages section of the alphabetic directory.

A classified directory, or yellow pages, lists telephone subscribers under headings for types of businesses, such as "Office Supplies or Laboratories—Medical." Classified directories also contain advertising for subscribing businesses and sometimes contain local street maps and ZIP Code listings.

There are also many directory services available on the Internet—for example, Switchboard.com, whitepages.com, yellowpages.com, B2B (Business-to-Business) Yellow Pages, and many more. These directories use search engines to locate phone numbers, addresses, and e-mail addresses locally, in the United States, and in some foreign countries.

A personal directory is used for phone numbers that are frequently called by the office staff. The personal directory should be kept near the phone for easy access and should include a list of the following phone numbers:

- Hospitals
- Insurance companies
- Laboratories
- Medical supply companies
- Pharmacies
- Hospital emergency room
- Specialists for referrals made to patients

Most phone systems are equipped with an automatic speed-dial feature that allows the user to store multiple phone numbers electronically. A frequently dialed number can be stored under one or two digits to save time in dialing. If speed-dial numbers are used, they can be listed in a separate column or table in the personal directory.

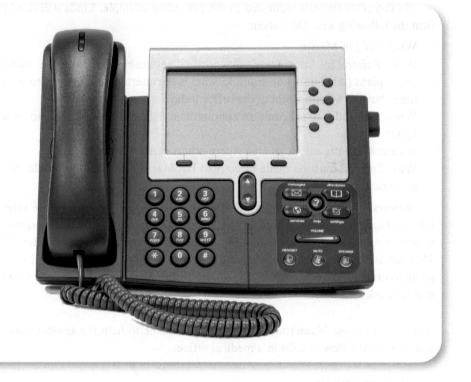

Other Automated Features

Desk phone systems today, such as the one shown in Figure 4.5, are designed to provide automated features such as call pickup, call forwarding, call transfer, automatic hold recall, and automatic call distribution. They can also be programmed to place a call at a set time or to notify the user when a previously dialed busy line is open. Voice mail, voice mail to e-mail, and conference calling are other popular features of a telephone system. Recorded messages and/or music can be played while a caller is on hold. This beneficial feature can provide information to patients, such as when flu shots will be available.

Placing the Call. When you have the proper information and are prepared to place a call, use the following procedures:

- Identify yourself and the physician's office. If you are calling for the physician, identify the physician.
- State the reason for the call.
- Provide the necessary information.
- Ask tactfully for information.
- Listen carefully and make notes as needed.
- Verify information.
- If the person you are trying to reach is unavailable, leave a message for that person to call you back. Remember to follow the confidentiality guidelines of the office.

Using the Fax Machine. A facsimile (fax) machine may be used to send or receive information about patients. The physician must develop and follow guidelines for faxing information about patients. A patient's confidentiality must be protected—the fax machine should be located where only authorized personnel have access to it and checked frequently for incoming faxed documents and transmittal notice of outgoing documents. Federal and state laws must be followed for maintaining medical records. Generally, follow these guidelines:

- Contact the receiver before transmitting the information. This serves two purposes: (2) to inform the receiver of the impending transmitted fax and (2) to verify the fax phone number.
- Send a release of information—if needed for reasons others than TPO—with a facsimile cover letter (see the example in Figure 4.6).
- File the original cover letter and other documents, if applicable, in the chart if other than a direct copy of a patient's PHI was faxed.
- Request a signed return receipt of the faxed information.
- Photocopy documents received on thermal fax paper before placing them in a patient's chart because thermal fax paper deteriorates over time. Scan faxed documents into a patient's electronic chart.

KAREN LARSEN, MD

2235 South Ridgeway Avenue   312-555-6022
Chicago, IL 60623-2240   Fax: 312-555-0025

FACSIMILE COVER LETTER

DATE: _____ TIME: _____ A.M./P.M.

TO: _____
_____(name)_____

_____(facility)_____

_____(address)_____

FAX NUMBER: _____

RE: _____

FROM: _____
_____(name/department)_____

    KAREN LARSEN, MD

Number of pages including cover letter: _____

NOTICE OF CONFIDENTIALITY: The faxed document or documents contain confidential information. The information is only for use by the above-named receiver. Use of the information in any form is strictly prohibited if you are not the intended receiver. Please notify our office immediately if you received this fax in error. Contact our office by telephone to arrange for the return of the original fax document.

RETURN RECEIPT: Please complete the following statement and return it to the above-stated fax number.

I, _____, verify that I have received _____ pages
          Authorized Receiver
from _____.
        Sending Facility

Figure 4.6

Facsimile Cover Letter with Return Receipt

Even with faxing safeguards in place, the advances in software capabilities create challenges when verifying the authenticity of a faxed request. Consider the following:

> *Your male patient is in the process of a divorce. Because of the past relationship, both parties know a substantial amount of personal information and history about the other, such as medical and financial issues. The wife phones the office, posing as her husband's attorney, and requests that his medical records be faxed to "her" office. She is advised that a faxed release of information from the husband is needed before the data may be released. The wife creates a fake letterhead using an online template, and she forges her husband's signature to a false release-of-information form. After reviewing the faxed request, the office manager gives the approval for the records to be faxed to the "attorney" using the fax number on the release. Through this illegal disclosure of information, the wife learns that the husband had contracted a sexually transmitted disease and had disclosed the name of a partner from whom he may have received the disease. It was not his wife.*

Double-checking with the patient prior to faxing the information and checking the authenticity of the law firm might have prevented the disclosure. Also, using a predetermined password for releasing information may deter illegal requests. For example, when completing registration paperwork, include a field called "Release-of-Information Password." All requests for disclosure of PHI must contain this password. Additionally, the implementation of electronic health records will help eliminate the need to fax sensitive medical information. Electronic health records will be discussed in more detail in a later chapter.

Faxing may be done using stand-alone equipment—not connected to any other machine—or through fax software on a computer. Some printers function as both printers and stand-alone fax machines. Newer faxing systems use computer-based services and Cloud-based services. Documents may be faxed over telephone lines or the Internet. Many medical practices have dedicated fax lines, which means that the fax machine is connected to a separate phone line reserved only for sending and receiving faxes. With a dedicated fax line, the fax machine is available 24 hours a day to receive or send faxes.

Following Through on Calls. Proper handling of telephone calls does not end after the call has ended. The administrative medical assistant must follow through on all requests made and instructions provided in the conversation. See Figure 4.7, Figure 4.8, and Figure 4.9 for examples of follow-through methods.

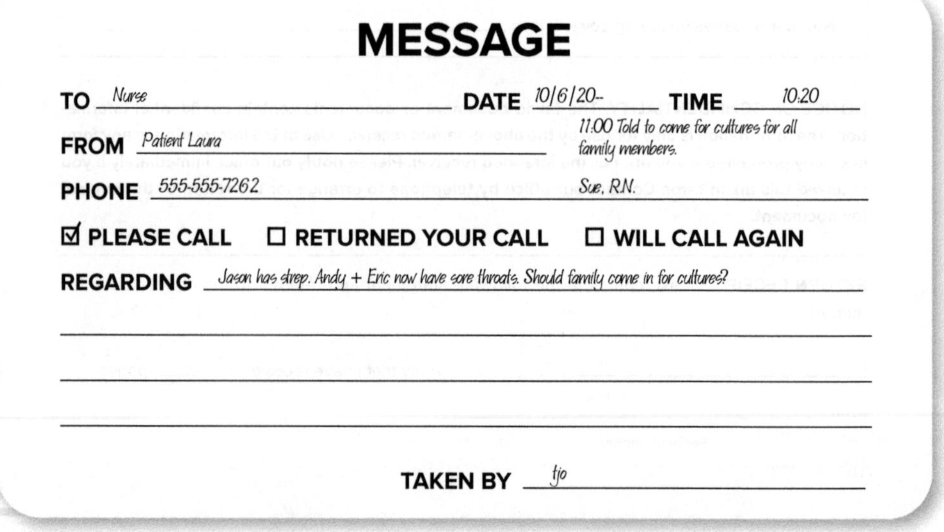
MESSAGE

TO Nurse DATE 10/6/20-- TIME 10:20

FROM Patient Laura

11:00 Told to come for cultures for all family members.

Sue, R.N.

PHONE 555-555-7262

☑ PLEASE CALL ☐ RETURNED YOUR CALL ☐ WILL CALL AGAIN

REGARDING Jason has strep. Andy + Eric now have sore throats. Should family come in for cultures?

TAKEN BY tjo

Figure 4.7

Follow-Through Notation Made Directly on a Telephone Message Slip

MEMO TO: Karen Larsen, MD
FROM: University Hospital
DATE: September 25,20--
SUBJECT: Dr. Dean Ashcroft's seminars

The University Hospital telephoned at 4 P.M. today about a series of four seminars titled "Educating Caregivers."

1. Early Care: Prenatal
2. Prevention of Accidents Involving Household Poisons
3. Early Abusive Behaviors
4. Addicted Caregivers

Dr. Ashcroft is the sponsor of the series. Please let me know if you would like to register for any of these seminars.

TJO

Figure 4.8

A Telephone Call

TO-DO LIST

Date ___7/24/20--___

RUSH	ITEMS TO DO	DONE
	~~Send records to Dr. Peters re: Jill Sommers.~~	7/26
	~~Reserve conference room 7/31 at 8 a.m.~~	7/26
	Remind Dr. Larsen to get slides for 7/31.	
*	Call Patient Brent 7/23 re: disability form at 555-555-7287.	

Figure 4.9

Follow-Through Notation on a To-Do List

All telephone messages (and other messages) from or concerning a patient should be entered into the patient's medical record. In such cases, the message slip can be taped or filed inside the chart after it has been verified as completed. Another option is to make a chart notation of the telephone call information, or the physician may make a chart entry. All entries must be signed and dated (see Figure 4.10 for an example). If using electronic medical records, the message should be transferred or keyed directly into the patient's electronic record. Some offices have a page in the patient's record specifically for messages.

Figure 4.10

Telephone Message Notation Made on a Patient's Chart

CHART NOTE

```
Patient Dan
DOB: 07/27/19--

July 20, 20--, 8:30 A.M.
TELEPHONE CALL

From Nurse Wicks, RN, at Wilcox Nursing Home. Patient complained of
difficulty hearing. Nurse Wicks checked his ears and found them to be
plugged with wax. Called for directions. I told the nurse to irrigate the
patient's ears. If the patient is not better in a day, an appointment
should be made.
```

Karen Larsen

K. Larsen, MD/tjo

Using Electronic Mail (E-Mail). Messages and files can be transmitted in digital form using e-mail. It is critical to note that e-mail must be subject to the same strict privacy rules as other forms of communication. The medical office adopts guidelines to protect the confidentiality of patients' electronically transmitted medical data. E-mail is becoming a popular method for communicating appointment confirmations and other forms of nonspecific patient PHI. Currently, e-mail is not the preferred method of communicating medical information. The potential for unintentional disclosure of PHI is high. A possibility exists that PHI can be read by someone other than the patient.

However, this does not mean that a provider cannot communicate via e-mail or through other electronic channels, such as texting, if reasonable safeguards are applied. If the patient initiates communication to the physician via e-mail, then the physician may reasonably assume that this is an acceptable form of communication with the patient. The minimal amount of information necessary needed to respond to the patient's request should be used. Additionally, if e-mail or other electronic forms of communications are to be used for tasks, such as confirming appointments, the use of such communication channels should be stated in the Notice of Privacy Practices, for which the patient will acknowledge that he or she has received, read, understood, and agreed to its provisions.

In an office using electronic communication channels, the patient will need to supply to the medical office an e-mail address or number for texting. An area within the patient's initial registration information should be provided to ask for electronic contact data. Prior to communicating via e-mail or text, the physician should verify the e-mail address and phone number. One way to do this is to send a confirming message to the recipient to verify the address using the contact information supplied by the patient during registration with the medical office. If the patient asked to have information sent to a different communication e-mail address or texting phone number, offer to send the information via a more traditional method (such as to the mailing address supplied by the patient), and ask the patient to come to the office and update his or her contact information.

When communicating electronically, patients should be made aware of the dangers of sending PHI using unencrypted channels. If a patient states that he or she does not wish to use electronic methods to communicate medical information such as appointments and test results, other routes of communication should be used. For example, a reminder notice may be sent to the patient. Any requests by the patient for alternate channels of communication must be noted in the patient's chart and followed.

Current government initiatives mandate the implementation of electronic health records, which will be discussed in a later chapter, and the transmission of electronic medical data. A much higher level of electronic security will need to be developed before e-mailing of medical information is considered secure.

4.2 SCHEDULING

Scheduling appointments is one of the principal duties of the administrative medical assistant. To be able to do so efficiently and intelligently is an important skill. Appointments are commonly entered into a computer scheduling system. Some offices may use a hardcopy appointment book. The assistant is responsible for collecting the necessary data for an appointment, such as the patient's name, phone number, insurance coverage, and reason for making the appointment.

To help in juggling patients' appointment preferences with the policies of the physician and the availability of office personnel and equipment, a number of scheduling methods are used. Changes in scheduled appointments, such as cancellations, must be indicated and the time slot used for another patient whenever possible. The physician's outside appointments should be listed, and if necessary, the physician reminded of them in advance. Clear and accurate communication between the administrative medical assistant and the physician yields beneficial results for both the practice and the patients.

Following the Physician's Policy

The physician's policy for seeing and treating patients is the initial guideline in scheduling. Policy may be affected by the physician's office hours, the physician's specialty, how quickly the physician works, the treatment or procedure to be performed, the available office personnel and equipment, and the type of facility.

Office Hours. Before appointments can be made, the administrative medical assistant must know the basic schedule of the physician's office. The physician may need to make rounds to see patients at one or more hospitals on certain days and at certain hours. Office hours, therefore, may vary on different days. Some physicians have office hours in the evenings and on weekends. If there are several physicians in the practice, the hours of each physician may be different. The administrative medical assistant should be aware of each physician's hours as well as how and where each physician can be reached at other times. While office hours may differ depending on the requirements of the practice, a thorough understanding of specific policies within a practice contributes to greater efficiency.

Length of Time Required for Appointments. The length of time required for different types of appointments is based on the procedure, the equipment used, and the amount of time usually spent with a patient. The assistant must be aware of the range of possibilities. A complete physical examination takes longer than a routine blood pressure checkup, for example. The physician may also specify to the assistant when certain types of procedures are best scheduled. For example, the physician may ask the administrative medical assistant to schedule lengthy appointments, such as complete physicals, as the first appointment available in the morning or afternoon, or not to schedule them on certain days or at certain times of the day.

Other Policies, Preferences, and Obligations of the Physician. Most physicians treat patients only in their specialty field of practice. The administrative medical assistant must be familiar with the types of patients the physician sees. For example, the physician may not see patients under age 16. Other preferences the physician has that affect the daily schedule may include a preferred lunchtime, as well as times for meetings or appointments attended on a regular basis. A primary consideration in scheduling is allotting time for the physician's hospital rounds. Hospital visits at set hours should be noted on the schedule.

Once the basic schedule of the office is set, specific guidelines are used to schedule appointments for patients.

Types of Scheduling

An efficient scheduling system reduces the waiting period for patients, makes the best use of the physician's time, and takes advantage of available personnel and facilities. Many providers have added evening and weekend appointment times to their schedules in order to accommodate the changing work needs of their patient population. Scheduling methods must also provide flexibility during high-patient season, such as seasonal allergy periods and the beginning of school. A number of traditional and newer scheduling systems are commonly used.

Fixed Office Hours Appointment Scheduling. Many physicians' offices and clinics use a **fixed office hours** scheduling system in which each patient is given a set appointment time—that is, an approximate time the patient will be seen by the physician. Fixed scheduling is also referred to as *time-specific* or *streamed scheduling*. This system decreases the waiting time for the patient and gives the office staff more control over the flow of patients in the office. Also, because the reason for each patient's visit is known in advance, the staff can make the best use of office facilities, equipment, and medical staff time. Abbreviations for the **chief complaint (CC),** the reason for the visit, are used when making appointments. Equipment, time, and other resources necessary to provide medical care can be prepared when the CC is known prior to the patient's arrival.

Open Office Hours Appointment Scheduling. Patients who are in need of a same-day or next-day nonemergency appointment often turn to healthcare facilities offering an **open office hours** scheduling system. Other names for open office hours scheduling are *open-access scheduling* and *easy-access scheduling*. In a true open office hours scheduling system, specific appointment times are not made and patients are normally seen on a first-come-first-seen basis. Patients who are in need of immediate attention are given first priority. Two disadvantages of this system are that (1) the patient's chief complaint is not known prior to his or her arrival and (2) the flow of patients may be inconsistent—very busy on one day but extremely slow on another. Therefore, healthcare providers may turn to a combination of scheduling methods.

Open and Fixed Office Hours Appointment Scheduling. Many clinics use a combination of **open and fixed office hours** during which the physician is in the office and available to see patients. Patients arriving during open hours, for example, from 8 A.M. to noon, will sign in with the receptionist and are seen in the order in which they arrive. Other patients are scheduled at specific/fixed appointment times, for example, from 1 P.M. to 4 P.M., and are seen at or close to their scheduled appointment time. This system allows patients the freedom to come to the clinic when they wish, but it also has several drawbacks:

- The reason for the patient's visit during open office hours is not known until the patient arrives at the office.
- It is difficult to control the flow of patients during open office hours. Thus, many patients may arrive at the same time, causing crowding and long waits. Patients who arrive at the same time and have a longer waiting period may become irritated. At other times, there may be no patients, causing the physician's and staff's time to be used inefficiently.
- Equipment and office facilities may be used inefficiently.

Wave Scheduling. Another scheduling method used is called **wave scheduling,** also known as **cluster scheduling.** In an office using wave scheduling, the administrative medical assistant arranges for a certain number of patients (such as four) to come between 9 A.M. and 10 A.M., then arranges for the next four patients who call to arrive between 10 A.M. and 11 A.M., and so on throughout the day. Wave scheduling gives patients the flexibility of open office hours while allowing the assistant more control over the flow of patients. This method works well in practices such as dermatology and endocrinology, in which the physician often does not need laboratory and x-ray results in order to diagnose and treat the patient.

A modification of wave scheduling is to schedule a patient with a complex problem on the hour (for example, 10:00 A.M.) and to schedule short routine exams for the remainder of the hour.

Shared Medical Appointments. Many appointments are made for the chief complaint of follow-up or routine care. **Shared medical appointments,** also called *group appointments or visits,* are voluntary for patients. Patients with the same condition(s) meet in a group setting, with typically 8 to 15 patients, with a multidisciplinary medical team. Healthcare providers, such as physicians, nurse practitioners, physician assistants, dietitians, and so on, meet with the group to provide routine care to a group of patients. Vitals are taken and prescription updates are accessed. Shared medical appointments are typically appropriate for

- patients needing follow-up or routine medical care (e.g., type 2 diabetic patients).
- patients who are stable but chronically ill (e.g., pancreatic cancer patients).
- patients who may otherwise require more one-to-one physician time (e.g., "healthy well" patients).
- patients who come in for frequent medical visits (e.g., allergy immunization patients).
- patients who are seeking more information about a certain health condition or issue (e.g., patients seeking information concerning a localized outbreak of spinal meningitis).

In a shared medical appointment environment, patients can gain encouragement—they realize they are not alone in their medical struggles. Through interaction among the patients, they see examples of how other patients are managing their health issue. Information is shared among group participants. If a patient learns through the group that a certain pain management method has worked for others, group participants are prompted to try the pain management method for themselves. At all times, the group discussions are under the supervision of healthcare providers. Other advantages of shared medical appointments include

1. decreased waiting time. Shared medical appointments tend to start promptly.
2. more time with the physician. A multidisciplinary team is working together to provide medical care, which allows each of the providers more time to discuss issues with patients. This also allows for a more relaxed pace of medical care.

3. confidentiality. Each patient and guest must sign a privacy and confidentiality agreement before attending the shared medical appointment.
4. support. Individual patients may bring a support person with them to the appointment.

Many practices and their patients benefit from shared medical appointments. However, not every practice is suited for patient group appointments. Practices may lack the necessary resources, such as time, space, and staff, to run group appointments. Additionally, smaller practices or practices that can accommodate patients' requests for individual appointments may prefer not to offer shared medical appointments.

EXAMPLES: SHARED MEDICAL APPOINTMENTS

A pediatrician offers shared medical appointments twice per week for the month before school begins. During this appointment, the pediatrician and two nurses conduct school physicals for students entering kindergarten.

An immunologist has a large Spanish-speaking patient population, and many have diabetes. A shared appointment is scheduled on the first Tuesday of each month. During this shared medical appointment, diabetic, Spanish-speaking patients meet together to have fasting blood glucose tests performed, vitals taken, and wounds on feet checked. A dietitian also attends the appointment to offer suggestions and answer questions. The caregiving team uses Spanish during the appointment to communicate with patients.

Patient Online Scheduling. As technology has grown and provided electronic features for use by the medical office, technology is also providing features to patients. Web services, such as ZocDoc, allow patients to search for and schedule appointments with physicians. Patients can electronically look into the physician appointment book and schedule a medical visit. Other features enable patients to rate and read reviews on physicians and to fill out medical forms that would normally need to be completed when arriving at the doctor's office. Patients can search for doctors by different methods, such as ZIP Code, specialty, or insurance carrier.

Another Web service estimates the wait time a patient will have when arriving at the office. Appointment timing features estimate if the patient will be seen at the scheduled appointment time or if there is a delay. Patients are electronically notified prior to their appointment time, such as 30 minutes prior.

Patient portals allow patients secure 24/7 online access to their personal health information. One of the features of a patient portal is online scheduling. A patient may select a convenient appointment date and time. Many other features are available through patient portals and may be more or fewer depending on the portal provider. Features include a summary of healthcare visits/procedures, medication listings, discharge summaries, e-mail access to providers, online payments, educational materials, and many more.

Double-Booking. When the schedule is full and there are more patients who need to be seen, some offices use the method of **double-booking appointments.** Depending on the method of scheduling, the extra appointments are entered in a second column beside the regularly scheduled appointments. In some cases, triple columns are used for triple-booking of appointments. Double-booking can be done efficiently; however, most double-bookings occur simply because too many patients were scheduled in a given time frame, which is the result of an inefficient scheduling method. Knowing the chief complaint of the patient and the resources, including room, equipment, and personnel to provide for the encounter, will help the assistant know when and how many patients to schedule in a given time.

EXAMPLE: DOUBLE-BOOKING APPOINTMENTS

An allergist sees both new and established patients in his practice. Eight rooms and two nurses are available. Each new patient takes approximately 2 hours to assess, and a follow-up visit takes 15 minutes. New patients are scheduled as the first appointment and every half hour beginning at 9 A.M. Follow-up visits are also scheduled during the same time frame. After the 9 A.M. new patient is taken to the exam room and assessed, the first follow-up appointment arrives at the scheduled 9:15 A.M. appointment. By this time, the nurse has finished taking the new patient's history and is now available to prepare the follow-up patient. Only four new patients are scheduled in the morning and four in the afternoon. Follow-up patients are scheduled each 15 minutes during the same time frame.

See Figure 4.11 for examples of appointment pages using various scheduling methods.

Computer Scheduling. Most medical offices use electronic scheduling systems to set up and maintain appointments. These systems have many features that are not available with hardcopy appointment books. For example, with electronic scheduling, an administrative medical assistant can print a daily list of appointments for the physician. Having schedules available in a quick and easy-to-read format is helpful for everyone in the medical office. Figure 4.12 shows an electronic appointment schedule.

In addition to a printout of the daily schedule, most scheduling software can generate reports of attended appointments, cancellations, and no-shows. A **no-show** is a patient who, without notifying the physician's office, fails to show up for an appointment.

Electronic schedules enable available appointment slots in a physician's schedule to be easily located. Most scheduling software allows the user to search for the next available slot for the amount of time needed and other resources, such as a specific room and/or equipment, desired locations (such as an outreach clinic), or requested physician. For example, suppose a patient needs to schedule three 15-minute appointments during the next 3 weeks but is available only on Tuesday and Thursday afternoons and needs to be seen at the Outreach Clinic. The assistant enters a set of criteria in the scheduler, and the computer locates the first available slot that matches the criteria. The first appointment is made, and then the search continues for the next available appointment meeting the criteria. This saves the assistant time by not searching through several weeks of appointments in a paper appointment book.

Another advantage is efficient rescheduling of appointments. With a hardcopy appointment book, first the assistant locates the appointment that needs to be changed. Once the appointment is found, it has to be crossed through and a new entry made. With electronic scheduling, the assistant enters the patient's identifying criteria, such as name or date of birth, in a search box, and the computer locates the appointment in seconds. Old appointments can be deleted with a single keystroke, and the new ones keyed into the computer. It is also easy to move an appointment to a different time, day, or month.

Electronic scheduling can also be used to keep track of providers' time away from the office, such as for medical conferences, surgical procedures performed in the hospitals,

Tuesday, September 26

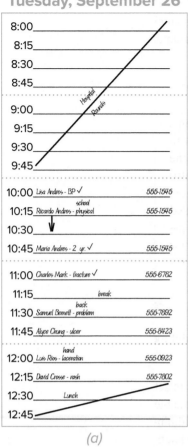

(a)

Tuesday, September 26

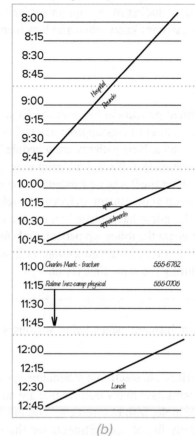

(b)

Tuesday, September 26

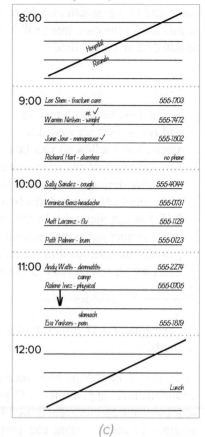

(c)

Figure 4.11

Appointment Books
Showing (a) Scheduled
Appointments, (b) Open
and Fixed Appointment
Hours, (c) Wave Schedule,
and (d) Double-Column
Schedule

Tuesday, September 26

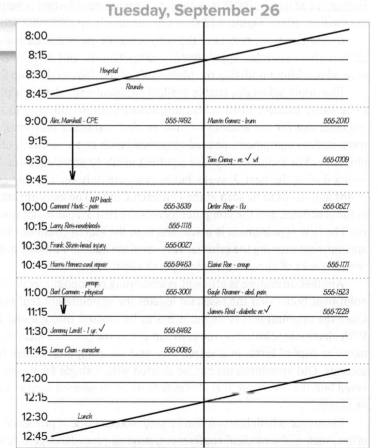

(d)

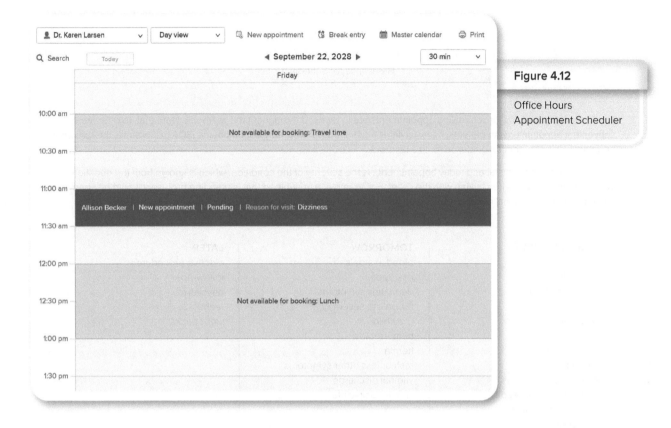

Figure 4.12

Office Hours
Appointment Scheduler

and days when the physician is not available for appointments. Reminder notices and telephone calls that need to be made to patients before appointments also can be automatically generated.

Screening Patients' Illnesses

When scheduling an appointment, the administrative medical assistant must use good judgment to determine how soon a patient needs to be seen. This process is called screening, or **triage** (tree-áhj). Some patients must come to the office *stat* (the term used in healthcare to mean "immediately"), some may be scheduled for later the same day or the following day, and others may be scheduled at a later time that is convenient for both the physician and the patient.

Figure 4.13 lists the appointment scheduling guidelines that are to be used throughout this text. Many offices have their own protocol for scheduling; thus, an administrative medical assistant on the job must adapt to that office's scheduling guidelines.

The difference between stat and today appointments depends on the severity of the condition, which is determined by questions developed by the clinical staff to be used by administrative staff and the answers received when triaging the caller. Many offices use a flowchart method of triage, similar to the method used by 911 dispatchers. When a patient calls the office, the assistant will begin with a low-complexity medical question, such as "How high is your fever?" or "Are you having difficulty breathing?" Based on the patient's answer to each question, the assistant will progress to the next question or appropriate response. At all times, the assistant must remember that he or she is administrative, not clinical, personnel and cannot practice medicine by giving medical instructions. If, after triage, the situation is considered an emergency, the patient should be immediately brought to the office, instructed to call 911, or sent directly to the emergency department.

Figure 4.13

Guidelines for Scheduling

The following guidelines for scheduling appointments are to be used throughout this textbook. Note that, to offer more convenient appointments to patients, many facilities have adopted same-day appointments (SDAs); therefore, the following breakdown is just a general guideline for this textbook.

The difference between stat and today appointments is the severity of the condition, which is known from the questions and answers received when talking with the caller. For example, a nosebleed that is bleeding profusely would be seen sooner than an occasional nosebleed. It is also always better to make an appointment sooner than to leave a critical condition until later.

STAT and/or TODAY	TOMORROW	LATER
abdominal pain	blood in stools	elective procedures
blurry vision	cast repair	follow-ups
breathing difficulty	dermatitis symptoms	physicals
burn	flu, unless severe or in	rechecks
chest pain	a child	well checks
croup	hemorrhoids	
foreign bodies	hernia	
head injury	rash unless other symptoms	
laceration	vaginal discharge	
migraine/severe headache	vague complaints	
nausea and vomiting		
nosebleed		
pain when urinating		
possible fractures		
pregnancy with		
cramps/bleeding		

It is imperative to understand that a tomorrow appointment can change to an emergency situation with the addition of another symptom; for example, cast repair would become a today appointment if the patient stated that there was swelling around the cast, change in the color of skin, and/or moisture drainage.

Considering Patients' Preferences

The trend is to offer more convenient appointments to patients. As a result, many facilities have adopted same-day appointments (SDAs). Figure 4.13 provides a general guideline. Be aware that an appointment for tomorrow can change into an emergency situation with the addition of another symptom. For example, skin rash would become a today appointment if the patient stated that there was a sudden temperature spike and onset of vomiting.

Some patients prefer to be seen at a certain time or on a certain day of the week. Work schedules vary from the traditional "9 to 5" schedule. Physicians must consider the demographics of their patients and service area. In a community with a high factory-employee population, the practice may offer more evening hours. In a "college town," Saturday and Sunday hours may be more popular than morning hours. Try to schedule appointments according to patients' preferences if the schedule allows, taking into consideration the urgency of the appointment situation. Some physicians have office hours on certain evenings, such as every other Thursday evening, to better accommodate their patients' work schedules.

Necessary Data

When patients' appointments are scheduled, all necessary data should be collected and recorded. In general, this includes some or all of the following information:

- Patient's first and last names
- Telephone number
- E-mail address for electronic communications
- Address
- Date of birth (DOB)
- Reason for the appointment
- Patient status: **new patient (NP)** (a patient who has *not* seen the physician or a physician of the same specialty in the same practice in the last 3 years); **established patient (EP)** (a patient who *has* seen the physician or a physician of the same specialty in the same practice in the last 3 years); or referred by another physician
- Referring physician
- Insurance provider
- Notations regarding any laboratory tests or x-rays required before the examination

Always verify the patient's name and its spelling and repeat contact information—telephone number(s) and/or e-mail address. A practice may have patients with duplicate names. Careful attention must be used to be sure the correct patient is scheduled. In cases such as twins, the patient should be asked for an individually identifiable piece of information, such as a driver's license number, insurance ID number, or other individually identifying factor. Confirm the appointment time by repeating it to the patient—for example, "Sara, your appointment with Dr. Larsen is for Wednesday, July 16, at 2:15." When the patient arrives in the office, the information taken when the appointment was scheduled should be verified. New patients are asked to arrive at least 15 to 30 minutes early to complete the registration process. To save time, the forms may be mailed or e-mailed to the patient prior to the appointment. The patient should bring the completed form(s) with him or her. Established patients are asked at least once a year whether any information previously given has changed. If the information has changed, the patient should be asked to fill out updated registration forms. If the information is the same, the patient should be asked to sign and date a verification, stating that the information has not changed.

If a practice uses electronic medical records, the administrative medical assistant can verify and update patient information without the patient completing new paperwork. Caution must be used to protect the patient's PHI when verbally verifying patient information. When a website is used by a medical practice, forms can be printed and completed by patients and brought to the office. Or, if the website allows, patients can complete and submit forms electronically via the medical office's website.

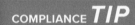

WP | **Mc Graw Hill connect** | **GO TO PROJECTS 4.2, 4.3, AND 4.4 AT THE END OF THIS CHAPTER**

Keeping to the Schedule

Any number of situations arise in the course of a day that require the administrative medical assistant to cancel and reschedule appointments or to work an appointment into the existing schedule. In addition, the assistant must adjust the schedule for any emergencies that arise, as well as set up next appointments for patients currently in the office who need a follow-up encounter with the physician.

Irregular Appointments. Occasionally, a patient walks in without an appointment. If the physician is busy and it is judged that the walk-in patient should be seen at that time, you may explain that the physician will see the patient for a few minutes when the patient can be worked into the schedule.

A patient with a true emergency should be seen on arrival. The administrative medical assistant should notify the nurse or physician of the emergency and escort the patient to an available examination room. The assistant must tactfully explain, without revealing PHI, the presence of walk-in and emergency patients to other waiting patients who have made appointments that will now be delayed. If a physician outside the office calls to request that a patient be seen that day by one of the physicians in your office, that patient should also be worked into the day's schedule.

On days when the schedule is full, and after the assistant has completed triage, the office nurse may help determine whether a patient is truly an emergency case and will ask the physician for further instructions or whether the case is urgent, and the patient may wait to see the physician. In some cases, the physician may request that emergency patients who telephone be referred to the emergency room. Do not refer the patient to another physician or clinic unless you are directed to do so by your employer.

In addition to appointments for patients, physicians have hospital commitments, seminars, lectures, meetings, and personal appointments that may change at the last minute. All these changes must be logged into the appointment calendar to avoid schedule conflicts later on.

Late Patients

The entire schedule may be thrown out of balance because a patient is late. Patients who are late for appointments may be asked to wait until the physician has seen the next patient or until a treatment room is available. It is not the administrative medical assistant's place to criticize a patient for tardiness, but most physicians wish to be notified of a patient who is habitually late because it is an inconvenience to other patients. Sometimes the patient who is late must be asked to reschedule.

For patients who are habitually late, a notation should be entered in the patient's record. Such patients should be scheduled either in the last appointment slot for the morning or during the last appointment slot of the day. It is also a good practice to ask habitually late patients to arrive 15 to 20 minutes prior to their scheduled appointment.

Extended Appointments

Schedules also fall behind when either the physician or the patient loses track of the time during an examination, causing the appointment to go past the allotted period. The physician may have to be reminded if the visit runs over the scheduled time. The administrative medical assistant can use the intercom or knock on the examination room door and hand the physician a written reminder when the physician comes to the door. For physicians who use electronic methods for recording patient data, an electronic message may be sent, reminding the physician that the next patient is ready. The physician can then decide whether or not to conclude the visit with the current patient.

Out-of-Office Emergencies

The schedule may also be disrupted when the physician is called out of the office for an emergency. Certain specialties, such as OB/GYN, tend to have more out-of-office situations than other specialties. The administrative medical assistant should explain the situation to waiting patients and ask patients whether they wish to wait for the physician or reschedule their appointments.

Assistant: Dr. Larsen has been called out on an emergency. She is expected to be out for at least an hour. Would you like to wait for her to return, reschedule your appointment, or leave and come back in 1 hour? If you choose to leave and come back, you can leave me your contact phone number, and I will text you when Dr. Larsen is expected to return.

As a courtesy, patients should also be informed if the physician is running late as a result of unforeseen interruptions. The administrative medical assistant may explain as follows: "Dr. Larsen is running behind schedule by about 30 minutes. Would you like to wait, or shall I reschedule your appointment?" Do not offer to reschedule if the schedule is behind by only a few minutes.

Registering Arrivals. Registering patients (asking them to sign in) on arrival at a physician's office or clinic is the duty of the administrative medical assistant. The assistant should then verify the patient's name, address, and other information with the patient's record. If a computerized scheduling program is being used, it is all the more important to verify the spelling of each patient's name, since an exact spelling will help locate the patient's appointment time and information quickly.

When an appointment is made for a new patient, many offices ask the patient to arrive a few minutes early to complete information forms. At this time, the practice's payment policy is explained to the patient. Preparing new patient packets with information about the practice, insurance coverage accepted, payment policy, privacy practices, and similar items will save time in the schedule. If the practice has a website, new patient information can be loaded and accessed electronically by the patient.

Patients' identities, which are part of their PHI, must be protected. This includes the sign-in methods used for registering patients' arrivals. If using a sign-in sheet, minimally necessary patient data should be collected to prohibit unintentional disclosure of patient PHI. An example would be to only ask for the patient's last name and appointment time. If it is a multi-physician practice, ask which physician the patient is to see or what service is to be performed. A simple way to protect PHI is by using a dark, broad-tipped marker to strike out the patients' information. Another method is to use peel-off labels. Electronic sign-in pads can also be used by patients to sign in upon their arrival. The goal is to protect the PHI of patients.

When the patient has signed in, the administrative medical assistant leaves the medical file for the nurse or physician's assistant, indicating that the patient is ready to be seen. If an appointment book is used, a check mark is entered to show that the patient has arrived. It is the assistant's responsibility to see that the patient's chart is in order and that all forms are completed before the physician sees the patient.

Electronic health records allow the assistant to electronically show the status of the patient—in waiting room, in exam room, for instance. Other medical office team members can see when a patient moves through the medical office and update the patient's status by using this feature. Programs can use different colors to show where the patient is in the office. Green may indicate the patient is in the waiting area, and blue may indicate the patient is in the exam room.

The registration record can be checked periodically against the appointment schedule to make sure that a patient who has arrived has not forgotten to sign in. Many offices post a sign, asking that patients notify the front desk if they are still waiting 20 minutes past their appointment time.

COMPLIANCE *TIP*

It is important to ensure that patients' names on an office sign-in sheet remain confidential.

Canceling and Rescheduling Appointments. Almost every patient will cancel an appointment at one time or another; some patients, however, make it a habit. When a patient calls to cancel an appointment, a new appointment time should be suggested. A notation regarding the cancellation is also entered into the patient's medical record (especially if the cancellation is made on the same day as, or the day before, the scheduled appointment).

If a manual schedule is kept, cancellations are noted by drawing a line through the appointment and entering the new appointment. As changes in the appointment book are made throughout the day, the assistant must remember also to make the changes on all hardcopy schedules used by the physician and nurse. In electronic scheduling systems, the administrative medical assistant must locate the appointment and reschedule it. The appropriate cancellation code should be used to show the reason for the cancellation and whether it was rescheduled.

The office policy for cancellations and rescheduled appointments should be posted in areas accessible to patients, such as the waiting area or examination room. Registration packets for new patients should also contain the written policy. If a patient habitually cancels appointments (e.g., three sequential appointments), the physician may dismiss the patient from his or her care. A certified letter should be sent, informing the patient of the dismissal and the reason.

No-Shows. The administrative medical assistant should also make a notation in a patient's hardcopy and/or electronic medical record if the patient fails to keep an appointment and does not call to cancel. Since medical records are legal documents, all notations of no-show appointments should be entered into the record, signed, and dated. Figure 4.14 shows an example of a chart note recording a no-show appointment.

The physician will decide what action to take if a patient repeatedly makes appointments but does not keep them. Specialty practices sometimes charge patients for no-show appointments or canceled appointments when notification is not made 24 hours in advance. Collection of no-show charges is difficult and typically causes bad public relations. Insurance carriers' policies for charging no-shows should be consulted. Since it is considered fraud to charge for a service that was not rendered, charging an insurance carrier for no-show fees is discouraged. However, it is the physician's decision to pursue the collection of no-show fees.

Next Appointment. Before a patient leaves the examination room, the physician will tell the patient when to return. When the patient stops at the checkout area, the administrative medical assistant should inquire whether another appointment is needed. In many offices, the need for another appointment—often referred to as a "recall"—is noted on the encounter form or in the patient's medical record, which the patient gives the assistant after the appointment. If using electronic health records, the patient's record should also be consulted for follow-up information.

Figure 4.14

Chart Notation for a No-Show Appointment

August 14, 20--
Patient failed to show for appointment. Called the nursing home and left a message for the head nurse to call our office.

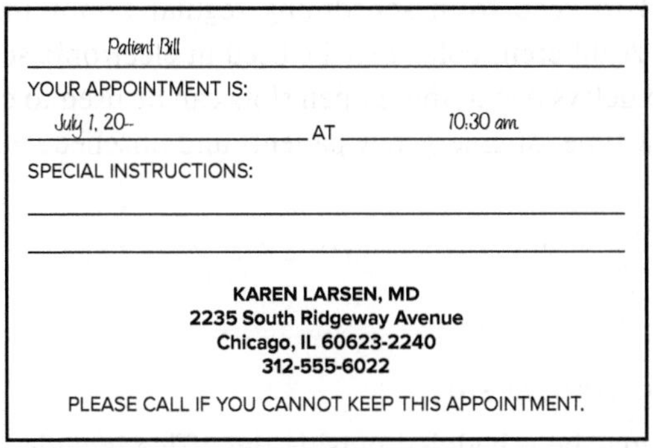

Patient Bill

YOUR APPOINTMENT IS:

July 1, 20– AT 10:30 am

SPECIAL INSTRUCTIONS:

KAREN LARSEN, MD
2235 South Ridgeway Avenue
Chicago, IL 60623-2240
312-555-6022

PLEASE CALL IF YOU CANNOT KEEP THIS APPOINTMENT.

Figure 4.15

Appointment Card

In most cases, the physician will give the patient instructions such as "Return in 10 days" or "Return in 3 weeks." The assistant should schedule the patient's next appointment for a convenient time as close as possible to the suggested return date.

Never trust an appointment time to memory with the intention of entering it later, no matter how hectic the office is. Make it a habit to enter the information into the appointment book or computer immediately, and then write an appointment card, which will serve as a reminder for the patient. See Figure 4.15 for an example of an appointment card.

Many offices use a system of follow-up telephone calls to remind a patient of an appointment for the next day. If the follow-up appointment is several months in the future, the patient may be asked to complete a postcard with the patient's address before leaving the office, so that the card can be sent as a reminder to the patient. File the reminder card in a chronological (by month) filing container and mail the self-addressed reminder card to the patient prior to the next appointment. Mail the card at least 1 or 2 weeks prior to the first day of the month in which the appointment is scheduled. If the office uses a computerized scheduling system, the computer can print reminders to be sent to patients scheduled for follow-up visits.

As electronic medical records continue to increase in use, the ability to contact patients electronically will become the norm. Currently, variations of the electronic format for patient communications are being used. Web-based, automated, practice-initiated message delivery systems are being used to notify patients of appointments. As previously discussed, patient portals are used by many patients to schedule and verify appointments. When agreed to in writing by the patient, e-mail and text message reminders can be sent to remind patients of upcoming appointments. The patient will supply the e-mail address or number to be used for text messaging. Examples of secure messages include health maintenance information, lab results, and financial information, such as past due notices. Nonsecure information, such as flu shot notices, may also be sent to the patient.

As discussed earlier in this chapter, the method or methods used to communicate medical information, such as appointment reminders, must be stated in the Notice of Privacy Practices and acknowledged by the patient by his or her signature on the Acknowledgment of Receipt of Notice of Privacy Practices form.

Open Slots for Catching Up. No matter how carefully appointments are scheduled, crowding is sometimes unavoidable and appointments fall behind schedule. Leaving a 15- or 20-minute interval free in the late morning and again at the end of each day will help you straighten out a delayed schedule. Place a label, such as "WORK-INS," in the appointment slot(s) to keep from scheduling regular appointments in the empty, available time slots. A different color may be used in electronic scheduling to indicate "work-in" slots. If no delays occur, these open slots can be used to complete other work. Open slots also allow time for emergency patients and unscheduled patients.

 Mc Graw Hill connect   **GO TO PROJECT 4.5 AT THE END OF THIS CHAPTER**

Out-of-Office Appointments

Appointments that may be scheduled outside the office include hospital admissions, surgery, and diagnostic or other special procedures. Follow basic scheduling procedures for such appointments, obtaining the necessary patient data required for each type of appointment. Many electronic medical records allow scheduling patients for outside service appointments from within the electronic record. When this feature is used, patient information is available for the administrative medical assistant to complete the outside service appointment or to submit a request for the appointment.

Hospital Admissions. The following information is needed for hospital admissions:

- Complete name of patient
- Patient's information: age, DOB, address, and telephone number
- Diagnosis or problem (usually submitted with an *ICD-10-CM* code)
- Preferred date of admission
- Preferred accommodations
- Previous admissions
- Insurance coverage information

Surgical and Diagnostic Procedures. The following information, in addition to the preceding information (excluding "Preferred accommodations"), is needed for surgery or for diagnostic or other procedures:

- Surgery or other procedure to be performed
- Length of time needed for surgery (if known)
- Approximate date and time desired
- Specific surgical assistants required
- Type of anesthesia to be used and person administering it
- Special requirements, such as diagnostic testing required before the patient undergoes the procedure

Other considerations for scheduling are

- scheduling the appropriate time required by the physician in each situation.
- giving patients clear and simple instructions for hospital admission.
- scheduling fasting tests in the morning so the patient does not need to go without eating longer than necessary. Inform patients about any preparations that are required before undergoing a surgical or diagnostic procedure (for example, informing them that they are to have nothing to eat or drink after midnight of the night prior to the procedure and/or how and when to complete pretesting, such as x-rays).
- confirming that any requested assistants and/or anesthesiologists are available.

 Mc Graw Hill connect   **GO TO PROJECT 4.6 AT THE END OF THIS CHAPTER**

PROCESSING INCOMING MAIL AND PREPARING OUTGOING MAIL

Every physician receives an enormous amount of mail every day, so the efficient handling of correspondence is vital. As an administrative medical assistant, you must learn to distinguish quickly between the types of mail most often received. Use sound judgment to sort mail according to its importance. The mail generally falls into these categories:

- Important items, such as those sent by Express or Priority Mail, or mail that is registered or certified (or sent via overnight services, such as Federal Express)
- Regular first-class mail
- The physician's personal mail
- Periodicals and newspapers
- Advertising materials
- Samples

Processing Guidelines for Incoming Mail

Use the following guidelines to process incoming mail. Sort the items by category, depending on their importance.

1. Open all letters except those marked "Personal" or "Confidential," unless you are authorized to open all mail. If a mailing marked "Personal" or "Confidential" is opened accidentally, the assistant should reseal the correspondence with clear tape, note "Opened by Mistake" on the envelope, and place his or her initials by the notation.
2. Check the contents of each envelope carefully.
3. Stamp the date on each item to show when it was received.
4. Attach enclosures to each item.
5. Carefully put aside checks from patients to be recorded and deposited later. Verify whose bill is being paid; the name on the check may not be the same as the patient's name.
6. Check to be sure the envelope is empty and is not needed before discarding it. If evidence of a postmark is needed, retain the envelope.
7. Write a reminder on the calendar or in the follow-up (tickler) file about material that is being sent separately.
8. Attach the patient's chart to correspondence regarding the patient. If using electronic medical records, correspondence can be scanned into the patient's record. Place such correspondence in a high-priority area on the physician's desk.
9. If a business letter responds to a request, pull the relevant file and attach the letter to it.
10. Set aside correspondence that can be answered without the physician's seeing it, such as payments needing receipts, insurance forms or questions, bills, and other routine business matters.

In some offices, the assistant is required to **annotate** communications. That is, the assistant skims an item and writes necessary or helpful notes in the margin or on an attached self-stick note.

It may save time if the items that require the physician's attention are placed on the desk in the order of importance. Medical journals are placed on the physician's desk with other mail. Medical samples should be unpacked and placed in the physician's supply cabinet if they can be used. Notify the physician of the new samples.

For out-of-date and unused medication, the FDA (U.S. Food and Drug Administration) suggests taking these medications to a community "drop-off" or "take-back" event in your area. Also, out-of-date or unused medications can be taken to a centralized location for proper disposal. Contact city or county government agencies or state/local law enforcement for information on drug "take-back" events. Additionally, ask the pharmaceutical representatives who bring medications to the office how to dispose of the unused medications. Samples should not be thrown in the trash.

Best Practices for Safe Mail Handling

Since the anthrax mailings in 2001 and subsequent suspicious mailings since then, businesses have realized they may be at risk for mail threats and have implemented steps to protect the mail handlers and the business. The U.S. Department of Homeland Security has issued *Best Practices for Safe Mail Handling,* which sets in place best practice procedures for federal agencies. The following are some of the standards issued by Homeland Security. The complete document can be found at www.dhs.gov or http://about.usps.com. At the site, search for "Best Practices for Safe Mail Handling."

- *Centralize mail handling.* Centralizing mail handling and processing operations contains the risk to the business or provider.
- *Wear personal protective equipment.* Gloves should be worn when sorting mail. Surgical gloves are readily available in the provider's office and should be used. Other protective equipment includes masks, protective/safety glasses, and smocks. It is during the initial contact with incoming mail that suspicious items can be identified.
- *Maintain a list of suspicious indicators for handlers.* Establish and use a listing of suspicious package indicators, such as a "grainy" feel to the contents of the envelope. Personnel should receive initial and ongoing training to help them identify suspicious mailings.
- *Develop isolation/emergency procedures.* Policies and procedures regarding the steps to isolate a suspicious mailing should be posted in the centralized incoming mail area, so that they can be read easily and quickly. Emergency procedures should also be posted. Included in the emergency procedures should be emergency phone numbers, including the phone number and/or contact number for the local hazardous materials (HAZMAT) team.

As with most situations, it is better to be prepared and proactive than to be unprepared and reactive.

Preparation of Outgoing Mail

Outgoing mail consists of professional, business, and personal correspondence. Professional correspondence concerns patients, clinical matters, and research. Business correspondence relates to the management of the office and may concern insurance companies, lawyers, supply houses, and bills to patients. Personal correspondence pertains to the physician's personal rather than professional life, such as notes to friends or letters about the physician's personal business interests.

Mail Classifications. For mail to be handled in the most efficient and cost-effective way, the assistant must know the various classifications of mail and services offered. The United States Postal Service (USPS) provides excellent information in easy-to-use formats.

The USPS website (www.usps.com) has a complete listing and description of services and rates. The site is an easy reference for ZIP Codes and correct state postal abbreviations, as well as for all domestic rates and fees; it has postal rate calculators and information on new rates and mailing rules. The local Post Office can also supply leaflets describing USPS services. The assistant must always be aware of current postal rates, requirements, and services.

The following are mail classifications specified by the USPS:

- **First-class mail** includes all correspondence, whether handwritten or typewritten; all bills and statements of accounts; and all materials sealed against postal inspection and weighing 13 ounces or less. Postcards may be sent first class and must be rectangular in shape.
- **Priority Mail** offers 2- to 3-day service to most domestic destinations. Items must weigh less than 70 pounds. This is the cheapest way to send heavier items. Rates depend on the weight when the charge is calculated by postal zone. Another option is to send any item or items that fit into the priority shipping container and pay one fee. Priority Mail items are insured up to $50.
- **Priority Express Mail,** the fastest service, offers 1- or 2-day expedited delivery to most destinations. Priority Express Mail deliveries are made 365 days a year, including Saturdays, Sundays, and holidays. All items must weigh less than 70 pounds and be less than 108 inches in combined length and girth. Up to $100 in insurance is included with Priority Express Mail. If a signature verifying receipt is needed, a return receipt service can be added. The charge depends on weight. There is pickup service. For all materials that can be sent in a flat-rate envelope (provided by the USPS), there is one, single fee for all items.
- **Retail Ground and Package Service** is a collective term that includes three subclassifications of mail: Bound Printed Matter, Media Mail, and Library Mail. It is used for mailing certain items weighing up to 70 pounds and no more than 130 inches in length and girth. The charge depends on weight, distance, and shape of the container. Many extra services, such as a Certificate of Mailing and a Signature Confirmation of Delivery, can be added to Parcel Post.

Mail Services. The following services are available through the USPS:

- **Certified Mail** provides the sender with a mailing receipt. The USPS keeps a record of delivery and requires a signature upon delivery. Certified Mail service is available with first-class or Priority Mail. The USPS issues unique article numbers, which allow senders to track online the delivery status of the mailing. The recipient's signature (required upon delivery) is maintained by the USPS. The sender has the option to purchase a Return Receipt, either electronic or hardcopy, as evidence of delivery. When it is important to verify the mailing of materials, such as a patient termination letter, Certified Mail may be used to maintain evidence that the correspondence was mailed.
- **Insured Mail** is used to cover mailings for loss or damages. Coverage is available for up to $5,000. First-class mail, Parcel Post, and Media Mail may all be insured for rates determined by the declared value of the mailed item(s).
- **Registered Mail** provides the greatest security for valuables. The sender gets a receipt at the time of mailing, and a delivery record is kept by the USPS. The mailing Post Office also maintains a record of mailing. Only first-class and Priority Mail may be registered. Postal insurance is provided for articles with a declared value of up to $50,000. The charge is determined according to the declared value of the item(s).
- **Collect on Delivery (COD)** allows the sender to have the USPS collect the recipient's payments and, if necessary, postage. Items are insured up to $1,000. COD may be used on domestic deliveries; however, it may not be used on international shipments and mailings sent to military Post Office addresses (APO/FPO).

- **Delivery Confirmation** provides proof by the date, ZIP Code, and time of delivery. If the delivery was not successful, the date and time of the attempt are recorded. This service is both in the traditional hardcopy detail format or through the electronic USPS Tracking System. Six classifications have USPS Tracking as part of their service: first class (parcels), Express, Priority Express, Retail Ground, Media, and Library Mail.
- **Special Handling** should be used when shipments are unusual or require extra care, such as live poultry. Items that are breakable normally do not require special handling. Adequate packing should be used, and "FRAGILE" should be marked on the package.
- **Return Receipt** provides the sender with evidence of delivery. The recipient's signature is required upon delivery and can be viewed by the sender online or by receipt of a postcard showing the recipient's signature. Return Receipt is available for all mail classifications. Some classifications require insurance of the item(s) before a Return Receipt can be purchased.
- **Certificate of Mailing** is a certificate that provides only proof of an item's having been mailed. It does not provide proof of delivery. It must be purchased at the time of mailing and is kept by the sender.
- **Signature Confirmation** is used to provide proof (confirmation) of the date and time of delivery or attempted delivery. This service may be purchased only at the time of mailing. A similar service, Adult Signature Confirmation, requires someone 21 years of age or older at the recipient's address to sign for delivery of the item.
- **Restricted Delivery** permits a sender to authorize delivery only to the addressee or the addressee's authorized agent. The addressee must be specified in the address by name. An ID may be requested of the recipient. Restricted Delivery is available only as an additional service to Certified Mail, COD, Insured Mail over $500, Registered Mail, or Signature Confirmation.

ZIP Codes. Before sending any outgoing mail, the ZIP Code or the ZIP+4 should be placed as the last item in the mailing address. **ZIP** (Zone Improvement Plan) is a standardized, numeric code that is assigned by the USPS and designates a special delivery area. In 1983, the USPS expanded the ZIP system to include a four-digit extension to the original ZIP Code. This system is known as **ZIP+4.** The four-digit extension provides very specific details for delivery, such as a building number, floor number, office number, or other identifying unit that can be used to pinpoint more precisely the delivery destination.

Though the use of ZIP+4 is not mandatory, it provides more efficient delivery of mail by reducing the number of handlings. Fewer handlings by humans and/or machines reduce the number of inaccurate deliveries and, consequently, reduce cost. Though mail can be processed by humans, cards and other first-class mail are primarily processed by an **optical character reader (OCR),** which reads the address. **POSTNET** (a bar code consisting of a series of long and short vertical lines) is placed on the lower portion of the mailing. POSTNET is an interpretation of the ZIP Code or the ZIP+4. Often the delivery point is added. The delivery point could be the last two digits of the destination address or the PO box number. Most word processing software packages have the ability to print the POSTNET onto the envelope.

If you do not know the ZIP or ZIP+4, visit the ZIP Locator at www.usps.gov.

4.1 Explain how proper screening and triage of patients during a phone conversation can assist the office environment.	• When patients call the medical office, they must be properly assessed in order to meet their needs. By asking a predetermined sequence of questions (triage), the assistant can determine if the situation is an emergency. • By having the information available, the patient can be given proper instruction, such as "Go directly to the emergency department" or "Make an appointment in the near future." • Assessing/triaging better uses office resources by determining the time, equipment, and personnel needed to assist and properly direct the patient.
4.2 Recall and explain two different types of scheduling options and provide examples of practices that would be most suited to each of the schedules.	• Two methods of scheduling appointments are (1) open and fixed hours and (2) wave hours. — Open and fixed scheduling: The physician sees patients during nonscheduled times, such as noon to 2 P.M. Patients are seen in the order in which they arrive. During the remaining hours, the physician sees patients by appointment. Outreach clinics are well suited for open and fixed hours scheduling. — Wave scheduling: Groups of patients are asked to arrive usually on the hour. For example, 10 patients are asked to arrive at 9 A.M., and another group of 10 is asked to arrive at 11 A.M. Larger clinics with multiple physicians may use this method of scheduling.
4.3 Recall the steps in processing incoming and outgoing mail and discuss related safety recommendations.	• When processing incoming mail, the assistant should follow the practice's policies and procedures for handling incoming mail. Examples of the procedures are — opening all incoming mail, except those marked "Personal" or "Confidential," and carefully removing all contents. — date-stamping each item and attaching any enclosures to the items. — double-checking the envelope for any missed content. — setting aside checks to be processed in a central, secure location. — attaching the patient's chart or other office record to correspondence.

	• Many best practice procedures for handling incoming mail have been implemented by Homeland Security.
	— Protective equipment, such as gloves and masks, should be worn by individuals processing incoming mail to provide for personal protection.
	— Centralizing receipt and processing of incoming mail will reduce the threat risk to the practice by localizing the possible effect.
	— Providing a list of suspicious indicators to mail handlers can reduce the possibility of a threat being carried out. This increased awareness will help them identify possible threats in the initial processing stage. As soon as a threat is suspected or confirmed, the local authorities should be notified.
	— Providing a list of all emergency contact information and procedures will reduce the employees' response time.

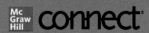

Project 4.1 (LO 4.1) Taking Messages

Today's date is October 10, 2028, and Dr. Larsen is not available for telephone calls. Using Working Papers 10–17 (WPs 10–17), take complete messages for the following situations:

- Jane Kramer at 312-555-1913 calls at 9:30 A.M., stating that her 8-year-old son, Jeffrey, a patient of Dr. Larsen's, has been complaining about a sore throat and an earache for 2 days. They are unable to come to the office for an appointment today. Jeffrey has no fever, is on no medications, and has no allergies. Is there any OTC medication they can use until they can make an appointment?
- Sara Babcock, an established patient, calls at 9:45 A.M. Her telephone number is 312-555-5441. She would like to have her Ortho Tri-Cyclen birth control medication refilled at Consumer Pharmacy (312-555-1252). It was last filled 1 year ago.
- At 9:50 A.M., Wanda Norberg, MD, calls to set up an appointment with Dr. Larsen. Dr. Larsen has hired Dr. Norberg to work part-time, starting in January. She can be reached after 5:30 P.M. at 312-555-1322.

Put the remaining message slips in your Supplies folder.

Project 4.2 (LO 4.2) Scheduling Decision Making

Using Working Paper 18 (WP 18), choose the appropriate answer for each situation. Be prepared to discuss your answers in class.

Project 4.3 (LO 4.2) Setting Up Dr. Larsen's Practice

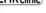

If you are instructed to complete this project using EHRclinic, your instructor will assign you the project as part of a Connect assignment.

Information about Dr. Larsen's appointment schedule is found on Working Paper 19 (WP 19). Working Papers 20–35 (WPs 20–35) are Dr. Larsen's appointment calendar pages.

You will use WP 19 through WP 35 throughout most of the course, entering, canceling, and rescheduling patients' appointments, as well as Dr. Larsen's other appointments. Prepare a binder or folder to use as your Appointment Calendar. Remove WPs 19–35 and secure them in your appointment calendar binder or folder. Place WP 19 as the first page of the binder or folder you will use for your appointment calendar.

Today's date is October 7, 2028. Check the calendar for the week of October 9, noting that Dr. Larsen is attending an all-day seminar at the University on October 9. Some appointments have been preset on your calendar.

Enter Dr. Larsen's following commitments on the appropriate pages:

- October 13, University Hospital Accreditation Meeting from 5 P.M. to 6 P.M., Whitman Hall, Rosewood Room

- October 20, 5 P.M. to 6 P.M., University Hospital Dining Room, dinner meeting with Wanda Norberg, MD
- October 25, 7 P.M. to 8 P.M., lecture on resident requirements, Dr. Margo Matthews at University Hospital, Whitman Hall, Room 203

Project 4.4 (LO 4.2) Scheduling Appointments

EHRclinic If you are instructed to complete this project using EHRclinic, your instructor will assign you the project as part of a Connect assignment.

Today's date is October 9, 2028. On your Appointment Calendar, enter the following appointments. Dr. Larsen's policy is to enter the first and last names of the patient, the reason for the visit, and the patient's telephone number. The amount of time needed for the appointment (15 minutes, unless otherwise noted) is blocked out with arrows.

Appointments

- October 11, 11:00 A.M., Gary Robertson, established patient, urinary problems, 312-555-9565
- October 11, 11:15 A.M., Laura Lund, established patient, cramps, 312-555-4106
- October 11, 11:45 A.M., Charles Jonathan III, established patient, knee pain, 312-555-3097
- October 12, 10:30 A.M., Ardis Matthews, established patient, nausea, 312-555-3178
- October 16, 10:30 A.M., Jack Kyser, established patient, wheezing, 312-555-8901
- October 16, 10:45 A.M., Cynthia Kyser, established patient, cough, 312-555-8901
- October 17, 10:30 A.M., Thomas Baab, established patient, CPE (1 hour), 312-555-3478
- October 17, 11:45 A.M., Doris Casagranda, established patient, rash, 312-555-1200
- October 18, 11:00 A.M., Sara Babcock, established patient, CPE (1 hour), 312-555-5441
- October 19, 11:15 A.M., Ana Mendez, established patient, sore throat, 312-555-3606

Project 4.5 (LO 4.2) Rescheduling Appointments

EHRclinic If you are instructed to complete this project using EHRclinic, your instructor will assign you the project as part of a Connect assignment.

WP

Dr. Larsen's policy is to draw a single line through canceled appointments. Cancel and reschedule the patients' appointments listed here.

Appointments

- Thomas Baab calls to ask if he can cancel his appointment on October 17 at 10:30 A.M. and reschedule it for this week. You inform him that 11:00 A.M. on Thursday, the 12th, is available. He agrees to that time. Make the appropriate changes.

- Charles Jonathan III stops in to change his October 11 appointment. You reschedule him for October 18 at 10:45 A.M. Complete an appointment card using the form on Working Paper 36 (WP 36). Make the appropriate changes. Place the unused appointment cards in your Supplies folder.

Project 4.6 **Project 4.6 (LO 4.2) Out-of-Office Scheduling**

Using Working Paper 37 (WP 37), choose the appropriate answer for each situation. Be prepared to discuss your answers.

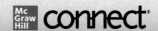

Ability to Communicate (LO 4.1)

A person is only as effective as his or her communication skills. Learning how to communicate effectively will increase your confidence, make you more comfortable with other people, and fine-tune your information incoming and outgoing skills. The ability to communicate well often starts with a good vocabulary. Without good communication skills, you may find yourself not being understood. Communication skills, in short, give you the ability to relate information effectively, with little or no chance for misunderstanding. This is especially important in healthcare. **Explain why the ability to communicate well is so important**.

USING TERMINOLOGY

Match the term or phrase on the left with the correct answer on the right.

_____ 1. [LO 4.3] Certified Mail

_____ 2. [LO 4.2] Established patient

_____ 3. [LO 4.2] Chief complaint

_____ 4. [LO 4.1] Urgent

_____ 5. [LO 4.2] Shared medical appointment

_____ 6. [LO 4.2] Stat

_____ 7. [LO 4.2] Triage

_____ 8. [LO 4.2] Wave scheduling

_____ 9. [LO 4.2] Open/fixed hours scheduling

_____ 10. [LO 4.3] Return receipt

a. Systematically assessing a patient to determine when the patient can be scheduled

b. A method of scheduling patients that combines times during which patients may be seen without a prearranged appointment and scheduled appointment times

c. A method of scheduling patients that has the advantage of patient interaction

d. The main reason a patient seeks medical services

e. Medical condition that requires treatment as a result of an unforeseen illness, injury, or condition but that is not defined as an emergency

f. A method of seeing multiple patients during a block of time—usually patients arrive at or close to the same time

g. Classification of a patient who has seen the physician or a physician of the same specialty in the same practice within the last 3 years

h. Immediately

i. Provides the sender with evidence of delivery

j. Provides the sender with documentation of mailed materials

CHECKING YOUR UNDERSTANDING

Select the most correct answer.

1. [LO 4.1] Which of the following is *not* an appropriate, professional ending for an administrative medical assistant to use when finishing a telephone call?

   a. Thank you for calling, Mr. Rodriguez, and goodbye.
   b. I will leave your message with Dr. Larsen's nurse. Goodbye, Mr. Rodriguez.
   c. We will see you for your appointment on Monday, October 31. Goodbye, Mr. Rodriguez.
   d. Thank you for calling, Mr. Rodriguez, bye-bye.

2. [LO 4.2] Which of the following methods of scheduling appointments would be beneficial for established patients in Dr. Larsen's practice who have been diagnosed with ovarian cancer and need frequent follow-up appointments and medication checks?

   a. Shared medical appointments
   b. Wave scheduling
   c. Open appointment scheduling
   d. New patient scheduling

3. [LO 4.3] While opening mail for a medical office, the administrative medical assistant scans the correspondence and places a sticky note on items needing the physician's attention. This is called

    a. first-class mail handling.

    b. date-stamping the mail.

    c. annotating.

    d. reading the mail with an optical character reader.

4. [LO 4.1, LO 4.2] While triaging a patient over the phone, the AMA learned the patient had "a really deep cut on the inside of the upper thigh and there was blood everywhere." The patient stated he was not able to stop the bleeding. The patient should be advised to

    a. come to the office since the wound may become infected.

    b. go immediately to the emergency department because he may have cut into an artery.

    c. elevate the leg above his heart and see if the bleeding decreases.

    d. schedule an appointment for the following morning.

5. [LO 4.2] During the monthly office meeting, the method of scheduling appointments was discussed. The patients frequently had wait times in excess of 2 hours and were very upset by the time the physician saw them. The practice is a large community clinic that uses wave scheduling. Which of the following scheduling methods may be a better alternative for the clinic?

    a. Scheduled appointments in the morning for call-in patients and open hours in the afternoon

    b. Wave scheduling with double- and triple-booking of patients at the top of each hour

    c. There is no better scheduling method.

    d. Seeing fewer patients

6. [LO 4.3] When processing incoming mail, the assistant should do all of the following except

    a. date-stamp the correspondence.

    b. attach needed patient data to correspondence.

    c. refrain from opening the physician's mail marked "Confidential."

    d. place received checks in different locations.

7. [LO 4.3] Kendra works in an abortion clinic and has been asked to develop a proactive plan for safe mail handling. Her recommendations include receiving all mail in one location, developing a list of risk identifiers, and establishing protocol for suspicious mail. Based on *Best Practices for Safe Mail Handling,* which of the following should be added to Kendra's plan?

    a. Remove all coffee cups from the mail-receiving area.

    b. Establish a uniform time for processing mail.

    c. Open all mail, regardless of whether or not it is marked "Personal" or "Confidential."

    d. Require all mail handlers to wear protective gear, such as surgical gloves, goggles, and masks.

8. [LO 4.1] When faxing PHI, which of the following should the medical office assistant do prior to faxing the documents?

    a. Send a release of information with the fax cover document.

    b. Contact the entity to whom the transmitted information is to be faxed.

    c. Request a signed return receipt of the faxed information.

    d. All of these.

9. [LO 4.2] Alianna has missed four consecutive appointments with Dr. Larsen without notifying the office or rescheduling. Documentation in Alianna's chart should show a(n) _____ notation.

a. no-show
b. new patient
c. established patient
d. triaged patient

10. [LO 4.2] Faith called the office to schedule an annual exam with Dr. Larsen. Her last visit was 4 years ago. Faith should be scheduled as a(n)

a. established patient.
b. no-show patient.
c. new patient.
d. reestablished patient.

THINKING IT THROUGH

These questions cover important points in this chapter. Using your critical-thinking skills, play the role of an administrative medical assistant as you answer each question. Be prepared to discuss your responses.

1. [LO 4.3] State four important procedures in opening and sorting the mail.
2. [LO 4.3] What steps would you take to investigate the lowest-cost shipping method for a small package that must be delivered overnight?
3. [LO 4.1] A patient calls at 11:15 A.M. on a Tuesday morning to say that she has slipped on the ice while going out to get her mail and may have fractured her wrist. There is a good deal of pain and swelling. Her son is available to drive her to the office. You check today's schedule and find that it is full. What is the best way to respond to the patient?

Chapter 5

Managing Health Information

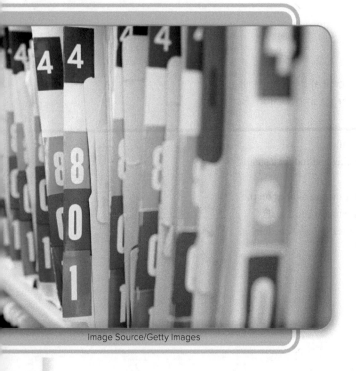

Image Source/Getty Images

LEARNING OUTCOMES

After studying this chapter, you will be able to

5.1 classify various uses of computer technology.

5.2 recall reasons for maintaining a medical chart and documents that comprise the medical chart.

5.3 discuss the advantages and challenges of electronic health records.

5.4 list three commonly used medical abbreviations and three medical abbreviations targeted for nonuse by the Joint Commission.

5.5 discuss various input technologies used to create medical documentation.

5.6 identify components of a paper-based medical record and explain how the same components will be compiled in an electronic health record format.

5.7 distinguish among active, inactive, and closed files.

5.8 differentiate among records management systems that may be used in a medical office.

KEY TERMS

Study these important words, which are defined in this chapter, to build your professional vocabulary:

accession book	coding	folders	laptop
active files	color-coding	graphics application	lateral files
AHIMA	cross-reference sheet	guide	mainframe
alphabetic filing	database	history of present	Meaningful use
application software	dead storage	illness (HPI)	medicolegal
ARMA	diagnosis (Dx)	impression	microcomputer
assessment	electronic health	inactive files	micrographics
CHEDDAR	records (EHRs)	indexing	minicomputer
chief complaint (CC)	e-mail	inspecting documents	mobile-aisle files
closed files	family history (FH)	Internet	networking
cloud computing	file server	label	numeric filing

objective
online
open-shelf files
operating system
out guide
output device
password
past medical history (PMH)
physical exam (PE)
plan

problem-oriented medical
   record (POMR)
records management
release mark
retention
review of systems (ROS)
rule out (R/O)
scribe
SOAP
social history (SH)

sorting
spreadsheet programs
storing
subject filing
subjective
supercomputers
tab cuts
tabs
template
transcription

vertical carousel files
vertical files
virus (computer)
voice-recognition
   technology
wireless communication
word processing program

ABHES

3.d. Define and use medical abbreviations when appropriate and acceptable.

4.a. Follow documentation guidelines.

4.b.1. Institute federal and state guidelines when releasing medical records or information.

4.f. Comply with federal, state, and local health laws and regulations as they relate to healthcare settings.

4.f.3. Comply with Meaningful Use regulations.

4.h. Demonstrate compliance with HIPAA guidelines, the ADA Amendments Act, and the Health Information Technology and Economic and Clinical Health (HITECH) Act.

5.f. Demonstrate an understanding of the core competencies for interprofessional collaborative practice (i.e., values/ethics; roles/responsibilities; interprofessional communication; teamwork).

5.h. Display effective interpersonal skills with patients and healthcare team members.

7.a. Gather and process documents.

7.b. Navigate electronic health records systems and practice management software.

10.b. Demonstrate professional behavior.

www.abhes.org/accreditationmanual

The ABHES standards appear with permission of The Accrediting Bureau of Health Education Schools

CAAHEP

V.C.8. Discuss applications of electronic technology in professional communications.

V.C.16. Differentiate between subjective and objective information.

V.P.3. Use medical terminology correctly and pronounce accurately to communicate information to providers and patients.

V.P.8. Compose professional correspondence utilizing electronic technology.

V.P.11. Report relevant information concisely and accurately.

VI.C.4. Define types of information contained in the patient's medical record.

VI.C.5.a. Identify methods of organizing patient's medical records based on problem-oriented medical record (POMR).

VI.C.5.b. Identify methods of organizing patient's medical records based on source-oriented medical record (SOMR).

VI.C.6.a. Identify equipment and supplies needed for medical records in order to create.

VI.C.6.b. Identify equipment and supplies needed for medical records in order to maintain.

VI.C.6.c. Identify equipment and supplies needed for medical records in order to store.

VI.C.7. Describe filing indexing rules.

VI.C.8. Differentiate between electronic medical records (EMRs) and a practice management system.

VI.C.11. Explain the importance of data backup.

VI.C.12. Explain Meaningful Use as it applies to EMRs.

VI.P.3. Create a patient's medical record.

VI.P.4. Organize a patient's medical record.

VI.P.5. File patient medical records.

VI.P.7. Input patient data utilizing a practice management system.

X.C.11.b. Describe the process in compliance reporting errors in patient care.

X.P.2.a. Apply HIPAA rules in regard to privacy.

X.P.2.b Apply HIPAA rules in regard to release of information.

X.P.3. Document patient care accurately in the medical record.

X.A.2. Protect the integrity of the medical record.

2015 Standards and Guidelines for the Accreditation of Educational Programs in Medical Assisting, Appendix B, Core Curriculum for Medical Assistants, Medical Assisting Education Review Board (MAERB), 2015.

INTRODUCTION

There are three main categories of records found in medical facilities: (1) hardcopy (paper) and electronic medical records of the patient's state of health, (2) correspondence pertaining to the field of healthcare, and (3) documents related to the business and financial management of the practice. Management of these records is the topic of this chapter.

5.1   COMPUTER USAGE

Today's medical environment requires an administrative medical assistant to possess skill and knowledge of computer functions and related programs. Following are five areas where computers are commonly used in the medical office:

- Scheduling
- Creation and maintenance of patients' medical records
- Communications
- Billing, collections, claims, and financial reporting
- Clinical work

Scheduling

Electronic maintenance of the medical office schedule provides advantages over paper appointment books. Ease of searching for and scheduling/rescheduling appointments, daily appointment list printouts, and tracking no-show patients are just a few examples. Computerized scheduling is discussed in detail in the Office Communications: Phone, Scheduling, and Mail chapter. Figure 5.1 shows an electronic appointment schedule.

Creation and Maintenance of Patients' Medical Records

A medical record contains all the office's information about a patient, such as medical history, physician notes, medical reports, x-rays, charts, and correspondence. Medical practices use computers to handle some or all parts of patients' medical records. In most medical offices, the records are completely electronic. With electronic health records, there are no actual paper records. All data about a patient, including x-ray images, lab test results, medical history, and so on, are created and stored on a computer. Electronic health records will be discussed later in this chapter.

Communications

Computers are used in the medical office to handle many communications tasks. An assistant needs to be familiar with the use of the following:

- Word processing
- E-mail
- Computer networks
- The Internet
- Wireless communication

HIPAA *TIPS*

HIPAA regulations require medical offices to prevent unauthorized users from accessing office computers. Virus detection and elimination software, firewall technology, and intrusion detection tools will all assist in serving this purpose by keeping unauthorized users from violating HIPAA.

Why is it important to never share your password with other employees?

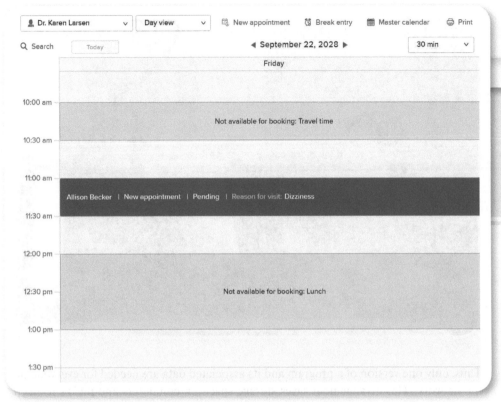

Figure 5.1

Electronic schedulers like EHRclinic are used in many medical offices. *In what ways do such programs make the administrative medical assistant more efficient?*

Word Processing. A **word processing program** is used to enter, edit, format, and print documents. A word processor can handle all the written correspondence an assistant usually creates: referral letters, consultation reports, routine letters about appointments or test reports, interoffice memorandums, and standard forms and reports. In addition, the assistant may use a word processor in conjunction with a dictation machine to transcribe medical records, letters, reports, and articles.

A development in computer application programs that directly affects word processing and medical dictation is the improvement of voice-recognition software, which is discussed later in this chapter.

E-Mail. A second communications tool widely used in the medical office is electronic mail, or **e-mail,** a telecommunications system for exchanging written messages through a computer network. E-mail is discussed in the Office Communications: An Overview of Verbal and Written Communication chapter.

Computer Networks. A third type of communications tool used in a medical office is a computer network. A network links local (not Internet-based) computers together, so that software, hardware, and data files can be shared. **Networking** provides a means of communicating, exchanging information, and pooling resources among a group of computers. A user who goes **online** is connecting to a computer network. Networks provide

- simultaneous access to programs and files.
- a simple backup process.
- sharing of computer devices.

In a network, a central computer, called a **file server** (or, simply, a *server*), stores the computer programs and data to be shared by all the computers in the network. Network versions of software programs provide users simultaneous access to programs and data.

COMPLIANCE *TIP*

Protecting confidentiality when releasing information through e-mail is as critical as with any other communication method. The assistant should check that a current release is on file for the information that is being shared.

Figure 5.2

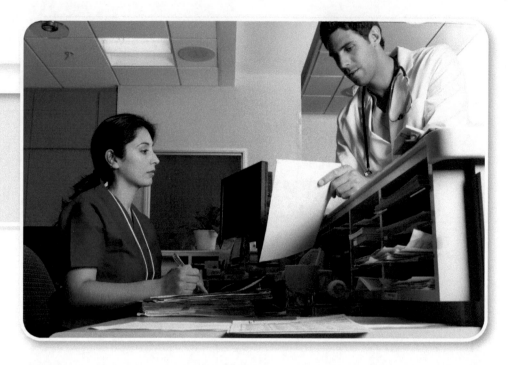

Thus, only one version of a program and its associated data are needed for everyone on the network. This arrangement saves storage space on computers and makes it much easier to keep track of information, because all information is stored in one place. In addition, computer data, such as patient billing information, can be used by more than one person at a time. If the computers are not linked together in a network, only one person can access a file at a time. In a large office that manages a high volume of data, this would be highly inefficient. Similarly, at the end of the day, an extra copy of all data for safekeeping (a backup copy) can be obtained by creating a duplicate of the data on the file server, rather than on many separate machines. This procedure saves time and introduces fewer errors, because one person, usually the file server manager, is in charge of all backups.

Computers in a network are also able to share external devices, such as printers. Normally, every computer that does not operate within a network has its own external devices. If the computers are connected through a network, several computers can share the same equipment. This arrangement is less expensive for the office.

The Internet. An administrative medical assistant should also be familiar with the use of the Internet as a communications tool. The **Internet** is an enormous computer network that links computers and smaller computer networks worldwide. The Internet connects millions of computers around the world, making it possible to exchange information in seconds. The information that is shared can be text, graphics, sound, video, and even whole computer programs.

Use of the Internet in the medical office continues to expand. Transmitting health claim information, accessing third-party insurance websites to determine a patient's coverage, researching medical data, obtaining travel fares, and ordering medical supplies are just a few of the unlimited uses of the Internet. Assistants use Internet search engines, such as Google, Bing, Twitter, and Yahoo!, to locate information they need. Key words and phrases are used to retrieve data from various Internet sources. Online medical databases are used to educate physicians concerning conditions and treatment regimens. Patients are also able to research medical topics and educate themselves as consumers of healthcare.

Another aspect for Internet usage is **cloud computing.** The "cloud" is similar to the Internet. Data and programs are accessed and linked (also known as *synched*) through an Internet-based application. Multiple people can use the information on the cloud to perform needed tasks. Cloud-based applications can be used anywhere and anytime as long as Internet connection is available. It can be used for processing data within the cloud and/or for storing, backing up, and synchronizing data, such as for backing up local computer information to cloud storage. Many cloud applications utilize all of these tasks. Examples of cloud-based applications include Office Online, Dropbox, GoogleDocs, and Apple iCloud.

Medical offices also used cloud-based applications to perform clinical, as well as administrative, tasks. Prior to using a cloud-based medical office application, or any cloud program housing PHI, verify that the program meets national specifications, criteria, and standards to be certified by the Office of the National Coordinator for Health Information Technology (ONCHIT; usually abbreviated just *ONC*) and that the program is HIPAA compliant. An example of an ONC-certified medical office cloud program is Practice Fusion.

EXAMPLES: CLOUD COMPUTING

Example 1

At 11 A.M., Dr. Larsen asked you to update the patient information form to include the patient's e-mail and mobile phone contact information and preferred communication language. She also listed several other changes to be made on the form. She needs to view the changes by 3 P.M. today. You previously scheduled to be out of the office all afternoon in order to attend your child's Parent Luncheon. After the luncheon, using a cloud-based program, you make all the changes. Dr. Larsen views the changes using the same cloud-based program and makes comments on other needed changes. You and Dr. Larsen are able to communicate on the changes simultaneously, and the 3 P.M. deadline is met.

Example 2

You are sick and cannot come to work today. Using an ONC-certified, cloud-based medical office program, you are able to view patients' appointments, Dr. Larsen's clinical notes (to validate medical codes), and today's charges; verify patient insurance coverage; and process medical insurance claims from home. No time is lost in the revenue cycle due to sickness.

Wireless Communication. All networks require some type of material to send data from one computer to another. In network communications, these materials are referred to as *media.* Types of media currently in use include twisted-pair wire, which is made of copper, and fiber-optic cable, made of a thin strand of glass that transmits pulsating beams of light. A newer form of communications system, referred to as **wireless communication,** or wireless connectivity, uses radio waves, rather than wires or cables, as the medium for transmitting data. Cell phones and wireless Internet connections, known as WiFi, are examples of wireless communication. Wireless communication networks should be password-protected to prohibit unauthorized users from accessing the wireless network. To better protect PHI, public domain WiFi should not be used to access patient data. Wireless communication will be discussed in more detail later in this chapter.

Billing, Collections, Claims, and Financial Reporting

Computers are used in medical offices to manage financial records. Computers were originally invented as tools for working with numbers. This makes them well suited for managing financial accounts. Computers are often used in the medical office for

- billing and collections.
- electronic transmission of insurance claims.
- financial records relating to the operation of the office, such as employee records, payroll, accounts payable, and legal financial data.

Billing and Collections. Most medical offices use a medical billing program to keep track of patients' accounts. It is important for any business to keep track of its funds. Accurate financial records are required for tax reporting and are critical for the practice's success. Without them, the business's owners do not know whether they will meet their financial obligations each month and whether the business is working at a profit or loss.

It is the administrative medical assistant's job to see that every patient is billed appropriately and that insurance claims are submitted for patients who have health insurance. It is also the responsibility of the assistant to see that payments received from patients and insurance carriers are properly recorded. A medical billing program is designed to keep track of the constant flow of bills and payments between patients, the medical practice, and insurance companies. Figure 5.3 shows a Patient Account Ledger report.

Although different medical offices use various types of software to keep track of patient accounts, all medical accounting systems require certain types of information. They are designed to use **databases,** which are collections of related data, such as the following:

- *Patient data.* The program's patient database contains information about each patient.
- *Transaction data.* The program's transaction database contains information about each patient's visits.

Electronic Transmission of Insurance Claims. One of the most important tasks of an administrative medical assistant is the creation of health insurance claims. When a patient with health insurance visits the office, a health insurance claim must be submitted

---

Figure 5.3

A Patient Account Ledger provides information about a patient's charges. *What kinds of numerical errors can be eliminated by using a computer program?*

Karen Larsen MD
Patient Account Ledger
As of October 31, 2028

Show all data where the Date From is between 10/1/2028, 10/31/2028

Entry	Date	POS	Description	Procedure	Document	Provider	Amount
AA001 Monica Armstrong				(312)555-4413			
		Last Payment: 0.00	On:				
218	10/17/2028	11		99212	1310310000	1	44.00
219	10/17/2028	11		80048	1310310000	1	51.00
220	10/17/2028	11		83001	1310310000	1	97.00
221	10/17/2028	11		85025	1310310000	1	25.00
222	10/17/2028	11		81001	1310310000	1	24.00
						Patient Total:	241.00
AA003 Sara Babcock				(312)555-5441			
		Last Payment: 0.00	On:				
226	10/18/2028	11		99395	1310310000	1	136.00
227	10/18/2028	11		85018	1310310000	1	13.00
228	10/18/2028	11		80061	1310310000	1	72.00
229	10/18/2028	11		88150	1310310000	1	33.00
230	10/18/2028	11		81001	1310310000	1	24.00
						Patient Total:	278.00
AA008 Doris Casagranda				(312)555-1200			
		Last Payment: 0.00	On:				
233	10/17/2028	11		99212	1703160000	1	44.00
						Patient Total:	44.00

to the patient's insurance company, describing the date of the visit, the diagnosis, the procedures performed, the cost of each procedure, payments made by the patient, and so on. On the basis of this information, the insurance company determines how much, if anything, the insurer owes the practice and/or the patient. A medical billing program helps the assistant generate health insurance claims and can be used to send the claims to insurance companies electronically. Filing claims electronically costs less than mailing printed forms, allows almost instantaneous submission, and creates an audit trail of submitted claims from the provider. The receiver (insurance payer) transmits a report of received claims back to the provider. Missing electronic claims can then be retransmitted to the insurance payer. Faster payments from insurance payers are received through electronic fund transfers (EFTs) into the provider's account.

Financial Records Relating to the Operation of the Office. In addition to keeping track of patients' accounts, computer programs can be used to keep track of office operations. Like any business, a medical office must keep employee records, pay its employees (payroll) and suppliers, and maintain financial legal files. Computer programs are available to help in the creation and management of such records.

Clinical Work

Clinical use of computers in the medical office is changing rapidly. Even simple procedures, such as recording a patient's pulse, blood pressure, or weight or conducting a simple auditory test (which used to be performed by a doctor using handheld instruments), are now carried out with the help of computerized equipment. The variety of computers used in the field of radiology alone is staggering, from simple x-ray machines to specialized equipment designed to improve data gathering, such as digital mammography (x-rays of the breast).

Medical labs, such as pathology labs and blood labs, also rely heavily on computers. Computers are required for administering tests, extracting results, and outputting test data. Indeed, the use of electronic medical records has been a natural outgrowth of the widespread clinical use of computers in the health industry.

Physician research today also takes advantage of computers. Physicians conduct research to help with patient care, to prepare papers for lectures, and to write articles for journals. In the past, physicians conducting research turned to medical textbooks, journals, case studies, and other materials found in a medical library. Today, much of the same material can be accessed with the help of a computer.

Each office should have an acceptable use policy (AUP) for equipment, time, and other resources, including the computer. Acceptable use policies should be written and included in the office's policy and procedure manual. However, the policy may be unstated. It is best practice to recognize that all hardware, software, and connectivity belong to the practice. Personal use of company-owned resources should be avoided.

Computer Categories

Many of the specifications that have usually separated one type of computer from another are becoming harder to define. The smallest computers used today have processing powers that rival the processing powers of the largest computers made less than a decade ago. The terms used to describe the major categories of computers—*supercomputer, mainframe, minicomputer,* and *personal computer*—have remained the same, but the capabilities of each group continue to change dramatically.

Supercomputers. **Supercomputers** are the most powerful computers available. They are designed to process huge amounts of data. Because of their ability to process intensive computations, supercomputers are used in fields such as weather forecasting, government security, and molecular modeling. Supercomputers are extremely expensive, costing many millions of dollars.

Mainframe Computers. **Mainframes** are used in large businesses, hospitals, large clinics, and government organizations. They store massive databases, which many users can access at the same time. Mainframes are most often used in conjunction with computer terminals. A mainframe computer terminal is a workstation that consists of a keyboard and screen. A computer terminal does not have its own processing unit or storage, since it uses the processing unit and storage of the mainframe to which it is connected, which may be close or miles away.

Minicomputers. **Minicomputers** have less power than mainframes. Some minicomputers are designed for single users, but many operate with tens or even hundreds of terminals. In size and shape, minicomputers resemble a large file cabinet. They are popular in all kinds of businesses because they have many of the features of a mainframe but are not as big or nearly as expensive.

Microcomputers. Most computer users are more familiar with the microcomputer than with any other type. **Microcomputers,** also called personal computers (PCs), come in many sizes and shapes. Those that are designed to sit on a desk are called desktop computers. To save space on the desktop, some models, called *tower models,* are designed so that the system unit stands vertically on the floor. Portable or mobile models that are designed to fit into a briefcase or pocket are notebook computers, personal digital assistants, tablet PCs, or **laptops.** These mobile devices have the popular feature of being able to run on plug-in current or batteries. "Smart" devices are also making their presence known in the medical environment. Smartphones are being used to transmit medical data from patient to physician and to conduct a virtual office visit. Other applications are used by the patient to take his or her own electrocardiogram (ECG), interpret the results, and send a report to the physician. Blood pressure readings can be measured using a smart device, such as a smart watch or wristband. In the future, smart devices will be used more extensively in the medical environment. Figure 5.4 illustrates a physician using a portable device.

Ergonomics

Ergonomics is the science of designing the work environment to meet the needs of the human body. Ergonomics theories are finding practical application in computerized offices because of the number of injuries associated with working long hours on computers. The physical ailments that can result from long hours at a computer are known as *cumulative trauma disorders* or *repetitive stress injuries.*

Two hardware components—the keyboard and the monitor—are especially problematic. Figure 5.5 shows an ergonomic keyboard. A person who spends long periods at a computer performing repetitive movements should take frequent breaks. It is also a good idea to stretch the wrists and upper body at given intervals to avoid such problems as carpal tunnel syndrome and frozen shoulders. Following are a number of ergonomic tips to help computer users avoid the stress and strain that often result from working on a computer:

- Position the monitor at or below eye level, between 2 and 2.5 feet away, to avoid unnecessary neck strain and eyestrain.
- Use a copyholder to hold up any papers you need to refer to, and place it at eye level, a comfortable distance from your eyes (about 1.5 feet away), to avoid neck strain and eyestrain. Do not place papers flat on the desk, which forces you to keep your neck bent for long periods of time.

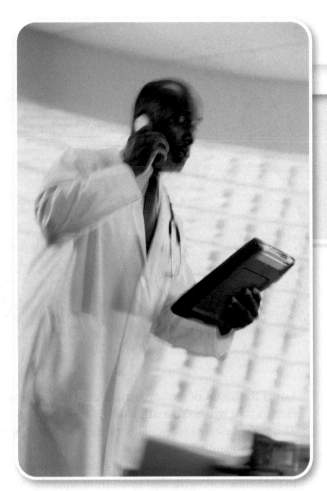

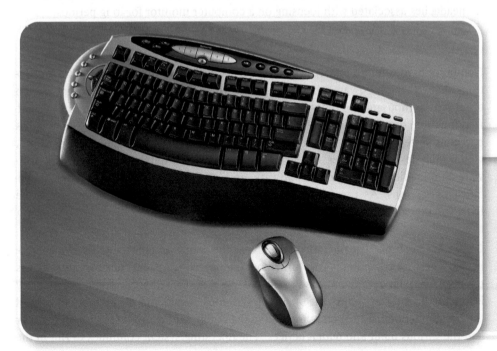

Figure 5.6

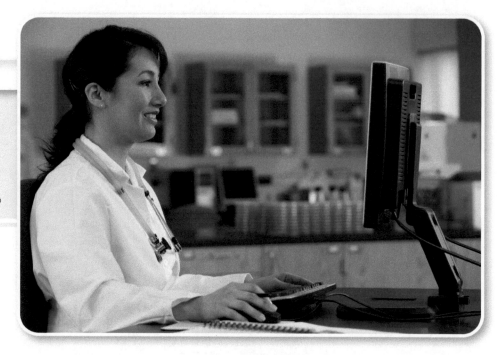

Maintaining the correct position for keyboarding reduces strain. *How can incorrect keyboarding techniques affect a computer user?*
Huntstock/Alamy Stock Photo

- Lower the height of the keyboard, if necessary, so that your hands are at the same level as your wrists. Your arms should be relaxed and forearms parallel to the floor. This is the best way to avoid injuring your wrists. Figure 5.6 is an example of proper keyboarding ergonomics.
- Hand and wrist supports are highly recommended to prevent the fatigue and stress to the hands and wrists that result from repetitive motions at the keyboard or with a mouse.
- Adjust the height and tilt of the chair, so that both feet are flat on the floor and your back is properly supported. Arm rests are recommended for office chairs.
- Focus your eyes on distant objects at regular intervals to avoid the eyestrain and headaches associated with focusing on a computer monitor for long periods.

Computer Software

Computer hardware, no matter how powerful, is useless without software, the instructions that tell the hardware what to do. Since there are many things a computer can do, there are thousands of types of software. Before the software performs any specialized function, however, such as word processing or claims transmitting, the computer's **operating system** gets the computer running and keeps it working. **Application software,** which includes word processing, graphics, spreadsheet, database management software, and medical-office-specific software, applies the computer's capabilities to specific applications. As previously discussed, application software programs may be local (on the computer's network system) or cloud-based.

Operating System. The operating system tells the computer how to use its own components. When the computer is first turned on, the operating system runs various self-tests to check what devices are attached to the computer and whether the computer memory is functioning properly. Next, the operating system is loaded into the memory to control the basic functions of the computer, telling the computer how to interact with the user and the various input and **output devices.** The operating system continues to run in the background until the computer is turned off. The administrative medical assistant who uses computers regularly should know what operating system the computer uses, in case technical help is required. It is also important for the assistant to keep up-to-date with new versions of the operating system and learn how to take advantage of them.

Word Processing Programs. Most computer users are familiar with word processing programs. Microsoft Word, Corel WordPerfect, and Apple iWork Pages are examples of popular word processing programs. In addition to allowing the user to enter, edit, and format text quickly and easily, a word processor can be used to create templates. A **template** is a standard version of a document that is used over and over. It is altered slightly for each new document and saves the assistant the time required to key and format each document anew. Word processors also have features for checking spelling and grammar. Spell-checkers are used to verify the spelling of words in a document before proofreading. The assistant can add words, such as uncommon medical terms for a given specialty that come up often in a physician's notes and/or dictation, to a customized dictionary in the computer. The spell-checker will include these words each time it checks a document for spelling errors.

Graphics Applications. A **graphics application** allows the user to manipulate images. Some graphics programs, called *paint or draw programs,* allow the user to create illustrations from scratch electronically. Others are designed to mix and match already created images, text, video, sound, and animation.

Another type of graphics application, which is more likely to be used in a medical office, is presentation software. Microsoft PowerPoint, Corel Presentation, and Apple iWork Keynote are examples of presentation software. It can be used to create professional-looking visual aids for presentation to an audience. These aids include photographic transparencies; paper printouts, such as cover sheets, colored graphs, and charts; and computer slide shows.

Spreadsheet Programs. **Spreadsheet programs,** such as Microsoft Excel and Apple iWork Numbers, are designed to imitate paper bookkeeping ledgers. An electronic spreadsheet is a grid made up of rows and columns. Each box on the grid is a cell, and each cell has an address. For example, the address for the cell at the intersection of Column D and Row 3 is D3. By keying a combination of text labels, numeric data, and mathematical formulas into the cells, the user controls which calculations are to be carried out where in the spreadsheet. The result is that any number of calculations can be carried out at great speed. Anyone in charge of creating and maintaining a budget will find a spreadsheet program indispensable.

In a medical office, spreadsheets can be used for any activity involving numbers—for example, to keep track of supplies or to prepare budgets. Personnel departments often use spreadsheets to track wages and salaries paid to employees.

Database Management Software. Database management software helps the user enter data into a database and then sort the data into useful subsets of information. A number of database management programs are popular for personal computers, such as Microsoft Access and Oracel Database. Organizations that handle specialized data require custom-made database management programs to meet their needs.

The four categories of application software discussed—word processing, graphics, spreadsheets, and database management—are perhaps the most widely used of all computer applications. Each type of software may be purchased separately, or an integrated software package—also called an "office suite"—may be bought. An integrated package combines several application programs.

Other categories of software generally include desktop publishing software, entertainment and education software, utilities software, and communications software. Utilities software helps with the upkeep and maintenance of the computer. Communications software is used to set up a network, for example, or connect to an Internet service provider.

Computer Security and Patient Confidentiality

Although everyone working in a medical office must maintain the strict confidentiality of patients' medical records, proper treatment and billing often require information from these records to be released to insurance companies, other medical facilities, or other physicians. Because much of the information used in healthcare is stored and accessed using computers, special care must be taken to preserve the confidentiality of computerized patient information and to maintain HIPAA Security Rule compliance. Following are ways a medical office can take to safeguard computerized information.

Screen Savers. Assistants and other office workers should not leave their desks and allow a computer screen showing information about a patient to remain visible. If a worker must be away from the desk for short periods of time regularly, a screen saver can be used to protect data from being seen by others. Screen savers are programs that display moving images on the screen if no input is received for several minutes. As soon as input resumes, the moving images disappear.

Passwords for Limited Access. The use of electronic health records raises questions about who should have access to such files and how the information in them can be safeguarded, so that it does not end up where it does not belong. Often, the information in an electronic health record is highly confidential, since it contains all the details of a case, including a patient's medical history, the patient's ledger, insurance information, and other patient PHI.

One security measure for safeguarding computerized information is the use of passwords. **Passwords** are assigned to limit the number of individuals who have access to particular computer files and to help users create a computerized audit trail. They are changed on a regular basis to assist with maintaining security and should never be shared.

Virus Checkers. A **virus (computer)** is a program written with the intent of damaging another user's data, software, or computer. Generally, the virus is buried in a legitimate program or file. By running the program or using the file, the user unknowingly activates the virus. Viruses can be programmed to do many things, such as destroy data or erase an entire hard drive. One way of contracting viruses is by downloading unknown programs or files from the Internet. Trojans, viruses hidden inside a seemingly safe file (like the mythical Trojan horse), are activated when the "safe" file is used. A worm virus will "eat" its way through a computer program or system. Trojans and worm viruses are examples of *malware* (malicious software).

A virus checker is a utilities program that periodically searches a computer system for viruses. Antivirus software is designed to root out a virus before it does damage. Antivirus programs check every file on a storage drive and can be set up to check periodically or continuously. If they find infected files or suspicious programs, they attempt to remove them. Because so many viruses are sent through the Internet as e-mail or attached files, it is best to set up the virus checker to receive updated virus-detection information from the manufacturer's Internet site at least once per week. The virus checker automatically downloads information on new viruses that have been identified and runs the check to detect their presence on the computer system.

Safeguards for Electronic Claims Transmission. Online systems should use a form of encryption to safeguard data that are being transmitted electronically. Encryption is a method of turning data into unintelligible gibberish during transmission. The recipient of the data must have a method of decrypting in order to read the medical data, such as a password or secret key. Encrypted data is referred to as *cipher text;* unencrypted data is referred to as *plain text.*

Electronic signature systems should also be used to maintain the security of transmitted data in a medical practice. Electronic signature systems, which are regulated by state authorities, are used with electronic health records and electronic prescriptions, as well as for electronic claims transmission. Similar to a password system, an electronic signature system identifies the sender and the recipient of the data being sent. It locks the document, so that it can be opened only by the intended recipient, who has the unlocking key.

One way of protecting data transmitted over the Internet is to use a firewall. A firewall is a software program developed specifically to prevent outside parties from gaining access to particular areas of an organization's computer files. Another means of protecting files is the use of some combination of passwords, encryption, and electronic signatures.

Standard Release-of-Information Forms. Electronic health records must be kept as confidential as any other type of medical record. Therefore, a signed and dated release-of-information form must be on file before an electronic record can be transmitted or disclosed for purposes other than TPO. As with paper-based records, the release of information should be limited to the purpose mentioned in the request, so that only the portion of the medical records specifically requested is transmitted. Similarly, any conditions about when the permission expires, such as "permission expires in 60 days," must be carefully met. Further discussion of release-of-information forms can be found in the Medical Ethics, Law, and Compliance chapter.

Full Disclosure Policy. It is a good practice for the medical office to display a written policy on who has access to patients' medical records, as well as what that level of access is. Informing patients of such a policy protects the medical practice from potential lawsuits.

Inspection of Audit Trails. Another security measure that is used with computerized patient data is the periodic inspection of a data entry log. The inspection is usually done by the chief compliance officer or the practice manager. Whenever new information is entered or existing data in a database are changed, the computer records the time and date of the entry, as well as the name of the computer operator. This computer record creates an audit trail that can be used to trace unauthorized actions to the responsible person.

Backing Up Data. There are many unpredictable ways computer files can be lost or destroyed. A hard drive failure, power surge, or destructive computer virus can wipe out weeks of work. Every computer system should have a regular procedure for backing up data to safeguard against lost or corrupted files. On a network, the person in charge of managing the file server takes charge of backing up files. System backups should be made through a specialized program and stored off-site, through an online backup storage service, or in the cloud. On stand-alone (independently operated) computers, each user is responsible. On a personal computer, for instance, a full backup copy of all files should be made no less than once or twice a month. Partial backups of files that have been worked on in the course of a day should be made at the end of every day. External storage devices may be purchased and used to back up personal computers. As with system backups, personal computer backups should be stored off-site. Backup can also

COMPLIANCE *TIP*

The medical practice's data entry log should be examined on a regular basis to check for any irregularities or suspicious activity. This procedure is particularly important if the computer used for data entry is part of a network, since people outside the medical office may be able to gain access to the information and alter it. Evidence of data entry log compliance should be recorded in the Compliance Plan.

be done through the Cloud. Cloud storage capacity varies and can be changed as the needs of the medical practice change. Although backing up files this often may seem extreme, it is important to consider the potential loss.

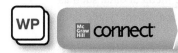

GO TO PROJECT 5.1 AND PROJECT 5.2
AT THE END OF THIS CHAPTER

5.2 THE MEDICAL RECORD

The patient medical record, also referred to as the patient's "chart" or "file," is the source of information about all aspects of a patient's healthcare. Accurate, up-to-date medical records are vital to a medical practice. Current records are necessary for enabling a continuum of care for patients, for financial and legal success, and for research purposes. It is not surprising, therefore, that one of the most important skills an administrative medical assistant can demonstrate is the ability to maintain accurate, complete medical records. In working with medical records, the assistant should be familiar with

- medical records as legal documents.
- the types of reports and information typically found in a medical record.
- the importance of well-maintained medical records for the practice.
- the method for making corrections to a medical record.

Medical Records as Legal Documents

A patient's medical record constitutes the legal record of the medical practice. On occasion, patients' records may have to be produced in court, either to uphold the rights of the physician if the physician is involved in litigation or to substantiate a patient's claim if the physician is called as a witness. In malpractice cases, the content and quality of a medical record can be pivotal, leaving a greater impression on a jury, it is said, than even the physician's credentials, personality, or reputation. For this reason, medical files are often referred to as **medicolegal** documents, providing documentation of medical care and being admissible in a court of law. If the data in a medical record are incomplete, illegible, or poorly maintained, a plaintiff's attorney may be able to make even the best patient care appear negligent. Therefore, it is important for the administrative medical assistant to help the physician maintain medical records as carefully as possible. The assistant should bear in mind that any record could become a vehicle for defending a clinical course of action down the road.

What Is in a Medical Record?

A patient's medical record holds all the data about that patient. Medical records generally include the following items.

- *Chart notes:* A chronological record of ongoing patient care and progress, chart notes are entries made by the physician, the nurse, or another healthcare professional regarding pertinent points of a given visit or communication with the patient. The chart notes for a new patient may be extensive, often containing the details of a comprehensive medical history and physical. Thereafter, chart notes may simply describe changes in the patient's condition or treatment plan. Figure 5.7 is an example of a simple chart note, entered by a registered nurse, regarding a phone call from a patient. Additionally, chart notes forwarded by other providers are included in the patient's records (e.g., immunization record from a previous pediatrician).

```
                           CHART NOTE


        Jackson, Alma
        DOB: 09/06/19--
        AA014


        8/3/20--
        Patient called today regarding lab results from last week.
        Explained to patient that the lab tests were sent to an
        outside lab, and Dr. Larsen will contact her with the results
        when they are received.



        Karen Latter

        Karen Latter, RN
```

Figure 5.7

Chart Note Regarding a
Phone Call from a Patient

- *History and physical (H&P): History* refers to the patient's complete medical history (usually obtained by the nurse, assistant, or physician during an interview with the patient on his or her first visit); *physical* refers to the objective evaluation of relevant body areas or systems based on the patient's medical history.
- *Referral and consultation letters:* Copies of letters sent to or received from other physicians referring the patient for specific examinations, tests, and so on are part of the medical record.
- *Medical reports:* Lab reports, x-ray reports, and reports from procedures such as electrocardiograms are kept in the medical record. The type and number of medical reports in the file depend on the patient's condition and the specialty of the attending physician. After the physician has reviewed the medical report, he or she must sign and date it to document the physician's review of the data.
- *Correspondence:* Copies of all correspondence with the patient, including letters, faxes, and notes of telephone conversations and e-mail messages, are part of the medical record.
- *Clinical forms:* Forms such as immunization records and pediatric growth and development records are included.
- *Medication list:* A list of all medications prescribed, including dosage and dispensing instructions, and a list of the patient's known allergies to medications are in the medical record.
- *Advance directives and other legal forms:* Advance directives, such as a DNR (Do Not Resuscitate) order, living will, and/or a durable power of attorney (medical, financial, or both) are critical components to express the patient's intent for his or her care should the patient not be able to make those decisions for himself or herself. Other legal forms, including legal custody documentation for a minor patient, are also important to maintain in a patient's medical record.

In addition to medical data, the patient's record contains administrative information, such as the patient's personal data (including insurance and billing records), as well as data on the release of information and the assignment of benefits. Medical documents and documentation are typically maintained in reverse chronological order—the most current document on top. Electronic medical documentation is maintained chronologically by the operating system date, which should be the current date.

Reasons for Maintaining Medical Records

Medical records provide the practice with complete information regarding the patient. Thus, they are used as

- the main source of information for coordinating and carrying out patient care among all providers involved with the patient.
- evidence of the course of an illness and a record of the treatment being used, thereby providing a record of medical necessity.
- a record of the quality of care provided to patients.
- a tool for ensuring communication and continuity of care from one medical facility to another.
- the legal record for the practice.
- the main record to ensure appropriate reimbursement.
- a source of data for research purposes—for example, as background material for preparing a lecture, an article, or a book.

Because the medical record is the basis for so many activities in a practice, every effort should be made to maintain it well. The following procedures should be used. Each time the patient is seen by a provider—such as for a blood pressure check or a return visit for a medication, whether in the office or at another location—an entry must be made in the patient's medical record. Entries in a paper-based medical record must be keyed or handwritten in ink. As the sample chart note in Figure 5.7 illustrates, every entry should contain (1) patient identifying information—name, date of birth, and a patient identifier, such as an account number (Social Security Numbers, or any part thereof, should NOT be used in the patient account number); (2) the date of the patient's visit or communication; and (3) the signature and title of the responsible provider or other healthcare professional. If an entry is transcribed, it is signed with the name of the dictator, followed by the initials of the transcriptionist. Two or three lines of space should be left on the record for the dictator's handwritten signature. A signature log should be maintained with the policy manual and updated as employees either leave or join the practice. Physicians in medical offices using electronic medical record entry methods should affix an electronic signature to all chart entries. Electronic signatures should contain the date and the time stamp of when the electronic signature was affixed to the record or document. Phrasing such as "Electronically signed by" or "Reviewed and verified by" usually accompany the electronic signature.

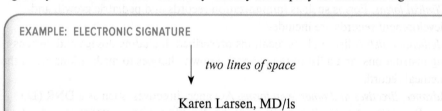

EXAMPLE: ELECTRONIC SIGNATURE

two lines of space

Karen Larsen, MD/ls

Electronically signed by Karen Larsen, MD, 10-23-2028 @ 11:30 A.M.

Entries should be made in a compact way, without leaving large gaps between notes. This eliminates the possibility of someone's tampering with the record later and ensures that the entries will be sequential. It is also important to make entries in a medical record promptly. Frequent delays in making entries will reflect poorly on the provider. Finally, the items should be placed within each section in a consistent chronological order, either ascending or descending.

Making Corrections in Paper-Based Medical Records

Because medical records are legal documents, it is not permissible to correct paper-based records with an eraser or correction fluid or to scribble out entries. Such methods could present the appearance of fraud. The original chart entry must remain legible. If you make an error in a paper-based medical record while recording an entry or discover an error in a paper-based medical record, use the following method to correct it:

- Use the strike-through feature in the word processing program or draw a single line through the incorrect statements in the medical record (making sure the inaccurate material is still legible).
- Enter the word *error* or *mistaken entry* next to the deleted statement or other reason for the correction.
- Write your initials and the date next to the correction.
- Enter the correct information above or below the inserted line in the medical record.

Methods of making corrections in an electronic medical record are discussed in the next section.

COMPLIANCE *TIP*

Remember that no part of a record should be altered, removed, deleted, or destroyed. Only proper correction procedures may be used. Great care must be taken when entering data to ensure that they are inserted in the correct chart. If an error or a discrepancy is discovered in a medical record at a much later date, the physician may dictate an addendum to the record to correct the discrepancy. Remember, any alteration of a medical record may constitute the appearance of fraud, and proper correction procedures should always be followed.

 McGraw Hill connect

GO TO PROJECTS 5.3, 5.4, AND 5.5 AT THE END OF THIS CHAPTER

5.3 ELECTRONIC HEALTH RECORDS (EHRs)

The need to store large amounts of medical data and to protect those data efficiently is a primary concern of the medical and governmental communities. Laws have been passed and large sums of money have been and are being invested in the implementation of healthcare reform. Mandatory implementation of **electronic health records (EHRs)** is part of national healthcare reform. Billions of dollars have been directed to be used as incentives for implementing the use of EHRs. Advances in technology and their subsequent affordability make EHRs accessible to healthcare facilities and physicians' practices. It is estimated that nearly 90 percent of medical offices have adopted and are using some form of an electronic health record system. However, the percentage of healthcare providers using an ONC-*certified* electronic health record system drops to almost 80 percent.

Electronic health records are the assimilation and interoperability (electronic systems working together) of various healthcare databases compiled over the course of different patient encounters. In other words, an EHR is an electronic record kept over the lifetime encounters of a patient. An electronic medical record (EMR) is the record on *one* encounter. Multiple EMRs compile the EHR. However, in the medical environment, *EMR* and *EHR* are often used interchangeably.

Patient demographics, clinical assessment data, lab and other reports, medication lists, progress notes, and other medical data are entered into a software program and then stored electronically, either locally or in cloud storage. The medical database of the patient is retrieved and updated at each patient encounter. The encounter may be face to face, such as when a child comes to the office for an immunization or when the

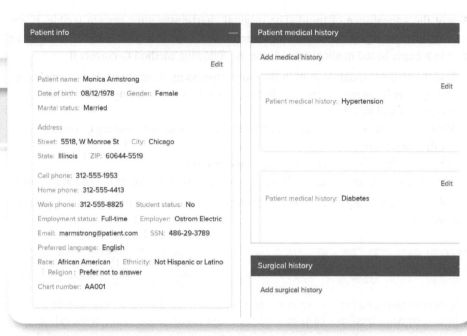

Figure 5.8

EHR Chart Summary Screen

physician visits the patient in a hospital setting, or a virtual encounter, such as when the physician in his or her office uses electronic applications to access a patient who is at a remote location. It may also be a nonvisit update of the patient's database, as when a patient calls to have a prescription refilled. Figure 5.8 shows an example of a chart summary screen within an EHR, and Figure 5.9 is an example of a patient progress note.

Laptops may be in each exam room and/or workstation, or the medical team members may carry a handheld mobile device with them from station to station. Templates and drop-down menus are used to input clinical data into the EHR, with menus providing other selections for administrative office personnel. Space is provided for additional notes and comments. As an example, "blurred vision and headache" may be entered into the

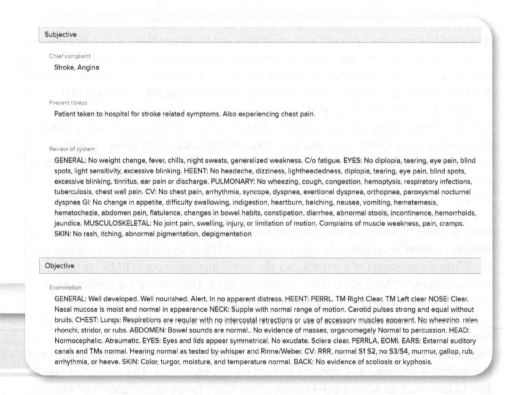

Figure 5.9

EHR Patient Progress Note

chief complaint screen and a drop-down menu of related symptoms may appear. From that point, a screen for review of systems for the cardiovascular system may be provided.

Advantages of Electronic Health Records

EHRs have many advantages over paper-based systems, including accessibility for both medical care personnel and patients. More than one medical team member may use the stored data at the same time. Paper-based records can create a backlog of work when the same patient chart is needed to complete a task for different medical team members. Each medical team member has access to electronic data using an individually assigned password. The password allows the medical personnel access to all, or a limited amount, of the medical database. For example, nurses may have access to all areas of patient assessment but not have authorization to view insurance claim information. Using passwords will also create a usage log and an audit trail of individuals accessing medical data, which will increase record security. As more medical records become accessible through the Internet, patients will have access to areas of their EHR. The following are additional advantages offered by EHRs:

1. Easy and quick updating of medical records
2. Automatic verification of medications
3. Fewer medical misinterpretations due to poor handwriting
4. Higher level of data security by use of passwords, encryption, and frequent backup of medical data; minimum backup requirement is to perform a daily backup, with some practices conducting backups throughout the work shift
5. Greater amount of time spent in patient care as a result of less time spent updating medical records
6. Faster questions and answers related to patient medical information
7. Electronic input and submission of orders and prescriptions
8. Electronic reminders sent either directly to patients or to office personnel for follow-up
9. Access to electronic medical records from multiple locations

Challenges of Electronic Health Records

The advantages of converting from paper-based medical records to electronic health records are many, but making the conversion is not without challenges. For many facilities and private practices, the cost of EHRs is still prohibitive. Initial cost and contract fees can be too costly for healthcare providers. When evaluating EHR software, update of the system should be a consideration. As the field progresses, technologies advance, and government regulations change, it would be cost-effective for the medical practice to be contracted with a software vendor that will provide the mandatory updates to the system for a contracted amount or as part of the initial cost. Before investing in an electronic health records system, seek information from others who have used or are using the system.

Frequent and ongoing training for medical team members is imperative to ensure the integrity of the input data and the security of the system. New computer and other technology is introduced to society at a fast pace, and healthcare providers must look to cutting-edge technology for medical records storage. Policies and procedures for updating medical personnel and evidence of the training should be placed in the Compliance Manual.

Converting paper-based records to electronic health records requires the scanning of paper records into the electronic database. This task can be costly and time-consuming—many healthcare providers have chosen to create a position specifically for scanning documents. Even after all office medical documents have been scanned into the system, hardcopy lab reports, consultation letters, and so on may still be received and will need to be scanned into the patient's electronic record.

Time spent by the provider on capturing medical information from the patient and entering it into the EHR is time taken away from patient care. As more EHRs are used in the medical field and a higher level of documentation is required, a physician may be spending less face-to-face time caring for the patient and spending more face-to-computer time entering the patient's information. **Scribes** are being trained and employed to meet the need for entering data into the EHR, allowing the physician more time for face-to-face assessment of the patient. In addition to entering new patient data into the EHR, other duties of scribes may include navigating the EHR to locate previous patient data, researching data as requested by the provider, and responding to the provider's requests and messages. A scribe must only enter patient data in the presence of the provider or at the provider's request. All scribe entries must be signed, dated, and time stamped. Physicians must also document their presence when the data were recorded and must time, date, and verify the accuracy of the patient data.

Making Corrections in an Electronic Health Record

As in a paper-based medical record, errors will occur in an electronic health record. Examples of errors are transposition of letters and numbers, omission of patient information, and confusing data entries. After a patient encounter, the electronic medical data should be reviewed and proofread for errors. Medical transcriptionists are skilled in grammar, punctuation, medical terminology, anatomy and physiology, and format. Their expertise provides a needed second look at the documentation.

Policies and procedures for correcting electronic medical documentation should be in place to maintain the integrity of information. It is not good business practice to delete information so that it is nonrecoverable. Overwriting the original entry in the electronic health record may be interpreted as improperly altering the medical data; therefore, the original entry should be viewable. It may be suppressed but should still be viewable. Erroneous medical data should be flagged and a notation made to notify users of corrected data and their location.

Suspected errors in a medical record should be verified with the physician or other original entry clinician to confirm that the information is truly erroneous. Recommendations for correcting electronic medical data include the following:

1. Add an amendment to *clarify/correct the original entry.* All amendments should be completed in a timely manner (as stated in the practice's policies and procedures) and should be electronically signed (with credentials) and time/date-stamped. The reason for the amendment should be noted. If a hardcopy was printed from the original electronic medical data, the hardcopy should also be corrected.

> **EXAMPLE: AMENDMENT TO MEDICAL RECORD**
>
> A patient presented to the physician for an annual physical examination. When entering the patient's age, the physician transposed the numbers. Instead of keying that the patient is a "52-year-old patient," the physician keyed "25-year-old patient" into the electronic medical record. The title "Amendment" was keyed and information entered into the electronic medical record for the date of the visit correcting the patient's age. The original data ("25-year-old patient") were flagged with the note, "See amendment correction."

2. Add a late entry to *add missing or omitted information.* Normally, a late entry is made only to direct documentation, such as physician orders or nursing assessments. When the missing information is noted, the additional information should immediately be documented into the electronic medical record. Title the entry

"Late Entry" and enter the data. As with an amendment, electronically sign and time/date-stamp the entry. Some EHR programs will not permit late entries—the late entry should then be entered as an amendment.

> **EXAMPLE: LATE ENTRY TO A MEDICAL RECORD**
>
> A nurse was triaging a morning patient and was called away for an emergency phone call and forgot to enter the patient's review of systems. When the nurse returned to work after lunch, he realized the record was incomplete and entered a late entry for the missing review of systems information.

3. Add an addendum to *insert new information in an original electronic medical record entry.* There are situations when information should be added to the original entry, but the additional data were not available when the original entry was made. When the information is received, it should be added under the title "Addendum." Addendums should be made in a timely manner and should also state the reason for additional data being added to the original entry. Entries should be signed and time/date-stamped.

> **EXAMPLE: ADDENDUM TO A MEDICAL RECORD**
>
> A child is brought to the pediatrician with a sprained wrist and numerous bruises. The parent states the child fell down the front porch stairs. The physician makes the documentation in the electronic medical record. At the follow-up visit, a discussion with both the child and the parent reveals the child was abused by the older sibling. The physician returns to his original note and completes an addendum to indicate the abuse.

Depending on the electronic health record program and the provider's policies and procedures, an electronic medical record may be corrected with an electronic strikethrough or changing of data if the record has not been locked (that is, it does not contain a final signature of the provider). Some programs do not consider edits made prior to locking the record to be a correction. Policies and procedures should clearly state protocol for corrections made prior to locking a record.

Meaningful Use/Promoting Interoperability Program (PI) and Electronic Health Records

As discussed previously, electronic health records have many advantages for both the provider and patient. Benefits, however, depend on how the EHR is used. The overall goal of using EHRs is to provide better patient care, and the goal of Meaningful Use/Promoting Interoperability Program (PI) in providing better patient care has five broad areas:

1. *Accurate and complete information.* EHRs provide complete demographic and medical information, which allows the provider to provide the care that is best suited to the patient. Benefits of using a certified EHR include improving the quality and safety of patient care, increasing efficiency, and reducing errors.
2. *Improved access to information.* EHRs allow providers not only to access the patient's medical information but also to go from within the EHR to Internet links, such as pharmaceutical information sites, which allows for better diagnosis and treatment. As discussed earlier in this section, multiple providers can access the EHR and

share patient and medical information. Being able to view and exchange patient information through EHRs provides for better and faster coordination of care.

3. *Patient empowerment.* EHRs will allow patients to be more active in their medical care. Patients can electronically receive copies of their medical records and communicate electronically with the provider. Patients and their family members can be more engaged in their healthcare.

4. *Improve public/population health.* Through EHRs, health trends can be easily tracked and addressed.

5. *Protect the privacy and security of PHI.* Through various methods, such as using passwords and logging access, patients' PHI can be secured within an EHR.

Under the Health Information Technology for Economic and Clinical Health Act, better known as HITECH, providers who demonstrate that *certified* EHRs are being used in a meaningful way are eligible to receive financial incentives through 2017. The Centers for Medicare & Medicaid Services established a set of standards known as **Meaningful Use,** which define the use of *certified* electronic health records and how incentives are earned. In 2019, CMS changed the name from Meaningful Use to Promoting Interoperability. There are three implementation stages (Stages 1–3) of Meaningful Use/Promoting Interoperability, each stage requiring eligible providers to meet a set of core objectives and a set of menu objectives. Specific objectives for each stage of Meaningful Use/Promoting Interoperability can be found at www.cms.gov. Each stage builds on the previous stage and federal incentives can be earned by the provider.

STAGE 1 (ALREADY PAST)

PRIMARY FOCUS: CAPTURING AND SHARING DATA

Implementation:

Capturing medical information in a standardized format
Using information to track clinical conditions
Coordinating care by electronically communicating patient information
Reporting on certain clinical quality measures and information for public health
Using electronically captured patient medical information to engage patients in their care

STAGE 2 (ALREADY PAST)

PRIMARY FOCUS: ADVANCING CLINICAL PROCESSES

Implementation:

Increasing health information exchange (HIE)
Increasing e-prescribing
Incorporating lab results
Using electronically transmitted patient care summaries between many different settings
Providing more venues for patients to control their own medical data

STAGE 3 (2019-2021)

PRIMARY FOCUS: IMPROVING PATIENT HEALTH OUTCOMES

Implementation:

Protect PHI
Electronic prescribing
Clinical decision support
Computerized provider order entry
Patient electronic access to health information
Coordination of care through patient engagement
Health information exchange
Public health and clinical data registry reporting

When a provider must demonstrate that its EHR has met criteria for a certain stage depends on when the provider implemented the EHR. The time frame for implementation of and demonstration that the EHR has met Stage 1 and Stage 2 requirements for Meaningful Use/Promoting Interoperability of the certified EHR program is already past. Providers must meet Stage 3 requirements 2019 through 2021. As new information and possible revisions are made, they will be released by the Centers for Medicare & Medicaid Services.

5.4 MEDICAL TERMINOLOGY AND ABBREVIATIONS

In medical documents, care must be taken with the use of medical terminology and abbreviations. It is important to use only standard, approved abbreviations. A listing of the approved medical abbreviations used within the medical environment should be listed both in the Compliance Plan and in the medical environment's Policies and Procedures Manual. Table 5.1 contains a list of abbreviations commonly used in

Table 5.1 Abbreviations Commonly Used in Medical Records

a.c.	before meals	HEENT	head, eyes, ears, nose, throat	PMH	past medical history
AP	anteroposterior			p.o.	per os (by mouth)
b.i.d.	twice a day	HPI	history of present illness	p.r.n.	as desired or as needed
BP	blood pressure	HS	hour of sleep	PSA	prostate-specific antigen
BUN	blood urea nitrogen	I&D	incision and drainage	RLQ	right lower quadrant
C&S	culture and sensitivity	ICU	intensive care unit	R/O	rule out
CBC	complete blood count	IM	intramuscular	ROS	review of systems
CC	chief complaint	IV	intravenous	RTC	return to clinic
cc	cubic centimeter	kg	kilogram	RUQ	right upper quadrant
cm	centimeter	L	liter	Rx	prescription
CNS	central nervous system	LLQ	left lower quadrant	SDA	same day appointment
CPE	complete physical exam	LMP	last menstrual period	SH	social history
D&C	dilation and curettage	LUQ	left upper quadrant	S/P	status post
DS	double strength	m	meter	stat or STAT	immediately
DTR	deep tendon reflexes	mcg	microgram		
Dx	diagnosis	mEq	milliequivalent	STD	sexually transmitted disease
ECG	electrocardiogram	mg	milligram		
EEG	electroencephalogram	mL	milliliter	T&A	tonsillectomy and adenoidectomy
EENT	eyes, ears, nose, throat	mm	millimeter		
ENT	ears, nose, throat	n.p.o.	nothing by mouth	t.i.d.	three times a day
EOM	extraocular movements	OB	obstetrics	TM	tympanic membrane
ER	emergency room	OTC	over-the-counter (as in medications)	TPR	temperature, pulse, respirations
FH	family history				
F/U	follow-up	P&A	percussion and auscultation	UA	urinalysis
FUO	fever unknown origin			UC	urine culture
Fx	fracture	p.c.	after meals	URI	upper respiratory infection
g or gm	gram	PE	physical exam	UTI	urinary tract infection
GI	gastrointestinal	PERLA	pupils equal, reactive to light and accommodation	VD	venereal disease
gr	grain			VS	vital signs
GU	genitourinary			wbc	white blood cell
GYN	gynecology	PERRLA	pupils equal, round, reactive to light and accommodation	WBC	white blood count
h	hour			WNL	within normal limits
H&P	history and physical				

Official "Do Not Use" List[1]

Do Not Use	Potential Problem	Use Instead
U (unit)	Mistaken for "0" (zero), the number "4" (four), or "cc"	Write "unit"
IU (International Unit)	Mistaken for IV (intravenous) or the number 10 (ten)	Write "International Unit"
Q.D., QD, q.d., qd (daily)	Mistaken for each other	Write "daily"
Q.O.D., QOD, q.o.d., qod (every other day)	Period after the Q mistaken for "I" and the "O" mistaken for "I"	Write "every other day"
Trailing zero (X.0 mg)*	Decimal point is missed	Write X mg
Lack of leading zero (.X mg)	Decimal point is missed	Write 0.X mg
MS	Can mean morphine sulfate or magnesium sulfate	Write "morphine sulfate" Write "magnesium sulfate"
MSO_4 and $MgSO_4$	Confused for one another	Write "morphine sulfate" Write "magnesium sulfate"

[1]Applies to all orders and all medication-related documentation that are handwritten (including free-text computer entry) or on preprinted forms.

Exception: A "trailing zero" may be used only where required to demonstrate the level of precision of the value being reported, such as for laboratory results, imaging studies that report size of lesions, or catheter/tube sizes. It may not be used in medication orders or other medication-related documentation.

Source: The Joint Commission, 2013.

medical records. The list includes the following types of abbreviations, arranged in alphabetic order for ease of use:

- Weights and measures (mainly medication dosages and lab values)—for example, *mL* (milliliter)
- Designations of times and methods—for example, *b.i.d.* (twice a day)
- Terms typically found in chart notes—for example, *TPR* (temperature, pulse, respirations)

It is also important to keep up to date on medical abbreviations that are obsolete or are targeted for nonuse, as shown in Table 5.2.

5.5 TECHNOLOGIES FOR DATA INPUT

The one thing employees can count on to be consistent is that change will happen. Desktop computers are being replaced by laptops and handheld devices, and physicians and other healthcare personnel are using smart devices to enter patient data, research medical resources, and keep in contact with other team members. Newer technologies, when used effectively, can help improve productivity and efficiency. Traditional methods of inputting medical data are being integrated, updated, and, in some cases, replaced. As an administrative medical assistant, you must be open to learning new skills and technologies, such as voice recognition for data input, to enhance patient care and increase office productivity.

Traditional Data Input

Electronic recording and storage of medical data are rapidly becoming the preferred methods of documenting medical data. Prior to electronic storage, medical data were—and for some offices still are—maintained through verbal recordings, then typed/keyed.

Transcription. Some offices today continue to input medical data using the **transcription** method. The physician, or other provider of medical care, dictates the medical data into a recording device (tape recorder or phone recording system) to be transcribed by a keyboardist who specializes in medical data keyboarding. The transcriptionist will listen to the dictation, either from tapes or from other recorded media, and transcribe the verbal medical data into keyed format. Medical offices may employ their own transcriptionist or may use a transcription service.

A thorough knowledge of grammar and punctuation, medical terminology, anatomy and physiology, and accurate keyboarding skills are required. Medical transcriptionists must also be able to proofread medical documents with a high level of proficiency. Mistakes in medical documentation can lead to a vast array of consequences. Misdiagnoses can take place when medical decisions are made based on errors in transcribed documents. Consider what would happen to a patient who was directed to take 5 mg of a prescribed medication when the amount should have been 0.5 mg.

Transcriptionists use templates to input medical data. Different formats include a history and physical format for general practitioners, radiologic reports for radiologists, and cardiovascular evaluations for thoracic surgeons. Although medical specialties may adjust formats to meet their documentation requirements, generalized rules for transcribing materials should be used. A sampling of these guidelines can be found in the Appendix.

The future of transcription is changing. As electronic health records are implemented in the medical field, transcriptionists may proofread and edit documentation. They may be employed as scribes to assist the physician EHR data entry. Different input technologies, discussed in the next section, allow physicians to input data directly into medical records. However, proofreading and editing medical documentation for errors, such as punctuation, will still be a much-needed skill. The high cost of implementing electronic health records makes the highly skilled transcriptionist a valued medical team member.

Newer Input Technologies

Voice-Recognition Technology. A technology being used in medical and other offices for data input is **voice-recognition technology.** Using voice-recognition software, the dictator speaks into a headset that has been specifically trained for his or her voice. As the dictator speaks, data are input into the medical record. Some refer to this as "typing on the fly." Software efficiency varies. Some software requires the dictator to dictate all punctuation, while in other software punctuation is based on the next given command, such as "new paragraph." Voice-recognition technology provides a hands-free input method that can reduce the possibility of keyed errors. With practice, data that are input with voice-recognition technology can be recorded at a faster rate than keyed words per minute, and individuals can multitask. This is not always an advantage, however, as errors can occur with dictation when attention is diverted to other tasks. Noise-filtering headsets should be used to filter out unwanted noise in the surrounding environment. Another disadvantage is that different lingual accents may "confuse" the software and produce flawed documentation.

Wireless Technology. Wireless technology, such as that in smart devices, is used not only for social networking and communication but also for medical data input. Physicians may use these technologies to access and update patient and other medical office information. Wireless technologies allow medical team members to retrieve items such as e-mail and calendars through electronic devices. Patient information can be retrieved through Internet or cloud-based medical records, and medical decisions can be made without the need for the physician to return to the office. Current technologies

Figure 5.10

Wireless Smartphone
Device Tolgart/iStock/
Getty Images

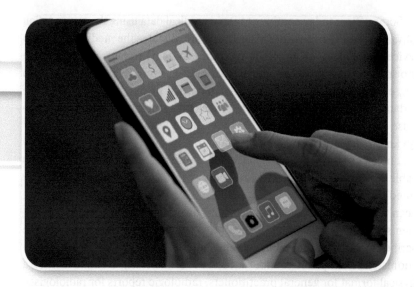

for wireless devices require Internet accessibility through WiFi or an Internet service plan. Physicians also use portable laptop and handheld wireless devices for data input. Both are small and portable, making them convenient for mobile and remote data entry. Wireless devices are illustrated in Figure 5.10 and Figure 5.11.

Remember, change will happen. As electronic health records are fully implemented in the medical environment, assistants must be flexible and willing to learn new technologies and to integrate the old with the new. It is an exciting time to be part of such a progressive environment.

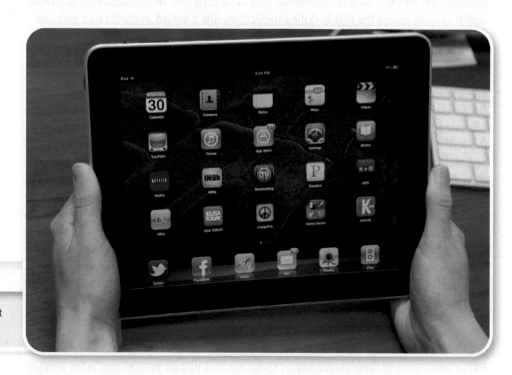

Figure 5.11

Portable Wireless Tablet
Mark Dierker/McGraw-Hill

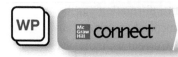

WP Mc Graw Hill **connect**

**GO TO PROJECTS 5.6 and 5.7
AT THE END OF THIS CHAPTER**

DOCUMENTATION FORMATS

The **SOAP** method is the most common system for outlining and structuring chart notes for a medical record. It facilitates the creation of uniform and complete notes in a simple format that is easy to read. The acronym *SOAP* stands for the following headings that are used to structure the chart notes: *Subjective, Objective, Assessment,* and *Plan.* Each of these headings contains a specific type of information, as follows. The CHEDDAR format breaks down the components of a patient encounter into seven detail-oriented sections: chief complaint, history, exam, details of problem, drugs/dosages, assessment, and return information. Problem-oriented medical records (POMR) and the source-oriented medical records (SOMR) are two other common documentation formats.

The SOAP Method

Subjective Findings. **Subjective** findings are the patient's description of the problem or complaint, including symptoms troubling the patient, when the symptoms began, external or associated factors, remedies tried, and past medical treatment. The subjective information (patient's description of the reason for the encounter) in a SOAP record may include any or all of the subheadings that follow:

- **Chief complaint (CC):** The reason for the visit, or why the patient is seeking the physician's advice. All records must contain a chief complaint.
- **History of present illness (HPI):** Information about the symptoms troubling the patient—location, quality, severity, timing, duration, context, modifying factors, and any associated signs and/or symptoms. The patient should be asked questions such as when the symptoms began, what affects them (things that make the symptoms

S O A P
Subjective Findings

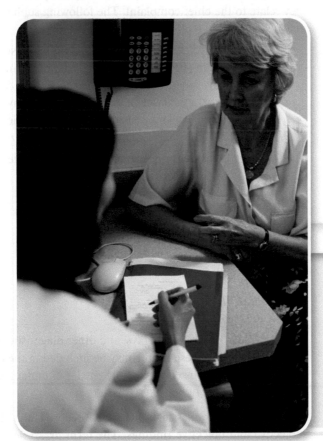

Figure 5.12

During a new patient's first visit, the physician usually takes note of the patient's complete medical history. *Why is it important for patients' medical histories to be placed in their charts promptly?* Ryan McVay/ Photodisc/Getty Images

better or worse), what may have caused the symptoms, any remedies the patient has tried, and any medical treatment already given.

- **Past medical history (PMH):** A listing of any illnesses the patient has had in the past along with the treatments administered or operations performed. This history also includes a description of any accidents, injuries, congenital problems, or allergies to medicines or other substances.
- **Family history (FH):** Facts about the health of the patient's parents, siblings, and other blood relatives that may be significant to the patient's condition. For example, family history is especially important in treating hereditary diseases.
- **Social history (SH):** The patient's social history and marital history, especially if they are pertinent to the patient's treatment. Information regarding the patient's eating, drinking, or smoking habits; the patient's education; the patient's occupation; the patient's sexual activity and sexuality; and the patient's interests may also be included in this section.
- **Review of systems (ROS):** The physician's review of each body system or the body systems related to the chief complaint with the patient (for example, the respiratory system and the genitourinary system). The physician asks specific questions about the functioning of the system and reviews information in the patient's record.

In some chart notes, the three subheadings *PMH, FH,* and *SH* (for *past medical history, family history,* and *social history*) may be combined into one subheading, *PFSH.*

Objective Findings. The **objective** findings (the physician's verifiable data) in a SOAP record are the physician's assessment after an examination of the patient. Results of the examination may be recorded under the heading **physical exam (PE).** The exam may be a complete physical examination, in which the findings for each of the major areas of the body are included, or it may cover only the pertinent body systems for that visit as they relate to the chief complaint. The following subheadings cover body systems that may be included in a physical exam:

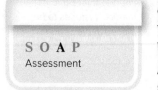

SOAP
Objective Findings

> *VITAL SIGNS (VS):* The patient's temperature, pulse, and respirations (TPR); blood pressure (BP); and height and weight are included in this category. This heading may also be labeled *CONSTITUTIONALS.*
>
> *GENERAL:* A general description of the patient may be, for example, "This is a well-developed, well-nourished, 27-year-old female."
>
> *HEENT:* This abbreviation stands for *head, eyes, ears, nose,* and *throat.*

The following body areas my also be included, contingent on the chief complaint:

> *NECK*
> *HEART*
> *CHEST*
> *LUNGS*
> *ABDOMEN*
> *PELVIC*
> *RECTAL*
> *EXTREMITIES*
> *NEUROLOGICAL*

The results of lab tests, x-rays, and other diagnostic procedures are also part of the objective findings. These results may be included in the corresponding body system review, or they may be listed as separate entries or under a separate heading, such as *LAB,* usually after the list of body systems.

SOAP
Assessment

Assessment. The **assessment** in a SOAP record is the physician's interpretation of the subjective and objective findings. The term *assessment* is used interchangeably with

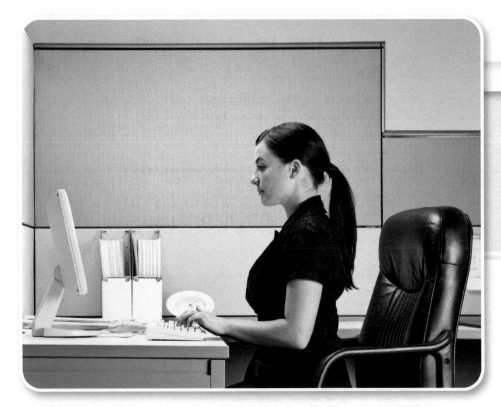

Figure 5.13

Findings from the physician's examination must be recorded accurately in the patient's chart. *How can the administrative medical assistant ensure that the transcription is accurate?* Avava/Shutterstock

the terms **diagnosis (Dx)** and **impression** and gives a name to the condition from which the patient is suffering. Sometimes the assessment is tentative, pending further developments. Occasionally, the physician uses the phrase **rule out (R/O)** before a diagnosis, meaning that the diagnosis, while possible, is not likely and that further tests will be performed for confirmation.

Plan. The **plan,** or treatment, section lists information regarding the physician's treatment of the illness. Following are examples of information which may be included in the plan:

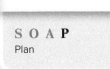

S O A P
Plan

- Prescribed medications and their exact dosages
- Instructions given to the patient
- Recommendations for hospitalization or surgery
- Any tests that need to be performed
- Referral to a specialist
- Patient education/counseling

Figure 5.14 and Figure 5.15 contain examples of chart notes that incorporate the SOAP format. In Figure 5.14, although not all the SOAP headings are spelled out, the entries clearly follow the SOAP format. The subjective findings begin with *CC* (chief complaint) and continue to *PHYSICAL EXAM,* which contains the objective findings. The assessment and plan follow with their own headings.

In Figure 5.15, the SOAP format is more apparent, with the addition of a *LAB* heading after the objective findings. Notice that the level of detail contained in the entries in Figure 5.14 is much greater than that in Figure 5.15. This is because the patient described in Figure 5.14 is a new patient, and therefore a complete history and physical have been performed. The patient described in Figure 5.15 is a returning patient who is visiting for help with a specific illness.

As can be seen from an examination of Figure 5.14 and Figure 5.15, the SOAP format can accommodate many variations. The value in using the SOAP outline, or a variation of it, is that, by following the simple formula of the acronym, the person writing, dictating, or

HISTORY AND PHYSICAL REPORT

Patient, Laura
DOB: 03/01/19--
Patient ID: AA096

3/6/20--
CC: Annual female exam for this 44-year-old black patient.

PMH: Tonsillectomy at age 3; wisdom teeth pulled at age 29.

ALLERGIES: SULFA.

CURRENT MEDICATIONS: None.

FH: Father died at age 70 of multiple problems, including carcinoma of larynx, stroke, and pneumonia. Mother, age 66, is in good health. No siblings.

SH: Laura completed high school, plus one to two years of college. Patient works at a dry cleaner, pressing machine and front desk. Does not smoke or use alcohol. She was never on birth control pills or any other major medication.

MARITAL HISTORY: Husband, age 46, is in good health. They have been married 24 years and have three children in good health.

ROS:
SKIN: Negative.
HEENT: Patient wears glasses with last eye exam 3 months ago. She has occasional sinusitis.
CHEST: No chest pain or palpitation.
RESPIRATORY: Negative.
ABDOMEN: Negative.
PELVIC: LMP 3 weeks ago. Gravida 3, para 3. Patient uses OTC birth control products.
MUSCULOSKELETAL: Occasional stiffness of elbow.
NEUROLOGICAL: Negative.

PHYSICAL EXAM:
GENERAL: Alert black female in no acute distress. BP, 116/82. Pulse, 86. Respirations, 24. Height, 64 inches; weight, 128 pounds.
HEENT: Normocephalic. Ears, TMs normal. Eyes, PERLA; EOMs, intact. Nose, patent. Throat, within normal limits.
NECK: Supple. Thyroid, not enlarged. Carotids, equal without bruits.
BREASTS: Fine lumps bilaterally; nothing suspicious.
HEART: Regular sinus rhythm without murmurs.
LUNGS: Clear to A&P.
ABDOMEN: Soft; without masses, tenderness, or scars.
PELVIC: Cervix, clean. Uterus, anteverted and smooth. Adnexa and vagina, WNL. Rectovaginal confirms.
EXTREMITIES: Within normal limits with fine varicosities bilaterally.
NEUROLOGICAL: Cranial nerves II-XII, intact.

ASSESSMENT: Generally healthy female.

PLAN: 1. Schedule mammogram.
         2. Routine screen labs.
         3. UA.
         4. Hemoccults x 3.

Karen Larsen

Karen Larsen, MD/ls

electronically recording the note is more likely to cover all the important issues. In addition, the logic of the format lends itself well to displaying the provider's thought processes in deciding on a course of treatment. Having such a record improves communication for all those involved in the care of the patient. It also minimizes the provider's exposure to legal risk.

The CHEDDAR Method

Another format used for medical documentation is called **CHEDDAR.** This method of entry uses the same information as the SOAP method and places it under seven headings:

C (chief complaint)
H (history of the present illness and other pertinent histories)
E (examination)
D (details of problems and complaints)
D (drugs and dosage—past and current medications)
A (assessment)
R (return visit or referral to a specialist)

An example of a chart note using the CHEDDAR documentation format is shown in Figure 5.16.

CHART NOTE

Patient, Harriett
DOB: 07/29/19--
Patient ID AA097

March 6, 20--

SUBJECTIVE: Patient presents with mild urinary urgency and frequency. Patient has also had frequent lower abdominal pain, but no abnormal vaginal symptoms.

OBJECTIVE: Temperature, 98.6°. Pulse, 76 and regular. Respirations, 20. Abdominal exam reveals mild suprapubic tenderness; otherwise, exam is unremarkable.

LAB: Urinalysis is negative; urine culture is pending.

ASSESSMENT: Suspect urethritis.

PLAN: Patient placed on 7-day course of ciprofloxacin 500 mg b.i.d. She was reminded to drink at least 8 glasses of water daily. RTC if not improving.

Karen Larsen

Karen Larsen, MD/ls

Figure 5.15

Chart Note in the SOAP Format

Problem-Oriented Medical Records (POMR)

Another form of record keeping revolves around a list of the patient's problems. A record organized in this way is referred to as a **problem-oriented medical record (POMR).** In a problem-oriented medical record, there are four essential components: the Database, the

CHART NOTE

Patient, Erin
DOB: 07/31/20--
Patient ID AA098

07/07/20--

CC: Patient's mother stated daughter has developed a red, itchy skin rash on her right arm.

H: Patient began complaining of an "itchy" arm after returning from a school outing 2 days prior in a park with poison oak. The patient fell into the poison oak when attempting to retrieve a ball. Soon after the itching began, the patient developed a red, pinpoint rash on the arm. Mother stated she used OTC ointments on the rash with no relief.

E: General: Patient is a WD, WN 9-year-old female with no history of rashes. BP 110/75; WT 82 lbs., Pulse 80.

Skin: Smooth, red rash on the right inner and outer forearm. No discharge noted.

HEENT: Normocephalic. Ears, TMs normal. Eyes, PERLA. Nose, Patent. No deviation noted. Throat, within normal limits.

D: Patient has dark red, nonpustule rash on right inner and outer forearm. Rash appears irritated.

D: Mother gave patient OTC Benadryl 4 hours prior to being examined. Patient is currently on no other medication.

A: Dermatitis due to contact with poison oak.

R: Patient is to continue to use OTC antihistamine. If rash has not subsided in 2 days, return to office. Otherwise, prn.

Karen Larsen

Karen Larsen, MD/ls

Figure 5.16

Chart Note in the CHEDDAR Format

Master Problem List, the Initial Plan, and the Notes. Some providers may choose to include Notes in the Initial Plan section.

Database. The Database consists of the patient's complete history, including the problem, history of present illness, past medical history, family history, social history, and review of systems, followed by information derived from a complete examination and routine diagnostic and laboratory tests.

Master Problem List. The Master Problem List is a running account of the patient's problems. Each problem is the conclusion or a decision based on information obtained in the Database. The Master Problem List functions as an index for the remainder of the POMR. Active, inactive, temporary, and potential problems are recorded in the Master Problem List. It is referred to and updated at each clinic visit. This procedure helps ensure that all problems are considered during a visit. Using the list, the physician can, at a glance, learn what problems the patient has had, how often they have appeared, and the treatment prescribed. This list saves time in that the physician does not have to study the patient's entire chart before obtaining relevant information.

Generally, the SOAP format is used for organizing entries within the Master Problem List. The SOAP format may also be used to outline the history and physical for the Database section. Figure 5.17 is an example of a problem-oriented medical record.

CHART NOTE

```
Patient, Ian
DOB: 08/02/19--
Patient ID AA099

March 7, 20--
PROBLEM 1: Tonsillitis.

CHIEF COMPLAINT: Sore throat times 2 days.

S: Sore throat, difficulty swallowing.
O: Temperature 101°. Pharyngitis with exudative tonsillitis.

PLAN: 1. Throat culture.
      2. 1.2 units Bicillin C-R
      3. Recheck in 10 days.

Karen Larsen

Karen Larsen, MD/ls

March 14, 20--
PROBLEM 1:

S: Recheck. Patient feels better.
O: Temperature, normal. No problem with swallowing.
A: Problem 1 resolved.
P: Gargle with warm salt water if necessary. Pharyngitis with exudative
   tonsillitis resolved.

Karen Larsen
Karen Larsen, MD/ls

June 11, 20--
PROBLEM 2: Chip fracture lunate, left.

S: Pain in instep and tarsal bones.
O: Swelling and ecchymosis, left foot.
A: X-ray shows questionable undisplaced chip fracture of lunate.
P: 1. Continue supportive shoes.
   2. Referred to orthopedics for further evaluation.

Karen Larsen

Karen Larsen, MD/ls
```

Figure 5.17

Chart Note for a Problem-Oriented Medical Record (POMR)

Notice how each entry begins with the date of the patient visit, followed by a reference to the problem being treated—*Problem 1, Problem 2,* and so on.

Initial Plan. Each problem listed in the Master Problem List is named and described in the Initial Plan section. Medical documentation is typically in the SOAP format. The physician begins a course of treatment and details the results in either narrative or flowchart format. A discharge assessment summary of the treatment progress is included for each problem.

Notes. All providers of care include progress notes under the Notes section. Physicians, nurses, radiologists, and others all place progress notes in this section. For continuity, the SOAP format is recommended as the documentation format. Discharge information may also be included in the Notes section or placed as a separate section after Notes.

Source-Oriented Medical Record (SOMR)

Another method of organizing medical documentation within a record is to organize the data by the source or supplier of the information. Notes from physicians, nurses, laboratory reports, and so on would each have their own section and are recorded within the section in reverse chronological order. Each entity is responsible for maintaining and updating its individual section within the SOMR. An advantage of an SOMR is the ease of reviewing all documentation from a single source at one time. However, it is difficult to gain a complete picture of a patient's current status from the SOMR without going to each individual section and reviewing notes and dates. This becomes time restrictive.

 OWNERSHIP, QUALITY ASSURANCE, AND RECORD RETENTION

Every medical practice has a variety of files that need to be preserved. Patient medical records, in particular, require special attention because of their importance to the practice and their value as legal documents. All medical records should be kept until the possibility of a malpractice suit has passed. This time period is determined by each state's statute of limitations. Although most medical records are, in fact, kept permanently, they are generally removed from an active file (pertaining to current patients) to an inactive file or closed storage (for patients who have died, moved away, or terminated their relationship with the physician).

Every provider should have guidelines for transferring patient medical records from one classification to another. These guidelines should specify the information that is to be kept and, if possible, the type of storage medium to be used. It is important for an administrative medical assistant to be familiar with these guidelines, since their application will help protect the physician and the practice from potential legal complications.

Ownership

The ownership of medical records is addressed by the American Medical Association Council on Ethical and Judicial Affairs. According to the Council, medical notes made by a physician—the actual chart notes, reports, and other materials—are the physician's property. The notes are for the physician's use in the treatment of the patient.

The provider may deny, in writing, a request for a copy of medical records if it is determined that, if the patient had a copy, they might misinterpret the data, harm themselves, or harm others. Psychotherapy notes are an example of notes that are normally not released to the patient.

However, the physician cannot use or withhold the information in the record according to his or her own wishes. For example, the physician is ethically obligated to furnish copies of office notes to any physician who is assuming responsibility for care of the patient. Even though, under the TPO portion of HIPAA, a signed release of information from the patient is no longer required, some practices still ask their patients to sign a release of information prior to releasing PHI to another physician for the continuity of the patient's care. It is understood that, even though the physician's notes are the physician's property, the information in the record—the nature of the patient's diagnosis and so on—belongs to the patient. For example, Patient A is seen by Dr. Smith for a routine office visit. The medical information given by the patient and recorded about the patient (history, exam, etc.) belongs to the patient, but the paper record or electronic medical record on which it is recorded belongs to the physician. For this reason, patients have the right to control the amount and type of information released from their medical record, with the exception of legally required information, such as a birth record. Furthermore, patients alone hold the authority to release information to anyone not directly involved in their care, such as an attorney or a spouse. A fee may be charged for furnishing copies of complex medical reports; however, information should not be withheld because of an unpaid fee. State laws should be referenced when determining if a patient may be charged for copied medical documents and, if so, how much may be charged.

More and more patients are using mobile devices and apps to send and receive PHI. Blood glucose and heart rate readings can be monitored by mobile devices. When a patient requests PHI to be sent from a provider to a mobile device, the physician is not liable for how the mobile device app secures or uses the patient's PHI.

Quality Assurance

The medical record is the best measure of the quality of care given a patient. The assistant helps the physician maintain high standards of care by paying attention to the data entered in the medical record.

COMPLIANCE *TIP*

Credibility of the record is called into question when there is delayed filing of reports and physicians' notes, or when there are incomplete files, illegible records, or alterations in the record.

To ensure that files are complete, a standard office procedure should be used to follow up on pending reports for x-rays and other diagnostic procedures. A separate file marked "Pending Work" may be used, or a reminder may be placed in a tickler file. In an EHR, pending items may be noted by using a different color, such as red, to indicate needed action.

If the assistant is unsure about a word written or dictated (for example, it may be unclear whether the physician means *"15"* or *"50"* milligrams), the item should be flagged for the physician's attention. The assistant should not interrupt the physician if he or she is attending to other tasks at that time.

The assistant should make sure that each record contains the following:

- Dated notations describing the service received by the patient
- Notations regarding every procedure performed
- Accurate notations; an addendum by the physician should be made if a discrepancy occurs (for example, a previous notation about a condition may have stated "left side," while the latest notation states "right side")
- Justification for hospitalization
- If necessary, a discharge summary regarding hospitalization before the patient arrives for a follow-up visit

Patients also have the right to inspect their medical documentation. If they feel an entry error has occurred, they should notify the provider, in writing, and ask that the correction be made. The provider must respond to the request. If the healthcare team reviews the documentation and, in fact, an error has occurred, a correction should be made in the chart and the patient notified of the correction. The correction should be made using the previously discussed method. If the corrective entry is longer than would fit either above or below the correction line, an addendum or an amendment should be made in the medical record. However, if the physician does not feel an error has occurred, he or she cannot be forced to make a corrective entry. In this situation, the patient should submit his or her own version of the encounter, which should then be included in the medical record.

Retention of Records

Every medical practice has files from previous years and all types of information. For example, patient medical records include files for patients who are currently being treated by the physician, those who have not seen the physician for some time, and those who are no longer patients.

For management purposes, these files are classified as

- **Active files,** pertaining to current patients.
- **Inactive files,** related to patients who have not seen the physician for a stated period of time, such as 3 years or longer. Depending on the medical specialty, this time period may be shorter or longer. For example, a file may be considered inactive in a family medical practice after 3 years of inactivity; however, a file in an OB-GYN practice may be considered inactive after 5 years of nonactivity. A practice may choose to classify a file as inactive when the patient is no longer an established patient (has not seen the physician or a physician of the same speciality in the same practice within the last 3 years).
- **Closed files,** those of patients who have died, moved away, or terminated their relationship with the physician.

Each office sets the criteria and time frames for placing files in one of the categories. This policy is part of a larger policy for record **retention**—the length of time records must be retained and the proper disposition of them when they should no longer be stored. Record retention policies protect physicians from exposure to legal problems.

Legal Requirements. Federal law does not regulate retention time frames for patients' medical records, other than for federal agencies (i.e., the Department of Veterans Affairs). Many states, however, have specific requirements for the length of time, such records must be kept. Existing state laws and regulations must always be observed. Record retention may also depend on the medical speciality or on the patient's condition. Healthcare providers who receive payment under the federal Medicare program must also comply with CMS's conditions for record retention. Currently, those regulations for providers and healthcare entities that provide services to Medicare beneficiaries is to retain the record for a minimum of 5 years. For providers who provide services to Medicare beneficiaries under a Medicare managed care program, the patient's record is to be maintained for a minimum of 10 years. State record retention laws should be used to determine the retention schedule for Medicaid beneficiaries.

In 2013, the American Health Information Management Association **(AHIMA)** proposed the following guideline in a practice brief:

At a minimum, a records retention schedule must

- ensure patient health information is available to meet the needs of continued patient care, legal requirements, research, education, and other legitimate uses of the organization.

- include guidelines that specify which information is kept, the time period for which it is kept, and the storage medium on which it will be maintained (e.g., paper, microfilm, optical disk, magnetic tape).
- include clear destruction policies and procedures that include appropriate methods of destruction of each medium on which information is maintained.

Retention Time Frames. In the absence of either federal or state retention guidelines, the following time frames for retention may be used (the retention time period should be considered as the minimum time to maintain a record):

- *Patient health records (competent adults):* 10 years after patient's most recent encounter
- *Patient health records (incompetent adults):* (a) until the patient becomes competent, then following the guideline for a competent adult; (b) 7 years after the patient's death; or (c) indefinitely
- *Patient health records (minors):* age of majority (varies between 18 and 21 years of age) plus statute of limitations on malpractice (some states require the provider to maintain a minor's medical record for 10 years past the state's age of majority)
- *Diagnostic images (such as x-rays):* 7 to 10 years or permanently
- *Master patient index, register of births, register of deaths, register of surgical procedures:* permanently

The office policy should include a variety of other records related to the physician's practice management:

- *Insurance policies:* Current policies are kept in safe storage in an accessible file. Professional liability policies are kept permanently.
- *Tax records:* Tax records for the 3 latest years are kept in a readily accessible file. Under certain circumstances, such as filing a tax claim with bad debt reduction, the IRS can ask for tax records for the latest 7 years. The remaining records may be kept in a less accessible storage area.
- *Receipts for equipment:* Receipts for both medical and office equipment are kept until the various pieces of equipment are fully depreciated—that is, until the value of the equipment has completely diminished.
- *Personal records and licenses:* Professional licenses and certificates are kept permanently in safe storage. Banking records, such as statements and deposit slips, are kept in the file for 3 years. They may then be moved to a storage area. Other personal records, such as noncurrent partnership agreements, property records, or other business agreements, are also kept permanently in a storage area.

Individual state statutes should be referenced when determining how long to maintain medical and business-related records.

Paper Versus Micrographic Medical Records. To save space, paper records can be stored through a process called **micrographics,** in which miniaturized images of the records are created. These images are usually in a microfiche (sheet of film holding 90 images) or ultrafiche (compacted film holding up to 1,000 images) format and are viewed on readers that enlarge the images. Micrographic records may be stored in card files or binders. With the increased use of the large memory capacity afforded by computers, paper records may also be scanned and stored on space-saving electronic or digital storage media such as CDs. Digital storage of medical records may be used in conjunction with electronic medical records.

As electronic health records become the norm, traditional hardcopy patient records must be scanned directly into the practice program. This is a time-consuming task, and some practices have created employee positions for the sole purpose of scanning paper documents into the electronic health record program. Other medical practices have contracted with an outside agency to scan documents. Scanners may work during hours when patients and employees typically are away from the office. Using off-hours to scan documents makes patient medical data available to medical personnel as patients are being seen. All electronically stored records must be kept according to the same retention schedule as that for paper records.

Disposition of Records. Records that have been closed and those that must be kept permanently—patient records, personal records, and business records—may be transferred and are said to be in **dead storage,** a storage area separate from the area where active files are kept. Dead storage need not be easily accessible and can be in a location other than the office. The storage area should provide a secure, safe area for records.

There are financial and storage considerations for every practice. All records cannot be kept indefinitely. Some states have laws related to the destruction of records and even specify the method of destruction. General guidelines include the following:

- Appropriate ways to destroy paper records include burning, shredding, and pulping. Records must be destroyed so that there is no possibility of reconstructing them.
- When destroying computerized data, suggested methods of destruction include overwriting data or reformatting the disk, pulverizing, incinerating, cutting, degaussing, electronic or solid state shredding, and so on. The method used must ensure that the information cannot be recovered or reconstructed.

The HIPAA Security Rule addresses the destruction of medical records. Covered entities are required, under HIPAA, to have policies and procedures in place to state how the media on which PHI is stored are to be destroyed and how the PHI is to be removed from the electronic media before the media are reused.

When medical data are destroyed, it is the practice's responsibility to maintain a record/log of the destruction. The destruction log should include

- the date and method of destruction.
- a description of the record (patient name, contents, etc.).
- the date range of records destroyed (i.e., January through December 2028).
- signatures of the the individual(s) who destroyed the records and of the individual(s) who witnessed the destruction.
- a statement saying that the medical records were destroyed as part of normal business operations.

If destruction of records is outsourced, a Certificate of Destruction is issued and maintained by the outsourced company.

Mc Graw Hill connect   **GO TO PROJECT 5.8 AT THE END OF THIS CHAPTER**

5.8 FILING SYSTEMS

Records management is the systematic control of records from their creation through maintenance to eventual storage or destruction. Records may be managed electronically or manually (paper records). To handle these tasks, administrative medical assistants have a source of helpful information in the Association of Records Managers and Administrators **(ARMA).** This international organization's members include information managers, archivists (those who specialize in control of records storage), librarians, and educators. One of the major purposes of the organization is to set standards for the filing and retention of records. Although ARMA standards are voluntary, rather than set by the government, following them makes it possible for medical offices to manage records more efficiently.

ARMA
INTERNATIONAL
11880 College Blvd.
Suite 450
Overland Park, KS 66210
Phone: 913-341-3808
or 800-422-2762
Website: www.arma.org

Medical offices may use the ARMA guidelines as a basis for records management procedures and adapt the guidelines to fit individual office records management needs. For consistency, it is important to include written policy and procedures for records management in the office manual. A good question to ask is, "Using the medical office records management policy, can the correct medical record be retrieved in a timely manner by a medical team member and data given to the right individual to make informed medical decisions?"

Recorded information in any form—whether in a paper, electronic, or digital format—is considered a record. In medical offices, the three main types of records are (1) patient medical records, (2) correspondence related to healthcare, and (3) practice management records.

1. *Patient medical records.* The central responsibility of the physician's practice is patient care. For this reason, the proper handling of the patient medical record is critical. This contains chart notes, all medical and laboratory reports, and all correspondence to, from, and about a patient.

2. *Correspondence related to healthcare.* General correspondence includes items about the operation of the office, such as orders for medical supplies. It also includes physicians' research reports; articles from medical journals related to new procedures or treatments; and correspondence, newsletters, and announcements from professional organizations.

3. *Practice management records.* Materials about the business and financial management of the practice must also be carefully kept. These documents include insurance policies, income and expense records, copies of tax returns for the practice, financial statements, and leases or contracts related to office space or the premises. Also kept are copies of managed care contracts and the office's compliance program and privacy policy. Personnel and payroll records are also part of practice management.

Two broad categories of files are centralized files and decentralized files. Centralized files—those kept in one central location—must be used by many people in the medical office. Thus, ease of access is necessary. Information of use to only one staff member, such as a physician's correspondence, is stored in a decentralized file convenient to the user. The kinds of filing equipment and supplies that best suit a medical office depend on how records are used and who needs to use them.

Filing Equipment

Filing Cabinets. Many kinds of filing cabinets are available. The best choice for a particular office will be based on available space, cost, and level of security that is desirable. All filing cabinets should be locked to secure records and should be fireproof and waterproof.

Open-Shelf Files. **Open-shelf files** are bookcase-type shelves that hold files, as shown in Figure 5.18. These shelves may be adjustable or fixed and may extend from floor to ceiling. Folders are placed in the files sideways with identifying tabs protruding.

The need to conserve space has made open-shelf files popular in many offices. They take up less floor and aisle space and are less expensive to purchase than most other kinds of filing equipment. Because staff members do not need to open drawers, these files also save time and labor. However, open shelves do mean that records are less secure than if they were held in closed steel drawers. The records are also more vulnerable to accidents, including fire and water damage. Therefore, open-shelf filing equipment should have doors that can be closed and locked to protect medical records from theft and natural disasters, such as fire or flood.

Vertical Files. Drawer files, called **vertical files,** are contained in cabinets of various sizes. These letter-size cabinets, meant for documents that are 8½ by 11 inches, are usually metal. They vary in capacity from one to five drawers; files are arranged from front

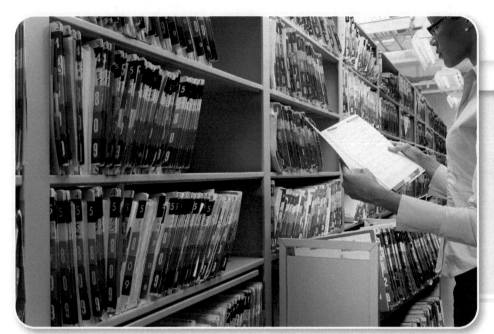

Figure 5.18

The assistant must understand the ways in which the office files are used, the organization of the files, and the principles and procedures for accurate filing. *How can an assistant get help in learning the filing procedures of a specific medical office?*
Image Source/Getty Images

to back in each drawer. Vertical files, shown in Figure 5.19, are popular because they provide a large amount of filing space. Vertical files can be moved fairly easily compared to open-shelf files. However, because these cabinets have drawers that must be opened and closed, using vertical files takes more of an assistant's time in filing and retrieving records. The space required to open the drawers is also a consideration in planning efficient use of storage and aisle space.

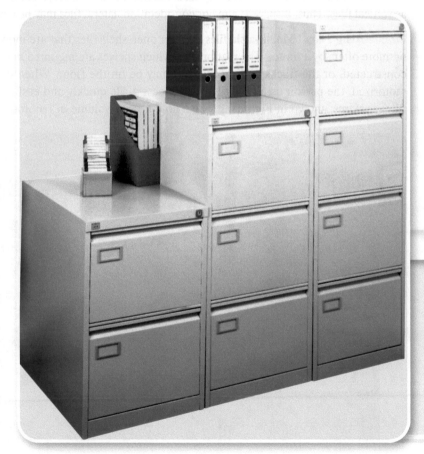

Figure 5.19

Vertical file cabinets are commonly used to store business documents and files. *Do business documents need to be more or less accessible to medical personnel than medical records do?*
Ingram Publishing/Alamy Stock Photo

Figure 5.20

Drawers open horizontally in lateral file cabinets to provide easy access. *How important is it for the assistant to have easy access to files?* Jacobs Stock Photography/BananaStock/Getty Images

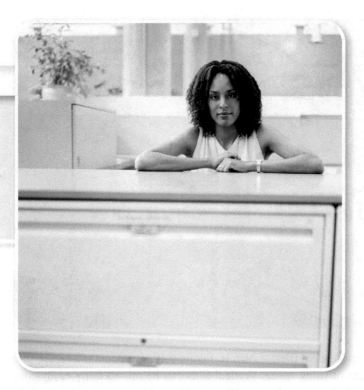

Lateral Files. In **lateral files,** the drawers or shelves open horizontally and files are arranged sideways, from left to right, instead of from front to back. Lateral files, as shown in Figure 5.20, may have standard drawers or doors that are rolled down from the top of the shelf and retract when the shelf is being used. Lateral files do not project as far into an aisle as vertical files. Thus, if space is a major consideration, lateral files may be a good choice.

Mobile-Aisle Files. **Mobile-aisle files** contain open-shelf files that are moved manually or, more often, by a motor. The platform on which shelves are mounted may be specially constructed, or the tracks and mechanism may be on the floor. When these files are motorized, the person using the files may access a file quickly and easily. Mobile-aisle filing systems, shown in Figure 5.21, also hold a large volume of records. Because this

Figure 5.21

Mobile-aisle files save space and are easily accessible. *Which kinds of files seem most suitable for a single-physician office? A multi-physician office? A clinic? A hospital?* ERproductions/Blend Images/Getty Images

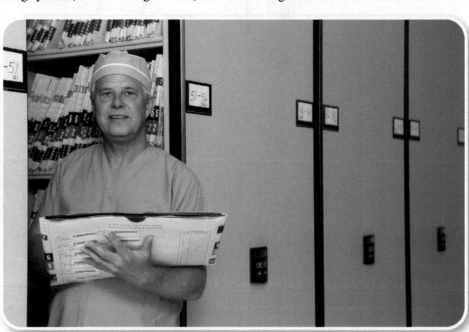

system holds so many records and because the system is mechanized, safety features, such as an electronic eye to sense when someone is using another portion of the files and to prevent movement of the files and the amount of weight the files will safely hold, are important factors in the decision to install this system.

Vertical Carousel File. Vertical carousel files allow the user to bring the drawer forward using a carousel-like motion. The motor rotates the unit containing file drawers and brings the selected drawer forward to the desired height. Since the height can be selected by the operator, a person may stand or sit when retrieving files. Figure 5.22 shows an example of a vertical carousel file unit.

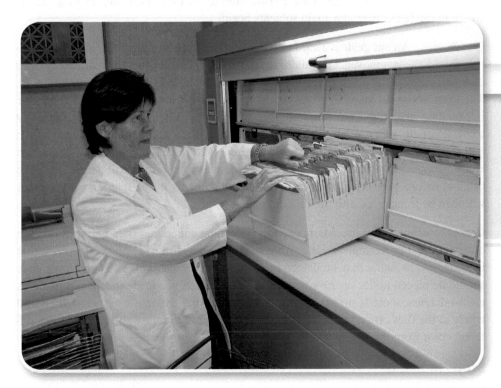

Figure 5.22

Carousel storage units require fewer footsteps to retrieve stored information. Why is this an important feature in a medical environment? Courtesy of Kardex Remstar, LLC

Filing Supplies

Folders, tabs, labels, and guides are all designed to make the location of and access to files efficient. Important considerations in choosing filing supplies are the durability of the material and the uses of color and positioning within a file to make the user's task easier. Out guides and cross-reference sheets help track record usage and location.

Folders. File **folders,** which may be open on one, two, or three sides, hold the items that are stored. Folders may be purchased in various colors, styles, weights, and tab cuts. **Tabs** are the projections that extend beyond the rest of the folder, so that the folder can be labeled and easily viewed. **Tab cuts** are the positions of the tabs. For example, the first cut creates a tab at the left; a center cut, at the center. The most popular position of a tab for a patient chart is a third-cut tab, which places a tab at the right of the chart. Folders are filed in such a way that tab cuts, with the accompanying labels, are read in an orderly fashion from left to right.

Labels. Oblong pieces of paper, frequently self-adhesive, are called **labels.** Once the person establishing the file has keyed in a descriptive title or subject on the label, it is used to identify a file. (Handwritten labels are to be avoided, as they are hard to read.) Labels are available in perforated rolls or on self-adhesive strips. Many assistants use a computer and printer to key in file titles and print out the required labels. Labels with a color band on top for ease of identification are also available. Scanners and bar codes may be used to identify patient charts. Codified data, such as patient names or numbers, are placed in a bar code and read by the programmed scanner, similar to purchasing items at a store and having them scanned for purchase.

Guides. **Guides** are rigid dividers placed at the end of a section of files to indicate where a new section or category of files begins. Because guides are made of rigid material, they support folders and are visual cues to the user of the file, showing exactly where in the file drawer new main subjects begin.

Out Guides. An **out guide** is a card or sheet that is placed as a substitute when information from a file is removed. Out guides are particularly useful when there are many users of a particular set of files. Everyone always knows where information may be found. The front of the out guide has lines to record the name of the person who is taking the information, the date it was removed, the material that was removed, and the date it is to be returned. When the information is returned, these annotations are crossed out and the out guide is removed and may be reused. Out folders may be substituted for an entire patient chart when it is removed. They serve as a temporary storage unit until the original record is returned. Any accumulated documents in the temporary out folder will then be transferred into the original patient chart.

Cross-Reference Sheets. Many documents can be coded and filed under more than one heading. For example, a letter from the physician's Internet provider service that has changed its name may be placed in more than one location. The correspondence should be placed under the new name and a cross reference made for the old name. A **cross-reference sheet** is prepared to indicate where the original material is filed and where in the files other copies may be found. The cross-reference sheet may be in a different color from the file folders to make identification simpler.

Steps in Filing

Following logical, consistent, systematic steps in preparing materials for filing enables the assistant to file accurately, to find materials quickly, and to refile documents efficiently.

The following are the steps in filing:

1. Inspecting documents
2. Indexing
3. Coding and if, necesary, cross-referencing
4. Sorting
5. Storing

Inspecting Documents. The assistant is responsible for **inspecting documents** received for filing. Each document should be in good physical condition, and the information should be complete. For example, if an attachment is indicated, it should be present. If the document says that an action should be taken—such as a form letter should be sent to an insurance company—the item relating to the action should be present or there should be an indication, such as a check mark, that the action was taken. The document must also bear a release mark. A **release mark** is an indication, by initial or by some other agreed-upon mark, that the document has been inspected and acted upon and is ready for filing. Note that a release mark is different from a time-date stamp, which is documentation of the time and date a correspondence or document was received.

Indexing. Once a document has been released, it is ready to be indexed. **Indexing** is the *mental* process of selecting the name, title, or classification under which an item will be filed and arranging the units of the title or name in the proper order. For example, information about a patient named *José Gomez* would be filed under *G* for *Gomez*. Selecting the proper classification for an item is critical to finding the document when it is needed.

Coding. **Coding** is *physically* placing a number, a letter, or an underscore beneath a word to indicate where the document should be filed. For example, in the correspondence of José Gomez, the name *Gomez* would be underscored or coded in some way. Or the code might be written on the document, usually in the upper right-hand corner.

If the document could be requested by a name or subject that is different from the name or subject under which it is actually coded and stored, cross-referencing the document is required. The cross-reference sheet is filed under the cross-reference location. For example, a cross-reference sheet for *José Gomez* may be found under *José*. No documents are filed under the name *José,* but the cross-reference sheet will instruct the medical team member to see *Gomez Jose* to find the patient's medical record. Types of patient names that should be cross-referenced are

- *similar names* (Bayes, Bays, Bazes). Original record is stored under BAYES with two cross-references made—one for BAYES SEE ALSO BAYS, BAZES; and one for BAZES SEE ALSO BAYS, BAYES.
- *hyphenated surnames/last names* (Mrs. Susie Williams-Ortigo). Original record is stored under WILLIAMSORTIGO SUSIE MRS with one cross reference made for ORTIGO SUSIE WILLIAMS MRS SEE WILLIAMSORTIGO SUSIE MRS.
- *unusual names* (Mr. William James). Original record is stored under JAMES WILLIAM with one cross reference made for WILLIAM JAMES SEE JAMES WILLIAM.
- *alternate names* (Susie Patient is also known as Mrs. John Patient). Original record is stored under PATIENT SUSIE with one cross reference made for PATIENT JOHN MRS SEE PATIENT SUSIE.

Sorting. The assistant working with a number of items prepares them for the file by **sorting** them, or arranging them in the order in which they will be filed. Before they can be sorted, documents must be indexed and coded. When the assistant is indexing the item, the code should also be chosen and recorded on the record.

Storing. **Storing,** or filing, is the actual placement of an item in its correct place in the file. When the item is placed in the folder, the top of the item should be to the left. Documents are placed in the folder with the most current document on top (reverse chronological order). The folder is then placed in the record storage unit.

Follow-Up Procedures. Many items that have been stored may require some further action to be taken. For example, even though the correspondence relating to José Gomez has been filed, Mr. Gomez may require a reminder to return for his annual checkup, which can be done with the use of a tickler file.

A useful tickler (reminder) file should be consulted daily. An arrangement of index cards by months of the year and, within each month, by days of the month is practical. Notations of actions to be taken are placed on cards behind specific dates of the month. At the end of the current month, new cards are placed behind each date of the next month. There are also electronic monthly calendars available in most software application suites, as shown in Figure 5.23. If actions to be taken are entered on specific dates of the electronic calendar, the software will provide an automatic tickler—a message on the screen—on the appropriate date. The assistant may find this system more efficient and easier to use.

Figure 5.23

An automatic tickler serves as a reminder for follow-up tasks and appointments. *What kinds of items may be noted?*

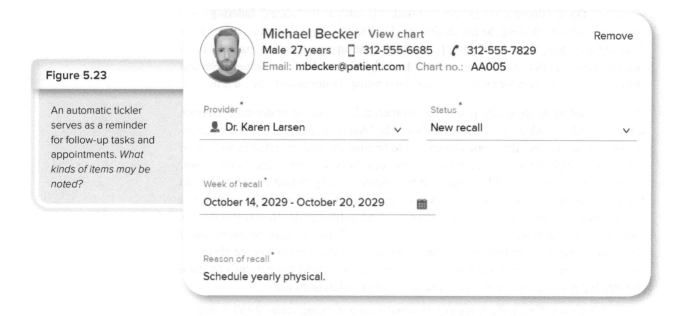

Michael Becker View chart   Remove
Male 27 years 📱 312-555-6685 📞 312-555-7829
Email: mbecker@patient.com | Chart no.: **AA005**

Provider*
👤 Dr. Karen Larsen   ⌄

Status*
New recall   ⌄

Week of recall*
October 14, 2029 - October 20, 2029   📅

Reason of recall*
Schedule yearly physical.

Another way to be reminded of a follow-up action is to use a colored index tab clipped to a patient's record. The colored tab indicates that action is required. Different colors may be assigned to stand for different kinds of actions.

Filing Methods

Effective records management requires records to be filed in the way they will be accessed. Most offices use more than one filing method to organize their different types of information. The major filing methods are alphabetic, numeric, and subject. Each method has advantages as well as disadvantages.

Alphabetic Filing. The most popular filing method is **alphabetic filing,** the arrangement of names, titles, or classifications in alphabetical order. This method is popular because it is based on the familiar letters of the alphabet. It provides a direct reference—if the name is known, the record can be located. An alphabetic method enables a user to find a misfiled paper document easily and has low setup and maintenance costs. It is commonly used by word processing and database software to organize lists of files. Most programs include a sort feature, which automatically alphabetizes a list of entries (Figure 5.24).

There are, however, several disadvantages to alphabetic filing. Because the method is so simple and so easily recognizable, there is much less confidentiality. File labels may be easily seen and read; computer files can be quickly searched. It is also possible that similar names will be confused or that a letter will be transposed and the document misfiled. A typing error can cause a patient's information to be filed incorrectly. An alphabetic method for paper records offers limited filing space and makes expanding the system difficult when folders labeled alphabetically are full.

The assistant must thoroughly understand the basic rules for alphabetizing and indexing in order to accurately manage records. ARMA's general rules for alphabetic filing, which are the standard for medical offices, are described in this section.

General Filing Rules

- Each filing segment is considered a unit.
- Alphabetize units by comparing letter by letter within that unit.
- Ignore all punctuation marks.

COMPLIANCE TIP

To protect the confidentiality of medical records and patient PHI, medical charts should be placed backward in holding areas. The label containing the patient's name will not be visible to anyone walking past the chart.

KAREN LARSEN MD
PATIENT LIST
09/12/2028

Figure 5.24

Alphabetized Patient List

Chart	Name	City, State, Zip Code	Phone
AA001	Monica T. Armstrong	Chicago, IL 60644-5519	312-555-4413
AA002	Thomas R. Baab	Chicago, IL 60625-1220	312-555-3478
AA003	Sara Babcock	Chicago, IL 60644-4455	312-555-5441
AA004	Allison Becker	Chicago, IL 60632-1979	312-555-6685
AA005	Michael Becker	Chicago, IL 60632-1979	312-555-6685
AA006	Paul Burton	Chicago, IL 60641-6730	312-555-7292
AA007	Randy T. Burton	Chicago, IL 60641-6730	312-555-7292
AA008	Doris L. Casagranda	Chicago, IL 60632-1406	312-555-1200
AA009	George Casagranda	Chicago, IL 60632-1406	312-555-1200
AA010	Joseph W. Castro	Chicago, IL 60634-3727	312-555-1020

- File "nothing before something." In a letter-by-letter comparison of two terms, if one term has nothing and the other has an "a," the term with nothing is put first.
- Arabic and Roman numerals are filed sequentially before alphabetic files, with Arabic numerals coming before Roman numerals.

Rule 1: Order of Indexing Units. Patient names: Index individual names in the following order: surname (last name), given name (first name), and then middle name or initial.

Business names: Index business names as they are written using the letterhead as a guide. Each word within the business name is to be considered as a separate indexing unit. When a personal name is used within a business name, it is still indexed as it is written. Do not transpose the name.

Names	Indexing Order		
	1	**2**	**3**
Wade R. Benje	Benje	Wade	R
Wayne Benje	Benje	Wayne	
Wayne Benje Clinic	Wayne	Benje	Clinic

Rule 2: Symbols and Minor Words. Business names: Each article, conjunction, preposition, and symbol is considered as a separate indexing unit. When indexing a symbol, spell the symbol and use it as the indexing unit. If the word *The* is the first word of a business name, move it to the last unit position.

Names	Indexing Order		
	1	**2**	**3**
A Imaging	A	Imaging	
#s Away Clinic	Pounds	Away	Clinic
The Sleep Clinic	Sleep	Clinic	The

Rule 3: Punctuation. Personal names: Disregard all punctuation.
Business names: Disregard all punctuation.

Names	Indexing Order	
	1	**2**
Julia Smith-Cline	SmithCline	Julia
South-End Diagnostics	SouthEnd	Diagnostics

Rule 4: Shortened Forms and Abbreviations. Personal names: Abbreviated and shortened forms of personal names are not spelled out. Use the abbreviation or shortened

form. Make sure the patient states his or her legal name. Initials within a name are a separate indexing unit.

Names	Indexing Order		
	1	2	3
Bill J. Wicks	Wicks	Bill	J
Geo. Lester Wilson	Wilson	Geo	Lester

Business names: Compound expressions are treated as written—if there is a space between terms, the terms are separate units. Single letters are indexed as written—if they are separated by a space, then they are separate units. Spell out symbols (&, #). Acronyms and call letters (for TV and radio) are single units. Abbreviated words and names are indexed as a single unit regardless of spacing.

Names	Indexing Order			
	1	2	3	4
A B C Clinic	A	B	C	Clinic
A&D Surgical Supplies	AandD	Surgical	Supplies	
A-B-C Clinic	ABC	Clinic		
Clinic On Main	Clinic	On	Main	
The Free Clinic	Free	Clinic	The	
John St. Claire Clinic	John	Stclaire	Clinic	
KARE TV Station	Kare	TV	Station	
South West Clinic	South	West	Clinic	
Southwest Clinic	Southwest	Clinic		

Rule 5: Titles and Suffixes. Personal names: Professional or personal titles (*Dr., Mr., Mrs., Ms., Prof.*), professional suffixes (*MD, DDS, Ph.D., CPA*), and seniority designations are the last indexing unit. When a name has both a title and a suffix, the title is the last unit. If you have only a title and one name, index the name as it is written. Numbers are filed before letters; therefore, in seniority terms, the sequence is numbers (*2nd, 3rd*), Roman numerals (*I, II*), and then *junior (Jr.)* and *senior (Sr.)*.

Business names: When a title appears in a business name, index the business name as it is written. Remember, *The* is moved to the last indexing unit.

Names	Indexing Order		
	1	2	3
Alan Berg MD	Berg	Alan	MD
Matthew Blue 2nd	Blue	Matthew	2
Charles Jonathan III	Jonathan	Charles	III
Charles Jonathan Jr.	Jonathan	Charles	Jr
The Ladies II	Ladies	II	The
Sister Mary-Margaret	Sister	Marymargaret	
Sister Mary-Margaret Smith	Smith	Marymargaret	Sister

Rule 6: Prefixes. Personal and business names: Prefixes are considered part of the surname, not separate units. Some prefixes are *Aba, Abd, a la, D', Da, De, Del, De la, Den, Des, Di, Dos, Du, El, Fitz, ibn, La, Las, Le, Lo, Los, M, Mac, Mc, O', Saint, San, Santa, Santo, St., Te, Ten, Ter, Van, Van de, Van der, Von,* and *Von der.* Disregard the punctuation and close up the space.

Names	Indexing Order		
	1	2	3
Lorne Fitz-gerald	Fitzgerald	Lorne	
Esther Ann O'Reilly	Oreilly	Esther	Ann
David R. Van de Wan	Vandewan	David	R

Rule 7: Numbers. Business names: Arabic numerals (1, 2, 3, 4) and Roman numerals (I, II, III, IV) are considered a single unit and are filed in numeric order before alphabetic characters (*Arabic* comes before *Roman*). Roman numerals are indexed in ascending order by their value. Ignore ordinal endings *(st, d, th)*.

Names	Indexing Order		
	1	**2**	**3**
1-A Physical Therapy	1A	Physical	Therapy
5th Avenue Clinic	5	Avenue	Clinic
50+ Retirement Group	50plus	Retirement	Group
XXI Century Medical Group	XXI	Century	Medical Group
Sixty-Third Street Pharmacy	Sixtythird	Street	Pharmacy
South 36th Pharmacy	South	36	Pharmacy

Rule 8: Organizations. Business names: Committees, hospitals, universities, hotels, motels, and churches are indexed as written. Cross-reference items to ensure finding them.

Names	Indexing Order			
	1	**2**	**3**	**4**
Alexander Hotel	Alexander	Hotel		
Committee for Academic Affairs (Could be cross-referenced under *Academic Affairs Committee for*)	Committee	for	Academic	Affairs
St. Paul's Medical Center	StPauls	Medical	Center	
University of Illinois Hospital	University	of	Illinois	Hospital

Rule 9: Identical Names. When names are identical, index the names by city, state (spelled in full), street name, quadrant *(NE, NW, SE, SW),* and house or building number in numeric order (lowest number first). Zip Codes are not considered as an indexing unit.

Names

Emily Beck
1055 Maple Lane
Chicago, IL 60623-9623

Emily Beck
8275 Maple Lane
Chicago, IL 60623-9627

Indexing Order

1	2	3	4	5	6	7
Beck	Emily	Chicago	Illinois	Maple	Lane	1055
Beck	Emily	Chicago	Illinois	Maple	Lane	8275

Rule 10: Government. Government names are indexed first by the governmental unit (country, state, county, or city). Next, index the name of the department, bureau, office, or board. Words such as *Office of* and *Department of* are separate indexing units and are transposed.

Federal Government
The first three units of all federal government names are *United States Government*.

Names	Indexing Order				
	1	**2**	**3**	**4**	**5**
U.S. Department of Health and Human Services	United	States	Government	Health	and
	6	**7**	**8**	**9**	
	Human	Services	Department	of	

State and Local Governments

Names	Indexing Order				
	1	**2**	**3**	**4**	**5**
City of Anoka Health Department	Anoka	City	of	Health	Department
Anoka County Health Department	Anoka	County	Health	Department	
Illinois Bureau of Health	Illinois	Health	Bureau	of	

Foreign Governments

Names	Indexing Order				
	1	**2**	**3**	**4**	**5**
Republic of Sweden Health Department	Sweden	Republic	of	Health	Department

Numeric Filing. Offices with a large volume of patient records may use a **numeric filing** system, that is, one in which each patient is assigned a number. The patient number is assigned from an **accession book,** which is a book or electronic log of consecutive numbers indicating the next available number to be assigned. A cross-index is then prepared to match the numbers with the names. Many electronic medical database programs automatically assign the next available number from within the program's database. In order to access a patient's file, the assistant must first locate the patient's number, and then, using the patient's number, access the patient's records. This is considered an indirect access method of locating records. Larger medical facilities maintain a master patient index (MPI), which identifies all patients who have received care at the facility. Patient information can be accessed only after retrieving the assigned patient number from the MPI.

There are several ways to assign numeric values. Two of the most frequently used ways are straight-numeric filing and terminal-digit filing.

1. *Straight-numeric filing:* The straight-numeric system uses ascending numbers in consecutive order. For example, File 125203 would be filed after File 125202 and before File 125204.
2. *Terminal-digit filing:* The terminal-digit system uses the terminal (last) digit, or set of digits, as the indexing unit. The file numbered 33-52-12 would be filed in Section 12 (the last unit) behind 52 (the guide number) and would be the 33rd item in sequence.

Another filing method combines both alphabetic and numeric characters. The alphanumeric system is commonly used in medical settings to assign patient numbers. Figure 5.25 provides an example of an alphanumeric listing.

Numeric filing is a very accurate method of filing. It is more difficult to misfile or to lose files. Therefore, there is speedier storage and retrieval. It is a method that helps maintain confidentiality of files. In a numeric filing system, expansion is unlimited, depending only on the next unassigned number in the sequence.

Although numbers provide accuracy, there is still an opportunity to transpose numbers, especially if the sequence is a long one. More guides are required, and there is a need to consult and maintain an alphabetic cross-index. Using the system efficiently also requires a thorough training program for staff members. A patient's Social Security Number or any part of a Social Security Number should not be used as the patient number.

Subject Filing. **Subject filing** is the placement of related material alphabetically by subject categories. It is a useful method for keeping nonpatient correspondence, research

Patient name	SSN	Chart number	Date of birth	Gender
Monica Armstrong	486-29-3789	AA001	08/12/1978	Female
Thomas Baab	581-57-0376	AA002	10/06/1974	Male
Sara Babcock	987-87-3759	AA003	12/20/2007	Female
Allison Becker	470-55-8533	AA004	01/27/2003	Female
Michael Becker	581-66-9644	AA005	08/31/2001	Male
Paul Burton	333-90-7182	AA006	10/22/1999	Male
Randy Burton	567-89-0123	AA007	01/16/2026	Male
Doris Casagranda	890-29-5649	AA008	09/01/2012	Female
George Casagranda	497-27-3367	AA009	11/22/1991	Male
Joseph Castro	876-91-3629	AA010	11/02/2009	Male
Lena Crac	616-58-7513	AA011	09/11/1996	Female
Theresa Dayton	767-90-1128	AA012	03/13/2006	Female
Todd Grant	399-11-2939	AA013	05/18/1996	Male
Alma Jackson	195-75-2316	AA014	09/06/1968	Female
Charles Jonathan III	444-02-4422	AA015	11/29/1990	Male
Andrew Kramer	747-22-3401	AA016	12/31/1998	Male
Jeffrey Kramer	981-42-5167	AA017	04/22/2020	Male
Jack Kyser	567-89-0123	AA018	08/17/2019	Male
Cynthia Kyser	223-09-4012	AA019	04/11/1989	Female

Figure 5.25

EHRclinic Screen Showing Patient Account Numbers

articles, practice management files, and other material of a general nature. A computer database is also organized by subject. For example, in many electronic health record programs, databases are set up for patients, insurance companies, physicians, and guarantors. (A *guarantor* is the person who is responsible for payment to the physician.) In each database, the entries are listed alphabetically.

Subject categories depend on the specific needs of the physician and on the amount of material to be filed under each heading. Manuscripts are filed alphabetically under the title of the article or book. Reviews of, and references to, the physician's own writing are also filed under the title of the article or book. Abstracts of research articles, excerpts, and other reviews may be clippings from magazines or newspapers. Whether these are filed by the author's name or by the subject depends on how the physician plans to use the items. Figure 5.26 illustrates a relative subject index with a sample of headings that may be used in subject filing.

When all items pertaining to the same subject may be found in one location, as they are with subject filing, valuable time is saved. Statistics and other types of information are easily accessible. The relative subject index is easy to expand. However, when there is a great amount of material, subject categories may overlap or extensive cross-referencing may be required for complex topics. It can become time-consuming, even for those who are experienced in filing, to file and retrieve materials.

Color-Coding. **Color-coding** is used in many medical offices. In a color-coded system, typically the first two or three letters of the surname are placed on the tab. Each letter of the alphabet is a different color; for instance, A is green, B is blue, and so on. All folders within the A section of the files should have a green first label. Therefore, a folder containing a yellow label in the first position would be a misfiled chart. Using this system, it is easy to locate misfiled charts.

Multi-physician practices may use color-coded patient charts. Each physician's patients' charts are identified by color. Differentiating between charts becomes more efficient using this method.

Figure 5.26 Relative Subject Index

Advertisements
Drugs
Medical
Office

Automobile
Insurance
Maintenance

Clinic Property
Building
Inventory
Maintenance
Medical Equipment
Office Equipment

Collections
Accounts Receivable
Agency Contracts
Form Letters

Education
Doctor's Continuing
Employee
Patient

Entertainment
Financial Information
Annual Financial
Banking
Monthly Financial

Forms
Applications
Consent
Release from Work
Release of Information

Hospital
Policy
Reports
Staff Meetings

Insurance
Clinic
Fire
Liability—Doctor's

Patients
Index Control File
Patient Billing List

Personnel
Applications—Inactive
Benefits and Policies
Current Employees
Doctor's Personal File—Diplomas,
    Licenses, Publications

Referral Information
Society Information
American Medical Association
Seminars
State Medical Society

Subscriptions and Publications
Drug Companies
Lobby Magazines
Medical Magazines
Newspapers
Professional Library

Supplies
Inventory
Medical
Office
Order Forms

Taxes
Payroll
Personal (Doctor's)
Property

Travel
Expenses
Pending

Utilities
Electricity
Gas
Telephone
Water

Another use of color-coding indicates different functions. Different-colored files are used for various documents, such as lab reports, signature files, or imaging results. Special-colored folders may also be used to forward information for insurance specialists, nurses, office managers, and so on.

Locating Missing Files. Even in a well-organized office, paper documents will occasionally be lost or misfiled. Here are a number of suggestions for locating a missing file:

- Look directly behind and in front of where the item should be filed.
- Look between other files in the area.
- Look in the bottom of the file drawer and under the file folders if they are suspended.
- Check for the transposition of first and last names—for example, *Wheng, Hart* instead of *Hart, Wheng.*
- Check alternate spellings of the name—for example, *Thomasen* and *Thomason.*
- In a numeric filing system, check for transposed numbers—for example, *19-63-01* instead of *19-01-63.*
- In a subject filing system, check related subject files or the *Miscellaneous* file.
- With the permission of those who have used the file recently, search the desk or work area of previous users of the file.
- Check with other office personnel.

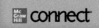 **GO TO PROJECTS 5.9, 5.10, 5.11, AND 5.12 AT THE END OF THIS CHAPTER**

5.1 Classify various uses of computer technology.	• Computer usage in a medical environment has increased tremendously in recent years. Office tasks that traditionally were completed by hand are now done with a high degree of efficiency by using a computer:
	— Scheduling: Appointment availability can be quickly accessed and schedules can be completed. Past, current, and future appointments can be viewed, created, and changed within specific computer menus.
	— Medical data entry: Patients' medical records can be created electronically. Patient data can be input into the electronic health records, prescriptions may be electronically prepared and either given to the patient or sent directly to the pharmacy, and orders for lab tests and procedures can be automatically processed.
	— Communications: Information is transmitted via the Internet within the office or across the globe. The ease, cost-effectiveness, and speed of e-mail have made it the leading form of intraoffice and interoffice communications.
	— Research: Physicians can research medical conditions, search for drug interactions, conduct webinars, and perform other clinical tasks through the use of technology.
	• Computers have integrated all phases of the medical community and will continue to be an asset to patient care.
5.2 Recall reasons for maintaining a medical chart and documents that comprise the medical chart.	• Medical records are used as the main source of medical data for patients, and they provide for continuity of care. They supply health information and protected health information, such as diagnoses and treatments for patients. Medical charts are legal documents.
	• Examples of documents that may be found in a medical chart are
	— chart notes.
	— history and physicals.
	— clinical forms.
	— medical reports.
	— communications with the patient or with other medical personnel concerning the patient.

5.3 Discuss the advantages and challenges of electronic health records.	• As the mandatory use of EHRs quickly approaches, many advantages may be gained from implementation: — Multiple users at the same time — Data protection through passwords, encryption, and backup — Quick and easy update of records — Automatic verification of prescriptions — Fewer errors due to handwriting — More time spent with patients — Faster access to data — Electronic submission of orders and prescriptions — Electronic reminders to patients • Implementation also presents challenges: — Updating of system — Ongoing training — Scanning of hardcopy documents into the system — Avoiding typographical errors
5.4 List three commonly used medical abbreviations and three medical abbreviations targeted for nonuse by the Joint Commission.	• Three commonly used medical abbreviations are BUN, Dx, and HPI. • Similar medical abbreviations may contribute to a misdiagnosis or misinterpretation. The Joint Commission has distributed a listing of "Do Not Use" abbreviations. Four examples follow: — U for unit — IU for international unit — Q. or q. for every — MS for either morphine sulfate or magnesium sulfate
5.5 Discuss various input technologies used to create medical documentation.	• Newer input technologies, such as voice-recognition software and wireless devices and cloud computing allow the input of data with greater speed and mobility. This, in turn, allows more time for patient care. — Voice-recognition software enables the dictator to train the program to his or her voice, and data are input by speaking into the trained device.

	— Wireless and cloud technology allows the input of medical data into extremely small, portable devices, such as smartphones. WiFi connection is now available at many locations, allowing data to be input directly into a patient's electronic health record. A physician visiting a patient in the hospital can research medical contraindications from his or her wireless device without the need to leave the patient's room or the facility.
	— Traditionally, transcription has been used for medical data input. Physicians dictate data into recording devices, and transcriptionists key in transcribed documents for the physician's verification and signature. The field of transcription is evolving, just as technology continues to evolve. Transcriptionists will be needed to edit medical data entered through electronic devices, such as voice recognition. Opportunities for "scribes"—individuals who input patient medical data into electronic storage as the physician dictates or provides data—exist for individuals with transcription training and/or experience.
5.6 Identify components of a paper-based medical record and explain how the same components will be compiled in an electronic health record format	• Notes from the patient encounter, such as the chief complaint, history, examination, impression/diagnosis, and treatment plan, are documented in a patient medical chart using various formats, such as SOAP. Lab reports, nurses' assessment, dietitian plans, and so on are placed into the chart either by encounter or by category—for instance, all nurses' assessments would be placed in a section.
	• Electronic input of these and other medical chart components is completed through main screens and drop-down menus. As data are input into the electronic health record, other options may be presented or additional space will be provided for comments.
	• Electronic health records can be quickly searched for data, and information from encounters can be compared.

5.7 Distinguish among active, inactive, and closed files.	• In a medical environment, a large number of medical records must be managed. Records are often classified by their activity. Three broad classifications are
	  — active files—medical records for current patients.
	  — inactive files—medical records for patients who have not seen the physician in a predetermined amount of time, such as 6 months to a year.
	  — closed files—medical records for patients who have moved away, have terminated their patient-physician relationship, or are deceased.
	As each medical specialty has its own requirements, a retention schedule should be developed by the practice based on its needs and state statutes.

5.8 Differentiate among records management systems that may be used in a medical office.	• Commonly used records management systems are alphabetic, numeric, and subject:
	  — Alphabetic filing—traditionally, the most frequently used system. This system manages records based on the alphabet, and it is easy to train office personnel in its use. However, the lack of confidentiality (the patient's name is on the label) makes this system vulnerable to unintentional disclosure of PHI.
	  — Numeric filing—uses a combination of numbers, not a Social Security Number, to maintain patient information. Because the patient's name does not appear on the label, this system provides a higher level of protection for PHI. Numeric filing is widely used in medical environments. Indirect access and employee training are two disadvantages of numeric filing.
	  — Subject filing—classifies records by subject titles, such as Invoices or Journals. This is useful when a group of similar data needs to be filed together. Indexes must be used for both the subject and numeric systems.

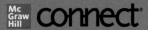
Project 5.1 — (LO 5.1) Computer Terms

Working Paper 38 (WP 38) contains computer terms and definitions. Match each definition to the correct term.

Project 5.2 — (LO 5.1) Computer Technology

Working Paper 39 (WP 39) contains statements that refer to computer technology in the medical office. Mark each statement with either "T" for *true* or "F" for *false*. For *false* statements, state why the statement is *false*. Be prepared to discuss your answers.

Project 5.3 — (LO 5.2) Preparing Patient Files

Dr. Larsen maintains a file folder (chart) for each patient. The patient information forms are available on Connect, labeled project 5.3 documentation. Print out each form and begin an alphabetic file folder for each patient. Note that each patient should have an individual file folder/chart. If you have already created a patient file folder, such as for SHERMAN FLORENCE in Project 3.1, do not create a duplicate folder. Material that pertains to each patient should be filed chronologically within that patient's file folder/chart, with the most current medical documentation on top. Prepare a chart note and new folder whenever a new patient arrives for an appointment. Prepare the identifier on the label by using either the patient's name—last name, then first name (i.e., SHERMAN FLORENCE)—or by using the patient's account/chart number. The account/chart number is a unique number that identifies each patient. Patient account/chart numbers are listed on WP 87.

Prepare the chart note in this way: Center the words "CHART NOTE" on the first line. Triple-space; then key information about the patient as shown in the following example. Save the document on your external storage device by the patient's last name, followed by the first initial.

CHART NOTE

JACKSON, ALMA
DOB: 09-06-19--
AA014

Update information on the patient information form as necessary. You will need to save this updated form to your own storage device. Place the alphabetized patient folders in your expandable portfolio.

Project 5.4 — (LO 5.2) Chart Entries

Dr. Larsen instructs you to make the following chart notations for her signature. Both should be dated October 10. Use WP 87 to locate patient account/chart numbers.

- Sara Babcock: Patient called for refill of Ortho Tri-Cyclen®. She has a physical scheduled for October 18, and we will deal with the prescription renewal at that time.
- Jeffrey Kramer: Father called for OTC help for Jeffrey for sore throat and earache. I advised the father to make an appointment as soon as possible. Patient to gargle with warm salt water every 3–4 h and be given Children's Tylenol® for pain relief p.r.n.

Project 5.5 — (LO 5.2) Lab Message Entries

The following lab results were received by telephone message. Dr. Larsen instructed you to make notations in the charts for her signature. Each chart note should be dated October 13. Dr. Larsen saw Gary Robertson (EP) on October 11 in the office, and Erin Mitchell (NP) was seen on October 11 in the ER. Laboratory tests were ordered for both patients. The remainder of Dr. Larsen's October 11 patients will be seen in Simulation 1. Key in a chart note for each patient's chart. Use WP 87 to locate patient account/chart numbers.

- October 13: Gary Robertson's urine culture results from October 11 show Enterobacter greater than 100,000 colonies, sensitive to sulfa. Left message for patient with results. Patient to continue Septra® and follow up in 2 weeks, sooner p.r.n.
- October 13: Erin Mitchell's urine culture results from October 11 revealed bacterial count greater than 100,000/mL. Talked with patient today. Patient to continue ciprofloxacin as directed. RTC if symptoms do not clear.
- *Note to Student:* Prepare a patient chart for Erin and place the chart note in the new patient folder.

Project 5.6 — (LO 5.5) Chart Transcription—Optional Project

Dr. Larsen has dictated most of her chart notes for patients seen on October 11 and 12. Dictated notes may be provided by your instructor. Audio files can be found on Connect. Use the chart note formats found in this chapter, and transcribe the dictation into each patient's medical record. Use WP 87 to locate patient account/chart numbers. *Note:* October 11 and October 12 are days 1 and 2 of Simulation 1, which is completed after Chapter 5. In order to gain transcription practice, chart notes for October 11 and October 12 are completed in this project. Additional dictation for patients seen on October 17 and October 18 (days 3 and 4 of Simulation 1) will be completed in Simulation 1.

Project 5.7 — (LO 5.3) Knowledge of the EHR

Working Paper 40 (WP 40) contains statements that refer to electronic health records. Write "T" or "F" in the blank to indicate whether you think the statement is *true* or *false*. If the answer is *false,* indicate what makes the statement *false.*

Project 5.8 — (LO 5.7) Internet Research: Using AHIMA as a Resource

AHIMA exists to serve health information management professionals. The organization offers credentials such as Registered Health Information Administrator. Like many professional groups, this organization also keeps those responsible for managing information current with the latest legislation and news and serves consumers of healthcare with topics of interest to them. Visit the AHIMA website at www.ahima.org. Follow the link from the home page to the page that allows you to search by key word. Key in the term *HIM Topics* or other key term assigned by your instructor and read one of the articles related to this topic. Be prepared to share the results of your reading.

Project 5.9   (LO 5.8) Cross-Referencing

Indicate the file and cross-reference entries for the following:

- Randolph Car Service (formerly Carl's Car Service)
- James Henry University
- File folders bought from Oliver Systems and Viking Office Supplies

Project 5.10   (LO 5.8) Using Subject Filing

On a plain sheet of paper, write the subject heading for each of the following items. Use Figure 5.26 as a guideline for your choices. Be prepared to discuss your answers in class.

- A copy of an article that Dr. Larsen had published in the *Journal of the American Medical Association (JAMA)*
- A new contract for employees' health insurance
- A bulletin about next month's continuing education seminar for the nursing staff
- The minutes from the hospital staff's last meeting
- A December itinerary for a symposium related to family practice physicians that Dr. Larsen will attend.

Project 5.11   (LO 5.3) Entering Patient Information

 If you are instructed to complete this project using EHRclinic, your instructor will assign you the project as part of a Connect assignment.

If you are instructed to use patient information forms, use Working Paper 41 (WP 41). Record the patient's information on the form. If the information is keyed on the form, save the document to your electronic storage device. Place a copy of the completed patient information form in the chart that was prepared in Project 5.5.

Erin Mitchell called Dr. Larsen's office today to give information to the office in preparation for her upcoming visit for a backache. Enter her patient information:

Name: Erin Jean Mitchell
Address: 5231 West School Street, Chicago, IL 60651-2248
Telephone: 312-555-8153
Spouse: Alan Mitchell
DOB: June 6, 1993
Employer: Unemployed
Alan's Employer: Computer salesperson at DataPlus, Wood Hills Plaza, 24614 W. 54th Avenue, Chicago, IL 60651-2268; phone 312-555-6141
Insurance: New York Mutual, Patient Insurance ID #304253B, Group #524S.
Alan's DOB: 12-01-19--
Erin's SSN: 470-25-6593
Note: *Erin's son, David, will also be seen by Dr. Larsen in Simulation 1.*

Project 5.12   (LO 5.3) Editing Patient Information

EHRclinic If you are instructed to complete this project using EHRclinic, your instructor will assign you the project as part of a Connect assignment.

WP

If you are instructed to use patient information forms, retrieve the electronically stored patient information form (WP 41 that was used in Project 5.11) and change the address. Resave the patient information form on your storage device. If you used a handwritten patient information form, retrieve the form from the patient's chart and make the necessary change by drawing a single line through the incorrect information and writing in the new information. Place your initials and the date the change was made beside the correction.

Erin Mitchell called the office to change Alan's employer name from DataPlus to DATAandMORE. The address and telephone number remain the same.

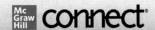
Teamwork (LO 5.3)

Effective teamwork can produce incredible results, but teamwork does not just happen. It takes a great deal of work and compromise. Knowing how to work on or with a team will be crucial to your success. Before we can reward teamwork and collaboration that integrates care, we need applications that let clinicians communicate patient information instantly and securely. **How can teamwork be beneficial to EHR and the medical office?**

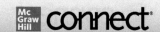
USING TERMINOLOGY

Match the term or phrase on the left with the correct answer on the right.

_____ 1. [LO 5.1] Word processing

_____ 2. [LO 5.6] SOAP

_____ 3. [LO 5.7] Active record

_____ 4. [LO 5.1] File server

_____ 5. [LO 5.8] Out indicator

_____ 6. [LO 5.3] Electronic health record

_____ 7. [LO 5.2] Medicolegal

_____ 8. [LO 5.6] ROS

_____ 9. [LO 5.5] Wireless communication

_____ 10. [LO 5.5] Voice-recognition technology

a. The use of radio waves to transmit data

b. A record of removed information

c. Records that provide proof of legal medical care

d. Software program used to enter, edit, format, and print documents

e. Technology used to input data using speech training

f. Heathcare databases that work together to compile complete patient healthcare records

g. Medical documentation format that includes subjective and objective data, assessment of data, and course of treatment

h. A subjective assessment of pertinent body systems

i. Records of current patients

j. Centralized storage of shared local network electronic data

CHECKING YOUR UNDERSTANDING

Select the most correct answer.

1. [LO 5.1] Maria works exclusively inputting data into medical records. She seldom takes a break from inputting and works 4 days per week, 10 hours each day. While driving, she noticed a change in her distance vision. Which of the following should she do to help ease eyestrain while working?

   a. Place her hands and wrists in horizontal alignment.
   b. Regularly focus on a distant object.
   c. Place source documents flat beside her computer.
   d. Frequently rotate her neck and shoulders.

2. [LO 5.2] Lori works for a medical practice that uses the first three letters of the patient's last name and the date of birth as patient numbers. When Lori was filing medical insurance claims, she noticed that a chart note had been made in the wrong paper-based chart. The physician sees twin females, and the chart for the wrong twin had been noted. To correct the error, she should

   a. eliminate the chart note with correction fluid.
   b. use a wide, permanent black marker to cross out the chart note.
   c. place a straight line through the entry, making sure it is still legible; mark it "error"; date her correction; and initial the correction.
   d. place a wavy line through the entry, making sure it is still legible; mark it "error"; date her correction; and initial the correction.

3. [LO 5.6] When Dr. Lee opened the EHR for his next patient, he was able to quickly view a listing of all the patient's current and previously treated medical conditions. Which documentation format does Dr. Lee use?

    a. SOAP
    b. CHEDDAR
    c. DATABASE
    d. POMR

4. [LO 5.7] After 10 years of practice, the administrative medical assistant observed that the medical charts container was full and hardcopy records were hard to retrieve and return due to overcrowding. No retention schedule had yet been developed. Which of the following strategies could be used efficiently to ease the overcrowding?

    a. Shred all records for patients who have not been seen in 3 years or more.
    b. Retrieve all the inactive folders, and place them in a corner.
    c. Remove and shred all files for deceased patients.
    d. Remove folders for inactive and closed files, and move them to a secure, secondary location.

5. [LO 5.8] Medical records in the office are marked with the patient number in the upper right-hand corner of the documents. This is known as

    a. inspecting a document.
    b. indexing a document.
    c. coding a document.
    d. storing a document.

6. [LO 5.3] Because of the high cost of EHR implementation and anticipated software updates, which of the following should not be considered when purchasing a program?

    a. A software program package that does not include future updates as part of the initial cost or at a stated cost
    b. Availability of ongoing software training by the manufacturer
    c. Ease of use
    d. Information from others who use the software

7. [LO 5.4] Which of the following is an acceptable chart notation for "as needed"?

    a. q.4h
    b. p.r.n.
    c. a.n.
    d. as ndd

8. [LO 5.5] Jamie does transcription for a local multi-physician practice. She has heard about the implementation of EHRs in her practice and is concerned about the future of her position. Which of the following would be beneficial for Jamie?

    a. Immediately resign from her position and return to school for training in a different field.
    b. Become involved in the selection process of an EHR program and contribute observations on the documentation template.
    c. Continue to update herself on grammar, punctuation, and format.
    d. Becoming involved in the selection process of an EHR program *and* continuing to update herself on format are both beneficial options for Jamie.

9. [LO 5.3] While triaging a pediatric patient, the administrative medical assistant noted the date of birth for the patient in the electronic medical record was incorrect. The patient's year of birth was stated as 2041 instead of 2014. Which of the following should be used to correct the electronic medical record?

   a. Addendum
   b. Late entry
   c. Amendment
   d. Strikethrough

10. [LO 5.3] When a correction or addition is made to a locked medical record, which of the following is *not* an acceptable method of editing or adding data?

   a. Deleting data
   b. Adding a late entry notation
   c. Adding an amendment
   d. Adding an addendum

MEDICAL VOCABULARY USED WITH OPTIONAL TRANSCRIPTION

Be sure that you are familiar with the following terms:

adnexa	accessory parts to the main structure
amoxicillin	an antibiotic
anginal	relating to constricting chest pain
bronchitis	inflammation in the bronchi
bruit	murmur
colonoscopy	visualization of the colon with a scope
costochondritis	inflammation of the cartilage between the ribs
dysmenorrhea	menstrual cramps
dysuria	painful or difficult urination
ecchymosis	black and blue or purple skin discoloration; bruise
exudative	relating to tissue material deposited as a result of infection
gallop	an abnormal heart sound
hepatosplenomegaly	liver and spleen enlargement
injection	inserting a solution under the skin (subcutaneously, intravenously, or intramuscularly) using a syringe or a needle
lymphadenopathy	enlargement of lymph nodes
malaise	feeling of uneasiness
normocephalic	relating to a normal-size head
ophthalmic	relating to the eye
otitis media	inflammation of the ear
PE tubes	polyethylene tubes
pharyngitis	inflammation of the throat
rhonchi	musical pitch heard on chest auscultation
sclera	the white of the eye

sitz bath	a type of bath that consists of soaking the area from the tailbone to the lower abdomen in a tub of warm water
supple	easily movable
tinea cruris	a fungal infection in the male perineal or groin area
tonsillitis	inflammation of the tonsils

THINKING IT THROUGH

These questions cover important points in this chapter. Using your critical-thinking skills, play the role of an administrative medical assistant as you answer each question. Be prepared to discuss your responses.

1. [LO 5.2] You are going through a patient's medical record to find information on a specific lab report, and you notice that several chart notes are not dated. What should you do?

2. [LO 5.2 and LO 5.6] How does the use of the SOAP format for organizing medical record data minimize a provider's exposure to legal risk?

3. [LO 5.4] You retrieve a patient's medical record and notice that the abbreviation *WDWNYM* is used several times in the chart notes. You know that this is not an approved abbreviation, though you eventually figure out that it stands for "well-developed, well-nourished young male." What do you do with this information?

4. [LO 5.6] You are asked to retrieve information regarding a patient's family history of intestinal cancer. The physician generally uses the POMR format. Where in the file should you look?

5. [LO 5.7] A former patient calls, hoping to locate x-rays taken more than 5 years ago. What should you say?

6. [LO 5.7] A patient calls and is moving out of town. She is concerned about her medical record. What would you suggest?

7. [LO 5.2, LO 5.3, LO 5.5] You are transcribing the physician's dictation and cannot understand several words in a chart note. What do you do?

Simulation 1

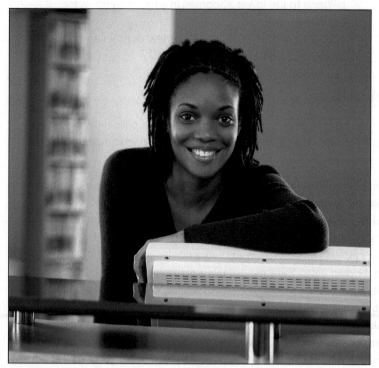

Air Images/Shutterstock

EHRclinic If you are instructed to complete this project using EHRclinic, your instructor will assign you the project as part of a Connect assignment.

YOUR ROLE

Welcome to the practice of Dr. Karen Larsen! You will continue to apply the skills you have learned in this text as you assume the role of Linda Schwartz, Dr. Larsen's administrative medical assistant.

Simulation 1 is the first of two simulations in the text. These simulations provide practical experience in working in a physician's office. You will discover how various tasks relate to each other. The daily events in the office are narrated on the Simulation Recordings that accompany this text. These recordings—as well as the other materials you will need for this simulation—are available in Connect in Simulation 1 (if your instructor assigned). As you listen to the recordings, you will handle various assignments as the assistant. Your simulation work will include making and canceling appointments, preparing messages, creating communications, preparing various medical forms, and following through on daily tasks.

BEFORE YOU START

The following suggestions apply to both Simulation 1 and Simulation 2.

1. Review the content of the previous chapters to ensure familiarity with procedures.
2. Prepare four file folders:
   a. Label as *Day 1 and your name.*
   b. Label as *Day 2 and your name.*
   c. Label as *Day 3 and your name.*
   d. Label as *Day 4 and your name.*
3. Assemble and organize necessary materials as listed under "Materials" (after the "Procedures" section).
4. Set priorities each day by organizing your work in order of importance and completing the work in that sequence. Any work left over from Day 1 should be carried over into Day 2, and so forth. The work left over from any previous day should be taken into account in setting the priorities for that day. It is also possible that you may have work left over from the final day. It is important to remember to complete major tasks each day.
5. Be prepared for interruptions. These occur frequently as they would in a physician's office. Do not let interruptions upset you—learn to rearrange priorities.
6. Develop shortcuts, easier procedures, and better ways of doing tasks.

PROCEDURES

Day 1, October 11

1. Check today's appointments. Pull chart folders for today's appointments. Keep them together.
2. Organize any other materials you will need. Arrange your desk in an orderly fashion, leaving room for you to work.
3. Use the *Telephone Log* form from Working Paper 44 (WP 44) to list the answering service and all incoming calls. Make only brief notations on this form, checking off items as you follow through on them.
4. Use your *To-Do List* from Working Paper 45 (WP 45), checking off tasks as you complete them.
5. The simulation begins with the call to the answering service. You will hear conversations between the assistant and the answering service, the patients, and other callers. (Remember, you are assuming the role of Linda Schwartz, administrative medical assistant for Karen Larsen, MD.) You will hear Dr. Larsen giving you directions and dictation. You will *not* hear the voices of all patients—only those who ask you to do something.
6. Dr. Larsen may give new directions. There may be additional telephone calls. Listen to the conversations continuously, stopping to obtain information, to have information repeated, and to obtain the appointment calendar, message blanks, and other items. Make appropriate notes as you listen.
7. As you complete tasks, place them in your Day 1 folder, organizing them as directed by your instructor. Place any incomplete work in the next day's folder.

Day 2, October 12
Day 3, October 17
Day 4, October 18

1. For the remaining days, follow the same procedures as on Day 1. Remember that some of the new items from Days 2, 3, and 4 may be more important than work left over from the previous day. Again, listen to conversations continuously, stopping as necessary.

Simulation 1

2. At the end of Day 2, put all your completed work in the Day 2 folder, following your instructor's directions, and repeat the same procedure with Days 3 and 4. Follow your instructor's advice with what to do with incomplete work.

MATERIALS

You will need the following materials to complete Simulation 1. If these materials are not already in the proper folders, obtain them from the sources indicated. If directed by your instructor, you may access all necessary materials via Connect and complete Simulation 1 there.

Materials	Source
Appointment calendar.	WPs 20–35
Supplies folder:	
Notepad	You provide
Plain paper	You provide
Letterhead	Available in Connect
Outside services	WP 5
Telephone message forms (blank)	WPs 10–17
Appointment cards	WP 36
Patient information forms	WPs 41, 42
Records release form	WP 43
Telephone log	WP 44
To-do list	WP 45
Patient Account/ Chart Numbers	WP 87

Note: All WPs are located within Connect and in the Working Papers section of this textbook.

To-Do Items

Note: If you have completed all the projects and do not have the following listed items, discuss the missing items with your instructor. Individual projects are not linked but can be found in the Chapter Projects section for each chapter by number.

Day 1 folder:
Place patients' charts for October 11.

Day 2 folder:
Place patients' charts for October 12.

Day 3 folder:
Place patients' charts for October 17

Day 4 folder:
Place patients' charts for October 18.

Miscellaneous folder:
Wanda Norberg, MD—message (Project 4.1) and interoffice e-mail (Project 3.2)

Patients' folders:
The following patients' folders (charts) should contain the patient information form, chart note (if one has been prepared), and any other items listed. If Optional Project 5.6 was completed, the transcribed chart note should be in the patient's chart.

Armstrong, Monica	
Baab, Thomas—transcribed chart note	(Optional Project 5.6)
Babcock, Sara—message and chart note	(Project 4.1 and Project 5.4)
Burton, Randy	
Casagranda, Doris	
Castro, Joseph—transcribed chart note	(Optional Project 5.6)
Dayton, Theresa	
Grant, Todd—transcribed chart note	(Optional Project 5.6)
Jonathan, Charles III	
Kramer, David—transcribed chart note	(Optional Project 5.6)
Kramer, Jeffrey—message, chart note, and transcribed chart note	(Project 4.1, Project 5.4, and Optional Project 5.6)
Matthews, Ardis—transcribed chart note	(Optional Project 5.6)
Mendez, Ana	
Mitchell, Erin—chart note	(Project 5.5)
Morton, Sarah	
Murrary, Raymond	

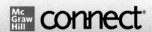
Phan, Marc—transcribed chart note   (Optional Project 5.6)
Richards, Warren
Roberts, Suzanne
Robertson, Gary—chart note,   (Project 5.5, Optional
    transcribed chart note   Project 5.6)
Sherman, Florence—referral
    letter, chart note, and envelope   (Project 3.1)
Sinclair, Gene
Sun, Cheng
Villano, Stephen

EVALUATION

You will be evaluated as follows:

1. Good judgment in establishing priorities: Did you use good judgment? Did you accomplish the most important tasks?
2. Quality of tasks completed: Are tasks accurate and neat?
3. Quantity: Did you complete a reasonable amount of work? Would a physician be satisfied with your rate of accomplishment?

Chapter 6

Office Management

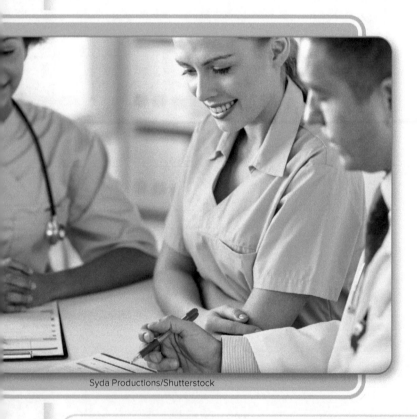

Syda Productions/Shutterstock

LEARNING OUTCOMES

After studying this chapter, you will be able to

6.1 design a medical office waiting area that exhibits the priority of patient comfort.

6.2 identify three stress triggers in your own life and define at least one method of reducing the associated negative stress.

6.3 differentiate among three common leadership/management styles.

6.4 explain why an administrative medical assistant needs to know how to collect and assimilate research data.

6.5 classify items into major categories of needed information when making travel and meeting arrangements.

6.6 justify why a policies and procedures manual should be developed and used in a medical office.

KEY TERMS

Study these important words, which are defined in this chapter, to build your professional vocabulary:

agenda	management qualifications	patient information brochure	Real ID Act
authoritarian/autocratic	meeting minutes		reprints
delegative/laissez-faire	outside services file	perfectionism	stress
ergonomics	participative/democratic	policies and procedures manual	travel agent
itinerary	patient education materials		visionary

ABHES

1.d. List the general responsibilities and skills of the medical assistant.

4.a. Follow documentation procedures.

4.e. Perform risk management procedures.

4.f. Comply with federal, state, local and health laws and regulations as they relate to healthcare settings.

5.e. Analyze the effect of hereditary and environmental influences on behavior.

5.h. Display effective interpersonal skills with patients and healthcare team members.

5.i. Demonstrate cultural awareness.

7.a. Gather and process documents.

7.f. Maintain inventory of equipment supplies.

7.g. Display professionalism through written and verbal communications.

8.g. Recognize and respond to medical office emergencies.

10.a. Perform the essential requirements for employment such as résumé writing, effective interviewing, dressing professionally, time management, and following up appropriately.

10.b. Demonstrate professional behavior.

www.abhes.org/accreditationmanual

The ABHES standards appear with permission of The Accrediting Bureau of Health Education Schools

CAAHEP

V.C.3. Recognize barriers to communication.

V.C.4. Identify techniques for overcoming communication barriers.

V.C.14.a. Relate the following behavior to professional communications: assertive.

V.C.14.b. Relate the following behavior to professional communications: aggressive.

V.C.14.c. Relate the following behavior to professional communications: passive.

V.C.15. Differentiate between adaptive and nonadaptive coping mechanisms.

V.P.4.a. Coach patient regarding policies.

V.P.5.a. Coach patients appropriately considering cultural diversity.

V.P.5.c. Coach patient appropriately considering communication barriers.

X.P.2.a. Apply HIPAA rules in regard to privacy.

XII.C.7.a. Identify principles of body mechanics.

XII.C.7.b. Identify principles of ergonomics.

2015 Standards and Guidelines for the Accreditation of Educational Programs in Medical Assisting, Appendix B, Core Curriculum for Medical Assistants, Medical Assisting Education Review Board (MAERB), 2015.

INTRODUCTION

The word *administrative* in the administrative medical assistant's job title refers to more than clerical or office tasks that contribute to the care of patients. The word also describes the management functions that assistants fulfill on a daily basis. In many practices, career advancement to office management may be an outgrowth of skills and abilities used every day on the job.

This chapter deals with management of the physical medical office environment; the types of management, such as stress and conflict management; and **management qualifications**—the skills, abilities, and responsibilities of the administrative medical assistant in the role of office manager, including

- helping with editorial research projects.
- making travel and meeting arrangements.
- evaluating, updating, and distributing patient information and instruction handouts.
- creating and maintaining office policies and procedures manuals.

6.1 PHYSICAL ENVIRONMENT

Analyzing the needs of the medical office and matching the overall medical office layout and design to those needs will contribute to a smoothly running office. An office design that is attractive, functional, and professional can assist personnel with meeting the healthcare needs of patients in a more productive manner. Patients, in turn, will be more satisfied with their care, and the medical office team will be positively motivated.

Patient Waiting Area

With the exception of the building exterior, the waiting area will give patients their first physical impression of the medical office team. On their arrival, patients may evaluate the professionalism of the staff based on the overall appearance and comfort of the waiting area. Reading material in disarray, trash on the floor, and tattered furnishings provide the impression that the office staff does not consider the comfort of patients to be a priority. Many patients are apprehensive when arriving for medical services, and the waiting area should provide a comfortable, clean environment. An already nervous patient should be made to feel as comfortable as possible while waiting for his or her medical encounter.

A waiting area should not be oversized. A smaller area that is well lit and clean and has drinking water and current applicable reading material will help a patient feel more at ease such as the patient seen in Figure 6.1. If children will be waiting in the area, provide a larger space and an area with quiet toys for them to use while they wait. Do not provide items that children can place into their mouth or that pose other hazards. A waiting area for sick patients should be separate from the waiting area for healthy patients. Remote controls for viewing media, such as a television, should be kept by the office staff. Maintain a station that has comfortable content, such as a travel or cooking station, and avoid viewing content that may contain questionable content (such as soap operas). DVDs for patient education are a good viewing choice.

Seats should be without tears and arranged to provide adequate walking space for patients. Leave enough room to allow for those using assistance devices, such as a walker or a wheelchair. Provide wall décor that is professional and will not create anxiety for patients. Calming scenes, such as a shoreline or mountains, are appropriate options; and soft, cool wall colors (neutrals, light pastels) are psychologically soothing. Also, a sound machine with relaxing selections could be soothing for apprehensive patients. The type of physician and patient base should be considered when selecting a sound. For example, a patient who arrives for an appointment with a psychiatrist to discuss and receive treatment for water phobia would be agitated by the sound of waves from a sound machine.

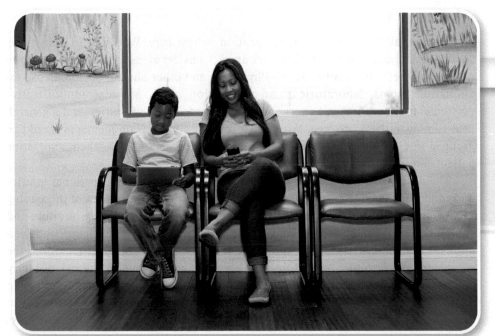

Live foliage helps purify the air and, when properly maintained, contributes to a comfortable waiting area. Beware of plants that may cause allergies for waiting patients or for office personnel. Water fountains may be provided for patient convenience. All decisions about the design of the waiting area should be made with the health and comfort of patients as the main goals. If necessary, consult an interior design professional.

Reception Area

Patient confidentiality should be the primary focus of the reception area. Patient information on the sign-in log should be visible only to the receptionist and should contain appropriately limited patient information. Having the patient list the reason for the visit on a sign-in log is a HIPAA violation. Office information is frequently displayed on walls close to the reception area. However, this can clutter the reception area. Consider placing office information in a patient brochure, or, if it needs to be displayed, place it on walls farther from the reception area. Placing office-related items in the examination room for patients to read as they wait can help eliminate clutter at the reception area.

Partitions are often used in the reception area to help eliminate the spread of germs and to protect PHI. However, if clear partitions are used between the reception area and the staff, unless they are soundproof material, conversations can still be heard, risking a breach of patient confidentiality.

HIPAA TIPS Using a cover sheet or a black marker to black out patients' names after their check-in may not meet HIPAA standards, if a patient's PHI can still be viewed after marking out the patient's data. Other sign-in methods exist that are HIPAA-compliant, such as electronically storing patient signatures.

Why is there a problem with patients being able to see the patient sign-in sheet?

Work Area

Fewer steps taken means more time spent on patient care. Workflow of individuals should be analyzed when designing work areas. Consider areas used by different components of the medical office team. Physicians and other clinical personnel use examination rooms, laboratories, and medication areas. Medical administrative personnel use reception and checkout areas, records storage facilities, and a generalized administrative work area. Work areas used by similar team members should be grouped in close proximity and provide little to no backtracking when completing patient care.

The design of furniture and equipment can help prevent occupational injuries and conditions, such as carpal tunnel syndrome. Individual body needs of those using the furniture and equipment are factors to consider when purchasing furniture and equipment: size, height, weight, and left- or right-handedness are primary considerations. **Ergonomics** attempts to match the individual's physiological factors to the equipment and furniture needed to complete tasks while reducing the risk of injury and hazards without decreasing output. Increased levels of stress may result when furniture and office equipment do not ergonomically meet the needs of the medical office team members. The next section discusses various items that can cause stress and how to manage them.

> **McGraw Hill connect** — GO TO PROJECT 6.1 AT THE END OF THIS CHAPTER

6.2 TYPES OF MANAGEMENT

Many things in life require individuals to be effective and efficient managers—stress, time, anger or conflict, and health, just to mention a few. As technology continues to change and provide faster methods of completing tasks, employees are expected to produce more in shorter amounts of time and with fewer resources. Effective management of self and other resources will allow an administrative medical assistant to be a valuable asset to the medical office team and its patients.

Stress

The word **stress** typically has a negative connotation. However, not all stress is negative. Stress can be a positive motivator for individuals. Why do students take this course or read this passage? For various reasons, individuals are learning new information to be applied in the medical office setting. This is a positive emotional or physiological response to an external requirement (achieving an educational goal, improving job performance, etc.). Good stress (eustress) is our body's nudge to maintain its function. For example, when you are feeling hungry, your body is experiencing eustress—go eat. However, when speaking of stress, the reference is normally to bad stress (distress), often referred to as the body's negative emotional and/or physiological reactions to external motivators. It can produce fatigue, sickness, and confusion, which negatively affect the medical office environment.

Everything in life is a choice, and an individual's reactions to external requirements are also a choice. Some may disagree with this statement, but please read on. Getting out of bed today—that is a choice. Taking a shower—that is a choice. Completing homework for class—again, that is a choice. Consider all the things individuals do or do not do each day. Many will say they did not have a choice, but there are choices.

Now, let's apply this to the medical office environment.

- As patients begin to come into the office, a member of the medical office team can either choose to greet them in a comfortable, professional manner or not.
- One of the medical team members may be in a particularly unpleasant mood—fellow team members can make the choice to respond in a similar demeanor or can choose a different, positive response. Sometimes that response is simply to *not* say what is truly being thought at that moment. Always consider what is best for the medical office team as a whole.

Before effectively choosing how to respond to stress, an individual must first learn to recognize possible stress triggers. The following are a few examples of stress triggers. There are many other external motivators for stress, and it is up to each person to learn what those are in his or her own personal and professional environment.

- *Workplace expectations.* Employees are expected to produce at a high level of efficiency, regardless of the position. This is a positive motivator, but emotional and physiological responses to work expectations can either propel employees forward in a positive manner, such as learning a new EHR program, hold an employee static, or even push an employee professionally backward. When was the last time you heard someone complain or perhaps you complained about an anticipated change? In the medical office environment, change is constant, and being adaptable to change will contribute to a positive work environment.
- *Single-parent provider.* Many employees are the sole family caregiver. This creates a tremendous amount of pressure on an employee. Often, a single-parent provider does not have others to help care for a sick child or children. In turn, a single parent may have a higher rate of absenteeism simply because he or she does not have help.
- *Caregiver to an aging family member.* As the aging population increases, many in the workforce are also caring for aging family members, such as parents, other relatives, and friends. This is a time-consuming responsibility, which takes an emotional toll on the caregiver. Employees who are also caring for aging individuals often deal with painful medical processes, such as dementia and Alzheimer's disease, and financial responsibilities and decisions. Many must make the decision whether to place a loved one in a long-term care facility. Many caregivers must miss work in order to take care of needed medical and financial business.
- *Multicareer family units.* When both individuals in a relationship have career and job responsibilities outside the home, balancing work and home responsibilities can be a stress trigger if individual, specific responsibilities are not clearly defined. Consider this—one individual may assume the other is responsible for dinner on Tuesday when, in fact, the other individual thinks just the opposite. The bottom line is that no one plans for dinner on Tuesday evening.
- *Multigenerational households.* Since 2000, the percentage of households in the United States in which three or more generations live together has steadily increased. According to data collected by the Census Bureau, and released in the 2009-2011 American Community Survey (ACS) report, 5.6 percent of all U.S. households had three or more generations living together under one roof. Later data collected, researched, and analyzed by Pew Research Center place the percentage of U.S. multigenerational households at 64 million or 20 percent of the U.S. population. The Pew Research Center, however, defines a multigenerational

household as two or more adult generations living together or a grandparent(s) and grandchild/children living together. Adjusting to the multigenerational lifestyle takes patience and cooperation. An advantage of cohabitation of generations is having multiple wage earners under the same roof. But even with this added advantage, multigenerational living may still be a stress trigger.

- *Financial pressures.* It is a fact: Today's money buys less than it bought just a few years ago. Individuals earn an income, but it just seems not to go as far. Whether this is due to a lack of sufficient income, poor financial choices, or just the inability to say no, financial pressures are a stress trigger for many, if not most, Americans.

As employees begin to recognize stress triggers, some of the following stress-reducing suggestions can be used to benefit from positive stress and reduce the emotional and physiological effects of chronic stress.

- *Get organized.* Make a to-do list of items to be completed. Make daily, weekly, and even monthly lists. Lists can be maintained in paper format or electronically such as in electronic organizers and calendars as seen in Figure 6.2. Set reasonable and achievable goals, and allow for flexibility and interruptions. Physically notate or check off items as they are completed—this provides a visual sense of accomplishment.

- *Set priorities.* What must be completed today? Which task(s) must be completed prior to the arrival of patients? Recognize your own limitations. Being a team member in a medical office environment means that many times administrative medical assistants say *Yes* to extra tasks. But when your resources (time, energy, knowledge, etc.) are limited and not sufficient to complete the tasks, ask for help or, if appropriate, respectfully seek another solution.

- *Develop a "whatever" category.* Know the items that create negative stress. If the situation can be changed effectively and constructively, then do so. If not, then let it fall into a positive, not negative, "whatever" category and choose to react positively. Focus attention on other needed tasks. Also, practice taking a deep breath before reacting. Remember, change will happen, interruptions will occur, and plans will

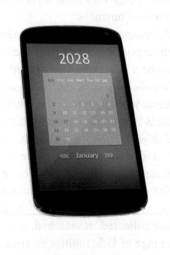

Figure 6.2

Electronic organizers through smart devices and e-mail options can be used to maintain schedules. *What are the pros and cons of electronic and paper-based organizers?*
Daniel Krason/Shutterstock

be revised. Adaptable employees will contribute to the smooth flow of the medical office environment.

- *Be an achiever, not a perfectionist.* **Perfectionism** is setting unrealistic expectations and goals and being dissatisfied with anything less. Perfectionists are often displeased with the end result. Achieving is accomplishing a goal or finishing a task.
- *Maintain your health.* Eat properly and exercise regularly. This will be discussed later in this chapter.
- *Balance both work and play.* Work hard while at work, but allow for the opportunity to play or relax. Watch a movie, read something just for fun, sing in the shower, or do any other activity that helps you reduce stress. If a medical team member does not take care of his or her physical and emotional needs, that member will find it difficult to be an effective, efficient part of the medical office team.

Time Management

Throughout the day, many people say, "I wish I had more time in the day," but is that what they really need? Everyone's day has 24 hours. If there were 28 hours in a day, individuals would simply fill all 28 hours and say, "I wish I had more time in the day." Time is a resource to be managed. Setting priorities and goals and creating to-do lists are two ways to manage time. Following are other time management tips:

- *Identify time wasters.* Keep a time log for a certain period, such as 1 full week (7 days). Record what you do, the time you started, and how long it took to complete the task. Nothing is too trivial for the log. Record when you wake up, take a shower, eat breakfast, watch the news, check social sites, and so on. It is important to account for all your time in the log. Prioritize tasks using a rating system, such as 1, 2, 3 or A, B, C. Evaluate the log for each day, and determine when the most productive and least productive times were to identify which tasks were time wasters.
- *Delegate tasks.* Everything cannot be accomplished by one employee. Sometimes it is necessary to ask others for help.
- *Use technology.* Technologies, such as computers and the Internet, allow tasks that traditionally needed to be completed using a greater amount of time—such as searching for the most efficient office furniture—to be completed by using search engines and websites. Using the telephone to call first before using time and other resources to physically go to a location is good not only for time management but also for the environment.
- *Defeat procrastination.* "When is the last day I can send in the lab work and still receive the results prior to the patient's appointment?" Procrastination is unnecessarily delaying the completion of a task. Employees delay completing a task for different reasons. Perhaps they are afraid of failing, overwhelmed (where do I start?), or upset at being asked to do the task. Or maybe it just isn't high on the employees' priority list. Also, technology failures may cause delays, and if an individual has already procrastinated and is almost at the deadline, this can disrupt the flow of the medical environment.
- *Use a calendar.* Many electronic calendars are available in various formats. Individuals also use traditional, printed calendars. Whatever format is preferred, choose one and use it consistently to record appointments, deadlines, and so on.

Anger and Conflict Management

Mismanagement of anger and conflict is one of the top triggers for producing negative stress. Consider the last time someone pulled out in front of you while you were driving. Did you consider why the person pulled out without regard to you, or did you just get mad? Choosing how to respond to internal anger motivated by external causes will help you avoid possible explosive situations and will reduce your negative emotional and physiological responses. Consider applying the following strategies when confronted with a possible conflict:

- *Distinguish between perceived and realistic situations.* How a situation is perceived may not be the reality of the situation. Determine facts and separate those from feelings.
- *Breathe.* When reacting to anger, bodies begin to exhibit physiological signs, such as tension in muscles, increased blood pressure, and/or a dry mouth. Deep breathing can help reduce the physiological effects of anger and allow an individual time to reconsider a different response. Rolling the neck and shoulders can reduce built-up tension in those areas.
- *Save the e-mail.* If responding to a communication such as an e-mail, do not click the Send button. Key in a response and either minimize it or save it—do not send the e-mail when angry. Allow time to gather more information and reevaluate your first response.
- *Leave/walk away.* Sometimes it is in the best interest of all involved to physically walk away from the conflict, allowing everyone time and space to calm down and/or rethink the situation. If physically leaving the area is not an option, emotionally take a walk. Count to 3 or 10, or imagine a comforting scene (mountains, beach, etc.) when the signs of anger begin to manifest themselves.

Health Management

Like a vehicle, when a body is not maintained and fueled properly, it does not function as it should. When the Check Engine light comes on, it is an indication that something is wrong and needs to be checked. A body has indicator lights as well. Some examples are chronic fatigue; changes in diet, sleep pattern, skin, or other physiological systems; or loss of interest. Many medical conditions cannot be avoided; however, choosing to maintain your body with a healthy lifestyle can contribute to your effectiveness as an administrative medical assistant.

- *Exercise regularly.* To exercise regularly does not mean joining a gym and spending 2 hours, 5 days per week exercising, although that is one option. Decide on an activity and do it. Walking, canoeing, biking, yoga, hiking, strength training, dancing—the list is as varied as there are individuals. The key is to be consistent with exercising and vary the activity (to avoid boredom). If you like to exercise with other people, find someone who shares your interest and hold each other accountable. Little changes can make a difference; park at the end of the parking lot instead of in the closest space to the door, or take the stairs instead of the elevator—there are many options.
- *Eat regularly and correctly.* The standard of three meals per day is still good. However, many health professionals recommend three main meals with small snacks—one snack between breakfast and lunch/dinner and another snack between lunch and dinner/supper. Still other health professionals recommend six smaller meals each day. But all agree. Eat. When the body is not fueled on a regular basis, it begins to conserve fuel (calories) instead of using those calories. Foods high in fat content can contribute to cardiovascular disease, one of the fastest-growing categories of disease in America.

- *Manage stress.* As discussed previously in this chapter, bodies can and do react to stress in physiological ways. Physiological reactions lead to decreased work efficiency and high absenteeism.

McGraw Hill connect   **GO TO PROJECT 6.2 AT THE END OF THIS CHAPTER**

6.3 THE OFFICE MANAGER'S ROLE

Advancing from the position of administrative medical assistant to office manager requires experience and specific skills and abilities. The experience ensures a broad and deep understanding of the many ways in which the medical practice is a business uniquely designed to serve people's most important and intimate needs. A high level of skill ensures a readiness to exercise initiative and to direct others.

The American Academy of Professional Coders (AAPC) offers an opportunity for an individual to become a Certified Physician Practice Manager (CPPM). Knowledge of general business processes, the revenue cycle, compliance laws and regulations, health IT, and human resources are examples of areas that a candidate must know to become certified. Detailed information on the CPPM credential is provided at the AAPC's website (www.aapc.com).

Moving into an office management position sometimes requires a change of duties. It always requires a change of emphasis in job responsibilities. While the employee working as an administrative medical assistant must have certain planning and management skills, the emphasis is most often on carefully following instructions, implementing plans made by the physician or other managers, and responding skillfully to a variety of situations. Office management requires the exercise of initiative that lets assistants act confidently because they grasp the goals and purposes of the practice.

Office management responsibilities involve the following managerial skills and abilities:

- *Being a team player:* It is important to understand the social fabric of the relationships in the office and to be recognized as someone who helps generously, listens to the thoughts and ideas of other team members, freely gives credit to other employees for their work, contributes to a pleasant atmosphere, and relates well to colleagues as well as to managers. Meetings provide an opportunity for medical office team members to practice these characteristics (Figure 6.3).
- *Increasing productivity:* Understanding how to complete tasks more efficiently—actually increasing output—is the mark of a good manager. Directing others so that they are able to get more tasks done more efficiently may be part of the office manager's responsibility. In addition to overseeing tasks performed by others, an effective manager delegates tasks. Thus, the manager's own development of time management skills and efficient ways of doing tasks is critical.
- *Planning strategically:* The office manager is expected to see beyond an immediate assignment, to view the whole business of the practice so as to contribute in ways that improve the daily operations of the office. This may involve anything from selecting a new electronic health records system to recommending the choice of a new supplier because of quality or price.

• *Using problem-solving skills:* The employer counts on the office manager to be able to analyze situations, determine the critical factors, apply knowledge gained in past working experience, and propose and implement solutions. Disputes and disagreements will develop between office team members, and the office manager must be able to remain impartial and to listen to all parties objectively. Using an organized approach to solving problems increases the likelihood of successful results. The following steps will assist in making decisions and solving problems:

1. Define the problem.
2. Set goals and/or results you want to achieve.
3. Gather needed information.
4. Brainstorm different solutions.
5. Select and implement a solution.
6. Evaluate the results of the solution and make any necessary changes.
7. Revise any of the problem-solving steps. You may need to start again!

• *Using available resources:* When physicians delegate the day-to-day management of the office, they may expect the office manager to get help from experts: an accountant, a lawyer, an insurance representative, and even a time management expert. Companies specializing in office management, known as medical management consultants, are available to assist the office manager. The consultant will spend time analyzing the accounting system, the appointment scheduling and flow of patients, the records management methods, and the work habits of everyone on staff, including the physicians. The consultant will then make recommendations for changes. Perhaps the appointment scheduling system will need to be changed to accommodate physicians or patients better. There may be ways that office expenses can be reduced. A consultant may also provide comprehensive training for office personnel. If the practice can afford the use of such a resource, the help may be very valuable, especially to a newly appointed office manager. Managers should use Internet search engines to research topics and gain information related to decisions they need to make.

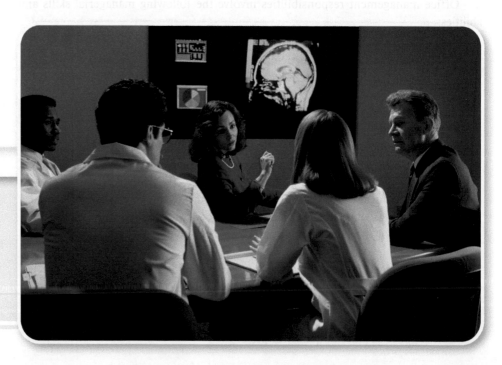

Figure 6.3

Medical office staff meetings provide an opportunity to share ideas. *What do you think are the most important aspects of effective meetings?* Comstock Images/Getty Images

The office manager is expected to see beyond an immediate assignment and view the business of the medical practice so that it contributes in ways that improve the daily operations of the office while improving the quality of care. This requires the quality of leadership. This quality enables the office manager to choose what to achieve, to plan for complex tasks, to prioritize time and tasks, and to motivate other employees to work effectively and efficiently.

Leadership Styles

A manager leads and motivates by example, either good or bad. Coaches motivate players, parents motivate children, and managers motivate employees. Before office managers can effectively manage situations, they must first know which management/leadership style is needed to meet the challenges and/or goals presented. Leadership styles fall broadly into the following categories, with varying degrees of styles within each category.

Authoritarian/autocractic. An authoritarian/autocratic leader provides clear and definitive expectations to his or her team members. Each member knows how and when a task is to be completed and who is responsible for each part of the project. The manager makes decisions with little or no input from others. This style works best when there is minimal time to make decisions, such as in emergency situations.

Example: While walking through the reception area, the office manager noticed she could hear the receptionist discussing PHI with a patient. The receptionist was behind a closed window and was using a speakerphone. The office manager made the immediate decision to discontinue using speakerphones and use headsets when talking with patients over the phone.

To replace the window with a soundproof option would be less cost-effective than to use headsets.

Participative/democratic. A participative/democratic leader offers advice but is also a participant in the team dynamics and seeks input from other team members. An atmosphere of "your input is important" makes this a positively motivating style of leadership. In both the participative and democratic styles of leadership, others have input. Democratic management involves others, not only with their input, but in the actual decision making. Conversely, in the participative style, the office manager retains authority to make final decisions. This style works best when an ample amount of time is available to make a decision. Other terms for management styles which seek input from others are *consultative* and *persuasive*.

Example: Office team members may be asked their preferences for redesigning the waiting room. The office manager will make the final decision on design.

Delegative/laissez-faire. A delegative/laissez-faire leader employs a "hands-off" policy and tends to allow other office team members to make their own decisions. Little guidance is given, and the manager becomes involved only when the situation makes it necessary.

Example: A committee may be formed to design an employee evaluation tool. The committee develops, edits, and has final approval of the form.

Visionary. A visionary leader concentrates on the overall goals/mission of the medical environment and encourages team members to all move together in the same positive direction. The manager normally does not become involved in the day-to-day functions but motivates the team members and trusts that they can work together to meet common goals. This style works well when a change is needed.

Example: The office is converting from a combination of hardcopy patient records and EMR to all EMR. The visionary manager would meet with employees to relate the conversion to EMRs to the overall goal of being compliant with HIPAA standards.

Good managers must be able to analyze the dynamics of each situation and implement the most appropriate leadership style. Using one style in all situations can lead to employee dissatisfaction and poor work efficiency.

EXAMPLE: PROBLEM-SOLVING AND LEADERSHIP STYLES

Competent and consistent services in offices are a necessity to today's medical industry. **(Problem)** During the summer vacation season, it is typical for the office manager to experience staffing challenges due to employees wanting to use vacation time. Additionally, the office manager must deal with the staff shortage this creates on a daily and weekly basis. Demand for professional administrative and clinical personnel can make or break an office. **(Goal)** Dr. Larsen's office manager makes it a priority to manage the summer season in a way that allows staff the opportunity to enjoy their vacation time while maintaining an adequate staff for efficient patient and administrative operations. **(Authoritarian Leadership Style)** The office manager prefers to make administrative decisions independently, without input from the medical team members, and has arrived at the following plan.

(Needed Information) To help offset the effects of the summer vacation season, the office manager used temporary employees. However, this plan proved unsuccessful to meet the standards for patient care and office coverage. Temporary employees were not paid an attractive wage by the temporary agency, and the employees were required to pay for uniforms. Additionally, temporary employees also had travel and parking expenses. To make matters worse, temporary employees were not guaranteed a certain number of hours by the agency nor did they receive any benefits. Consequently, they either paid for medical insurance coverage on their own or did not have coverage. All of these factors contributed to less-than-successful coverage of vacationing medical staff members.

(Brainstorm) After reconsidering the failed plan and other possible solutions, Dr. Larsen's office manager **(Select Solution and Participative Leadership Style)** decided to involve the medical office team in constructing a floating summer vacation schedule. **(Implement)** Each office member submitted their first two vacation choices for summer vacation leave time. Next, the office manager, Dr. Larsen, and the senior nursing staff member rated the choices in order by seniority. **(Evaluate)** Team members viewed this as a fair method of allocating valuable summer vacation time, and the office continued to flow smoothly.

Mc Graw Hill **connect**   **GO TO PROJECT 6.3 AT THE END OF THIS CHAPTER**

6.4   EDITORIAL RESEARCH PROJECTS

The physician may be involved with research in a wide variety of areas, including investigating clinical procedures, instruments, or drugs and conducting clinical trials. Perhaps the physician needs to prepare a medical case history of particular interest or an article summarizing findings to the scientific community. Whether it is for a lecture, an article, or a book, the administrative medical assistant may become involved in initial stages of research through obtaining material for the physician's reports at the library or from electronic resources. The administrative medical assistant will also keep copies of medical journals and will obtain and file reprints of articles in the physician's areas of interest or articles the physician has written.

Using the Library

In specialized medical libraries, such as those found in large medical centers or universities, librarians have educational qualifications in medical research and are prepared to be helpful to those who need to use the library. Public libraries have large computerized databases of materials in various medical specialties. These databases are quite simple to use because most of them include tips on how to search and are searchable by topic. If the document is located in another library, that information is also usually given. If the physician has given you only a topic and brief description, it may be efficient to print out those entries pertaining to the topic and ask the physician to check off those entries that seem most pertinent to the research. This will give direction to your search and will ensure that the most useful books or articles are provided.

Online databases are available in medical libraries and on the Internet; and information sites such as the Health Libraries, www.hlinc.org.au, or the Health Sciences Resources list, https://libguides.sullivan.edu/SUCOPDIC, are also useful. Other helpful resources are listed here.

- Dedicated websites—such as MEDLINE (https://medlineplus.gov), developed by the National Library of Medicine, and PubMed (https://www.ncbi.nlm.nih.gov/pubmed/)—provide MEDLINE software, which gives immediate access to abstracts and journals and allows the full text of journal articles to be retrieved online.
- Compact discs for use at home or in an office may contain whole medical books, periodicals, journals, or even interactive training (e.g., how to perform a particular surgery, complete with pictures, animations, photographs, and videos). Electronic resources can also be accessed from the cloud.
- Specialized e-mail and chat forums provide an opportunity for physicians to communicate publicly or privately with other physicians through e-mail messages.

Medical Journals

Most medical societies publish their own journals. The American Medical Association (AMA) publishes periodicals on special subjects. In addition, the AMA publishes the official publication of the society, the *Journal of the American Medical Association (JAMA)*. *JAMA* contains articles on all aspects of the field of medicine. Most medical specialties have their own journals. Physicians who receive hardcopy journals will find it useful to have them bound and stored. Many physicians find it more time- and cost-efficient to retrieve and read journals online. *JAMA* articles, archived and current, can be retrieved at http://jama.ama-assn.org. In addition to viewing articles, physicians can participate in forum discussions and listen to podcasts of guests presenting research and other information. These contain valuable information for reference and research. It is useful for you to know that each journal publishes a topical index at the end of a publishing cycle, although this cycle may not correlate exactly to a calendar year. Some research material that you may need may be found in the office storage area where these journals are kept.

Reprints

Physicians may inform their colleagues about their work by writing, lecturing, and publishing articles and papers on researched topics. If a physician presents a paper at a meeting of medical colleagues, the paper is usually published in the proceedings of the conference, in the organization's own publication, or in another medical journal. However, the physician may have submitted the article to a journal without having first presented it at a meeting.

Once the article is published, the author may receive a certain number of free copies of the article, called **reprints.** Additional copies or e-copies are usually available at cost. The physician sends these reprints to colleagues interested in the same field or allied fields. You should keep a record of the names and addresses of those who receive copies of the article and of those who have acknowledged receiving the article.

Mc Graw Hill connect   **GO TO PROJECT 6.4 AT THE END OF THIS CHAPTER**

6.5 TRAVEL AND MEETING ARRANGEMENTS

When the physician travels for professional or personal reasons, you will be involved in preparing for the trip. You need to know and understand the physician's preferences well to handle travel arrangements satisfactorily.

There are three general guidelines for handling travel:

1. Always consult with the physician in advance to be sure that the physician's preferences will be honored. Consider preferences in airline and airplane seating. First-class seating offers amenities such as larger seats, which are not available in coach-class seating. A traveler who is tall may prefer first class or, if traveling in coach class, an aisle seat. Other items to make notations of preferred choices are dietary needs or preferences in airplane meals; lodging requirements and the geographic relationship of the hotel to the meeting or conference site; car size, make, and model; car rental company of choice or other ground transportation; preferred times of travel; airport, if there is more than one in the departure or destination city; and any need for information about the city—places of interest or restaurants, for example.

   The assistant should maintain a travel folder (hardcopy or electronic) containing the physician's preferences, as well as other items relating to travel. This includes applicable discounts, such as membership discounts; financial items used to make reservations; and past itineraries for reference. When you are making travel arrangements, refer to this folder to save time.

2. Since the tragic events of September 11, 2001, travel requirements, especially when using airlines, have changed. Prior to traveling, the physician should be made aware of any changes made by the Transportation Security Administration (TSA) in traveling regulations. For example, as of the publication date of this text, the 3-1-1 Liquid Rule for carry-on items is applied. Liquid containers of 3.4 ounces or less may be placed in one 1-quart plastic ziplock bag, with one bag per traveler. The 3-1-1 Liquid Rule pertains to not only liquids but also gels, creams, pastes, and aerosols. However, due to the COVID-19 pandemic, the TSA has modified the 3-1-1 Liquid Rule until further notice. One liquid hand sanitizer container of up to 12 ounces may be placed in carry-on luggage. It will be screened separately from other liquids. All other items covered by the 3-1-1 Liquid Rule must still be 3.4 ounces or less. Larger liquid quantities, such as medications and baby formula, may be taken on board a plane. Items must be declared and will probably be opened and searched.

Another TSA feature available to travelers is the TSA Pre✓ program. Being approved through the TSA Pre✓ program means a traveler has applied for and paid a fee for a 5-year membership (after approval) to the program. Individuals complete an application and make an appointment at an enrollment center, which can be located through the TSA website. A background check and finger-printing of the applicant are completed during the appointment. If approved for the Pre✓ program, travelers are not required to pass through all requirements of security. Shoes, laptops, liquids, belts, and light jackets do not have to be removed by the approved traveler when going through security. This process shortens the time required to go through security. Standard guidelines for travel-ers is to arrive no less than 2 hours prior to departure for domestic flights and 3 hours prior to departure for international flights. Other trusted travelers' pro-grams recognized by the Department of Homeland Security include Global Entry, NEXUS, SENTRI, and FAST.

The bottom line is that a traveler and those making travel arrangements for the individual should consult the TSA's website (www.tsa.gov/traveler-information) for a complete, up-to-date listing of travel regulations and requirements. There is also an application (app) for smartphones and other mobile devices that allows a trav-eler to search for prohibited travel items for carry-on and checked luggage and other TSA regulations.

3. After September 11, 2001, another law was passed by Congress to set minimal stan-dards for verifying an individual's identification. This act, the **Real ID Act**, passed in 2005, established standards for state-issued identifications, such as driver's licenses, and prohibits federal agencies from accepting identifications which do not meet the Real ID standards. Airports are considered a federal agency. For most states, an enhanced driver's license which meets the Real ID Act standards will have a star in the upper corner, usually the right upper corner. However, not all states will place a star on the license. If there is not a star on the license, people who are traveling should check with their state's Department of Motor Vehicles (DMV) for the Real ID status of the license. If the license is not a Real ID en-hanced license, other forms of identification may be used to travel domestically. Examples of alternate travel identifications include a passport, a U.S. military identification, or a Department of Homeland Security trusted travelers card. For a complete listing of alternate forms of identification, go to the TSA website at https://www.tsa.gov/travel/security-screening/identification. Due to the COVID-19 crisis, the deadline date to have a Real-ID compliant driver's license was extended to October 1, 2021.

4. Use a skilled **travel agent** at a reputable agency or via the Internet to make travel arrangements. The travel agent does not charge the customer or may charge a small fee, and it is the agent's job to make all transportation, car rental, and lodg-ing arrangements requested by the traveler. Sightseeing and pleasure arrange-ments can also be made through the travel agent. Communicate the physician's preferences to the agent. Many agents require the completion of a written travel profile that states the traveler's needs and preferences. This is a valuable tool be-cause the physician does not have to take time to answer these questions every time a trip is planned.

Websites for travel companies, airlines, and airports are also a valuable time-saving tool for making travel arrangements. Using the websites allows for price comparison. Features such as room amenities and airline seat location can also be verified without making a reservation.

Reservations

If a travel agent is used, information should be supplied as early as possible so that the agent can research and obtain the best fare. Airline and travel websites may also offer lower fares for early booking of travel arrangements. Because many airlines use electronic tickets, called *e-tickets,* the airline provides a confirmation of the reservation and purchase, rather than a printed ticket. This confirmation may be used at curbside to check luggage and/or at the ticket counter to obtain a boarding pass. Boarding passes may also be printed within 24 hours of the scheduled flight. Airlines will provide a printed ticket if there is a specific request for one. Having a printed ticket makes changing airlines easier, should that be necessary during the trip.

Most travelers prefer to stay either at the meeting site or very close to it. A delay in making the needed hotel reservations could mean that the physician will not be able to stay at the meeting site. This could lead to increased transportation costs and require additional travel time to and from the site. Provide maps of the area with the travel documents to facilitate travel time and help provide directions. Internet services, such as Mapquest and other online direction services, can provide valuable and time-saving information. If it is anticipated or possible that the physician will arrive late, be sure the hotel has been notified. Hotels have a stated "late arrival time," such as 8 P.M.

Once all relevant travel arrangement information has been collected and confirmed, multiple copies of an **itinerary,** or daily schedule of events, should be prepared either by the assistant or by the travel agent. An itinerary should include flight times listed in the local departing and arrival destinations' times, flight numbers, hotel and car arrangements, and all pertinent addresses and phone numbers. Direct flights do not require the traveler to change planes but do have at least one stop before reaching their destination, and a nonstop flight is a direct flight with no stops. A sample of an itinerary is shown in Figure 6.4. In addition to the information shown in Figure 6.4, GPS coordinates or addresses should be placed on the itinerary for travelers who are renting vehicles and driving to destinations. As soon as you receive the itinerary, check to be sure that every arrangement is the same as what was originally requested or agreed upon. This itinerary, along with the confirmation ticket or airline ticket, should then be placed in a folder until the physician needs the information. However, you should notify the physician as soon as the itinerary arrives, so that the physician can supply a copy of the itinerary to the appropriate people and any others whom the physician specifies. One copy for reference should be kept in a convenient place in the office.

Changes in Travel Plans

Changes and delays sometimes occur in the physician's travel plans. Ordinarily, the physician will share with you information on how likely it is that the trip will occur. This is important because airplane tickets that are refundable or that may be used at another time are more expensive than nonrefundable tickets. However, it may be cost-effective to purchase a more expensive ticket or purchase travel insurance to allow for some flexibility in the physician's plans.

Because most hotel reservations are secured with a credit or debit card, it is also important to cancel a room reservation as soon as the travel plan changes. Each hotel has its own rules about cancellation without a financial penalty. The travel agent should be notified immediately, or you should call the hotel yourself to cancel the reservation. Request confirmation from the hotel that the reservation has been canceled. Confirmation is usually in the form of an e-mail or a cancellation confirmation number. If a charge is made mistakenly to the credit card, it will be easier to deal with the credit card company if there is a verification of cancellation.

```
                         ITINERARY

                    For Karen Larsen, MD

                      March 11-15, 20—


Friday, March 11

     5:00 P.M.    Depart Chicago, O'Hare International Airport,
                  American Airlines Flight 104, nonstop, 737

     8:00 P.M.    Arrive New York City, JFK International Airport

     Hotel:  Mariott Marquis
     1535 Broadway New York NY 10036
     212-555-5000
     Confirmation Number: GX476T02; nonsmoking room requested

Sunday, March 13

     7:00 P.M.    Depart New York, LaGuardia Airport, American
                  Airlines Flight 526, nonstop, 737

     8:01 P.M.    Arrive Boston, Logan International Airport

     Hotel: Sheraton-Boston Hotel
     39 Dalton Street, Boston MA 02199
     613-555-6789
     Confirmation Number: TZE32145, nonsmoking room requested

Monday, March 14

     Reminder:    Make restaurant reservations.

     7:30 P.M.    Dinner with Dr. and Mrs. Lawrence Carley

Tuesday, March 15

     6:45 P.M.    Depart Boston, Logan International Airport,
                  American Airlines Flight 175, nonstop, 737

     8:12 P.M.    Arrive Chicago, O'Hare International Airport


Travel and accommodations arranged by Linda Solomon, Chicago
Travel, 312-555-6777.
```

Figure 6.4

Travel Itinerary. *Why are travel itineraries important?*

Duties Related to the Physician's Absence

Be certain that you have instructions about how to handle phone calls, correspondence, and appointments in the physician's absence. Mark the days on the calendar when the physician will be away, so that no patients are scheduled. Notify those patients who are already scheduled that the physician will be away, and either make new appointments or refer the patients to the physician who will be substituting in the physician's absence. Failure to cancel or refer patient appointments, procedures, and so on to the covering physician could give the appearance of medical abandonment (covered in a different chapter). If the entire medical office is closed while the physician is gone, the answering service or office answering machine should provide patients with emergency medical direction, such as call 911 or go to the emergency department.

It is useful to keep a running daily summary of phone calls, incidents, and patient inquiries, specifying the action that was taken while the physician was away. While away from the office, most business travelers check e-mail and call the office on a regular or predetermined time schedule. Keep a log of important information to be discussed with the physician during calls, and organize your phone discussion beforehand to make this valuable time more productive.

Meeting Arrangements

Many physicians belong to the AMA. In addition, there are organizations related to all of the medical specialties. Most national organizations also have state and local levels, and physicians belong to the association at all three levels. These organizations provide a valuable way for physicians to exchange information, learn about new developments, continue their education, and contribute to their profession.

Participation in organizations may involve simply attending meetings or may consist of working on or chairing committees. Your responsibilities will vary, depending on the physician's responsibilities.

National and state societies hold meetings once or twice a year. The dates, times, and places of a national or state meeting are usually determined a year in advance. This information is printed several months in advance in the state or national journal and on the organization's Web page. Notices of the meeting are sent to organization members well in advance of the meeting. The notice should contain pertinent information about the meeting: who is to attend, what will be discussed, when the meeting begins and ends (including dates and times), where the meeting is being held (including directions, if needed), how many continuing education units (CEUs) will be earned, and information for guests to RSVP. Enter meeting information on the physician's appointment calendar as soon as notice of the meeting arrives. It is helpful to put a reminder in the tickler file, so that you can meet with the physician to find out about preferences in travel schedules and arrangements.

Local meetings are usually held on the same day of each month—for example, on the second Tuesday. Meeting dates and programs are published in the journal or newsletter. Mark the dates on the physician's appointment calendar, and send a memo or an e-mail to the physician several days before the meeting each month as a reminder.

Special meetings may be called to discuss important business matters pertaining to the organization. In these cases, an announcement of the meeting is sent to each member. A sample of such an announcement is shown in Figure 6.5.

Figure 6.5

Meeting Announcement

**THE CHICAGO MEDICAL SOCIETY
ELECTION OF OFFICERS MEETING**

Tuesday, October 3, 20--
8:00 P.M.

**UNIVERSITY HOSPITAL
5500 North Ridgeway Avenue
Room 254C**

Preparing for Meetings

A physician who is the chair of a committee or an officer of the organization may be responsible for making the arrangements for the meeting. In many cases, the physician will delegate that responsibility to the assistant. If the meeting is to be held locally, arranging for the meeting is simpler. However, contracting for a meeting room, food or other refreshments, and equipment will still be necessary.

The following arrangements need to be made:

- Once you know how many people are expected, contact several conference centers or hotels to price the arrangements. Most conference centers and hotels have catering managers or conference planners available to help you. Know whether or not meals or other refreshments will be required; what type of media support—computers and projectors, flip charts and pens, microphones, recording equipment, and so on—will be required; the length of time the room will be needed; whether or not a lectern or table should be at the front of the room; and whether chairs alone or chairs and tables will be needed for the audience. If the group is to take notes, the hotel may provide pads and pens. The hotel will also supply complimentary pitchers of ice water and glasses for the speaker and guests. Many facilities will fax you a worksheet for specifying all requirements, so that you can obtain the total cost.

- If there is to be a speaker, the physician will usually invite the person. However, you may need to confirm the person's attendance and the topic of the presentation. You may also need to make travel and hotel arrangements for the speaker. The administrative medical assistant should make reservations for ADA accommodations, if needed. The speaker should provide you with a brief *vita* (biographical and credentialing information), so that the physician can make a proper introduction. The vita should be placed in the physician's travel folder. You may also volunteer to prepare copies of handouts and to mail these to the meeting place. However, many handouts are presented in a more "eco-friendly" format. Presenters e-mail their presentation handouts in the form of an electronic file to the meeting facilitator. Attendees are then sent notification of the location of the handout. They may view it electronically or make a hardcopy for reference. Laptops may be used during the meeting to view the handouts and take notes.

- The physician may ask you to prepare an **agenda,** an outline of the meeting, that specifies the location, time, and major topics to be covered. A sample of an agenda is shown in Figure 6.6. Notice the large amount of white space, which enables attendees to make notes. Agendas are ordinarily sent out well ahead of the meeting to allow members to prepare for the business of the meeting.

- You will need to prepare and send, by either Postal Service or e-mail, an invitation to each person who is expected to attend the meeting. Those invited must also be told how and when to return their acceptance of the invitation. Frequently, travel directions to the meeting site are included as a courtesy. If the meeting is local, invitations should be sent at least 1 week, but not more than 2 weeks, prior to the meeting date. If the meeting is to be held in another city, invitations must be sent approximately 8 weeks before the meeting.

- Keep a record of the names, addresses, and telephone numbers of all those to whom you have sent invitations. It is also wise to keep a copy of the invitation and agenda in a convenient place. You will need to make copies of the agenda to hand out on the day of the meeting.

Figure 6.6

Meeting Agenda

"THE CHICAGO MEDICAL SOCIETY"

Agenda

Monthly Meeting
Tuesday, October 10, 20-- - 8:00 P.M.
University Hospital, Room 254C

1. Call to order

2. Reading of minutes of previous meeting (approved or changed)

3. Reading of correspondence

4. Reading of treasurer's report

5. Old business

   a. Choice of dates for state-level meeting for next year

   b. Arrangements for meeting room for monthly meetings

6. New business

   a. Reviewing plan for increasing membership

   b. Voting on increase of membership dues

7. Program: Thang Huai, MD, Urban Hospital Medical Center, Department of Oncology, "The Patient's Informed Decision About Radiation and/or Chemotherapy Treatment"

8. Announcements

9. Adjournment

Last-Minute Meeting Preparations. There may be times when you must personally visit the meeting room just before the meeting to ensure that everything has been provided and that the attendees will be comfortable. You may want to call the representative of the facility with whom you have dealt and ask that person to be available when you visit the meeting room. If food or other refreshments will be served, it is also a good idea to confirm the times of service and what is to be served. Be sure to check the meeting room for the following:

- Appropriate temperature
- Correct number of chairs
- Audiovisual and electronic equipment requested and in working order; many presenters prefer to use a pointing device to help them call attention to electronically displayed data, and the device is frequently combined with the ability to advance and reverse audiovisual slides during the presentation
- Microphone or other voice-amplifying device
- Lectern or table at the front of the room to accommodate the speaker and chairperson, along with a microphone if necessary
- Notepads and pens for note-taking
- Pitchers of ice water and glasses
- Name tags if required
- Copies of the agenda for the attendees

You may also be called upon to greet the guests when they arrive, and the physician may have requested that you remain so that you can record the minutes of the meeting.

Recording Minutes. The official record of the proceedings of a meeting is called the **meeting minutes.** Many meetings are conducted according to parliamentary procedure, and the minutes are then formatted in a formal way. Other meetings may proceed less formally. Minutes, therefore, may be formatted formally or informally, as shown in Figures 6.7a and 6.7b. Whatever the appropriate format, certain information is always included:

- Name of the organization or society holding the meeting
- Date, time, and location of the meeting
- Purpose of the meeting or indication that it is a monthly (quarterly, and so on) meeting

THE CHICAGO MEDICAL SOCIETY

Minutes

Monthly Meeting

Tuesday, October 10, 20--

The monthly meeting of the Chicago Medical Society was held on October 10, 20--, in Room 254C of the University Hospital. The meeting was called to order at 8:00 P.M. by Dr. Lee Wentworth.

The following members were present: Drs. Brian Cleary, Ernest Dodson, Jane Gunderson, Michael Pope, Yan Tuo, Lisa Twelvetrees, and Lee Wentworth.

The following members were absent: Drs. Roger Ahmed and Gloria Mahibir.

The reading of the minutes from the last meeting was waived.

The Treasurer reported that the Society's balance, as of October 1, 20--, was $1,257.72. There is one outstanding bill of $175.43 payable to the University Hospital Catering Service. A motion was made, seconded, and unanimously passed to pay this bill.

The next matter of business was the announcement of dates during which the state-level meeting will be held. Dr. Wentworth reported that the meeting was scheduled for December 4, 20-.

Dr. Gunderson reported that the University Hospital had renewed its agreement with the Society to allow the Society to use Room 254C for 2 more years.

A committee was formed to study ways to increase membership and will meet on November 1, 20--. Dr. Twelvetrees volunteered to chair the committee, and Drs. Cleary and Dodson agreed to serve as committee members.

For this month's program, Dr. Thang Huai, Urban Hospital Medical Center, Department of Oncology, gave a talk entitled "The Patient's Informed Decision About Radiation and/or Chemotherapy Treatment." A copy of the presentation is attached.

A motion was made to increase membership dues by $100 for the next year. It was seconded and unanimously carried.

The meeting was adjourned at 9:45 P.M.

_____   _____
Recorder   President

Figure 6.7a

Example of Formal Minutes

Figure 6.7b

Example of Informal Minutes

MEMO TO: Membership Committee of the
         Chicago Medical Society

FROM: Lisa Twelvetrees, MD
         Committee Chair

DATE: November 2, 20--

SUBJECT: Minutes of the Membership Committee
         Meeting of November 1, 20--

Present: Drs. Brian Cleary and Ernest Dodson

Absent: None

1. **Discussion of the Committee's objectives.** The Committee will explore ways to increase membership in the Chicago Medical Society. The Committee set a goal of attracting 10 new members for the next year.

2. **Discussion of courses of action.** The Committee discussed acquiring hospital mailing lists, sending an informational mailer to potential members, advertising in hospital bulletins, holding a hospitality evening for potential members, and offering incentives to current members who recruit new members.

3. **Actions to be taken.** Dr. Cleary agreed to research the cost of acquiring mailing lists and producing an informational mailer. Dr. Dodson agreed to get information on advertising and holding a hospitality evening. Dr. Twelvetrees agreed to speak with the Treasurer of the Society about incentives to current members for recruitment of new members. Committee members will report their findings at the next meeting of the Committee.

The next meeting of the Membership Committee will be held at 7:30 P.M., on December 12, 20--, at the office of Dr. Twelvetrees, University Hospital.

Lisa Twelvetrees, MD

rp

Distribution:

Dr. Brian Cleary
Dr. Ernest Dodson
Dr. Lee Wentworth

- Name of the presiding officer
- Names of the members in attendance and absent
- Order of business as it is taken up and any departures from the order as shown in the agenda
- Motions made and whether these were approved or rejected (some organizations state the names of the people who motioned and who seconded)
- Summaries of discussions

At certain meetings, portions of the minutes may need to be verbatim—that is, exactly as spoken. When this is necessary, the meeting is often taped and later transcribed.

It is usual for most organizations to have an assistant, sometimes called the "recorder." It is this person's responsibility to record the minutes of every meeting.

The recorder may request that you transcribe the minutes after the meeting. The minutes are signed by the recorder. Minutes are kept in an official book of minutes and are taken to every meeting.

In the absence of an official recorder, you may be requested to take the minutes. Be sure to familiarize yourself with the agenda, review the names of the attendees, and concentrate on the meeting. Sit next to the presiding officer if possible. Review and refer to the minutes of previous meetings. Do not hesitate to ask for clarification or the repetition of a point if you are unclear about what was said.

A laptop or notebook computer may be used to record meeting minutes. Tape recorders may also be used. If these are used, the assistant should consult the office policies and procedures manual to determine how and how long the tapes should be maintained. Minutes may also be taken by hand using a pen and notebook and transcribing them after the meeting.

6.6 PATIENT AND EMPLOYEE EDUCATION

Information intended to educate *patients* about the practice and about their own health-care is offered in many formats, including brochures, fact sheets, and newsletters. DVDs and in-person seminars are also used. Most practices display information on a Web page. You should work with the Web designer (webmaster) to include and update pages for patient education. Suggested topics to include in a patient information source are listed in the following section.

Information intended to educate and train *employees* is often gathered in an office policies and procedures manual. It contains key procedures about office operation. All patient information materials and employee education and training materials should be carefully proofread and be free of typographical errors.

Patient Information Brochure

A **patient information brochure,** or booklet, provides the patient with vital information that is particularly useful because it is in writing and can be kept in a convenient place in the patient's home or, if an electronic brochure is used, in an electronic file on the patient's electronic device. However, the brochure does not take the place of a personal orientation for new patients.

A patient information brochure can be used as a marketing tool for the medical practice, as well as a way to inform patients about the practice. Current and future patients should be well informed of the practice's policies and operations.

Deciding on the contents of the brochure is the first step that must be taken. Topics to be considered include

- a description of the services offered by the practice, including patient education classes and medical testing programs.
- a list of physicians' names, specialties, and qualifications.
- the names, functions, and contact information of the members of the office staff.
- instructions for scheduling appointments (be sure to list office hours and provide patients with instructions for emergencies, such as "Use 911 in life-threatening emergencies"; inform patients if the office has a 24-hour telephone service for emergency situations).

- policies and procedures related to physicians' fees and payment, prescription re-fills, and medical insurance and other forms.
- a statement of any other policies that are relevant and that you may be directed to include, such as the practice's Notice of Privacy Practices (NPP) and copy of the Patient's Bill of Rights.
- instructions for how patients can access their medical records.
- an expression of gratitude to patients for choosing the practice and for taking the time to read about the services it provides (include a statement such as "If you have any questions about our clinic, please telephone us at [phone number] or e-mail us at [address]").

Patient Education Materials

In some practices, depending on the size, specialties, and resources available, there may be an opportunity to provide other **patient education materials**—for example, descriptions of frequently ordered testing and surgical procedures along with an account of the restrictions on diet or activity that the procedures impose. A list of resources—agencies, DVDs, Internet sites, support groups—may also be useful to patients. A list of preventive actions or "tips" intended to promote good health may also be provided: getting regular checkups; limiting alcohol consumption; exercising regularly; avoiding tobacco; reducing stress, for example. A list of safety tips for avoiding injury at home and at work may also be appreciated.

Design Considerations

In many offices, the brochure is developed using a desktop publishing program. In others, this job is given to an outside resource.

There are many local businesses that specialize in designing and printing brochures, information sheets, and booklets. You will need to make clear to the professional who is assisting you the basic specifications of the piece you wish to create: length, quality of paper, and two-color (black ink and one other color for contrast) or full color. In addition, you will want to give the designer a sense of how you want the piece to look: visual appeal, use of photographs, and white (blank) space to make it easy to read. If you have friends who work in other practices, it would help you to evaluate the patient information brochures developed in their offices. This assessment will clarify the features you find effective. If this is not possible, you may cut out visually appealing magazine articles to show the designer and search the Internet for design and layout suggestions.

In addition to design considerations, there are issues of ease of understanding. Whether you or a professional writer creates the text, it must be easy to understand. The use of technical words should be minimal. You should also consider the cultural population in your service area and have the brochure written both in English and in other languages. If publishing the brochure to a website, American Disability Act guidelines should be followed. An example would be to post an audio version of the brochure.

Employee Policies and Procedures Manual

The **policies and procedures manual,** or employee handbook, is the reference that provides all employees with information about the work environment. Because employees are likely to refer to the manual often, it needs to be kept current and complete. The manual serves as a reminder of tasks to be done (referred to as *policies*) and how to complete the tasks (*procedures*). The office's Compliance Manual may be included as part of the policies and procedures manual, or it may be a completely separate manual. During an employee's temporary absence due to illness or vacation, the manual helps keep the office running smoothly. It is a great help in training new employees, substitutes, and successors. A signature page should be included for employees to sign and date attesting to the reading of and compliance to the policies and procedures manual. The completed signature page will be kept on file by the medical facility. When an update is made to the manual, employees should be asked to sign and date a new, updated signature page.

Format. A looseleaf binder with tab divisions is an ideal holder for a policies and procedures manual. Pages may easily be added or taken out. New topics only require additional tabs, inserted in a logical place. The only other format that offers as much flexibility is the computer. An electronic format, using a word processing program, would be easy to establish. Copies could be electronically sent to each employee. Updates or instructions about deletions could be sent the same way. It is important that every page be dated, so that the most recent update is easily identifiable. If the medical office maintains a website, the electronic manual may be placed on the website for easy access by employees.

Contents. Prepare an outline of topics that must be covered. The following suggestions for topics and the order of presentation will not address every situation. However, certain topics are common to almost all practices.

- *Office personnel directory:* This directory should contain the names, positions, physical locations, telephone or extension numbers, cell phone numbers, and pager numbers of everyone in the office, along with the numbers (business—not personal—cell phone numbers, unless a personal cell phone is used for business) for building services, such as maintenance and security. E-mail addresses should also be included for each individual and department.
- *Job descriptions:* This section lists the major responsibilities and duties of all employees other than the physicians—for example, administrative medical assistant, receptionist, technicians, billing specialists, nurses, and other medical office team members. A list of the names of the people currently holding the positions is often included, along with the name, e-mail address, and telephone number of a person to be contacted in case of emergency for each employee. Either in this section or in a separate section dealing with procedures, descriptions of how to perform the duties of the position are given. If job duties overlap, or if employees are expected to substitute for each other in case of absence or illness, that should be stated in this section of the manual.
- *Procedures:* Once the duties of the positions have been stated, a section on specific procedures may follow. Cross-training (training of employees to do other employees' tasks) of employees within an office helps eliminate lapses of services when an employee is absent. A current description of job responsibilities and procedures within the office can be a valuable tool to assist in cross-training. Forms may be included with the procedures for which they are used. Figures 6.8a and 6.8b show pages designed to describe procedures. Subsequent lists have examples of entries for the procedures section of the manual.

Section 4: HANDLING RECORDS

PATIENTS WHO HAVE MOVED

Procedure:

DECEASED PATIENTS

Procedure:

TRANSFER OF RECORDS

Procedure:

SUPERVISION OF FILING SYSTEM

Procedure:

Figure 6.8a

Page from a Procedures Manual Showing Form for Describing Administrative Procedures

Daily Routine

1. List duties to be performed that prepare the office each morning before patients arrive. These include checking the neatness and cleanliness of the office, calling the answering service or checking the answering machine for messages, checking e-mails, processing incoming and/or outgoing mail, pulling charts for the day's appointments (if hardcopy charts are used), preparing the appointment schedule, and checking to see that the examination rooms are ready to be used. Throughout the day, canceled and/or missed appointments should be recorded in the patient's record.
2. List other routine duties, including preparing correspondence and patient records, maintaining financial records, and completing insurance forms.
3. List the duties that must be done at the end of the day, including locking desks and files, turning off and covering certain equipment, verifying that all computers have been either logged off or shut down, and programming the answering machine for after-hours calls.

COMMONLY PERFORMED PROCEDURES

NAME OF PROCEDURE _____

USUAL TIME REQUIREMENT _____

SUPPLIES AND INSTRUMENTS:

PATIENT PREPARATION:

SPECIAL INSTRUCTIONS:

Figure 6.8b

Page from a Procedures Manual Showing Form for Describing Medical Procedures

Records Management: Creation, Use, Maintenance, Disposition

1. Describe the records management method used, and provide a diagram, if necessary, of the locations of sections—active, inactive, closed, transient.
2. Indicate the length of time for keeping records in active files (retention schedule).
3. If colors are used as a filing aid, explain what each color designates.
4. Describe the preferred order of documents in the patients' medical records (POMR, SOMR, CHEDDAR, etc.), including medication sheets, progress notes, laboratory reports, x-ray reports, special procedures notes, correspondence, and hospital summaries. This also includes the section and order in which electronic medical data are placed into EHRs.
5. List the types of medical reports that must be attached to a patient's chart or present in the electronic chart before a physician reviews it.
6. Describe follow-up procedures for test results.
7. Describe the steps to create a records inventory, a retention schedule, and a disposition (transfer to inactive storage, archive storage, or destruction) schedule for different categories of records.

Records Management: Transferring Patients' Records

1. State which staff member is responsible for handling the transfer.
2. List the rules for what can and cannot be transferred.
3. Describe the procedures for copying records to be transferred.
4. Describe the procedures for faxing records to be transferred.
5. Describe the procedure for recording when and what information was transferred.
6. Describe the procedure for filing the release-of-information form.

Scheduling Appointments

1. List the schedule commitments for each physician, including office hours, hospital hours, teaching or research schedule, and other nonpatient appointments. Follow office procedure for clarifying if the appointment is to be face-to-face or by electronic media.
2. Note which physicians have special scheduling requests, such as limiting the number of physical examinations to no more than two in the morning or scheduling no physical examinations on Monday mornings or Friday afternoons.
3. List the procedure for canceling and rescheduling appointments, including whether or not patients are called or notified electronically on the day before the appointment for confirmation.
4. List the information required from patients for scheduling an appointment.
5. List the standard length of time required for various procedures, such as 1 hour for a complete physical examination, 1/2 hour for school physicals, and so forth.

Orientation for New Patients

1. Describe the information to be provided to new patients and how it will be provided, including office hours and emergency care procedures.
2. List the hospitals affiliated with the practice and their addresses, telephone numbers, and visiting hours.
3. Describe the procedures for obtaining medication refills.

Telephone Procedures

1. Give the preferred greeting for answering the telephone.
2. Explain the triage procedure, covering what calls should be put through to the physician. Include a flowchart listing the questions to ask patients when they are being triaged.
3. List the ways in which questions should be phrased when obtaining information about patients over the phone.
4. Provide suggestions for referring a patient to a physician on call, to the hospital emergency room, to another facility, or to sources of financial assistance.

Patient Care

This section may be the most significant portion of the manual, covering everything from the level of interpersonal skills expected of the office staff to the specific ways to perform a variety of procedures.

Billing

1. Provide a sample patient statement, and explain the method of billing.
2. Note the name, address, and telephone number of any accounting service that is used.
3. If there is a billing specialist in the practice, state the procedures for disclosing and/or using information. If a BA (business associate) is used, state the procedures for HIPAA-compliant protection of PHI.

Collections

1. State and explain the steps established by the practice in the standard collection process.
2. Show sample collection letters, and provide a sample of the form used to track the collection process.

Processing Insurance Forms

1. Provide detailed instructions for handling each insurance account, for completing each type of form, for using and disclosing patient information to obtain third-party payment, and for billing patients who have insurance.
2. Provide the name of a contact person and the company's address, phone number, and e-mail address for each insurance carrier used within the practice.
3. List the approximate turnaround time for processing claims for each insurance carrier.

Forms and Supplies

If samples of forms, with instructions for completing them, have not been included in topical sections, a separate section should familiarize employees with all the forms used in the practice. Even if the forms are in an electronic format, a hardcopy should be included in the manual for reference and training.

Equipment/Materials

Include an inventory of all equipment. It is also useful to list equipment model and registration numbers. List the names, addresses, e-mail addresses, and phone numbers of equipment manufacturers, dealers, and local repair services.

Safety data sheets (SDS), formerly known as material safety data sheets (MSDS), which list the physical properties of substances, are to be kept for hazardous materials. OSHA-compliant SDSs provide medical office team members with the information needed to work safely with chemical substances.

Inventory and Ordering Procedures

1. Describe the rules for taking inventory and reporting on inventory levels. Include the required schedule for taking inventory—for example, every week.
2. State who is responsible for certain kinds of inventory. Nursing personnel may be responsible for medications, drugs, surgical gloves, and examination supplies. Administrative medical assistants may be responsible for desk, stationery, and maintenance supplies. Certain items, such as linens—laboratory coats, examination gowns, and towels—may be the property of the practice or may be rented from a linen supply company. Be sure to address how the linen supply is handled.
3. Provide the forms for ordering supplies and directions for completing them.

Employee Hiring Policies

1. Include a statement of nondiscrimination in hiring.
2. Describe hiring procedures, and indicate whose responsibility it is to interview and to recommend hiring for specific positions. If committees are used, indicate the positions that are to be on the committee—physician, office manager, administrative medical assistant. Positions on hiring committees will vary, depending on the vacancy being filled.

Employee Evaluation Policies

1. Indicate how often employees are evaluated and explain the process.
2. Define the rating system, if one is used, and the relationship of ratings to the amount of annual salary or hourly wage increase.

3. Include a copy of the blank appraisal form.
4. Describe the procedures related to unsatisfactory performance and the steps leading to job probation and/or termination of employment.
5. Describe the grievance or arbitration procedure in place that employees may use if they have a serious complaint.

Employee Benefits Policies

1. State the rules regarding vacations, sick days, personal leaves, bereavement leaves, jury duty, and the reporting of sickness or absence. The Family Medical Leave Act should be included in this section.
2. Describe the insurance benefits and the options employees may choose.
3. Describe any savings plans, 401k plans, and other retirement investment opportunities that are in place for employees.

Office Dress Code

State the rules related to professional dress established in the practice. If a dress code is in place (stated in the manual) before an employee is hired, and the employee is responsible for knowing the manual's content, the probability of charges based on dress code violation will be greatly reduced.

Meeting Schedule

1. List the established dates or days of staff meetings and committee meetings.
2. List the members for each committee and the purposes of the committee.
3. Describe the role and responsibilities or degree of involvement of the physician with each committee.

Maintenance, Safety, and Office Security

1. Describe the schedule of building maintenance along with the names, e-mail addresses, and telephone numbers of the building maintenance staff or of the custodial service with which the practice has a contract.
2. If the office staff has specific duties to help keep the office clean and tidy, describe the duties and who is to handle them.
3. List the guidelines for office safety. Employee safety training schedules and how this training is to be documented should also be included in this section. Policies and procedures for maintaining Occupational Safety and Health Administration (OSHA) compliance are included. How to handle, process, and dispose of medical waste and contaminants should be clearly outlined.
4. Describe implementation and documentation of Universal Precautions for blood-borne and airborne pathogens. A pandemic preparedness plan should be established, including assessment of potential risk factors.
5. Describe how building security works: requirements for identification badges and the security system itself—locks, alarms, and so forth. Include the rules for keeping doors locked or using buzzers for admittance. Provide the names of the security staff and their work telephone numbers and e-mail addresses. Include in this section reminders about securing personal property and demanding proper identification of strangers in the building.

Outside Services File

In addition to referring patients to other physicians, every physician must at times refer patients to agencies or businesses for help of various kinds, including health services and medical supplies. The policies and procedures manual should include an

outside services file containing the names, addresses, e-mail addresses, and phone numbers of those to whom the physician may refer patients for services, such as

- convalescent and nursing homes.
- dentists and dental specialists.
- health insurance organizations.
- home healthcare agencies and hospices.
- laboratories.
- medical specialists for referrals.
- pharmacies.
- medical supply companies.
- social services agencies.
- human services agencies.
- temporary agencies for staffing of medical personnel.
- website addresses of agencies and sites in your city that provide additional information and/or services.

Responsibility for Employee-Related Records

As an office manager, the assistant may be responsible for supervising other staff members and keeping records relating to their employment. Each employee will have a separate file containing information such as an application form and a cover letter, a résumé, a letter of employment agreement, performance evaluations, and an attendance record. These are confidential records and are stored in a locked drawer or secure electronic files.

Each physician will want to keep a personal file containing additional information regarding licenses—state license, narcotics license, workers' compensation registration, for example. Social Security information and insurance identification numbers should also be kept in this file. A file listing the physician's affiliations with medical societies, organizations, and hospitals is kept along with a list of continuing education requirements. A list should be kept, related to these files, that contains license and membership renewal dates, fees, and any necessary identifying numbers.

Office Manager's Resources

It can easily be seen by the extensive list of topics to be covered in the office policies and procedures manual that the assistant serving as office manager has an enormous amount of responsibility. Even though it is challenging to keep the manual current, the manual can be an extraordinarily useful tool. It makes the task of managing both daily routines and personnel less problematic. The routines are made explicit and directions are given for handling daily tasks. Staff members are able to thoroughly understand their job responsibilities. This knowledge, in turn, helps them understand the expectations that managers have of them.

Another extremely useful tool is the computer. The information available on the Internet is a great help. There are a number of search engines designed to assist in locating services, articles and books required for physicians' research, travel directions, medical organizations and societies, and contact information for companies and professionals.

Also, standard printed references and resources should be available in every office, including dictionaries (standard and medical); a thesaurus; English language usage references to provide formatting instructions, grammar rules, and writing style guidelines; drug references to provide information on medications, such as brand and generic names, manufacturers, contraindications, and dosages; and state and local medical directories to provide credential information about medical personnel—correct spelling of names, office addresses, and telephone numbers.

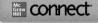 **GO TO PROJECT 6.5 AT THE END OF THIS CHAPTER**

6.1 Design a medical office waiting area that exhibits the priority of patient comfort.	• When considering the design of patient waiting areas in a medical office, consider each of the following: — Size of the area — Arrangements of chairs and walkways — Wall color, décor, and lighting — Available reading material and comforts (such as drinking water) — Separate areas for healthy patients, sick patients, and children — Visual, kinesthetic, auditory, or other forms of entertainment Patient confidentiality when registering on arrival is the primary focus of design.
6.2 Identify three stress triggers in your own life and define at least one method of reducing the associated negative stress.	• Stress triggers are as varied as there are individuals. Some of the most common stress triggers are associated with expected work productivity levels. Others include financial pressures and family-unit pressure (single parent, multicareer, caregiver of an aging family member). Health issues also cause stress. • Certain strategies will help reduce the negative effects of stress: — Analyzing how we use time and applying time management techniques — Managing our anger and reactions to conflict — Getting organized and setting priorities — Staying physically and mentally healthy — Taking time to relax
6.3 Differentiate among three common leadership/management styles.	• Managers lead and manage using different styles. The manager must choose the style best suited to meet the current situation. — Authoritarian/autocratic leaders make decisions with little or no input from others. — Leaders who prefer to seek advice and input from those involved are using the participative/democratic style of leadership. — A common leadership style is used by the manager who encourages team members to make their own decisions with little input or direction from the manager. This is known as delegative/laissez-faire management. An effective manager is able to analyze the situation and match it with the correct leadership style.
6.4 Explain why an administrative medical assistant needs to know how to collect and assimilate research data.	• Physicians often research medical cases and data to gather treatment protocol for a condition or disease, to keep up to date on medical trends, and to prepare articles for professional medical journals and presentations. The physician will often rely on

	the administrative medical assistant to collect data from medical libraries and other sources. Collating and preparing the information in proper, keyed format are also skills needed by an AMA.

6.5 Classify items into major categories of needed information when making travel and meeting arrangements.	• When making travel arrangements for yourself or for others, maintain a reference folder with the following preferences:
	— *Method of travel*—air or ground
	  • *Air travel*—airline, seat, meal, travel time, type of flight
	  • *Ground travel*—rental company, size/make/model, smoking or nonsmoking
	— *Lodging*—smoking or nonsmoking accommodations, room and bed size, proximity to event, room/resort amenities
	— *Membership discounts*—professional social affiliations
	— *Past itineraries*—use for reference
	— *Meeting location*—number of attendees, services offered, media support, ADA accommodations
	— *Speaker*—travel and hotel arrangements, meeting materials,
	— *Agenda and meeting minutes*—prepare and record

6.6 Justify why a policies and procedures manual should be developed and used in a medical office.	• Employees frequently need to be instructed on office policies and how to implement or complete tasks. A thorough and up-to-date manual provides a reference for current and new employees on topics related to all areas of the medical office. • When someone is absent, reference can be made to the manual for the completion of tasks; lost productivity because of someone's absence is reduced or does not occur. • When an employee has a question concerning office policy or procedure, reference can be made to the manual, thus reducing lost income due to errors. • Proof of compliance and employee training documentation can be maintained within the manual, reducing the possibility of financial penalties. • Time and money spent preparing and maintaining a policies and procedures manual are justified when compared with the cost of lost income due to errors, absence of employees, and noncompliance.

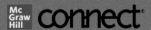
Project 6.1 — (LO 6.1) Designing a Waiting Area

The goal of waiting room design is to create a place where patients can relax—to allow them to collect their thoughts before seeing the physician and to calm their nerves to prepare them for their appointment. Patients will form their first impression of your office when they enter the waiting room. The look of the office could influence how likely they are to return for future care. Design a waiting room for a local physician's practice. Be sure to focus on the mechanics of patient flow and office efficiency.

Project 6.2 — (LO 6.2) Analyze Usage of Time

Keep a time log for 7 consecutive days. Document all 24 hours of the day—for example, 6:30 A.M. to 7:30 A.M.: got out of bed and got ready for school. 7:30 A.M. to 8:20 A.M.: drove to school. Determine the most and least productive times of the day and time wasters. Annotate the less productive time periods with ways to improve your time management skills.

Project 6.3 — (LO 6.3) Internet Research: Improving Office Management Skills

It is important to have some good resources for informational and motivational articles. Using your favorite Web browser, find articles on time management, prioritizing, problem-solving, initiative, strategic planning, and leadership. Choose at least two articles, and summarize the content. Be sure to address within your summary of each article the soft skills needed. Prepare a correctly formatted bibliography page for the Internet resources. Use either MLA or APA format for resources used. Be prepared to discuss your research.

Project 6.4 — (LO 6.4) Internet Research: Journal Articles and Patient Education Form

Dr. Larsen has asked you to search the Internet for recent articles (within the last year) on chickenpox (varicella) or mumps (epidemic parotitis). Design and prepare one patient education form (or brochure) containing both chickenpox and mumps, including (1) a complete description of the disease, (2) signs and symptoms, (3) precautions to be taken by the infected patient and by those caring for the patient, and (4) treatment(s). Differentiate for the reader between the two conditions. Include bibliographic data in either MLA or APA format for resources you used.

(LO 6.6) Internet Research: OSHA Compliance Plan for the Medical Office

Research various websites including the OSHA website (www.osha.gov), and collect information to develop and implement an OSHA Compliance Plan for Dr. Larsen's office. Prepare an outline that includes the five standards for a medical office, as defined by OSHA, that will help minimize incidents and protect employees in the medical office. Each standard should include OSHA requirements for the standard. For example, a requirement for the Emergency Exit Route standard is to provide ample safety routes, based on the number of employees, to allow safe and accessible exits from the medical office area.

The five OSHA standards are

1. Bloodborne Pathogens.
2. Hazard Communications.
3. Ionizing Radiation.
4. Emergency Exit Routes.
5. Electrical Standards.

Be prepared to discuss your research findings and your outline.

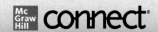
Adaptability (LO 6.2)

In today's business world, change is coming faster than ever before. Even minor change can be unsettling and intimidating. Stress and resistance will follow. This is especially true of the healthcare industry, where the only thing that remains the same is change. Change is important, and so is the way you react to it. During times of change, adaptability is required to foster progress and to help you remain effective and productive. **How well do you adapt to change? Describe a situation in the medical practice that would require you to make a change.**

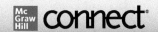
USING TERMINOLOGY

Match the term or phrase on the left with the correct answer on the right.

_____ 1. [LO 6.5] Travel agent

_____ 2. [LO 6.5] Itinerary

_____ 3. [LO 6.1] Ergonomics

_____ 4. [LO 6.3] Participative

_____ 5. [LO 6.2] Perfectionism

_____ 6. [LO 6.2] Stress

_____ 7. [LO 6.6] Patient information brochure

_____ 8. [LO 6.3] Delegative

a. "Hands-off" management style

b. Setting unrealistic goals; being dissatisfied with anything less

c. Management style in which a manager gives advice and participates in the decision process

d. Emotional and/or physiological reactions to external stimuli

e. Matching equipment/furniture and physical needs in order to complete tasks without decreasing productivity

f. Provides patient-related details of a medical practice

g. Daily schedule of travel events

h. Individual or agency used to assist with travel arrangements

CHECKING YOUR UNDERSTANDING

Select the most correct answer.

1. [LO 6.1] Which of the following is a HIPAA-compliant method for patient registration in the waiting area?

   a. Have patients sign their first and last names on a sign-in log.
   b. Ask patients to verbally state their full name to the AMA.
   c. Ask patients to sign a detachable label log, which is immediately removed prior to the next patient's signing the log.
   d. Have patients sign their names on a log and mark it out with a highlighter.

2. [LO 6.2] During the monthly office meeting, Carrie became defensive and angry when she received the news that all office staff would need to attend a 2-day training workshop on the new EHR software. She is behind on her work and being out of the office will just put her more behind. How can Carrie control her anger during the meeting without becoming a disruption?

   a. She can take a quiet, deep breath and reevaluate her perception of the news.
   b. She can walk out of the meeting.
   c. She can key in a quick comment on a social network.
   d. None of these are appropriate responses.

3. [LO 6.3] An effective office manager is one who has which of the following attributes?

   a. Understands the different roles of the office team members
   b. Delegates tasks and resources needed to accomplish them
   c. Manages available time
   d. All of these

4. [LO 6.4] Felicia, Dr. Gomez's AMA, needs to locate current information on fibromyalgia for a presentation Dr. Gomez will give at the next state medical conference. Which of the following would not be a credible source of information?

   a. Online medical journals
   b. Case studies
   c. Reprints from colleagues who published articles on fibromyalgia during the last 3 years
   d. Verbal information gathered during lunch break

5. [LO 6.5] Caitlin, an AMA, will continue to work in the medical office while Dr. Smith attends the American Medical Association National Conference. Dr. Smith will use her smartphone to receive and send information and to correspond through e-mail. In addition, Dr. Smith would like to talk to Caitlin on Tuesday and Thursday at 12:30 P.M. during a conference break. To prepare for the phone calls, Caitlin should

   a. wait to see what Dr. Smith wants to discuss and then retrieve the information.
   b. keep a log of important phone calls, mail, and messages, along with the related patient information, such as a chart or flagged EHR for quick reference.
   c. call other office staff and let them know when the doctor is going to call.
   d. take a nap prior to the call, so that she is refreshed.

6. [LO 6.6] When asked to design and construct a method to convey practice information to patients, Natalie was unsure of how to begin. She works for a new pediatrician, and the general parent population of their patients is below the age of 30. Which of the following would be a productive first step?

   a. Compile all the procedures and policies of the practice in a brochure format.
   b. Research local printing cost.
   c. Take a class on Web design.
   d. Conduct a survey of the patients' parents or legal guardian to determine their desired mode of delivery, such as electronic, written, or both.

7. [LO 6.3] Tension in the medical office has increased over the past 2 months. The receptionist and insurance biller each treated patients differently, and each felt the other was being rude to patients. As a result, patients began to ask questions of Dr. Larsen concerning the atmosphere between the two employees, and the office manager was instructed to fix the problem. The first step taken by the office manager is to

   a. brainstorm possible solutions.
   b. define the problem.
   c. fire both employees.
   d. implement a grievance policy.

8. [LO 6.2] MaKayla is normally an enthusiastic, happy employee. However, today she arrived to work in a quiet, sedate mood. She said that her son had lost his job, and he and his family, including two very young children, were now sharing MaKayla's home. She is thrilled to have her son, daughter-in-law, and grandchildren close to her. However, MaKayla may be experiencing adjustment stress due to which of the following?

   a. Single-parent provider
   b. Work expectation
   c. Lack of exercise
   d. Multigenerational household

9. [LO 6.5] Which type of flight should you book when the traveler does not mind a stop but does not want to change airplanes?

   a. Nonstop
   b. Connecting
   c. Direct
   d. First class

10. [LO 6.6] Under which heading in a policies and procedures manual would you likely find instructions on how to dispose of medical instruments that may contain bloodborne pathogens?

    a. Maintenance, Safety, and Office Security
    b. Employee Evaluation Policies
    c. Inventory and Ordering Procedures
    d. Collections

THINKING IT THROUGH

These questions cover the most important points in this chapter. Using your critical-thinking skills, play the role of an administrative medical assistant as you answer each question. Be prepared to discuss your responses.

1. [LO 6.1] In the following situation, show how you use these three qualifications for office management—being a team player, planning strategically, and increasing productivity: There are three physicians in the practice where you are employed. Each physician has an administrative medical assistant and a technician, and there is an office receptionist. As an office manager, you have just received approval to present a proposal for purchasing new waiting room furniture. How will you use your office management skills to handle this task?

2. [LO 6.3] Of the four main office management tasks discussed in this chapter, which one appeals to you most? Which task has the least appeal? Discuss reasons for your answers.

3. [LO 6.5] What are several things you can do to ensure that the physician's travel is as pleasant as possible?

4. [LO 6.5] The physician who is your employer is responsible for the next meeting of the local chapter of a professional association. What are three major tasks you must accomplish in making the arrangements for this meeting?

5. [LO 6.6] Prepare a rough draft outline—major points only—for a patient information brochure.

6. [LO 6.6] Design an office brochure to educate patients about your practice. This will be provided to new patients, and it should be functional for a physician's waiting room area. This brochure will represent the practice and the services provided. Patients retain only 20 percent of what they hear, so written information from a healthcare professional is very important. Keep in mind what you would want to know about a medical practice.

PART 3

Practice Financials

Part 3 discusses the important duties of the administrative medical assistant in managing the financial aspects of a practice. Presented are insurance and coding, billing, payments, and accounting tasks.

CONSIDER THIS: Financial duties are very important to a successful practice, and computers are primarily used to help handle this task. *How can you improve your computer-related skills?*

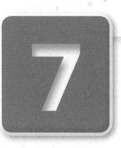

Chapter 7

Insurance and Coding

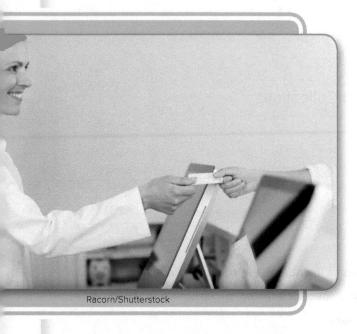

Racorn/Shutterstock

LEARNING OUTCOMES

After studying this chapter, you will be able to

7.1 identify and define the terminology related to medical insurance and medical coding.

7.2 explain the differences among the types of insurance plans.

7.3 compare and contrast PAR and nonPAR providers and the methods insurance companies use to determine how much a provider is paid.

7.4 apply *ICD-10-CM* conventions, symbols, abbreviations, and guidelines to properly code diagnoses in an outpatient setting.

7.5 apply *CPT* conventions and guidelines to properly code procedures and supplies in an outpatient setting.

7.6 explain the effects of coding compliance errors on the revenue cycle in the medical office setting.

KEY TERMS

Study these important words, which are defined in this chapter, to build your professional vocabulary:

accepting assignment
ACO (accountable care organization)
allowed charge
assignment of benefits
balance billing
birthday rule
Blue Cross Blue Shield Association (BCBSA)
capitation
carrier
CDHP (consumer-driven health plan)
Centers for Medicare & Medicaid Services (CMS)

CHAMPVA
code linkage
coinsurance
coordination of benefits (COB)
copayment (copay)
CPT
customary fee
deductible
Defense Enrollment Eligibility Reporting System (DEERS)
diagnosis-related groups (DRGs)
fee-for-service
gender rule
HCPCS

HMO (health maintenance organization)
ICD-10-CM
ICD-10-PCS
indemnity plan
insured
managed care
Medicaid
Medicare
participating (PAR) provider
patient encounter form
POS (point of service)
PPO (preferred provider organization)

preauthorization
premium
primary care provider (PCP)
provider
reasonable fee
referral
relative value scale (RVS)
resource-based relative value scale (RBRVS)
sponsor
third-party payer
TRICARE
usual fee
workers' compensation

ABHES

4.a. Follow documentation guidelines.

4.e. Perform risk management procedures.

5.c. Assist the patient in navigating issues and concerns that may arise (i.e., insurance policy information, medical bills, and physician/provider orders).

7.a. Gather and process documents.

10.b. Demonstrate professional behavior.

www.abhes.org/accreditationmanual

The ABHES standards appear with permission of The Accrediting Bureau of Health Education Schools

CAAHEP

V.P.3. Use medical terminology correctly and pronounced accurately to communicate information to providers and patients.

V.P.4.a. Coach patients regarding office policies.

VIII.C.1.a. Identify types of third-party plans.

IX.C.1. Describe how to use the most current procedural coding system.

IX.C.2. Describe how to use the most current diagnostic coding classification system.

IX.C.3. Describe how to use the most current *HCPCS* level II coding system.

IX.C.4.a. Discuss the effects of upcoding.

IX.C.4.b. Discuss the effects of downcoding.

IX.C.5. Define *medical necessity* as it applies to procedural and diagnostic coding.

IX.P.1. Perform procedural coding.

IX.P.2. Perform diagnostic coding.

IX.P.3. Utilize medical necessity guidelines.

IX.A.1. Utilize tactful communication skills with medical providers to ensure accurate code selection.

X.C.8.c. Describe the following type of insurance: personal injury.

2015 Standards and Guidelines for the Accreditation of Educational Programs in Medical Assisting, Appendix B, Core Curriculum for Medical Assistants, Medical Assisting Education Review Board (MAERB), 2015.

INTRODUCTION

Medical insurance, also known as *health insurance,* refers to insurance protection against medical care expenses. Administrative medical assistants must understand insurance in order to answer patients' questions about their health insurance policies and to process insurance claim forms properly, so that the physician receives compensation for services.

7.1   INSURANCE TERMINOLOGY

The administrative medical assistant must be familiar with basic insurance terminology in order to be helpful to patients and to process insurance claims.

The Medical Insurance Contract

Medical insurance is a policy, or certificate of coverage, between a person, called the policyholder, and an insurance company, or **carrier.** The policyholder pays a certain amount of money to the insurance company in return for benefits. The benefits are in the form of payments from the insurance company for the medical services received.

In the medical insurance contract, the insurance company agrees to carry the risk of paying for services required by the policyholder. The patient agrees to make regular payments to the insurance company to keep the policy intact. As with other types of insurance companies, medical insurance companies manage the risk that some individuals they insure will require very expensive services by spreading that risk among many policyholders.

Insured. The person who takes out the insurance policy is referred to as the **insured.** Since a medical insurance policy often covers the insured and the insured's dependents, in the strict sense of the term, *policyholder* refers to the person in whose name the policy is written (the person who is responsible for making payments) and the term *insured* refers to anyone, such as the policyholder or a spouse, covered by the medical policy.

Premium. The rate charged to the policyholder for the insurance policy is the **premium.** Premiums are usually paid by the policyholder on a regular basis—for example, monthly or quarterly.

Third-Party Payer. According to contract law, when a physician agrees to treat a patient who is seeking medical services, there is an unwritten contract between the two. The physician or other healthcare professional—the **provider** (the "first party")—agrees to treat the patient, and the patient (the "second party") assumes the legal responsibility of paying for the services received. If the patient has a policy with an insurance company, in which the insurance company agrees to carry the risk of paying for those services, the insurance company is referred to as the "third party" and is therefore called a **third-party payer.**

A patient who does not have insurance is referred to as a "self-pay." A self-pay patient is responsible for paying the physician directly for all services received.

Coordination of Benefits. The clause relating to **coordination of benefits (COB)** in an insurance policy provides that a patient who has two or more insurance policies can have only a maximum benefit of 100 percent of the health costs. If the insurance companies do not communicate with each other, there is the possibility that more than 100 percent of the cost of the covered services will be reimbursed.

Under the terms of the coordination-of-benefits clause, one insurance carrier is named the primary carrier. The clause explains how the policy will pay—whether as a primary or secondary carrier—if more than one insurance policy applies to the claim. For example, the primary carrier may pay up to 80 percent and the secondary carrier may pay up to 20 percent, not to exceed a maximum benefit of 100 percent.

The Birthday Rule and the Gender Rule. The **birthday rule** is used as a guideline for determining which of two parents with medical coverage has the primary insurance for a child. The rule states that the policy of the insured with the earlier birthday in the calendar year is the primary policy. The policy of the other parent, the secondary policy, may cover costs that are not covered by the primary policy. This ensures that the maximum benefit will not exceed 100 percent of the charge for covered services.

EXAMPLE: BIRTHDAY RULE

Both parents of a 6-year-old child have medical insurance. The child is covered under both policies. The mother's birthday is June 10, 1995, and the father's birthday is November 25, 1989. According to the birthday rule, the primary policy for the child would be the mother's policy because her birthday falls earlier in the year (June 10), and the father's policy would be secondary because his birthday falls later in the year (November 10). The birth year is *not* used when determining primary/secondary policies under the birthday rule, only the birth month.

If the mother's birthday was June 10, 1995, and the father's birthday was June 5, 1989, the father's policy would be primary because his birthday is earlier in the month of June.

An older method of determining coverage of a child is the **gender rule.** It states that when the mother and father both have coverage, the primary insurance is the father's insurance. If the child is covered under one policy that uses the birthday rule and one that uses the gender rule, the policy that uses the gender rule is primary.

EXAMPLE: GENDER RULE

Both parents of a 6-year-old child have medical insurance, and the child is covered under both policies. According to the gender rule, the father's insurance is primary.

If the mother's policy uses the birthday rule to determine coverage and the father's policy uses the gender rule to determine coverage, the father's policy is primary.

Types of Medical Insurance Coverage

Medical insurance coverage can be purchased in a variety of forms for different levels of coverage. The greater the coverage, the more expensive the plan. Insurance can also be purchased for a group or for an individual.

Under group insurance, one master policy is issued to an organization or employer, and it covers the eligible members or employees and their dependents. Thus, all the members or employees have the same healthcare coverage. Group insurance provides better benefits with lower premiums than does individual insurance.

Figure 7.1

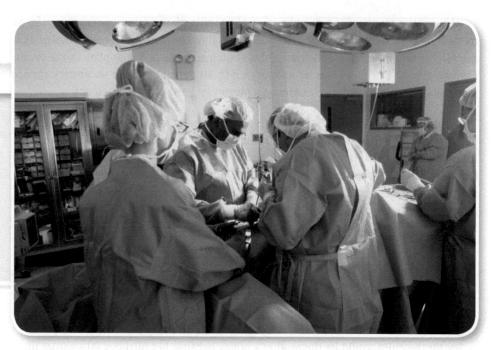

Medical insurance helps people pay for medical, surgical, and hospital costs. *Why is it important to both the patient and the provider for the administrative medical assistant to file insurance claims accurately and promptly?* Michael N. Paras/Pixtal/age fotostock

Individual insurance is usually purchased by people who are not eligible for group insurance, such as by those who are self-employed. Because it is not obtained at a group rate, the cost is higher than for group insurance.

The following are examples of the types of health insurance coverage that are available:

- *Basic:* A basic insurance plan generally includes coverage of hospitalization, lab tests, surgery, and x-rays.
- *Medical:* Medical insurance covers benefits for outpatient medical care. An outpatient is a person who receives medical care at a hospital or other medical facility but is generally admitted for less than 23 hours. The term *medical* refers to the physician's costs for nonsurgical services, whether in the office or in a hospital. Special provisions are made for pathology, x-ray, and diagnostic lab fees.
- *Hospital:* Hospital insurance provides protection against the costs of inpatient hospital care. It generally provides a room allowance (a stated amount per day for a semiprivate room) with a maximum number of days per year. Special provisions are made for operating room charges, x-rays, laboratory work, drugs, and other medically necessary items while the insured person is an inpatient. An *inpatient* is a person who is admitted to the hospital as a result of a documented admission order from a physician.
- *Surgical:* Surgical insurance provides protection for the cost of a physician's fee for surgery, whether it is performed in a hospital, in a physician's office, or elsewhere (such as in a surgical center). Charges for anesthesia generally are covered by surgical insurance. (See Figure 7.1.)
- *Major medical:* Major medical insurance offers protection from large medical expenses—such as extensive injuries from a car accident or those associated with a prolonged illness—that go above and beyond the maximum established by a regular health insurance policy.
- *Disability:* Disability insurance provides reimbursement for income lost because of the insured person's inability to work as a result of an illness or injury, which may or may not be work-related.

- *Dental insurance:* Dental insurance can be obtained, often under a separate policy, to cover all or part of the costs of dental care.
- *Vision care:* Vision insurance can be obtained, often under a separate policy, to cover all or part of eye care costs, such as eye exams and prescriptions for glasses and contact lenses.

 GO TO PROJECT 7.1 AT THE END OF THIS CHAPTER

7.2 INSURANCE PLANS: IDENTIFYING PLANS AND PAYERS

There are many medical insurance plans from which people can choose and many different insurance companies that offer them. Most insurance plans use one of two payment methods: fee-for-service or capitation.

Fee-for-Service

The first type of payment, **fee-for-service,** is made by the insurance carrier *after* the patient has received medical services. The insured pays for the medical services at the time of receiving them, and the insurance carrier reimburses the insured after receiving an insurance claim. Alternatively, the insured may instruct the carrier to pay the physician directly.

In a fee-for-service plan, fees are usually set by the physician. An insurance carrier and a physician may negotiate a *discounted fee-for-service* payment schedule. Under this schedule, a physician agrees to provide services for less than the usual charge. The physician makes up the difference in payment, at least in theory, by seeing more patients who have that insurance plan. The physician is paid for *each* individual service rendered, such as an office visit or a blood test, rather than receiving a single payment for services that are linked or bundled together. A disadvantage of the fee-for-service payment model is the possibility that the quantity of medical services rendered may become more important than the quality of the medical care.

Capitation

Under the second type of payment, **capitation,** a payment is made in advance. Capitation is the *prepayment* by the insurance carrier of a fixed (per capita, or per head) amount to a physician to cover the healthcare services for each member of one of its plans for a specified period of time, such as for a month. It is common for the payment to be based on categories such as patient gender and age. For the per member per month (PMPM) payment, the physician must provide all the care needed according to a predetermined set of services to each patient for which a capitation PMPM payment is made. In a capitated plan, the physician shares the risk with the insurance company for the cost and frequency of the services provided. For example, a physician may receive $80 per month for each male assigned patient between the ages of 35 and 50, regardless of the number of times the patient visits the physician during the month, or even if the patient receives no care that month.

Types of Plans

Most medical insurance plans fall into one of two categories, depending on their payment arrangements. Plans that use a fee-for-service payment arrangement are mostly indemnity plans. Those that use capitation are generally managed care plans.

Indemnity Plans. Under most **indemnity plans,** the insurance company reimburses medical costs on a fee-for-service basis. This type of plan pays for a percentage of the allowable cost, and the patient is responsible for the remaining portion. Patients receive medical services from the providers they choose, who usually file the required claims for payment on behalf of patients. Unlike other plans, the patient is not required to select and see a single physician for primary care needs, and a referral is not required for the patient to see a specialist. Therefore, indemnity plans provide patients with greater freedom of choice when seeking medical services.

For each claim, three conditions must be met before reimbursement is made:

1. The policy's premium payment must be up to date.
2. A deductible has been paid. A **deductible** is a certain amount of allowable or covered medical expense the insured must incur before the insurance carrier will begin paying benefits. Deductibles vary depending on the insurance plan. Annual amounts can range from smaller deductibles, such as $250 per coverage period (usually one year), to very high deductibles, such as $3,000. Plans may have both individual and family deductibles.
3. Any coinsurance has been taken into account. **Coinsurance** is the percentage of each covered claim that the insured must pay, according to the terms of the insurance policy. The coinsurance rate is expressed in terms of percentages, with the percentage the insurance company is to pay listed first. For example, a coinsurance rate of 80-20 means that the insurance company will pay 80 percent of the physician's allowable fee and the insured must pay the remaining 20 percent.

Managed Care Plans. **Managed care** plans generally use capitation as the basis for making payments to physicians. These plans are the predominant type of medical insurance in the United States. There are four main types of managed care plans—HMOs, PPOs, POSs, and CDHPs.

Health Maintenance Organizations (HMOs)
The oldest form of managed care, an **HMO (health maintenance organization)** is a medical center or a designated group of physicians that provides medical services to insured persons for a monthly or an annual premium. The insured is able to obtain healthcare on a regular basis with unlimited medical attention and minimal coinsurance payments. Thus, HMOs encourage insured persons to take advantage of preventive healthcare services in an attempt to make healthcare coverage more cost-efficient.

HMOs attempt to control costs by using a number of methods:

- *Restricting patients' choice of providers:* After enrolling in an HMO, members must receive services from the network of physicians, hospitals, pharmacies, and other healthcare providers connected with that HMO. The insurance will not cover visits to out-of-network providers, except for emergency care or in urgent situations when the member is away from home.
- *Requiring cost sharing:* Every time HMO members visit their physician, they pay a set charge called a **copayment (copay),** such as $10 to $20. Higher copayments are required when patients go to an emergency room or visit the office of a specialist.
- *Requiring preauthorization/precertification for services:* Often HMOs require **preauthorization,** also known as *precertification,* before the physician will deliver certain types of service. This enables the HMO to verify ahead of time that the service is medically necessary and is covered under the patient's policy. The HMO may also require a second opinion, from a different physician, about whether a planned procedure is necessary before granting authorization. Figure 7.2 shows an example of a precertification form.

PRECERTIFICATION FORM

PRECERTIFICATION FORM

Certification for [ ] admission and/or [ ] surgery and/or [ ] _____

Insurance carrier _____

Patient name _____

Street address _____

City/state/ZIP _____

Patient's date of birth _____ Telephone _____

Subscriber name _____

Employer _____

Member no. _____ Group no. _____

Requesting physician _____

Provider no. _____

Requesting physician's address _____

Requesting physician's phone number _____

Hospital/facility _____

Planned admission/procedure date _____

Diagnosis (*ICD-10-CM* codes and description) _____

Requested services (*CPT/HCPCS* codes and description) _____

Estimated length of stay _____

Complicating factors _____

Second opinion required [ ] Yes [ ] No If yes, [ ] Obtained

Corroborating physician _____

Insurance carrier representative _____

Approval [ ] Yes [ ] No If yes, certification no. _____

If no, reason(s) for denial _____

Figure 7.2

Precertification Form

- *Controlling access to services:* In most HMOs, patients are required to select a **primary care provider (PCP)** from the HMO's list of general or family practitioners, internists, and pediatricians. The PCP's role is to act as a gatekeeper, coordinating patients' overall care and ensuring that all services provided are, in the PCP's judgment, necessary. For example, HMOs require members to obtain a medical **referral** from the PCP before seeing a specialist or for hospital admission. The referral document names the provider the patient is to use and specifies the services the patient can receive. If a member visits a provider without a referral, the member is directly responsible for the full cost of the service. In addition to coordinating all medically necessary care, the PCP provides basic medical care to the plan member.

Preferred Provider Organizations (PPOs)

Another type of managed care plan, more popular now than HMOs, are PPOs. The **PPO (preferred provider organization)** contracts to perform services for PPO members at specified rates. These rates, or fees, are generally lower than the fees charged to regular patients. The PPO gives the insured a list of PPO providers from which to receive healthcare at PPO rates. If a patient chooses to receive treatment from a provider who is not in the PPO network, the patient has to pay more—usually a higher copayment or deductible or any difference between the PPO's rate and the outside provider's rate. This differs from an HMO, which does not pay a benefit if the patient seeks services from a physician or facility not within the HMO network.

PPOs, like HMOs, are managed care systems. This means PPOs use many of the same types of practices as HMOs to control the cost of healthcare. For example, they encourage members to use providers in their own PPO network, they usually require preauthorization for some procedures, and they require members to share in the cost of care by making copayments each time they have an encounter with a provider.

Unlike HMOs, PPOs do not generally require patients to choose a primary care provider to oversee their care. Nor are referrals to specialists required. As a result, however, premiums and copayments tend to be higher than those for HMO members.

Point of Service (POS) Plans

Another managed care option is the **POS (point of service)** plan. It is a combination of an HMO and a PPO. Like an HMO, the patient must select a primary care provider (PCP) who will manage all patient care within the network of HMO providers. Like a PPO, the patient can choose to either seek services from an in-network or out-of-network provider, paying a higher portion of the medical services when using an out-of-network provider. Therefore, each time or at a "point" when medical services are needed, the patient has greater flexibility through a POS plan option.

Consumer-Driven Health Plans (CDHPs)

Just as a consumer would shop and compare makes, models, and auto dealers when making a vehicle purchase, a **CDHP (consumer-driven health plan)** allows the patient to "shop and compare." When medical services are needed, the patient may choose the provider and treatment options based on his or her own research of cost, quality, convenience, and other factors important to the patient. By definition, a CDHP is a high-deductible, low-premium insurance plan that provides coverage for traditional medical services. For example, the CDHP may have a $3,000 annual deductible with monthly insurance premiums of only $50. After the patient has met the $3,000 annual deductible, the insurance plan then begins to pay benefits toward covered medical services.

CDHPs are typically paired with a specialized *Medical Savings Account* into which monies are deposited in order to pay for medical services while meeting the annual deductible. Typically, three types of accounts are used:

1. *Flexible Spending Account (FSA):* Monies are deposited into an FSA account by the employer and/or the employee to be used for eligible medical expenses. This is considered a "use-or-lose" account, in the sense that any money left in the FSA at the end of the year is returned to the employer. The money does not roll over and accumulate from year to year. For example, if the employer deposits $2,000 into an FSA, each time the patient receives a covered service, money from the account would be used to pay for the covered service. If the patient's annual deductible is $2,500, the patient would be responsible for out-of-pocket medical expenses of $500. However, if the patient uses only $1,500 of the $2,000 from the FSA for the year, $500 will be returned to the employer, regardless of who deposited the monies. Covered FSA items are established by the federal government. Most over-the-counter medications are not covered by FSAs unless the patient has a written prescription from a provider. Items typically paid using FSA dollars include deductibles, copayments and coinsurances, and medical equipment/supplies such as blood glucose monitors and bandages. Accounts are offered and administered by employers for employees to

contribute pretax dollars up to a federally stated amount. Employers may also contribute to the FSA but are not required to contribute.

2. *Health Reimbursement Account (HRA):* The HRA works like an FSA with the exception that any monies that remain at the end of the coverage period can roll over and accumulate. Additionally, only employers contribute to the HRA.

3. *Health Savings Account (HSA):* This account is similar to the HRA with the exception that any taxpayer (not just employers and employees) may contribute to the HSA.

An advantage of using an FSA, HRA, or HSA is that all dollars contributed are pretax dollars and, as a result, will lower the contributor's tax obligation. Contributions to the accounts are limited to a yearly maximum established by the federal government.

Accountable Care Organizations (ACOs). The Affordable Care Act established the concept of an **ACO (accountable care organization).** In an attempt to bring down healthcare costs, an insurance provider, such as Medicare, establishes an ACO, which brings together a network of physicians, hospitals, and other providers to provide patient care while minimizing unnecessary spending. Providers within the ACO communicate with each other to coordinate patient care and, consequently, eliminate duplicated procedures and medications. In this manner, members of the ACO share in the medical and financial responsibility of patient care.

Features of an ACO are similar to an HMO; however, in an ACO, members share in the financial savings by the insurance plan if they can provide evidence they are meeting the quality measurement standards set by the insurance provider. Patients may also choose to go to non-ACO providers.

Medical Insurance Payers

Medical insurance payers (plans), whether indemnity or managed care, are available through commercial insurance companies in the private sector, such as Aetna or WellPoint, Inc., or for eligible individuals through government-sponsored programs such as Medicare and Medicaid.

Private-Sector Payers. The private-sector market is made up chiefly of a few very large national firms that offer all the leading types of insurance plans. Although most of these payers are for profit, some are nonprofit, such as Kaiser Permanente, which is the largest nonprofit HMO.

The **Blue Cross Blue Shield Association (BCBSA),** one of the largest private-sector payers in the United States, has both for-profit and nonprofit components. As with many of the private-sector payers, BCBSA offers both indemnity and managed care plans, with many individual policy variations in each category. Its HMO network, HMO Blue Care Network, is one of the largest managed care networks in the country. BCBSA individual member plans, known as *Blue Cross Blue Shield (BCBS) plans,* offer many types of managed care programs, including an HMO, a PPO, and others.

There are also BCBS plans that make it easy for patients to receive treatment outside their local service area. The BlueCard Program enables members of a BCBS plan to obtain medical services when living or traveling in another BCBS plan's service area. Participating providers are linked together with other BCBS plans worldwide. Insurance claims for members who receive medical care when outside of their home plan area from a participating BCBS provider are submitted to the member's local BCBS plan for payment processing through a single electronic network.

Federal employees, retirees, and their families are covered under the Federal Employees Health Benefit Program (FEHBP). The BCBS Federal Employee Program, known as the *FEP,* has been part of the FEHBP since it began in 1960. Each year, the BCBS governing association negotiates with the U.S. Office of Personnel Management to determine the level of benefits and premiums for FEP members. Current figures state that FEP covers 5.3 million employees, retirees, and their families.

Medicare. **Medicare** is a federal health plan that provides insurance to citizens and permanent residents ages 65 and older; people with disabilities, including kidney failure; and spouses of entitled individuals. Medicare is divided into four parts—Part A, hospital insurance; Part B, medical insurance; Part C, Medicare Advantage; and Part D, prescription drug coverage.

Medicare Part A, also known as hospital insurance, covers lab tests, nursing facility, home health, hospice, surgery, and inpatient care. Those who are eligible for Social Security benefits are automatically enrolled in Medicare Part A. Medicare Part B, also known as medical insurance, covers outpatient services, services by physicians, durable medical equipment, some preventive services, occupational and physical therapy, and other services and supplies. Medicare Part B coverage is optional. Everyone eligible for Part A can choose to enroll in Part B by paying monthly premiums.

Medicare Part C, known as Medicare Advantage Plans, is available for individuals enrolled in Parts A and B. Under Part C, CMS (Centers for Medicare & Medicaid Services) contracts with private insurance carriers to offer Medicare beneficiaries Medicare Advantage Plans, which are competitive with the original Medicare plan, which includes Medicare Parts A and B. Medicare Advantage Plans must offer all the benefits covered in Medicare A and B but does not have to offer them at the same rate. In addition, Medicare Advantage Plans offer other coverage, such as hearing, vision, and dental, and lower deductibles.

Medicare Part D, known as the prescription drug coverage plan, provides voluntary Medicare prescription drug coverage for Medicare-eligible individuals. Part D plans are offered through private insurance plans, and most beneficiaries pay a monthly premium. Individuals who subscribe to a Medicare Advantage Plan including prescription coverage do not need Part D. Beneficiaries enrolled in the original Medicare plan and desiring prescription coverage may enroll in a Medicare Part D plan.

Each year all premiums and deductibles must be met before payment benefits begins. For example, in 2021 a yearly deductible of $203 is paid by Medicare Part B beneficiaries, and each month Medicare Part B beneficiaries pay a basic premium of $148.50. This premium may be adjusted for higher-income beneficiaries. Typically, individuals receiving Medicare Part A benefits (i.e. inpatient services) will not pay a premium. However, in 2021 beneficiaries pay a per inpatient hospital copay of $1484. In a traditional fee-for-service program (Part B), after the deductible has been met, Medicare pays 80 percent of approved charges and the patient is responsible for the remaining 20 percent. In a Medicare managed care program, the terms are different: Most managed care plans charge a monthly premium and a small copayment for each office visit but do not charge a deductible.

Medicaid. **Medicaid** is a health benefit program, jointly funded by federal and state governments, that is designed for people with low incomes who cannot afford medical care. Each state formulates its own Medicaid program under broad federal guidelines. As a result, programs vary in coverage and benefits from state to state. In some states, the program is known by a different name. For example, in California, Medicaid is called MediCal. Medicaid is known as the "payer of last resort"—all other insurance plans will be billed before Medicaid is billed.

The State Children's Health Insurance Program (SCHIP) was enacted by federal legislation in 1997. It offers states the opportunity to develop and implement plans that offer health insurance coverage for uninsured children. Children covered through SCHIP come from low-income families whose income is too high to qualify for Medicaid. Children up to 19 years of age may be covered.

TRICARE. **TRICARE** (formerly called *CHAMPUS*) is the Department of Defense's health insurance plan for military personnel (referred to as **sponsors**) and their families. Those eligible include active or retired members of the following uniformed services and their families: the U.S. Army, Navy, Marines, Air Force, Coast Guard, Public Health Service, and National Oceanic and Atmospheric Administration.

All military treatment facilities (MTFs), including hospitals and clinics, are part of the TRICARE system, which also contracts with civilian facilities and physicians to provide more extensive services to beneficiaries. TRICARE offers different health plans and options. TRICARE Select is a fee-for-service plan that also offers a Select Overseas option. TRICARE Prime is a managed care plan that also offers options including Prime Remote, Prime Overseas, and Prime Remote Overseas. Other plans include TRICARE Young Adult, TRICARE Reserve Select, TRICARE Retired Reserve, and US Family Plan. To be certain a patient is eligible, the administrative medical assistant checks the individual's military ID card and ensures that coverage is still valid by examining the expiration date.

If the eligible individual is not certain if he or she has coverage, the sponsor (the uniformed service member) may contact the **Defense Enrollment Eligibility Reporting System (DEERS)** to verify eligibility; the provider may not contact DEERS directly because the information is protected by the Privacy Rule.

TRICARE for Life (TFL) is secondary coverage available to TRICARE beneficiaries who have both Medicare Part A and Medicare Part B. It is available worldwide and does not require an enrollment fee. However, Medicare Part B monthly premiums must be paid. TRICARE for Life provides primary insurance coverage in all overseas locations. In the United States and its associated territories, Medicare is primary and TRICARE for Life is secondary. Once medical services have been rendered, an insurance claim form is prepared and submitted to Medicare; Medicare pays its portion and electronically forwards the claim to TRICARE for Life. Following is a summary of payment combinations for a TRICARE for Life beneficiary:

SERVICE COVERAGE	MEDICARE	TRICARE FOR LIFE
Services covered by Medicare and TFL	Pays first	Pays remaining coinsurance portion
Services covered by TFL only	Pays $0	Pays allowable amount and patient pays fiscal year deductible and any cost share responsibilities
Services covered by Medicare only	Pays allowable amount and patient pays fiscal year deductible and any cost share responsibilities	Pays $0
Services covered by neither Medicare nor TFL	Pays $0 and patient must pay the entire billed amount	Pays $0 and patient must pay the entire billed amount

CHAMPVA. **CHAMPVA,** which stands for Civilian Health and Medical Program of the Department of Veterans Affairs, is a government health insurance program that covers the expenses of the families of veterans with total, permanent, service-connected disabilities. It also covers surviving spouses and dependent children of veterans who died in the line of duty. Each eligible beneficiary possesses a CHAMPVA authorization card. Most CHAMPVA enrollees pay an annual deductible and a portion of their healthcare charges.

Workers' Compensation. Each state has its own **workers' compensation** laws to guarantee that an employee who is injured or who becomes ill in the course of employment will have adequate medical care and an adequate means of support while unable to work. The employer must obtain insurance against workers' compensation liability and is liable whether or not the employee is at fault for an accident or injury. Workers' compensation insurance operates under the jurisdiction of the state department of labor or an industrial commission.

The administrative medical assistant must verify with the employer that a patient who claims workers' compensation was indeed injured or became ill in the course of employment. The physician must submit a report, usually within 48 hours, to the workers' compensation insurance carrier, which notifies the Workers' Compensation Board. (The time period during which the physician must file the report varies by state and ranges from 24 hours to 10 days.) The report must include the patient's case history, symptoms, complete medical findings, tentative diagnosis, prescribed treatment, and length and extent of disability or injury. Work-related injuries are grouped into five categories, which are defined by the state and administered by its department of labor:

- Injury without disability
- Injury with temporary disability
- Injury with permanent disability
- Injury requiring vocational rehabilitation
- Injury resulting in death

COMPLIANCE *TIP*

Clinical notes of work-related illness or injury should be separate from other medical services and labeled "Workers' Compensation." A separate file should be kept for each workers' compensation case, even if the individual is an established patient. One reason for not mixing a patient's regular medical records with workers' compensation records is that workers' compensation claim information is not subject to the same confidentiality rules as private medical records. Most states allow insurance personnel and employers unrestricted access to the workers' compensation files. Copies of workers' compensation reports may be kept in the patient's regular medical record for future reference. Copies may be necessary to document the treatment provided by the physician if the dispute comes before an arbitration board or a court.

Progress reports on the case must be filed regularly until the physician releases the patient from care. The final report must be designated as such, indicating that the patient has recovered to the maximum capacity from the work-related disability.

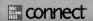 **GO TO PROJECT 7.2 AT THE END OF THIS CHAPTER**

7.3 PARTICIPATION AND PAYMENT METHODS

Physicians must decide with which insurance plans they want to participate. They judge which plans to join based on the types of patients they serve and the financial arrangements the plans offer them. Because more people are members of managed care plans than any other type of plan today, most physicians have contracts with a number of managed care plans in their area. Often, to avoid confusion, a medical practice displays a list of plans it participates in, so that patients know what to expect, given the insurance they have. Figure 7.3 is an example of such a list.

Welcome to our practice.

In order to make your visit as pleasant as possible, we have compiled a list of the most commonly asked questions regarding insurance and billing in this office.

With which insurance plans does the physician participate?

Aetna/US Healthcare Plans

CIGNA

Blue Choice FEP PPO: POS, PPO, Prestige, Select

Focus Workers Compensation PPO

Health Care Value Management, Inc.

Health Choice

Highmark

Kaiser Permanente

Medicare

Medicaid

National General

Oxford Health Plan

Physician Health Services

Prudential Healthcare

POS Plan

United Healthcare

Wellcare

What can I expect if the physician participates with my insurance?

We will file a claim with your insurance company for visit-related charges. Your insurance may require you to pay a copay at the time of service. You are responsible for any deductibles and noncovered services. You may need to obtain a referral from your primary care physician. Failure to obtain a referral may result in rescheduling of your appointment until you can obtain one.

What can I expect if the physician does not participate with my insurance?

Payment is expected at the time of service. You will receive a receipt for your visit charges and payments—use it to file a claim with your insurance carrier. As a courtesy, we will submit any surgery claims to your insurance carrier, but you are responsible for payment.

Figure 7.3

Example of an Insurance Plan Participation List

Plan Participation

A physician who joins an insurance plan is a **participating (PAR) provider** in that plan. As a participating provider, the physician agrees to provide medical services to the insurance plan members according to the plan's rules and payment schedules. The insurance carrier offers various incentives, such as faster payment, to participating providers.

A nonparticipating provider, or nonPAR, chooses not to join a particular insurance plan. A nonPAR physician who treats members of a plan does not have to obey the rules or follow the payment schedule of that plan. At the same time, a nonPAR physician will not receive any of the benefits of participation.

Fee Schedules

In a private managed care plan, contracts that set fees are often negotiated between the insurance company and the physician. In Medicare, the **Centers for Medicare & Medicaid Services (CMS)** are responsible for setting up the terms of the plan, referred to as the Medicare Fee Schedule (MFS). As an agency of the Department of Health and Human Services (HHS), CMS administers the Medicare and Medicaid programs to millions of Americans. Part of its role is to review managed care plans that want to become Medicare coverage providers.

Payment Concepts

Every health insurance plan has its own payment methods, rules, and regulations. An administrative medical assistant must keep up with the different options available in

each plan to be sure a patient has coverage for a given service and to process insurance claims for patients in a proper and timely manner. Succeeding paragraphs discuss basic concepts used in insurance contracts regarding methods of making
payments to providers.

Allowed Charge. When insurance companies set up the payment terms for an insurance contract, many set an **allowed charge** for each procedure or service a provider
performs. This amount is the most the insurance company will pay any provider for
that work and may or may not be the same as the charged amount. Insurance carriers
may refer to their allowed charge as the *allowed amount, allowable fee, covered service,* or
approved amount.

Balance Billing. If the physician is a nonPAR provider or if the service is not an allowable service, the patient should absorb the cost. The physician bills the patient for the
noncovered amount—a practice referred to as **balance billing.**

Under the PAR contracts, when the amount the physician charges is more than the
insurance company's allowed charge, the difference in cost must be absorbed by the
physician. Many insurance plans specify that a participating provider may *not* bill patients for balances. This means a PAR provider must accept the allowable charge of the
insurance carrier and payment from the insurance carrier and patient up to that amount
as payment in full for the procedure and not collect ("write off") the difference between
the physician's usual fee and the allowed charge. In other words, the physician subtracts
the unpaid amount from the patient's bill.

When a Medicare patient is to receive medical services that are not or may not be
covered by Medicare, the patient must complete a form (Advance Beneficiary Notice),
prior to services being rendered, which states the patient is aware that Medicare will not
or may not pay for the service(s). The noncovered amount is listed on the form, and the
patient may be billed for the service.

Accepting Assignment. A PAR provider who agrees to accept the allowed charge set
forth by the insurance company as payment in full for a service and not bill the patient
for the balance is **accepting assignment.** PAR providers must always accept assignment.

For some plans, such as Medicare, a nonPAR provider may decide whether to accept assignments on a claim-by-claim basis. A nonPAR provider who decides to accept
assignment on a given claim does not bill the patient for the balance. Conversely, if the
nonPAR provider decides not to accept assignment, the patient is billed for the unclaimed amount. This is discussed in more detail later in this section.

Assignment of Benefits. A physician who accepts an **assignment of benefits** agrees to
receive payment directly from the patient's insurance carrier. In this case, the patient
signs an assignment of benefits statement, usually on the patient information form, and
a notation is made on an insurance claim form that the patient has a signature on file

(SOF) for the assignment of benefits. If the provider is participating with the patient's insurance carrier and a direct payment of benefits is part of the participation agreement, the patient's signature for assignment of benefits is not needed.

When a nonPAR physician does not accept assignment on a claim, the patient is usually asked to pay for the service in full at the time of the visit, so that the medical office can avoid having to collect payment later. Some practices ask the patient to assign benefits for the claim at the time of the visit and then bill the patient later for any amount the insurance company does not pay.

Examples of PAR and NonPAR Provider Fees for a Medicare Patient. Suppose a patient whose primary insurance carrier is Medicare visits a physician for a procedure. Normally, the physician charges $120 for the procedure; the Medicare allowed charge for the procedure, however, is only $60. How much can the physician charge for the procedure, and how much will Medicare reimburse? Depending on whether the physician participates in the Medicare program, the amount the physician can charge will vary. PAR providers are reimbursed more than nonPAR providers. As part of its standard policy, Medicare sets the fees for nonPAR providers at 5 percent less than those for PAR providers for the same services.

Furthermore, depending on whether a nonPAR physician decides to accept assignment or not—and a charge limitation is imposed on a nonPAR provider who does not accept assignment, the amount Medicare pays varies. If a nonPAR provider decides not to accept the Medicare assigned amount as payment in full and decides rather to bill the patient for the balance, Medicare subjects the assigned amount to a limiting charge, thus limiting the amount of unpaid balance the physician can bill the patient. The limiting charge is 115% of the fee listed in the nonPAR Medicare fee schedule (MFS). For example, if the nonPAR amount for a covered service was $115.26, the limiting charge amount would be $132.55 ($115.26 × 115%). In effect, the limiting charge prevents the physician from balance billing the patient for the full unclaimed amount.

The following three fee structures illustrate the three possible scenarios:

Participating Provider

Physician's standard fee	$120.00
Medicare allowed charge	60.00
Medicare pays 80% ($60.00 × 80%)	48.00
Patient or supplemental plan pays 20% ($60.00 × 20%)	12.00
Provider adjustment ($120.00 − $60.00)	60.00

Nonparticipating Provider Who Accepts Assignment

Physician's standard fee	$120.00
Medicare nonPAR allowed charge ($60.00 × 95%)	57.00
Medicare pays 80% ($57.00 × 80%)	45.60
Patient or supplemental plan pays 20% ($57.00 × 20%)	11.40
Provider adjustment ($120.00 − $57.00)	63.00

Nonparticipating Provider Who Does Not Accept Assignment

Physician's standard fee	$120.00
Medicare nonPAR allowed charge	57.00
Limiting charge ($57.00 × 115%)	65.55
Patient billed	65.55
Medicare pays patient ($57.00 × 80%)	45.60
Total provider can collect	65.55
Patient pays balance ($65.55 − $45.60)	19.95
Provider adjustment ($120.00 − $65.55)	54.45

These examples can also be used to illustrate the different options for assigning benefits on Medicare claims. In the first and second scenarios, since the physician has agreed to accept the assigned Medicare amounts (PAR, $60, and nonPAR, $57, respectively) as reimbursement in full for the procedure, the physician would also accept an assignment of benefits, authorizing Medicare to pay the physician directly.

In the third scenario, since the provider has decided not to accept the Medicare assigned amount of $57 as payment in full for the procedure, the provider will also not accept an assignment of benefits for the claim. Instead, Medicare will send the payment directly to the patient (instead of directly to the provider), and the patient will be responsible for paying the bill in full up to the limiting charge.

Maximum Plan Dollar Limit. Prior to implementation of the Affordable Care Act (ACA) of 2014, insurers could set a limit on the maximum amount payable for covered expenses. This was a stated amount per coverage period, such as 1 year, or for a lifetime maximum dollar amount per episode of care. An amount was set for the insured individual and each covered dependent of the health insurance plan. A typical maximum plan dollar limit may be $1 million per covered individual.

The Affordable Care Act made it illegal for insurers to set maximum limits on essential healthcare services on new individual or small group policies. Categories defined as *essential services* are

* hospitalizations.
* laboratory services.
* emergency services.
* substance abuse/mental health treatment.
* maternity services.
* pediatric services.
* ambulatory/outpatient services.
* preventive care services.
* prescription drug orders.
* dental and vision care for children.
* rehabilitative services.

Medical insurance policies in place prior to January 1, 2014, are considered to be grandfathered policies and are not restricted by the ACA requirement.

Maximum Out-of-Pocket Expense. The maximum dollar amount a plan member is required to pay for out-of-pocket covered medical expenses during a coverage period is called the *maximum out-of-pocket expense.* Until the plan member reaches the maximum amount, the insurance carrier and the plan member share the cost of covered medical expenses. Once the maximum amount is reached, the insurance plan pays for all covered expenses. However, the insurance plan may set a maximum lifetime amount that would be paid.

Under the ACA, maximum out-of-pocket limits were set for the insurance policy coverage period. Included in the expenses are deductibles, copayments, and coinsurance. Not included as out-of-pocket expenses are premiums, cost-sharing for out-of network services, and payments for nonessential health benefits and noncovered services. The maximum out-of-pocket limit increases each year. In 2021, the maximum out-of-pocket limits were $8,550 for an individual and $17,100 for a family. These figures reflect a 4.9 percent increase from 2020 to 2021 out-of-pocket maximum.

Methods of paying up to the maximum out-of-pocket limit for medical expenses include (1) paying directly (out of pocket); and (2) using Medical Savings Accounts (MSAs), also referred to as *Health Savings Accounts (HSAs), Health Reimbursement Accounts (HRAs),* and *Flexible Spending Accounts (FSAs).* These options have been discussed previously in this chapter.

Setting Fees

Third-party payers use different formulas and systems for setting up fee schedules for the procedures and services they will reimburse. The most common types of payment systems are

- a list of usual, customary, and reasonable (UCR) fees.
- a relative value scale (RVS).
- a resource-based relative value scale (RBRVS).
- diagnosis-related groups (DRGs).

UCR Fees. To set fees for their services, providers establish a list of their usual fees for the procedures and services they frequently perform. In every geographic area, there is a normal range of fees for each procedure. Different practices set their fees at some point along this range. Third-party payers, to set the rates they pay providers, analyze providers' usual fees and establish a schedule of UCR (usual, customary, and reasonable) fees for each procedure.

- A **usual fee** is an individual provider's average charge for a certain procedure.
- A **customary fee** is determined by what physicians with similar training and experience in a certain geographic location typically charge for a procedure.
- A **reasonable fee** is one that meets the two previous criteria, or a fee allowed or approved by the insurance carrier for a difficult or complicated service.

Relative Value Scale (RVS). Another payment system is the **relative value scale (RVS).** A relative value scale sets fees for medical services based on an analysis of the skill and time required to provide them.

Resource-Based Relative Value Scale (RBRVS). The payment system used by Medicare is the **resource-based relative value scale (RBRVS).** The RBRVS, like the RVS on which it is based, is a scale that establishes relative prices for services. It is based on three factors: (1) the national relative value unit (RVU), which represents the amount of resources required (time, skill, overhead) to complete a service, (2) an adjustment factor for the geographic location, and (3) a national conversion factor.

Also, many private insurance companies use resource-based fee structures to establish what to pay for each procedure when company managers believe a resource-based fee structure more fairly reflects the real costs involved in providing medical services than the historical fees.

Diagnosis-Related Groups (DRGs). Another payment system, used by Medicare for establishing payment for hospital stays, is **diagnosis-related groups (DRGs).** Diagnostic groupings are based on the resources that physicians and hospitals have used nationally for patients with similar conditions, taking into account factors such as age, gender, and medical complications.

 WP | **Mc Graw Hill connect** | **GO TO PROJECT 7.3 AT THE END OF THIS CHAPTER**

To keep track of the many thousands of possible diagnoses and procedures and services rendered by physicians, and to simplify the process of verifying the medical necessity of each procedure, two coding systems are used:

- *Diagnostic coding:* Codes for reporting what is wrong with the patient, or what brought the patient to see the physician
- *Procedural coding:* Codes for reporting each procedure and service the physician performed in treating the patient

These systems are used to convert the physician's medical terminology into alphanumeric and numeric codes. In some medical practices, the physicians assign these codes; in others, a medical coder or a medical insurance specialist handles this task. Within an EHR, the assignment of codes must be verified; in other words, the documentation must support the assigned code. In whichever situation, an administrative medical assistant must be familiar with coding systems to work effectively with encounter forms and insurance claims. A **patient encounter form** is the form used in the medical office to record the diagnosis (or diagnoses) and the procedures performed during a patient's visit.

Accurate diagnostic coding gives insurance carriers clearly defined diagnoses to help them process claims efficiently. An error in coding conveys to an insurance carrier the wrong reason a patient received medical services. This causes confusion, a delay in processing, and possibly a reduced payment or denial of a claim. An incorrect code may also raise the question of fraudulent billing if the insurance company decides that, based on the diagnosis, the services provided were not medically necessary. Active diagnostic code databases can also provide statistics for medical researchers, physicians, and third-party payers about costs, trends, and future healthcare needs.

The *ICD-10-CM*

Diagnosis codes are found in the *ICD-10-CM,* the *International Classification of Diseases, 10th edition, Clinical Modification. ICD-10-CM* lists codes according to a system assigned by the World Health Organization of the United Nations. Diagnostic codes are used by government healthcare programs, professional standards review organizations, medical researchers, hospitals, physicians, and other healthcare providers. Private and public medical insurance carriers also use the codes.

The *ICD* has been revised numerous times. In the title, *ICD-10-CM,* the initials *CM* indicate that the edition is a clinical modification. For example, the *ICD-10-CM* is the clinical modification of the 10th edition of the *ICD.* Codes in this modification describe various conditions and illnesses with greater specificity and clinical detail than earlier *ICDs.* Beginning October 1, 2015, *ICD-10-CM* codes were required on insurance claim forms. In late spring of 2012, the Final Rule of the Administrative Simplification subtitle of the Health Insurance Portability and Accountability Act (HIPAA) changed the diagnosis-mandated Transaction Code Set from the previous *ICD-9-CM* code set to the *ICD-10-CM* code set. **ICD-10-PCS** *(International Classification of Diseases, 10th edition, Procedure Coding System)* replaced the previously used *ICD-9-CM, Volume 3,* which is used for inpatient hospital procedure coding. In this chapter, we will focus on *ICD-10-CM.*

ICD-10-CM Organization. *ICD-10-CM* is divided into sections. Mandatory coding rules are contained within the *ICD-10-CM Official Guidelines for Coding and Reporting.* These provide guidance on such topics as chapter-specific guidelines, how to determine the principal diagnoses, how to report additional codes, and how to report outpatient services. Guidelines are also located at the beginning of each chapter. These guidelines provide the foundation for effective coding and must be followed. The Alphabetic Index to Diseases and Injuries, Volume 2, provides an alphabetic listing of terms and their associated code(s). In addition to the alphabetic listing, there are two tables and another index: the Table of Neoplasms, the Table of Drugs and Chemicals, and the Index of External Causes of Injuries. Codes are listed alphanumerically in the Tabular List of Diseases and Injuries, Volume 1. This index is divided into 22 chapters based on body systems or conditions. Chapters in the Tabular List include the following:

Chapter 1—Certain Infectious and Parasitic Diseases
Chapter 2—Neoplasms
Chapter 3—Diseases of the Blood and Blood-Forming Organs and Certain Disorders Involving the Immune Mechanism
Chapter 4—Endocrine, Nutritional and Metabolic Diseases
Chapter 5—Mental and Behavioral Disorders
Chapter 6—Diseases of the Nervous System
Chapter 7—Diseases of the Eye and Adnexa
Chapter 8—Diseases of the Ear and Mastoid Process
Chapter 9—Diseases of the Circulatory System
Chapter 10—Diseases of the Respiratory System
Chapter 11—Diseases of the Digestive System
Chapter 12—Diseases of the Skin and Subcutaneous Tissue
Chapter 13—Diseases of the Musculoskeletal System and Connective Tissue
Chapter 14—Diseases of the Genitourinary System
Chapter 15—Pregnancy, Childbirth, and the Puerperium
Chapter 16—Certain Conditions Originating in the Perinatal Period
Chapter 17—Congenital Malformations, Deformations, and Chromosomal Abnormalities
Chapter 18—Symptoms, Signs and Abnormal Clinical and Laboratory Findings, Not Elsewhere Classified
Chapter 19—Injury, Poisoning, and Certain Other Consequences of External Causes
Chapter 20—External Causes of Morbidity
Chapter 21—Factors Influencing Health Status and Contact with Health Services
Chapter 22-Codes for Special Purposes

Categories, subcategories, and codes are contained in the Tabular List. All categories have three characters, which are alphanumeric. Subcategories contain either four or five characters. A complete code may be three, four, five, six, or seven alphanumeric characters. Because of possible confusion, some *ICD-10-CM* coding book publishers use the letter *O* to represent itself, and the number *0* is represented by Ø.

S91	Open wound of ankle, foot and toes	Category
S91.15	Open bite of toe without damage to nail	Subcategory
S91.151A	Open bite of right great toe without damage to nail, initial encounter	Code

ICD-10-CM allows for future expansion of codes. Within a code, a placeholder "X" is used within the structure of a code to allow for this expansion. Any code that requires an additional seventh digit(s) is considered an invalid code unless the additional digit is added. For example, the ❼ symbol indicates the requirement for a seventh digit. The following code example contains both a placeholder and a seventh digit.

EXAMPLE: *ICD-10-CM* PLACEHOLDER AND SEVENTH DIGIT

Subcategory T37.5X1D   Poisoning by antiviral drugs, accidental (unintentional), subsequent encounter

---

Codes used for long-term usage of drugs are located in Appendix A, and Appendix B is used to help locate symbols for codes requiring a seventh digit.

ICD-10-CM **Conventions and Symbols.** To help users correctly assign codes, certain abbreviations, punctuation, and notes have definitive meanings that affect the assignment of codes.

Abbreviations

In both the Alphabetic and Tabular Indexes, two abbreviations assist users to assign codes.

NEC means "not elsewhere classifiable." NEC codes are used to include specified conditions that cannot be classified with any other code in the code set. To simplify, the provider has supplied enough documentation for a clinically specific code, but a code does not exist.

NOS means "not otherwise specified." NOS codes are used when the documentation provided by the provider is insufficient to assign a code of greater specificity. If possible, the provider should be queried for more clinical detail.

Punctuation

Parentheses, brackets, colons, and dashes are used in both the Alphabetic Index and the Tabular List.

Parentheses ( ) are used in both the Alphabetic Index and the Tabular List to enclose nonessential modifiers or supplementary terms that may or may not be present in the diagnosis. The presence or absence of the supplementary terms does not affect whether or not the code can be used.

EXAMPLE: PARENTHESES

Alphabetic Index   Hemophilia (classical) (familial) (hereditary)

Tabular List   H44.611 Retained (old) magnetic foreign body in anterior chamber, right eye

---

Brackets [ ] are used in the Alphabetic Index to show manifestation codes. They are used in the Tabular List to enclose synonyms, alternative wording, or explanatory phrases.

EXAMPLE: BRACKETS

Alphabetic Index   Nephrosis, in amyloidosis E85.4 [NØ8]

Tabular List   BØ6 Rubella [German measles]

Colons (:) in the Tabular List are placed after an incomplete portion of a code description when more information is needed to make it a usable code. Choices to complete the diagnostic code follow the colon and are indented. These are primarily used with both "includes" and "excludes" notes, which will be discussed next. Colons are not used in the Alphabetic Index of *ICD-10-CM*.

EXAMPLE: COLON

Tabular List   N92.6 Irregular menstruation, unspecified

This code includes an Excludes 1 notation of

   Excludes 1   Irregular menstruation with:

In order to complete the code exclusion, one of the two choices that follow the colon (.) must be used. The complete code for the first Excludes 1 choice reads "Irregular menstruation with lengthened intervals or scanty bleeding (N91.3–N91.5)." The complete code for the second Excludes 1 choice reads "Irregular menstruation with shortened intervals or excessive bleeding (N92.1)."

Dashes (–) are used in the Tabular List to indicate an incomplete code—additional characters are needed to fully describe the condition using the character options. Dashes are used only in the Tabular List.

EXAMPLE: DASH

Tabular List   H90 Conductive and sensorineural hearing loss

  Excludes 1   noise-induced hearing loss (H83.3–)

The dashes in H83.3– provide typographical instructions that additional characters are needed to complete H83.3–. Choices for completion of the code include H83.3X1, H83.3X2, H83.3X3, and H83.3X9.

Eyes (👁) are used in the Tabular Index to instruct the coder to see the Official Guidelines for more coding and sequencing instructions.

EXAMPLE: EYE

Tabular List   E08 Diabetes Mellitus due to underlying condition.

👁 See Official Guidelines "Assigning and sequencing secondary diabetes codes and its causes" I.C.4.a.6.b.

Instructional Notes

Many instructional notes are used in both *ICD-10-CM* indexes. As users locate and use codes, all instructional notes should be read and followed. Each will provide further clarification on whether or not the code may be used, what conditions may or may not be coded with the code assignment, and reference to other locations for information. Figure 7.4 summarizes instructional notes used in the Alphabetic Index and the Tabular List.

One of the more extensive chapters in *ICD-10-CM* is Chapter 19. Injuries are grouped by major site, specific site, and by type of injury and are listed under the site where the injury occurred. For example, open wounds of the neck area are listed together in category S11 with subcategories for the specific site (i.e., pharynx and cervical esophagus), and type of injury (open wound). Code S11.25XA would be used to code an open bite of the pharynx and cervical esophagus, initial encounter.

Chapter 20 contains codes identifying the external causes of morbidity. In *ICD-10-CM,* the codes begin with V–Y. These codes should never be used as the first-listed code—they are intended to be used as a secondary code with a code from another chapter that indicates the condition. If a third-grade child fell off a swing during school recess and broke her left arm, the first-listed (primary) code would be for the broken left arm and a supplemental WØ9.1XXA code would then be listed to show how it happened.

Chapter 21 contains Z codes (previous V codes), which describe patients who receive medical services but may not have a definitive reason, such as an illness, for seeking medical services. Encounters when a Z code should be used are when

Chapter 22 contains U codes which are to be used for special purposes. Two code categories within this chapter relate to vaping-related disorders and COVID-19.

- a healthy patient is seeking services for a specific reason.
- a patient is receiving aftercare of a disease or of an injury.
- a patient presents with circumstances that are influencing the health status of the patient or that pose a potential hazard to community health.
- a patient is seeking services for birth status.

Figure 7.4

ICD-10-CM Conventions

INSTRUCTIONAL NOTE	MEANING
Includes	Defines or gives examples of the category.
Inclusion	Provides a list of terms included with the code.
Excludes 1	Provides a list of excluded conditions and codes that are NEVER to be used at the same time as the code preceding the Excludes 1 note.
Excludes 2	Provides a list of conditions that are not part of the code that is before the Excludes 2 note. However, the patient may have both conditions concurrently. It is acceptable to use both codes together if the patient has both conditions.
Code First	Instructs user to code the underlying condition first. This type of note is usually seen when two codes are needed to show the etiology (cause) of the condition and its manifestation (effects).
Use Additional Code	Instructs user to use an additional code to show the manifestation(s) of an underlying etiology.
And	Should be interpreted as "and/or."
With	Should be interpreted as "associated with" or "due to."
See	Instructs the user to go to the main term listed with the "See" notation for the possible code selection.
See Also	Instructs the user that another main term may be referenced to provide a more specific code selection.
Code Also	Instructs the user that two codes may be required to fully code the condition; however, no sequencing instructions are provided.

Examples of Z code usage would be for patients receiving immunizations, who have been or suspect they have been exposed to a communicable disease, who have a personal or family history of malignant conditions (cancer), who need adjustment of a medical device, or who are donating an organ or tissue. Z codes are also used on the maternal (mother's) record to indicate the weeks of gestation and the outcome of delivery.

Obtaining Documentation for *ICD-10-CM*. An insurance claim for a patient must show the diagnosis that represents the patient's major health problem for that encounter's claim. This condition is known as the "primary diagnosis." The primary diagnosis must provide the reason for medical services submitted on the claim. At times, there is more than one diagnosis because many patients are treated by a healthcare provider for more than one illness. The primary diagnosis is listed first on the insurance claim. After that, coexisting conditions may be listed. Coexisting conditions occur at the same time as the primary diagnosis and affect the treatment of or recovery from the primary condition. For example, a patient sustained a severe laceration on the right forearm and also has type 1 diabetes. The laceration is the primary condition and type 1 diabetes does affect the treatment and recovery of the laceration. Consequently, the patient's type 1 diabetes is a coexisting condition.

COMPLIANCE TIP

Using a seventh digit, when indicated, is required. When coding, always use the most specific code available. Most coding books have the ❼ symbol to direct the coder to use a seventh digit. If six prior digits are not assigned, use the "X" placeholder for missing digits.

Documentation for identifying a patient's diagnosis and any coexisting conditions is found in the patient's medical record. Notes about the patient's chief complaint may be entered in the patient's medical record by an administrative medical assistant, a nurse, or a physician. However, *only* the physician determines the diagnosis. A good rule of thumb to remember is "if it is not documented, it was not done" and, therefore, may not be coded. Thorough documentation by the provider is a must for accurate coding. The physician should be queried if there are questions concerning the medical documentation. All medical office team members who enter encounter data in the patient's medical record should make clear and complete medical entries. Ongoing training for all personnel is a key element in keeping the medical office team up to date on documentation guidelines and maintaining accurate medical documentation. All update training should be documented in the provider's Compliance Manual.

When the diagnosis is recorded in the patient's medical record and/or on the encounter form from the patient's visit, the written data are converted into *ICD-10-CM* code(s). In many medical offices, the encounter form lists the most frequently used diagnoses together with their procedure codes for the medical practice. If using a hardcopy encounter form, the physician can simply check off the appropriate diagnosis from the list of codes without the need to look up the code in the *ICD-10-CM* manual.

When a diagnosis code is not provided by the physician, the coder must know how to use the *ICD-10-CM* manual to look up and correctly code the physician's diagnostic statement. All medical codes should be coded to the highest level of specificity—in other words, coded to the most complete main category and subcategories base on documented patient information. Also, an administrative medical assistant may need to use the *ICD-10-CM* to verify a diagnosis code or to ensure the codes listed on the office's current encounter form are consistent with the annual *ICD-10-CM* updates. Encounter forms should contain the date on which the form was last updated to ensure the most current (current year's) codes are being used.

Basic Steps in Diagnostic Coding. Diagnostic coding is a multistep process:

Step 1 *Locate the diagnostic statement in the patient's medical record.* If necessary, determine the main term or condition of the diagnosis. In the diagnostic statement *peptic ulcer,* the main condition is *ulcer,* and *peptic* describes the type of ulcer. The main term could be a condition or a reason, such as Admission for, Encounter for, or Exposure to.

Step 2 *Find the diagnosis in the Alphabetic Index to Diseases and Injuries* of the ICD-10-CM. Look for the condition first. Then find descriptive words that make the condition more specific, such as the location or acute versus chronic. Read all references to check the possibilities for a term and its synonyms. Examine all subterms in the Alphabetic Index to be sure the correct term is found. Do not stop at the first code that "sounds right." **NEVER** code only from the Alphabetic Index. Always verify the code in the Tabular Index. Figure 7.5 is an example of a portion of the Alphabetic Index.

Step 3 *Locate the code in the Tabular List of Diseases and Injuries.* The codes are listed in alphanumeric order.

Step 4 *Read all category, subcategory, and subclassification information to obtain the code that corresponds to the patient's specific disease or condition.* Review the Official

Special attention should be given to the use of some V through Y codes because of their sensitive nature. For example, suicide attempts and assaults are likely to be highly confidential matters.

COMPLIANCE *TIP*

Atelectasis (massive) (partial) (pressure) (pulmonary) J98.11

    newborn P28.1Ø

    due to resorption P28.11

    partial P28.19

    primary P28.Ø

    secondary P28.19

    primary (newborn) P28.Ø

    tuberculous—see Tuberculosis, pulmonary

2021 edition

Figure 7.5

Example of the *ICD-10-CM* Alphabetic Index

Figure 7.6

Example of the *ICD-10-CM*
Tabular List

SØ6   Intracranial injury
Includes   traumatic brain injury
Code also any associated:
                open wound of head (SØ1.-)
                skull fracture (SØ2.-)
Excludes 1   head injury NOS (SØ9.9Ø)

The appropriate 7th character is to be added to each code from category SØ6
A   initial encounter
D   subsequent encounter
S   sequela

❺SØ6.Ø   Concussion
              Commotio cerebri
              Excludes 1 concussion with other intracranial injuries classified in
              subcategory SØ6.1- to SØ6.6-, SØ6.81- and SØ6.82- code to specified
              intracranial injury
    ❻   SØ6.ØX   Concussion
                         ❼SØ6.ØXØ-   Concussion without loss of consciousness
                         ❼SØ6.ØX1-   Concussion with loss of consciousness of
                                       30 minutes or less
                         ❼SØ6.ØX9-   Concussion with loss of consciousness of
                                       unspecified duration
                                       Concussion NOS

2021 edition

Guidelines for Coding and Reporting and Chapter Specific Guidelines for using and sequencing codes. Observe all conventions (abbreviations, symbols, punctuation, instructional notes) for help locating the exact code. For example, the code may be accompanied by ❼, which means the code requires a seventh digit. Figure 7.6 is an example of a portion of the Tabular List.

Step 5 *Record the diagnosis code in the medical record or on the insurance claim form.* Proofread the code for accuracy. As part of the proofreading process, a coder should always ask, Have all the numbers been entered in the right order? Are the codes complete? Has the code with the highest level of specificity been used?

Coding becomes easier with practice, but do not be tempted to take shortcuts. Every case is different, and additional terms or characters may be necessary to make a diagnosis code as specific as possible. If a step is skipped, such as not verifying the code in the Tabular List for the most specific code, important information may be missed. If more than one diagnosis is listed in the patient's medical record, work on only one diagnosis code at a time to avoid coding errors.

Crosswalks, resources that connect the previous code set *(ICD-9-CM)* with the current *ICD-10-CM,* are available to assist medical office personnel with translating codes from *ICD-9-CM* to *ICD-10-CM* and from *ICD-10-CM* to *ICD-9-CM*. At times, it may be necessary to research an older *ICD-9-CM* code. A crosswalk, a tool of the General Equivalence Mappings (GEMs), will be used by medical office personnel to relate the two coding systems. Figure 7.7 shows an example of a crosswalk. A GEM should be used as a guide and not as an absolute match. At times, the crosswalk will be a one-to-one match; other times, it will be a range of codes or multiple codes that should be consulted. Although the codes look different, the basic systems are very similar.

EXAMPLE 1

<u>ICD-9-CM</u> 896.2 Traumatic amputation of foot (complete) (partial) Bilateral, without mention of complication

<u>ICD-10-CM</u> Choose one of the following:

• S98.911A Complete traumatic amputation of right foot, level unspecified, initial encounter OR S98.921A Partial Traumatic Amputation of right foot, level unspecified, initial encounter   AND
• Choose one of the following:
• S98.912A Complete, traumatic amputation of left foot, level unspecified, initial encounter OR   S98.922A Partial traumatic amputation of left foot, level unspecified, initial encounter

Two *ICD-10-CM* codes are required for coding the bilateral amputation. The two codes specify both the bilateral amputation and whether the amputation was complete or partial. The *ICD-9-CM* code of 896.2 does not specify if the amputation was complete or partial.

EXAMPLE 2

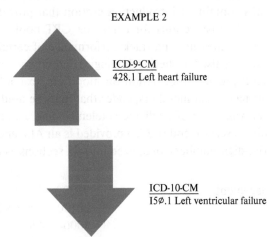

<u>ICD-9-CM</u>
428.1 Left heart failure

<u>ICD-10-CM</u>
I5Ø.1 Left ventricular failure

Notice that the new *ICD-10-CM* code provides the specific location of the failure—the left ventricle.

EXAMPLE 3

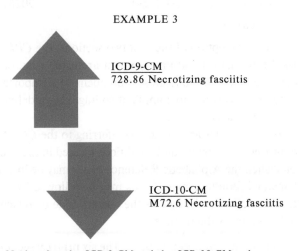

<u>ICD-9-CM</u>
728.86 Necrotizing fasciitis

<u>ICD-10-CM</u>
M72.6 Necrotizing fasciitis

ICD-10-CM, 2021 edition

Notice that the *ICD-9-CM* and the *ICD-10-CM* code descriptions are the same.

The procedural coding system classifies services rendered by physicians. Each procedure code represents a medical, surgical, or diagnostic service performed by a provider. A coding specialist in an insurance company compares the procedure codes with the stated diagnoses on every insurance claim to determine whether the procedures were medically necessary. An administrative medical assistant should be very meticulous in working with codes on encounter forms and insurance claims and applying the related guidelines, since accurate diagnostic and procedural coding is the only way to ensure that providers receive the allowable maximum reimbursement for services.

CPT-4

The most commonly used system of procedure codes is found in *Current Procedural Terminology,* fourth edition, a book published by the American Medical Association and known as the *CPT.* An updated edition of the *CPT* is published every year to reflect changes in medical practice. Newly developed procedures are added, and old ones that have become obsolete are deleted. These changes are also available in a digital file, because some medical offices use a computer-based version of the *CPT.*

CPT coding books contain an Introduction section that provides an overview of CPT coding and specific instructions for using the CPT book. Also included are Category II codes used to measure and track performance of certain procedures and care. Category III codes are used for new technologies that do not have a standard CPT code. Appendices A–P provide information on modifiers, examples of code usage, codes exempt from using certain modifiers, codes that must be used after other codes, and much more. A growing area of medicine is telemedicine. Appendix P provides a summary of telemedicine service codes. Also provided is an Alphabetic Index.

CPT codes are five-digit numbers, organized into six sections as follows:

Section	Range of Codes
Evaluation and Management	99202–99499
Anesthesiology	00100–01999, 99100–99140
Surgery	10004–69990
Radiology	70010–79999
Pathology and Laboratory	80047–89398, 0001U–0222U
Medicine (except Anesthesiology)	90281–99199, 99500–99607

Note: 2021 edition

With the exception of the first two sections, the *CPT* is arranged in numeric order. Codes for evaluation and management are listed first, out of numeric order, because they are used most often. Each section opens with important guidelines that apply to its procedures. It is critical to compliant coding that guidelines be checked carefully before a procedure code is chosen.

Procedure codes are located by referring to the *CPT* Alphabetic Reference Index, a list of procedures, organs, and conditions located in the back of the book. Depending on the publisher, the Alphabetic Reference Index may be located in the front portion of the CPT manual. Boldface main terms may be followed by descriptions and groups of indented terms. The coder selects the correct code by reviewing each description and indented term under the main term.

CPT Section Format and Symbols. The six primary sections of the *CPT* are divided into categories. These in turn are further divided into headings according to the type of test, service, or body system. Code number ranges included on each page are found in the upper right corner. This helps the coder locate a code quickly after using the Alphabetic Index.

In the *CPT* sections, symbols are used to highlight changes or special points. A bullet, which looks like a circle, black or red (●), indicates a new procedure code. A triangle (▲) indicates a change in the code's description. The triangle appears only in the year the descriptor (the description of the numeric code) is revised. When text, other than the code's description, is either new or revised, facing triangles (◆) are placed in front of the code. Appendix B (in the *CPT*) is a listing that contains all the new, deleted, and revised codes for the current year's edition. Appendix M (also in the *CPT*) supplies a crosswalk from the deleted code to the new code(s) to be used.

A plus sign (+) is used for add-on codes, indicating procedures that are usually carried out in addition to another procedure. For example, code 90471 covers one immunization administration, and code +90472 covers administering an additional vaccine. Add-on codes are never reported alone. They are used together with the primary code. When a product, such as a vaccine, is pending FDA approval, a thunderbolt symbol (⚡) is used. Once the product is approved, the symbol is removed, and the code may be used. The number symbol (#) precedes a code that has been resequenced or is an out-of-order code. Appendix N of the *CPT* lists all resequenced and out-of-order codes. Telemedicine codes, referring to services providing healthcare from a distance, are indicated with a star symbol (★). For example, this symbol would be used for physician evaluation and management of a patient at a distant location in a rural clinic. The physician is using real-time technology with minimum audio and visual capabilities.

The *CPT* uses a special format to show codes and their descriptions. The "parent code" description begins with a capital letter and may be followed by indented descriptive codes. The indented codes include the description of the parent code up to the semicolon, plus the indented information. See Figure 7.8 for an example of *CPT-4* code listings.

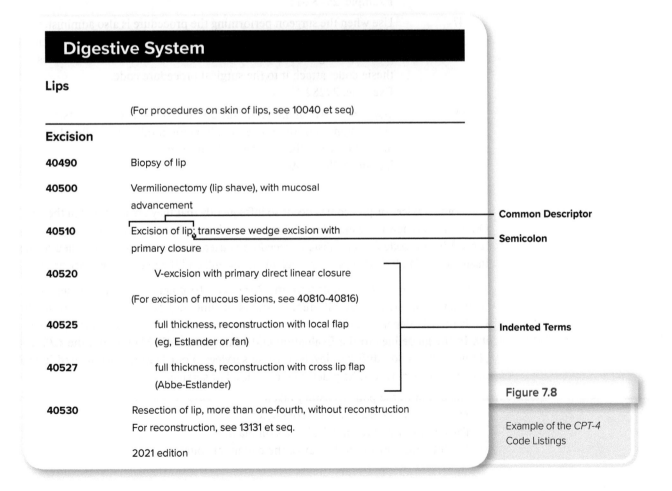

Digestive System

Lips

(For procedures on skin of lips, see 10040 et seq)

Excision

40490   Biopsy of lip

40500   Vermilionectomy (lip shave), with mucosal advancement

———— Common Descriptor

40510   Excision of lip; transverse wedge excision with primary closure

———— Semicolon

40520   V-excision with primary direct linear closure

         (For excision of mucous lesions, see 40810-40816)

40525   full thickness, reconstruction with local flap
              (eg, Estlander or fan)

———— Indented Terms

40527   full thickness, reconstruction with cross lip flap
              (Abbe-Estlander)

40530   Resection of lip, more than one-fourth, without reconstruction
         For reconstruction, see 13131 et seq.

         2021 edition

Figure 7.8

Example of the *CPT-4* Code Listings

Notes and Modifiers. *CPT* listings may also contain notes, which are explanations for categories and individual codes. Notes often appear in parentheses after a code. Many notes suggest other codes that should be considered before a final code is selected.

One or more two-character modifiers may need to be assigned to the five-digit main number. Modifiers are written with a hyphen before the two-character modifier. On an insurance claim form, a modifier is listed in its own area. Modifiers show that some special circumstance applies to the service or procedure the physician performed. They reduce (–53 Discontinued Service), increase (–22 Increased Procedural Service), or provide further description of the service, such as the physiological location of the service (–E1 Upper Left Eyelid) or the location of the service (–95 Synchronous Telemedicine). A quick reference of modifiers is typically printed on the inside front cover of the *CPT* book. Appendix A of the *CPT* provides a description of each modifier.

EXAMPLE: *CPT* MODIFIERS

Modifier	Meaning and Example
–73	Use when an outpatient procedure was discontinued before anesthesia was administered to the patient Example: 45378-73
–74	Use when an outpatient procedure was discontinued after anesthesia was administered to the patient Example: 45378-74
–T5	Use when the procedure was performed on the right foot, great (big) toe Example: 29282-T5
–47	Use when the surgeon performing the procedure is also administering either general or regional anesthesia. It is not to be used when administering local anesthesia and is not to be used with an anesthesia code; attach it to the surgical procedure code. Example: 29282-47-T5
–99	Use when two or more modifiers are needed to fully describe circumstances of the procedure. Specific modifiers are listed in a different area of the insurance claim form. Example: 29282-99

Some services or procedures occur so infrequently that they are not listed in the *CPT*. Others are too new to be included. Unlisted procedure codes are provided for these situations. When a code for an unlisted procedure is used, a report must be attached to the insurance claim. It describes the procedure, its extent, and the reason it was performed.

Coding Evaluation and Management Services. To diagnose conditions and plan treatments, physicians use different amounts of time and effort, as well as different kinds of skill, depending on the patient, the circumstance, and the physician's speciality. In the guidelines to the Evaluation and Management (E/M) section, the *CPT* explains how to code different levels of these services. Four factors documented in the patient's medical record help determine the level of service:

* The extent of the patient history taken
* The extent of the examination conducted
* The complexity of the medical decision making
* The total time spent on the day of the patient encounter

In addition to level of service, insurance carriers want to know whether the physician treated a *new patient* or an *established patient*. Physicians often spend more time during new patients' visits than during visits from established patients, so the E/M codes for the two types of patients are separate. For reporting purposes, the *CPT* considers a patient "new" if that person has not received professional services from the physician or a physician of the same specialty practicing within the same group in the past 3 years. Medical offices commonly use the abbreviation *NP* for a new patient. An established patient is one who has seen the physician or a physician of the same specialty within the same group in the past 3 years. (Note that the current visit need not be for a problem treated previously.) Medical offices commonly use the abbreviation *EP* for an established patient. Emergency patients are not classified as either new or established patients.

The *CPT* has a range of codes for new-patient or established-patient encounters. The lowest-level code is often called a Level I code (i.e., 99211); the codes continue to go higher, such as a Level V code (i.e., 99215). Annual physical examinations are located under the heading Preventive Medicine Services in the E/M section and are coded based on the age of new or established patients. For example, the procedure code 99385 (2021 edition), in the "new patient" category, covers the routine examination, with tests and counseling, of a patient between the ages of 18 and 39.

Location of the service is also important, because different E/M codes apply to services performed in a physician's office, a hospital inpatient room, a hospital emergency department, a nursing facility, an extended-care facility, or a patient's home.

Coders should also be familiar with the difference between a *referral* and a *consultation,* since codes connected with these services are different. Sometimes one physician sends a patient to another physician for examination and treatment. This transferring of the responsibility for the patient's care for that condition is called a *referral.* Standard E/M codes are used by the physician who assumes the responsibility. In contrast, a *consultation* occurs when an attending physician requests advice from another physician but retains responsibility for the care of the patient. The *CPT* E/M section lists several codes for consultations, depending on the level and location of the service.

Physicians providing consultation services to Medicare patients and billing the services to Medicare no longer use any of the consultation codes. The CMS does not distinguish between consultation codes and nonconsultation codes. Higher monies previously paid for the consultation codes will be redistributed among the office and hospital E/M service codes. For example, a physician who sees a Medicare-covered patient (who was sent by the patient's primary physician) and conducts a comprehensive history and examination using high-complexity medical decision making would have previously used code 99245. However, the physician now would use code 99205 if the patient is a new patient to the physician or code 99215 if the patient is considered established if the patient is a Medicare patient. Consultation codes may be used for other insurance carriers.

Coding Anesthesia Procedures. Services requiring the use of general, regional, supplemental, or other types of supportive anesthesia services for a procedure require codes. Code selections are based on the anatomical region on which the main procedure, such as an appendectomy, is performed. Time is also a factor when reporting anesthesia services. Time for anesthesia services begins when the anesthesiologist starts to prepare the patient for the induction of anesthesia services and ends when the patient is safely placed under postoperative care, and the anesthesiologist's services are no longer needed. Modifiers specific to anesthesiology services are used to indicate the physical well-being or status of the patient prior to anesthesia. Physical status modifiers range from P1 (a normal, healthy patient) through P6 (a declared brain-dead patient whose organs are being removed for donor purposes). Modifiers are also used to convey who actually administered the anesthesia. The modifier -AA indicates the anesthesia services were performed personally by the anesthesiologist, and -QX indicates that a Certified Registered Nurse Anesthetist administered the services under the medical direction of an anesthesiologist. Add-on codes, which can only be listed in addition to a primary code, are used to show any qualifying circumstances for the use of more than normal anesthesia services. Codes range from +99100 for a patient younger than 1 year or older than 70 years through +99140 to show anesthesia was complicated by an emergency condition. If the code description contains the qualifying circumstance, do not use the add-on code. Code 00326 contains the age qualifier of 1 year or younger; therefore, you would not use the add-on code 99100. If the patient was classified as a normal, healthy patient prior to the administration of anesthesia, the complete code would be 00326-P1.

Coding Surgical Procedures. In the Surgery section, a "separate procedure" is a surgical procedure usually performed as an integral part of a full surgical package (multiple services combined into one code). When the procedure is done independently, it may be reported by itself or with another procedure or service by adding the modifier -59 to the separate procedure code. In contrast to these procedures, most codes listed in the Surgery section include all routine elements. The Surgery section and all subsections have numerous guidelines for coding. All guidelines should be read and followed. Directional information is also listed in parenthetical statements after a code.

Coding Radiology Services. Diagnostic and therapeutic procedures may require the use of radiology. Many radiologic codes contain two components—the technical component and the professional component. Modifier -TC is attached to the code when the services being billed were for the actual performance, or doing, of the procedure. It typically is used to provide reimbursement for supplies, equipment, and clinical staff/technicians. An example would be billing for a radiologic examination (x-ray) of the skull, three views. In this example, the actual taking of the x-ray would be billed with modifier -TC (70250-TC). When the radiologist looks at the radiologic films, interprets what is seen, and prepares a written report (handwritten or electronic), the radiologist would bill the same procedure code (70250) but would attach the professional component modifier -26 (70250-26). If the radiologist took the x-ray (technical component) and interpreted and prepared the report (professional component), no modifier would be needed. Contrast materials may or may not be used with a procedure to show greater specificity of the area. If a contrast material is used, it is administered intravasculary (within blood vessels), intra-articulary (within a joint), or intrathecally (within the spinal canal). When a contrast material is administered either orally or rectally, it is *not* considered, for coding purposes, as being "with contrast." At times, the procedure (such as an MRI) is started without a contrast material being used and at a later point in the procedure a contrast material is injected. This is known as "without contrast materials followed by contrast materials."

Coding Laboratory Procedures. Organ or disease-oriented panels listed in the Pathology and Laboratory section of the *CPT* include tests frequently ordered together. An acute hepatitis panel, for example, includes tests for hepatitis A antibody, IgM antitibody; hepatitis B core antibody, IgM antibody; hepatitis B surface antigen; and hepatitis C antibody. Each element of the panel has its own procedure code. However, when the tests are performed together, the coder must use the code for the panel, rather than list each test separately.

Coding Medicine Procedures. Injections and infusions of immune globulins, vaccines, toxoids, and other substances require two codes—one for giving the route of administration (injection or intranasal/oral) and one for the particular vaccine or toxoid that is given. For example, for an influenza shot, the administration code 90460, 90471, or 90473 is used for the physical administering of the vaccine, along with one of the codes for the specific vaccine, such as 90653-90668, 90682-90694 (2021 edition). If a significant, separately identifiable E/M service was provided, the appropriate E/M code should also be reported in addition to the vaccine and toxoid administration codes.

HCPCS Codes

The *Healthcare Common Procedure Coding System,* commonly referred to as *HCPCS,* was developed by the CMS, and in 1996, HIPAA mandated the use of not only the *CPT* codes for billing and coding but also *HCPCS* codes. The *CPT* Level II codes, *HCPCS* (pronounced "hic-picks"), are a coding system that uses both all the codes in the *CPT* (considered *CPT* Level I codes) and additional codes that cover many supplies, such as sterile trays, drugs, and durable medical equipment (DME). *HCPCS* codes have five characters—numbers, letters, or both—and a different set of modifiers.

Some procedure codes are listed in both the *CPT* and the *HCPCS.* An example would be a screening mammography. In *CPT,* the code is 77067; in *HCPCS,* the code is G0202. When a Medicare patient receives services that are listed in both the *CPT* and the *HCPCS,* it is normally billed to Medicare using the *HCPCS* code. In medical offices where the *HCPCS* system is used, regulations issued by the CMS are reviewed to determine the correct code and modifier for claims. Examples of these codes follow.

Code Number	Description
G0104	Colorectal cancer screening; flexible sigmoidoscopy
V5299	Hearing service, miscellaneous

Basic Steps in Procedural Coding

Five steps are used for finding procedure codes in the *CPT* and in the *HCPCS,* as follows.

Step 1 *Become familiar with the* CPT. Read the introduction and main section guidelines and notes. For example, look at the guidelines for the Evaluation and Management section. They include definitions of key terms, such as *new patient, established patient, chief complaint, concurrent care,* and *counseling.* They also explain the way E/M codes should be selected.

Step 2 *Find the services that were provided.* The next step is to check the patient's encounter form to see which services were performed. For E/M procedures, look for clues as to the extent of history, examination, and decision making that were involved and the amount of time the physician spent with the patient.

Step 3 *Look up the procedure/service/equipment code.* First, pick out a specific procedure or service, organ, or condition. Find the procedure in the Alphabetic Index. For example, to find the possible code selection(s) for "burns, dressing," first look in the Alphabetic Index for the procedure. Then, turn to the procedure code(s) in the Numeric or Tabular List of the *CPT* to be sure the code accurately reflects the service performed. Although it may seem tempting to record the procedure code directly from the Alphabetic Index, resist the shortcut. Critical information is placed at the beginning of each chapter and sections within the chapter. Read all information prior to using a code. Explanations and notes in the guidelines and main sections more accurately lead to finding main numbers

If each test in a panel or procedure in a surgical package is listed separately, it will "unbundle" the panel or package. The review performed by the insurance carrier's claims department will rebundle the services under the appropriate code, which could delay payment. Note that when unbundling is done intentionally to receive more payment than is correct, the claim is likely to be considered fraudulent.

and modifiers that reflect the services performed. That is the only way to ensure reimbursement at the highest allowed level.

Step 4 *Determine appropriate modifiers.* Check section guidelines and the *CPT* Appendix A to find modifiers that elaborate on details of the procedure being coded. For example, a bilateral breast reconstruction requires the modifier -50. Find the code for "breast reconstruction with free flap": 19364. To show the insurance carrier that the procedure was performed on both breasts, attach -50: 19364-50.

Step 5 *Record the procedure code.* After the procedure code is verified, it is posted to the insurance claim form. If the patient has more than one diagnosis for a single claim, the primary diagnosis is listed first. Likewise, the corresponding primary procedure is listed first. The *primary procedure* is the main service performed for the condition listed as the primary diagnosis.

The physician may perform additional procedures at the same time or in the same session as the primary procedure. If additional procedures are performed, match each procedure with its corresponding diagnosis. If this is not done, the procedures will not be considered medically necessary, and the claim will be denied.

For example, Ms. Silvers, who saw Dr. Wellen for chest pain and shortness of breath, also has asthma. While the patient was in the office, Dr. Wellen renewed her prescription for asthma medication along with performing the ECG. If the ECG is mistakenly shown as a procedure for asthma, the claim will be denied, because that procedure is not medically necessary for that diagnosis.

Coding procedures become easier as the coder becomes more familiar with codes and with the layout of the manual. In fact, most medical offices use only a limited number of procedure codes.

7.6 CODING COMPLIANCE

On correct claims, each reported service is connected to a diagnosis that supports the procedure as necessary to investigate or treat the patient's condition. Insurance company representatives analyze this connection between diagnostic and procedural information, called **code linkage,** to evaluate the medical necessity of the reported charges. Correct claims also comply with many other regulations from government agencies and private payers.

Diagnostic and procedure codes are updated quarterly and annually. Current codes must be used to identify the diagnoses and procedures that are performed. Code numbers may be added or deleted, and code descriptions may be modified. Current-year coding books are available in October and January. Updates are also published quarterly on the CMS website. To not use the current year's code is considered noncompliant coding. When new codes go into effect, all hardcopy and electronic office resources, such as charge slips/encounter forms, must be updated to reflect the new codes. All EHR and coding software programs must be updated to reflect current codes.

Claims are denied because of lack of medical necessity when the reported services are not consistent with the symptoms or the diagnosis and when they are not in keeping with generally accepted professional medical standards. Correctly linked codes that support medical necessity meet these conditions:

- The *CPT* and *HCPCS* procedure codes match the *ICD-10-CM* diagnosis codes.
- The procedures are not elective, experimental, or nonessential.
- The procedures are furnished at an appropriate level.

Medical necessity rules are established by each third-party payer. For example, a Medicare carrier has its own guidelines for particular procedures and the diagnoses that must be linked for payment. Private payers may impose a different set of rules, and differences are common.

Common Coding Errors

There are many factors that contribute to coding errors. Some of the more common coding errors are listed here:

- Reporting diagnosis codes that are not at the highest level of specificity available
- Using out-of-date codes
- Altering documentation after the services are reported
- Coding without proper documentation to back up the codes selected
- Reporting services provided by unlicensed or unqualified clinical personnel
- Reporting services that are not covered or that have limited coverage
- Using modifiers incorrectly or not at all
- Upcoding—using a procedure code that provides a higher reimbursement rate than the code that actually reflects the level of service provided
- Downcoding—using a procedure code that is at a lower reimbursement rate than the code that actually reflects the level of service provided
- Unbundling—billing the parts of a bundled procedure as separate procedures

Most medical practices have a system, formal or informal, for evaluating coding errors in an effort to achieve better coding compliance. Some examples of efforts that can be made include the appointment of a compliance officer and committee, the use of regular training plans, and ongoing monitoring and auditing of claim preparation—all documented within the practice's Compliance Plan.

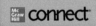 **GO TO PROJECT 7.4 AT THE END OF THIS CHAPTER**

connect **IF ASSIGNED, GO TO PROJECT 7.5 AT THE END OF THIS CHAPTER**

7.1 Identify and define the terminology related to medical insurance and medical coding.	• Administrative medical assistants should be familiar with basic terms and concepts of medical insurance, including coding and compliance. Insurance carriers may use different terminology, and medical office personnel need to know current terminology.
7.2 Explain differences among the types of insurance plans.	• Indemnity plans are usually fee-for-service plans that pay after services are provided. They offer benefits in exchange for regular payments of a fixed premium by the insured. In addition, the insured must also pay deductibles and coinsurance.
	• Managed care plans, in contrast, often use capitation payments, which are fixed, prospective payments made for services to be provided during a specified period of time. It is common to base capitation rates on gender and age. Managed care organizations contract with both patients and providers.
	• In an HMO, patients agree to receive services from providers who have contracts with the HMO; usually, a PCP coordinates the patient's care and makes referrals.
	• In a PPO, patients are offered lower fees in exchange for receiving services from plan providers but are usually not required to choose a PCP.
	• In a POS, patients must choose a PCP; however, the patient has the option of going out of network for services. In this manner, the POS is a combination of an HMO and a PPO.
	• In a CDHP, patients typically have a combination of a high-deductible health plan and a Medical Savings Account. Patients use pretax Medical Savings Account monies to pay for eligible medical expenses. After the deductible has been met, the health plan begins to pay benefits.
	• In an ACO, patients have the advantage of going to a network of providers who communicate with each other with the goal of reducing repetitive medical services. The ACO functions like an HMO; however, the providers within the ACO will share in any medical savings achieved by the insurance carrier, if the provider has met certain criteria.

7.3 Compare and contrast PAR and nonPAR providers and the methods insurance companies use to determine how much a provider is paid.	• PAR providers agree to render medical services to plan members according to the plan's rules and payment schedules; a nonPAR provider is not contractually obligated to abide by the rules or the payment schedule when treating members. • PAR providers receive a direct benefit payment from the insurance carrier through an agreed-upon assignment of benefits; a nonPAR provider collects payment from the patient at the time of service, and the patient receives payment from the insurance carrier. • Common types of payment systems used by third-party payers for reimbursing physicians are based on (a) usual, customary, and reasonable (UCR) fees; (b) a relative value scale (RVS); (c) a resource-based relative value scale (RBRVS); or (d) diagnosis-related groups (DRGs).
7.4 Apply *ICD-10-CM* conventions, symbols, abbreviations, and guidelines to properly code diagnoses in an outpatient setting.	• The *ICD-10-CM* is used to report patients' conditions (diagnoses) on their medical records and on insurance claims. Codes consist of three to seven alphanumeric characters and a description. The Alphabetic Index is used first to locate the approximate correct code for a diagnosis. Next, the Tabular List is used to verify and refine the final code selection. All conventions, symbols, abbreviations, instructional notes, and guidelines should be followed. The *ICD-10-CM* contains 22 chapters, each containing codes requiring high levels of specificity.

7.5 Apply *CPT* conventions and guidelines to properly code procedures and supplies in an outpatient setting.	• *CPT-4,* a publication of the AMA, contains the most widely used system for physicians' medical services and procedures. There are two levels of procedural codes: *CPT-4* and *HCPCS,* which include temporary codes. *CPT-4* codes are required for reporting physician services on insurance claim forms. Codes consist of five digits and a description. Modifiers may be used to indicate a change to the code description. *CPT-4* contains six sections of codes: — Evaluation and Management — Anesthesia — Surgery — Radiology — Pathology and Laboratory — Medicine These are followed by appendixes and an index. The Alphabetic Index is used first in the process of selecting a code; then the code number is referenced in the Tabular List. Notes, exclusions, inclusions, and other critical information are contained within the Tabular List. Therefore, *never* code directly from the Alphabetic Index without verifying the code selection in the Tabular List. • *HCPCS* codes are used to code supplies and equipment not listed in the *CPT-4.* Some procedures are also listed in *HCPCS. HCPCS* codes are selected the same way as *CPT-4* codes. Refer to the Alphabetic Index first, and then verify the code selection in the Tabular List. Within *HCPCS,* codes are alphanumeric.
7.6 Explain the effects of coding compliance errors on the revenue cycle in the medical office setting.	• Coding compliance is the process of coding using actions that satisfy federal official requirements and guidelines. Individual carrier guidelines must also be followed in order to be considered compliant.

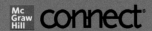

Project 7.1   **(LO 7.1) Insurance Terminology**

On Working Paper 46 (WP 46), match each insurance term in Column 2 with its definition in Column 1. Be prepared to discuss your answers.

Project 7.2   **(LO 7.2) Internet Research: The Medicare Website**

The official U.S. government website for Medicare provides information about Medicare basics, Medicare plan choices, publications, nursing homes, a participating physician directory for your area, a Medicare helpline, and more. Visit www.medicare.gov and look up information about the different Medicare plan choices available nationally, as well as what plans are available in your area.

Project 7.3   **(LO 7.3) Insurance Plans, Payers, and Payment Methods**

Working Paper 47 (WP 47) contains statements that refer to insurance plans and processing claims. Mark each statement with either "T" for *true* or "F" for *false*. For each *false* answer, document what makes the statement *false*. Also be prepared to share your answers.

Project 7.4   **(LO 7.4, LO 7.5) Identifying Diagnostic and Procedure Codes**

Refer to Working Paper 48 (WP 48)—*ICD-10-CM* diagnostic codes—and Working Paper 49 (WP 49)—patient encounter form for Janet Provost's annual exam—to answer the following questions regarding diagnostic and procedure codes.

1. **What is the *ICD-10-CM* diagnostic code for each of the following conditions?**
   a. Migraine headache   _____
   b. Chest pain   _____
   c. Lightheadedness   _____
   d. Annual physical exam, age 39   _____
   e. Family history of heart disease   _____
   f. Test for pregnancy, positive results   _____
   g. Osteoarthritis   _____
2. **Review Janet Provost's patient encounter form.**
   a. What is the diagnostic code for Janet Provost's visit? _____
   b. What is the description given in the *ICD-10-CM* for this code? _____
   c. What procedures did Dr. Larsen perform? List the *CPT-4* procedure codes for each: _____
   d. How much did Dr. Larsen charge for the complete blood count (CBC)? _____
3. **Do you think the *CPT-4* procedure codes marked off on the encounter form are in compliance with the *ICD-10-CM* diagnosis code given?** _____

Project 7.5 (LO 7.4, LO 7.5) Optional Diagnostic and Procedure Coding Exercises

If assigned, use the appropriate coding manuals to complete the following exercises.

1. **Provide the correct *ICD-10-CM* code(s) for each of the following diagnoses:**
   a. Swimmer's ear in the left ear _____
   b. Type 1 diabetes mellitus with diabetic nephropathy _____
   c. Labor, obstructed, due to a deformed pelvis _____
   d. Essential hypertension _____
   e. Alzheimer's disease _____

2. **Provide the correct *CPT* code(s) for each of the following procedures:**
   a. Circumcision using a clamp with regional dorsal penile block _____
   b. Office visit for an established patient requiring a detailed history, expanded problem-focus examination, and low-complexity medical decision making

   _____

   c. Anesthesia for a healthy, 10-month-old male patient having blepharoplasty (code only the anesthesia service—two codes are required) _____
   d. X-ray of the shoulder, one view _____
   e. Replacement during follow-up care of cast application of the left index finger

   _____

3. **Provide the correct *HCPCS* code(s) for each of the following procedures or supplies:**
   a. Breast prosthesis, mastectomy bra with integrated breast prosthesis form, bilateral _____
   b. Injection, tetracycline, 200 mg _____
   c. Injection, corticotropin, 30 units _____
   d. Food thickener, orally administered, 1 ounce _____
   e. Intraspinal catheter _____

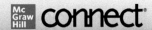
Time Management and Coding Compliance (LO 7.6)

How often do you find yourself running out of time? Many feel that there is just never enough time in the day to get everything done. When you know how to manage your time, you gain control. Effective time management helps you choose what to work on and when. This is important if you want to complete certain tasks, such as coding correctly and compliant. To start managing time effectively, you need to set goals. Consider setting a goal of correctly coding medical diagnoses and procedures at a rate of 98 percent or above for a given submission period (such as one workday). Without proper goal setting, your time will be wasted on the confusion of conflicting priorities. People tend to neglect goal setting because it requires time and effort. A little time and effort put in now save an enormous amount of time, effort, and frustration in the future. **Are your time management skills strong? Describe how your skills could be improved, or share how your skills have helped you become successful.**

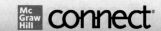
USING TERMINOLOGY

Match the term or phrase on the left with the correct answer on the right.

_____ 1. [LO 7.2] Capitation

_____ 2. [LO 7.3] PAR

_____ 3. [LO 7.1] Premium

_____ 4. [LO 7.3] CMS

_____ 5. [LO 7.5] Patient encounter form

_____ 6. [LO 7.1] Third-party payer

_____ 7. [LO 7.2] Managed care

_____ 8. [LO 7.1] Provider

_____ 9. [LO 7.5] *HCPCS*

_____ 10. [LO 7.2] Coinsurance

a. Stated amount an insured must pay for an insurance policy

b. Physician or other provider who agrees to treat the patient

c. Insurance payment that pays a prepaid, stated amount to the provider for covered services within a stated period of time

d. Percentage of a covered claim that the insured must pay

e. Provider who agrees to offer covered services per a plan's contract rules and regulations

f. Organization that administers Medicare and Medicaid

g. Used to record patient encounter diagnoses and procedures

h. Alphanumeric coding system used to record supplies and procedures

i. Insurance carrier

j. Most popular insurance plan in the United States

CHECKING YOUR UNDERSTANDING

Select the most correct answer.

1. [LO 7.1] Aubriella had a CBC and a PFT performed. Which type of insurance will cover the services?

   a. Major medical
   b. Surgical
   c. Basic
   d. Disability

2. [LO 7.2] Noelle's insurance policy states she has a coinsurance of 90/10 on covered services. When she received her notice from the insurance carrier, it stated that the charges for her last office visit were not allowed. How much of the charges is Noelle responsible for?

   a. 90 percent
   b. 10 percent
   c. 0 percent
   d. 100 percent

3. [LO 7.2] Under his insurance plan, Tyler is required to have prior approval for his upcoming knee replacement. Before the surgery, the surgeon must have which approval document from the insurance plan for the surgery?

   a. Informed consent
   b. Expressed consent
   c. Patient encounter form
   d. Preauthorization/precertification approval

4. [LO 7.2] Michelle and her husband, Drew, just had a baby. Michelle is laid off from her job, and Drew works part-time at a gas station. They are without insurance coverage. The administrative medical assistant should supply Michelle and Drew with the contact information for

   a. Medicare.
   b. Medicaid.
   c. TRICARE.
   d. CHAMPVA.

5. [LO 7.3] Dr. Abrams receives payment from BCBS for services rendered to patients covered by the plan. This is known as

   a. assignment of benefits.
   b. coordination of benefits.
   c. balance billing.
   d. preauthorization of services.

6. [LO 7.3] If the standard fee for a Medicare-covered service is $150 and the Medicare nonPAR fee schedule for the service is $142.50, what is the limiting charge for the service?

   a. $120.00
   b. $163.88
   c. $30.88
   d. $50.00

7. [LO 7.4] The insurance carrier has requested codes to indicate where its insured's injury took place. Which of the following code categories will be used?

   a. J codes
   b. *HCPCS* codes
   c. Evaluation and Management codes
   d. V–Y codes

8. [LO 7.5] Luke last visited his physician, who has a single-physician practice, in September 2016. He is at the office today for a sore throat and chest congestion. Since he was already a patient, the medical insurance coder submitted an established patient E/M code to Luke's insurance carrier for payment. The insurance carrier requested additional documentation on the visit. Which of the following may have been the reason?

   a. Luke's visit should have been coded from the *HCPCS* code selections.
   b. The medical insurance coder did not submit the claim to the insurance carrier on the actual day of Luke's visit.
   c. Luke's visit should have been coded from the new patient E/M category.
   d. There was no reason for the insurance carrier to request additional documentation.

9. [LO 7.5] During Luke's visit mentioned in Question 8, a CBC was performed. Which type of code(s) should be used for the service?

   a. Unbundled codes
   b. E codes
   c. Bundled code
   d. Medicine code

10. [LO 7.6] A claim was submitted with a diagnosis code for a stage 4 ulcer on the left foot and a procedure code for a hernia repair. Payment was denied. Which of the following is a reason for the denial?

    a. Using outdated codes
    b. Upcoding the procedure code
    c. Not submitting the proper modifier
    d. Lack of medical necessity

THINKING IT THROUGH

These questions cover the most important points in this chapter. Using your critical thinking skills, play the role of an administrative medical assistant as you answer each question. Be prepared to discuss your responses.

1. [LO 7.1] How would you explain to a patient who is unfamiliar with insurance terminology what is meant by the term *third-party payer*? How was the term derived?

2. [LO 7.2] Ellen Gold, a traditional-plan Medicare patient, does not understand her last month's medical statement. She already paid her deductible, yet the bill states that she owes $20 on a total bill of $100. How would you explain the bill to her?

3. [LO 7.3] Joe Cantinori inquires about his unpaid bill and asks whether the physician received payment from his insurance company. When you check his record, you find that your office submitted the insurance form on his behalf. However, the physician did not accept assignment on the claim, since he is not a PAR provider in that program. This means that the insurance company will send the payment directly to Joe. How would you explain this to Joe?

4. [LO 7.5] A patient complained of symptoms usually associated with arthritis. The physician ordered the following tests: rheumatoid factor, uric acid, sedimentation rate, and fluorescent noninfectious agent screening. The insurance claim submitted contained procedure codes for each test. You have not received any response from the insurance carrier, even though payments for other claims sent to the same carrier on that day have been received. What do you think accounts for the delay?

Chapter 8

Billing, Reimbursement, and Collections

LEARNING OUTCOMES

After studying this chapter, you will be able to

8.1 recognize and calculate charges for medical services and process patient statements based on the patient encounter form and the physician's fee schedule.

8.2 compare and contrast the process of completing and transmitting insurance claims using both hardcopy and electronic methods.

8.3 describe the different types of billing options used by medical practices for billing patients.

8.4 paraphrase the procedures and options available for collecting delinquent accounts.

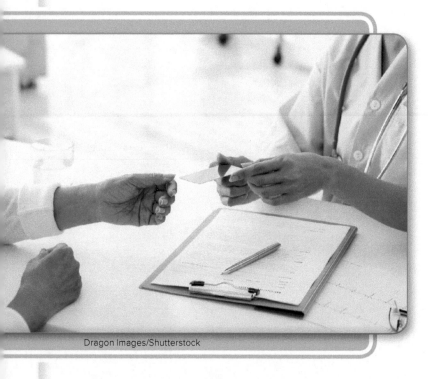

Dragon Images/Shutterstock

KEY TERMS

Study these important words, which are defined in this chapter, to build your professional vocabulary:

clean claim	collection ratio	explanation of benefits (EOB)	patient information form
clearinghouse	cycle billing		patient statement
CMS-1500 claim form	dependent	fee adjustment	scrubber program
collection agency	electronic claims	fee schedule	terminated account
collection at the time of service	electronic remittance advice (ERA)	guarantor	third-party liability
		monthly billing	write-off

ABHES

4.a. Follow documentation guidelines.

4.e. Perform risk management procedures.

5.c. Assist the patient in navigating issues and concerns that may arise (i.e., insurance policy information, medical bills, and physician/provider orders).

7.a. Gather and process documents.

7.c. Perform billing and collection procedures.

7.d. Process insurance claims.

10.b. Demonstrate professional behavior.

www.abhes.org/accreditationmanual

The ABHES standards appear with permission of The Accrediting Bureau of Health Education Schools

CAAHEP

V.P.3. Use medical terminology correctly and pronounced accurately to communicate information to providers and patients.

V.P.4.a. Coach patients regarding office policies.

V.P.8. Compose professional correspondence utilizing electronic technology.

VII.C.1.a Define the following bookkeeping term: *charges*.

VII.C.1.b. Define the following bookkeeping term: *payments*.

VII.C.1.e. Define the following bookkeeping term: *adjustments*.

VII.C.4.b. Describe types of adjustments made to patient accounts including: collection agency transaction

VII.C.4.c. Describe types of adjustments made to patient accounts including: credit balance.

VII.C.4.d. Describe types of adjustments made to patient accounts including: third-party.

VII.C.5. Identify types of information contained in the patient's billing record.

VII.C.6. Explain patient's financial obligation for services rendered.

VII.P.3. Obtain accurate patient billing information.

VII.A.1. Demonstrate professionalism when discussing patient's billing record.

VII.A.2. Display sensitivity when requesting payment for services rendered.

VIII.C.1.b. Identify information required to file a third-party claim.

VIII.C.1.c. Identify the steps for filing a third-party claim.

VIII.C.3.a. Describe processes for verification of eligibility for services.

VIII.C.3.b. Describe processes for precertification.

VIII.C.3.c. Describe processes for preauthorization.

VIII.P.1. Interpret information on an insurance card.

VIII.P.2. Verify eligibility for services including documentation.

VIII.P.4. Complete an insurance claim form.

2015 Standards and Guidelines for the Accreditation of Educational Programs in Medical Assisting, Appendix B, Core Curriculum for Medical Assistants, Medical Assisting Education Review Board (MAERB), 2015.

INTRODUCTION

Administrative medical assistants help maintain physicians' financial records. This includes billing patients, filing insurance claims, and collecting the appropriate fees. Billing, reimbursement, and collections are extremely important because the office depends on the cash flow generated by these functions. All the expenses of running the office, such as supplies, payroll, and liability insurance, depend on the revenue from patients' and insurance companies' payments. General rules for filing healthcare claim forms, billing patients, and implementing collection procedures are discussed in this chapter.

8.1 RECORDING TRANSACTIONS

Administrative medical assistants keep track of the services rendered and any payments made during a visit to the physician. After the patient completes the office visit, the administrative medical assistant updates the patient's hardcopy or electronic ledger to show the financial information for the encounter.

Patient Encounter Form

To facilitate the process of billing patients for physicians' services, medical offices may use a patient encounter form. A blank patient encounter form (also called a *charge slip, superbill, routing slip,* or *patient service form*) is attached to the patient's medical record for completion. It is used to record the details of patients' encounters for billing and insurance purposes. In particular, it is designed to record each procedure or the most common procedures the physician performs, the fee charged for each, and the diagnosis connected with the treatment. Offices using electronic health records may still use a hardcopy encounter form or may use an electronic encounter form for data entry.

Most encounter forms contain sections for recording the following information (see Figure 8.1 for an example):

- Patient's name, address, phone information, and type of insurance, as well as patient return information, such as 2 weeks, p.r.n.
- Date of service
- Diagnosis or diagnoses for the current visit
- Procedure information—a checklist of the most commonly administered examinations, lab tests, injections, and other procedures in that office and the physician's fee for each
- Financial information—the total fees for the day, payments made, and amount due for that visit (balances due from prior visits may also be listed on the encounter form)
- Physician identifying information—address, fax and phone numbers, National Provider Identifier (NPI), and Employer Identification Number (EIN)

Preprinted forms should be numbered to provide a higher level of audit control over the forms, thereby reducing the possibility of fraudulent claims. All numbered forms must be accounted for and any missing forms found. The word "VOID" should be written in large red letters across encounter forms that are not to be used (i.e., error on the form such as wrong patient name) and should be included with other daily encounter forms.

Procedural and diagnostic codes listed on the encounter forms should be updated annually and the codes verified with the current year's diagnostic and procedural codes. Documentation of the update is usually placed in the lower right corner, indicating when the form was last updated, such as "January 1, 2028."

The procedures listed on a patient encounter form are customized to represent the most commonly administered examinations, lab tests, injections, and other procedures for that practice. On some encounter forms, the fee for each procedure is printed beside

No.	Date	Description	Charge	Credit Payment	Credit Adjustment	Current Balance
	05/15/2028	Annual exam, HGB, UA	173.00	34.60	------	138.40

Patient Information

7911 Riverview Lane N.
Address

Chicago, IL 60632-1979
City, State, Zip

312-555-6685   312-555-3385
Home phone   Work phone

Alison Becker   self
Responsible person   Relationship

Real Insurance   BEC0127
Insurance   Patient Insurance ID

Patient _____ Becker, Alison _____

Date: 05/15/2028   Chart # AA004

Karen Larsen, MD   Diagnoses :
2235 S. Ridgeway Avenue
Chicago, IL 60623-2240   1. _ZØØ.ØØ_____

312-555-6022   2. _____

          3. _____
FAX: 213-555-0025
NPI: 1234567   4. _____

OFFICE VISITS

New Patient	Established Patient

Preventive Medicine

	____ 99381	under 1 year	____ 99391		
	____ 99382	1–4	____ 99392	____ 99211	
____ 99202	____ 99383	5–11	____ 99393	____ 99212	
____ 99203	____ 99384	12–17	____ 99394	____ 99213	
____ 99204	____ 99385	18–39	**136.00** 99395	____ 99214	
____ 99205	____ 99386	40–64	____ 99396	____ 99215	
	____ 99387	65+	____ 99397		

Hospital Visits
Initial:
____ 99221
____ 99222
____ 99223
Subsequent:
____ 99231
____ 99232
____ 99233
Discharge
____ 99238
____ 99239
Nursing Facility
Initial:
____ 99304
____ 99305
____ 99306
Other
____ 99318

Lab:
____ 80048 Basic
metabolic panel
____ 87110 Chlamydia
culture
____ 85651 ESR;
nonautomated
____ 83001 FSH
____ 82947 Glucose,
blood
____ 85025 Hemogram
(CBC) with
differential
____ 80076 Hepatic
function panel
13.00 85018 HGB
____ 86701 HIV-1
____ 83002 LH
____ 80061 Lipid panel
____ 86617 Lyme
antibody

____ 86308 Monospot
test
____ 88150 Pap
____ 85610 Prothrombin
time
____ 84152 PSA
____ 86430 Rheumatoid
factor
____ 82270 Stool
hemoccult x 3
____ 87430 Strep screen
____ 84478 Triglycerides
____ 84443 TSH
24.00 81001 UA with
microscopy
____ 87088 UC
____ 84550 Uric acid,
blood
____ 81025 Urine
pregnancy test

Injections:
____ 90471 admin 1 vac
____ 90472 each add'l
vac
____ 90716 Chickenpox
____ 90702 DT
____ 90700 DTaP
____ 90657 Influenza
0.25mL
____ 90658 Influenza
0.5mL
____ 90710 MMRV,
subcutaneous
____ 90707 MMR
____ 90649 4vHPV
____ 90713 Polio vac
inactivated (IPV)
____ 90714 Td
ECG:
____ 93000 ECG

Other
_____
_____

Return visit: Two weeks

Updated January 1, 2028

Figure 8.1

Completed Patient
Encounter Form

the procedure code. In most cases, however, because the physician's fees may change from year to year, and because they are sometimes adjusted or discounted for different patients and insurance plans, a space is provided before each code (as in Figure 8.1) for the administrative medical assistant to enter the appropriate fee at the time of the visit.

Following is the procedure for using a patient encounter form:

1. An encounter form is attached to the patient's file when the patient registers for the visit.
2. As the physician performs various procedures during the visit, check marks are made in the appropriate boxes on the encounter form (or the appropriate items on the form are circled). The diagnoses and corresponding codes are also recorded on the form.
3. At the end of the visit, the form is taken to the checkout area for the administrative medical assistant to record, or post, the necessary transactions in the office's billing system. The patient may be asked to validate the information on the encounter form by signing the form.

Practices using electronic health records (EHRs) will input data traditionally documented on an encounter form directly into the patient's EHR. Codes and charges will be linked to the documentation, and the patient's electronic account will be automatically updated and charged. A hardcopy encounter form may still be given to the patient to use during checkout.

Fee Schedule

Each physician or medical practice has a **fee schedule,** which lists the usual procedures the office performs and the corresponding charges. The administrative medical assistant should always refer to the practice's fee schedule in determining the total cost for each patient's visit.

Most medical practices have more than one fee schedule. For example, if a physician is a participating provider in a preferred provider organization (PPO), the procedures may be discounted for PPO members according to an agreed-upon amount between the physician and the plan.

While dealing with the office's fee schedule, the assistant should also be familiar with the policy of the office regarding financial arrangements: the charges when a reduction of the fee is possible, copayments and/or deductibles which are due, the acceptable minimal payment, and any other facts needed to deal efficiently with problems concerning patients' payments.

Patients who call to make a first appointment may inquire about the charges. Patients should be told that it is difficult to discuss exact charges prior to a visit because the charges will depend on the extent of the examination, the tests, and the type of treatment provided. Ideally, the patient should be told the approximate cost of the procedures before treatment begins. Many insurance carriers require that patients be given written notification of services that probably or certainly will not be covered by completing a form prior to having services performed. For Medicare beneficiaries, this form is called an Advance Beneficiary Notice (ABN). The form must contain specific information, such as a description of the noncovered services, amount, acknowledgment of patient payment responsibility, and the patient's dated signature. Without the completed document on file prior to services being rendered, neither the patient nor the insurance carrier may be charged for the service. Other insurance carrier contracts should be referenced for the proper procedure regarding noncovered services. Providing this information in advance will help avoid misunderstandings and will make collection of payments easier.

It may be necessary to explain the fee by calling attention to the time involved; the cost of medications or supplies; and the skill, knowledge, and experience of the physician. Either the physician or the administrative medical assistant can discuss the fee with patients. If the physician discusses the fee with a patient, the assistant needs to know what has been discussed.

It is a fair assumption that a patient who inquires about charges before a visit is concerned about the price and should be shown every consideration. If a definite amount is quoted and this amount seems to worry the patient, the administrative medical assistant can reassure the patient by saying that arrangements can be made to ease payment.

Patient Statements

The administrative medical assistant records all transactions—that is, charges incurred by the patient for office visits, x-rays, laboratory tests, and so on and all adjustments and payments made by the patient or the patient's insurance company—in the patient ledger. The patient's copy of the information stored in the patient ledger (hardcopy or electronic) is referred to as the **patient statement,** or patient bill.

Figure 8.2

Patient Statement

STATEMENT

Statement Date: 05/11/2028

Account Number: AA004

Any change or payments made after the statement date will appear on the next statement.

Amount Enclosed _____

Please remit all payments to:

Karen Larsen, MD
2235 South Ridgeway Avenue
Chicago, IL 60623-2240
312-555-6022   Fax: 312-555-0025

Responsible Person's Name

Alison C. Becker
7911 Riverview Lane N.
Chicago, IL 60632-1979

Service Date	Patient's Name	Procedure Code	Diagnosis Code	Service Description	Charge	Insurance Paid	Adj.	Patient Paid	Amount Due
03-15-28	Mike	99202	M79.1Ø	NP visit	73.00	-0-	-0-	-0-	73.00
04-01-28								73.00	-0-
05-15-28	Alison	99395	ZØØ.ØØ	Annual exam	136.00			34.60	101.40
			85018	HGB	13.00				114.40
			81001	UA	24.00				138.40
05-31-28				Real Insurance		138.40			-0-

ANY AMOUNT NOT PAID BY INSURANCE IS NOW THE PATIENT'S RESPONSIBILITY

ACCOUNT NUMBER	CURRENT	OVER 30 DAYS	OVER 60 DAYS	OVER 90 DAYS	OVER 120 DAYS	INSURANCE PENDING	AMOUNT DUE
AA004	-0-	-0-	-0-	-0-	-0-	-0-	-0-

Abbreviations

CBC (complete blood count)
ECG (electrocardiogram)
EP (established patient)

HV (hospital visit)
LAB (laboratory work)
NP (new patient)

UA (urinalysis)
UC (urine culture)

The patient statement shows the professional services rendered to the patient, the charge for each service, payments made, and the balance owed. Figure 8.2 shows an example of a patient statement. Notice that the statement contains transactions for two people—Alison and Mike Becker—since both are members of the same family and are under the same account.

Listing, or itemizing, the procedures on the statement reminds patients when they visited the physician and what services were performed. To save space on the statement, some common procedures are listed using procedure codes only, with no descriptions. The statement is generally sent to the patient who received treatment, although in some cases another person may be designated as the one responsible for receiving the statement and paying for the services. Most billing programs bill a single patient on each account; however, some may list multiple patients on an account, such as minor children on a responsible adult's account.

A copy of legal documents, such as a durable power of attorney and/or a medical durable power of attorney, should be maintained in the patient's medical documentation and notation made of the authorized individual(s). Careful attention must be used to prevent the unauthorized disclosure of PHI. In general, parents are responsible for the medical bills of minor children living in their home.

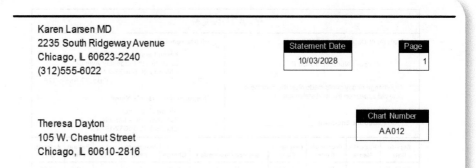

	Statement Date	Page
Karen Larsen MD 2235 South Ridgeway Avenue Chicago, IL 60623-2240 (312)555-6022	10/03/2028	1

	Chart Number
Theresa Dayton 105 W. Chestnut Street Chicago, IL 60610-2816	AA012

Date	Document	Description	Case Number	Amount
			Previous Balance:	0.00

Patient: Theresa Dayton   Chart #: AA012
Case Description: Physical Exam   Date of Last Payment: 9/30/2028   Amount: -20.00

Date	Document	Description	Case Number	Amount
9/21/2028	0309240000	Preventive, EP, 18-39 yrs.	7	136.00
9/21/2028	0309240000	Pap	7	33.00
9/21/2028	0309240000	Hemogram (CBC) with differential	7	25.00
9/21/2028	0309240000	UA with microscopy	7	24.00
9/21/2028	1310310000	Patient payment - check	7	-50.00
9/30/2028	0309240000	Insurance payment	7	-68.80
9/30/2028	0309240000	Insurance payment	7	-26.40
9/30/2028	0309240000	Insurance payment	7	-20.00
9/30/2028	0309240000	Insurance payment	7	-19.20

Computerized Billing

Most medical practices using an EHR system have the capability to handle patients' billing. If the EHR system does not have this capability, a separate software program may be used to handle the practice's financial tasks. Figure 8.3 shows an example of a electronic patient statement. In addition to generating itemized patient statements, a computerized billing system is usually used to produce the following reports for accounting purposes:

- A daily report, called a "day sheet," listing all charges, payments, and adjustments entered during that day
- Monthly reports summarizing the operation of the practice
- Aging reports, which list the outstanding balances owed to the practice by insurance companies or patients
- Lists of the amounts of money generated by various departments, such as laboratory, x-ray, and physical therapy
- Lists of the amounts generated by individual physicians in the practice
- Reports on the frequency of procedure codes reported by each physician in the practice

A patient billing program can also be used to print out blank patient encounter forms each day for patients who have appointments on that day. Medical billing programs are a valuable accounting tool for the physician, and the administrative medical assistant should be familiar with their use.

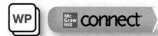 **GO TO PROJECT 8.1 AT THE END OF THIS CHAPTER**

Overview of the Process

When patients receive services from a medical practice, either they pay for services themselves or the charges are submitted to their insurance company or government agency for payment. Most medical practices complete an insurance claim form on behalf of the patient. The insurance claim form contains both clinical and financial information and is transmitted to the patient's insurance carrier for partial or full reimbursement of the services rendered.

Using the CMS-1500 Paper/Hardcopy Claim Form. The terms "paper" and "hardcopy" are used interchangeably, and both refer to a manually produced CMS claim form. The most commonly used paper or hardcopy claim form is the **CMS-1500 claim form** (formerly known as the *HCFA-1500 claim form*). See Figure 8.4 for an example. Accepted by private as well as government-sponsored programs, it is also called the

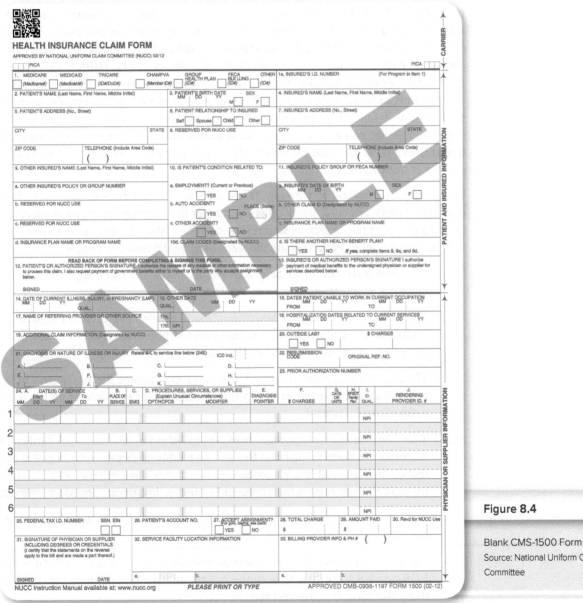

Figure 8.4

Blank CMS-1500 Form
Source: National Uniform Claim Committee

universal claim form. Two medical office forms are used to complete the CMS-1500 claim form: the **patient information form,** which is filled out or updated by the patient, and the patient encounter form. The patient information form may also include release-of-information and assignment-of-benefits statements. Prior to HIPAA, if a provider submitted a claim for a patient, a release-of-information statement had to be completed by the patient. Since HIPAA, the payment portion of TPO gives providers the authority to release claim-pertinent PHI to obtain third-party payment. If the patient decides to authorize a nonPAR provider to receive payments for medical services directly from third-party payers, an assignment-of-benefits statement must be signed by the patient and filed in the patient's medical record. For participating physicians, an assigned (direct) payment is one of the incentives for participation, and the patient's signature authorizing assignment of benefits is not needed. For convenience, some medical practices include these statements on the patient information form. Other practices prefer to use separate forms for each of them.

Submitting Paper/Hardcopy or Electronic Claims. Increasingly, medical offices are using computerized insurance claim forms, known as **electronic claims,** in place of paper claims. Electronic claims are prepared on a computer and transmitted electronically (from one computer to another) to an insurance carrier for processing. If necessary, an electronically prepared claim may be printed and a hardcopy claim sent to the carrier by Postal Service or other nonelectronic methods. The HIPAA 837, version 5010, claim is the standard format for electronic claims. Currently, HIPAA 837/5010 claim submissions are to be used by offices with 10 or more full-time employees or the equivalent of 10 full-time employees, such as 20 employees whose combined work status equals 10 full-time employees. Advantages of using electronic claims include immediate transmission, faster payment (Medicare claims are paid within 14 days versus 29 days), and easier tracking of claim status.

Processing by a Third-Party Payer. When the claim form arrives at the office of the insurance carrier, either on paper or as a computer file, the insurance carrier processes the claim. This entails a step-by-step review or adjudication process to determine the benefit payment level. Following are the steps used by the insurance payer:

Step 1 *The claim is received in the payer's system.* In Step 1, the claim is prescreened for any missing information, such as a date of birth.

Step 2 *The patient's eligibility and benefit level are determined.* In Step 2, the patient's benefit level, medical necessity, and covered/noncovered services are determined based on the patient's health plan.

Step 3 *The discount is applied.* In Step 3, the payer may reduce the physician's billed amount(s) based on the payer-provider contracted fee schedule or on the maximum allowed payment.

Step 4 *The claim edits and payer payment rules are applied to the claim.* In Step 4, further adjustments are made to the claim to allow for modifying factors, such as global payments, modifiers, and multiple procedures, which may either increase or decrease the payment amount. Noncovered services identified in this step are denied for payment.

Step 5 *The final payment is determined.* In Step 5, the auto-adjudication process is completed and the final benefit payment is calculated.

Step 6 *The EOB or ERA—or both—is generated and the payment is sent.* In Step 6, the EOB and ERA are sent to both the patient and the billing physician. Each of these is discussed in the next section.

A claim may be removed from the automated review cycle and submitted for a manual review if data for any of the above steps are missing or unclear.

Receiving an EOB or ERA. After the insurance carrier reviews the claim and makes a final reimbursement determination, it sends a remittance advice to the patient and to the provider with an explanation of its decision. The remittance advice also takes into account any deductibles or coinsurance the insured may owe. If the insurance company determines that there are benefits to be paid, a check for the appropriate amount is attached to the provider's report or an electronic deposit is made into the provider's financial account. In cases in which the benefits have not been assigned to the provider, the remittance is sent directly to the patient.

In the case of paper claims, the remittance advice sent by the insurance company in response to the claim is transmitted through the mail and is referred to as an **explanation of benefits (EOB)**. Figure 8.5 shows an example of an EOB for an office visit. In the case of electronic claims, the report is transferred from one computer to another and is therefore referred to as an **electronic remittance advice (ERA)**. As with an electronic claim, an ERA is typically not printed. When an ERA is sent electronically to the provider, a hardcopy EOB is sent to the patient. Although the formats used for the EOB and the ERA differ, the information conveyed in both types of reports is the same—both explain the amount of benefits to be paid to, or on behalf of, the insured and how that amount was determined.

Frequently, providers receive bulk payments—a single benefit payment that covers more than one submitted claim. For example, the insurance carrier submits one

Cross and Shield National Government Program
1290 Cimmons Road
Cincinnati, OH 45555

#FEI12398095643567#
Lena T. Crac
2520 Arizona Lane
Floyd, KY 41199-2520

Check sent to:	Karen Larsen, MD
Provider:	Karen Larsen, MD
Type.	PAR
Patient Name:	LENA CRAC
DOS:	03/23/20— to 03/23/20—
You Owe the Provider:	$20.00

EXPLANATION OF BENEFITS
This Is Not a Bill

ID Number:	R55559990
Claim Number:	R213213892308
Claim Paid On:	03/30/20--
Claim Received On:	03/25/20—
Claim Processed On:	03/30/20—
Claim Processed By:	Annie B.

Service Rendered	Submitted Charge(s)	Allowance	Codes	Deductible Amount	COB	Coinsurance or Copayment	Plan Payment	Patient Owes
OFFICE VISIT	100.00	61.15	160			20.00	41.15	20.00
TOTALS:	100.00	61.15		0.00		20.00	41.15	20.00

160-The charge submitted by the provider exceeds the allowable amount for this service. You are not responsible for the difference between the submitted charge and the plan allowance.

On this claim your out-of-pocket expenses are:	
Yearly Deductible:	0.00
Admission Copay:	0.00
Coinsurance Amount:	0.00
Copayment Amount:	20.00
Preauthorization Penalty Charge:	0.00
YOUR TOTAL:	20.00

	Yearly Ded	PAR	NonPAR
What You Have Paid:	34.91	0.00	0.00
Family:	34.91	301.00	301.00
Your Annual Max:	400.00	0.00	0.00
Family:	800.00	5,000.00	7,000.00

If you have a question concerning this claim, please call a customer service assistant. Refer to the Claims Section of your Service Booklet for disputed claims.

1-800-555-5555

Figure 8.5

An Example of an EOB

payment covering benefits for 15 Blue Cross Blue Shield patients instead of processing a single payment for each claim. Administrative medical assistants who process payments must be able to separate the bulk payments into individual claim benefits and post the payment and/or adjustments to the patient's account. The following is an example of three patient payments on one bulk statement. Using an 80/20 payment split, calculate how much should be credited to each patient's account from the insurance carrier and how much is left as patient responsibility. The provider is PAR.

Pt Name & Number	Submitted	Plan Allowance	Ins Pay	Deduct	Coins/Copay
PATIENT A (0012BA)					
09/16/20–	$ 80.00	$ 60.00	_____	$0.00	_____
09/23/20–	160.00	100.00	_____	0.00	_____
PATIENT B (0106SM)					
09/02/20–	80.00	60.00	_____	0.00	_____
PATIENT C (0219LS)					
09/15/20–	120.00	120.00	_____	0.00	_____
TOTALS	$440.00	$340.00	$272.00	$0.00	$68.00

Calculating the insurance payment and balance due from the patient using an 80/20 payment split:

Patient A
09/16/20–   Insurance payment of $48.00 and patient balance of $12.00
09/23/20–   Insurance payment of $80.00 and patient balance of $20.00

Patient B
09/02/20–   Insurance payment of $48.00 and patient balance of $12.00

Patient C
09/15/20–   Insurance payment of $96.00 and patient balance of $24.00

Patient A will require two entries into the payment system—one for each date of service. Also, since the provider is PAR, an adjustment will need to be made to each patient's account for the difference between the submitted amount and the plan allowance amount. What is the amount to be adjusted off each patient's date of service?

Patient A
09/16/20–   Adjustment amount   _____
09/23/20–   Adjustment amount   _____

Patient B
09/02/20–   Adjustment amount   _____

Patient C
09/15/20–   Adjustment amount   _____

Patient A adjustments are $20.00 and $60.00, respectively. Patient B will have an adjustment of $20.00, and Patient C will have no adjustment to the account.

Checking the Reimbursement Details. After the medical office receives the remittance advice (the ERA or EOB), the administrative medical assistant reviews it and checks it against the original claim. If all is in order, the report is filed with the patient's financial records. If a check from the insurance company is attached to the EOB, the payment received is posted to the appropriate patient's account, and the check is marked for deposit in the practice's bank account. Generally, if a claim is processed electronically, the method of payment is also electronic. In such cases, the payment attached to the ERA is deposited into the practice's bank account through an electronic funds transfer (EFT) rather than mailed in the form of a check to the medical practice.

Billing the Patient. If the patient still owes money to the medical practice after the EOB or ERA has been received—usually for charges that were not fully reimbursed by the insurance company, such as deductibles or noncovered services—the administrative medical assistant bills the patient for the amount due. If the patient is confused or has any questions about payments, the administrative medical assistant can try to help by going over the terms of the insurance plan with the patient. The administrative medical assistant may also need to call the insurance carrier and act as a patient advocate (go-between) for patients. Goodwill can be built for the physician's office by using problem-solving and communication skills to fulfill the role of patient advocate. Patients understandably get upset when they receive unexpectedly large bills or an incorrect payment. The administrative medical assistant is the patient's advocate with the insurance carrier. Sometimes explaining the solution again to the patient in different terms after speaking with the insurance carrier will help clear up the problem. Different forms of payment assistance may need to be explained to the patient. Examples include offering a payment plan or supplying information about local or governmental assistance agencies.

Patients may also accuse the medical office of billing incorrectly when they are unhappy with the benefits received. Use respect and care in solving any miscommunications or misunderstandings in such circumstances. It is important to separate the patient's feelings from the facts. When documented facts, such as EOB or ERA information, are professionally yet empathetically discussed with angry patients, the patient may be more accepting of the information. Be careful to avoid insurance and medical jargon; this will only add to patients' frustration.

Once the patient understands the terms of the payment due, the assistant follows up with the patient to see that the amount due is collected in a timely manner. When the patient pays the balance due, the account is listed as a zero balance, and the insurance claim process is complete.

Appealing Claims. If the physician thinks that the reimbursement decision is incorrect or unfair, the medical office may initiate an appeal. Appeals must be filed within a stated period after the determination of claim benefits or denial. Most insurance carriers have an upward structure for appeals, beginning at the lowest level and progressing upward. For example, the first step may be to submit a formal complaint. If the provider is not satisfied with the outcome, the second step may be to file an appeal. A grievance would be filed if the appeal did not produce the desired results. When making an appeal of an electronic claim, include the electronic claim number. Each insurance company has its own appeal process. A representative from the insurance company can instruct the assistant on the appeal process the insurer uses, if necessary. This information may also be available on the Internet by initiating a search from the insurance carrier's website.

Completing and Transmitting the Claim Form

Completing and transmitting the claim form accurately for a patient is one of the most important steps in successful claim reimbursement. Therefore, the administrative medical assistant should be familiar with the details of the process.

Verifying Insurance Information. The first step in processing a claim is to verify the patient's insurance information. With new patients, most practices routinely check insurance coverage before the patient's first appointment. Basic information about the patient and the patient's insurance is obtained over the phone when the first appointment is scheduled. The assistant then contacts the insurer by telephone, fax, Internet, or other electronic methods specified by the insurance carrier to verify that the patient is currently enrolled in the plan as specified and has paid all required premiums or other charges.

Checking the Accuracy of Essential Claim Information. Claim forms must be completed accurately. The following basic information is required on most claim forms:

- Contract numbers—that is, the group number and the insured's identification number from the insured's current insurance card
- The patient's complete name, date of birth, gender, and relationship to the insured
- The insured's complete name, address, date of birth, and employer
- Information on a secondary carrier—subscriber's name, date of birth, and employer
- Information about whether the condition is job-related or accident-related and whether it is an illness or an injury
- The patient's account number (if the facility assigns numbers to patients)
- Complete and current diagnostic codes for the submitted claim
- Information about the provider—name, address, identifying codes, NPI and other required identifiers, and signatures
- A statement of services rendered, which should include dates, procedure codes, charges, and total charges

The following is information presented on an insured's insurance card submitted to the provider through the registration process. Additional information, including important phone numbers, is listed on the back of the card. Always make a copy of both the front and back sides of an insurance card.

CROSS AND SHIELD PPO	www.crossandshield.org	
INSURED	Customer Service	1-800-555-5555
DAYS CATALINA S	Precertification	1-800-555-1234
ID NUMBER	Retail Service Pharmacy	1-800-555-5678
R123456789XX	Mail Service Pharmacy	1-800-555-9012
GROUP CODE DOC	Substance Abuse	
555 04-19-20—	Precertification	1-800-555-1235

EXAMPLE: CLAIM INFORMATION

Using the preceding insurance card information, a claim was submitted with the following information and the claim was denied. What is wrong with the submitted claim information?

Patient Name: Catalina S. Dayes

ID Number: R123456798XX

Group Code: 555

Before submitting claims, the assistant must carefully check every bit of information for accuracy. Typographical errors and transposition of numbers are two of the most common claim submission errors. This example contains two errors—a misspelled name and transposition of the numbers in the ID number.

Completing the CMS-1500 Claim Form. Most insurance companies accept the CMS-1500 for hardcopy/paper claims. However, the assistant may need to complete a specifically designed claim form for a carrier. Although the form may be different, the information required on most insurance claim forms is the same. If the assistant is familiar with the various fields on the CMS-1500 form, the same knowledge can be applied to other claim forms for successful completion.

Figure 8.6 shows a completed CMS-1500 claim form. Note that the form is divided horizontally into two parts: The top half contains patient and insured information (Items 1-13), while the bottom half contains physician or supplier information (Items 14-33). Table 8.1 presents the information that should be entered in each numbered blank (called a form locator). The table contains generalized information, and individual carriers, such as Medicare, should be contacted prior to completing

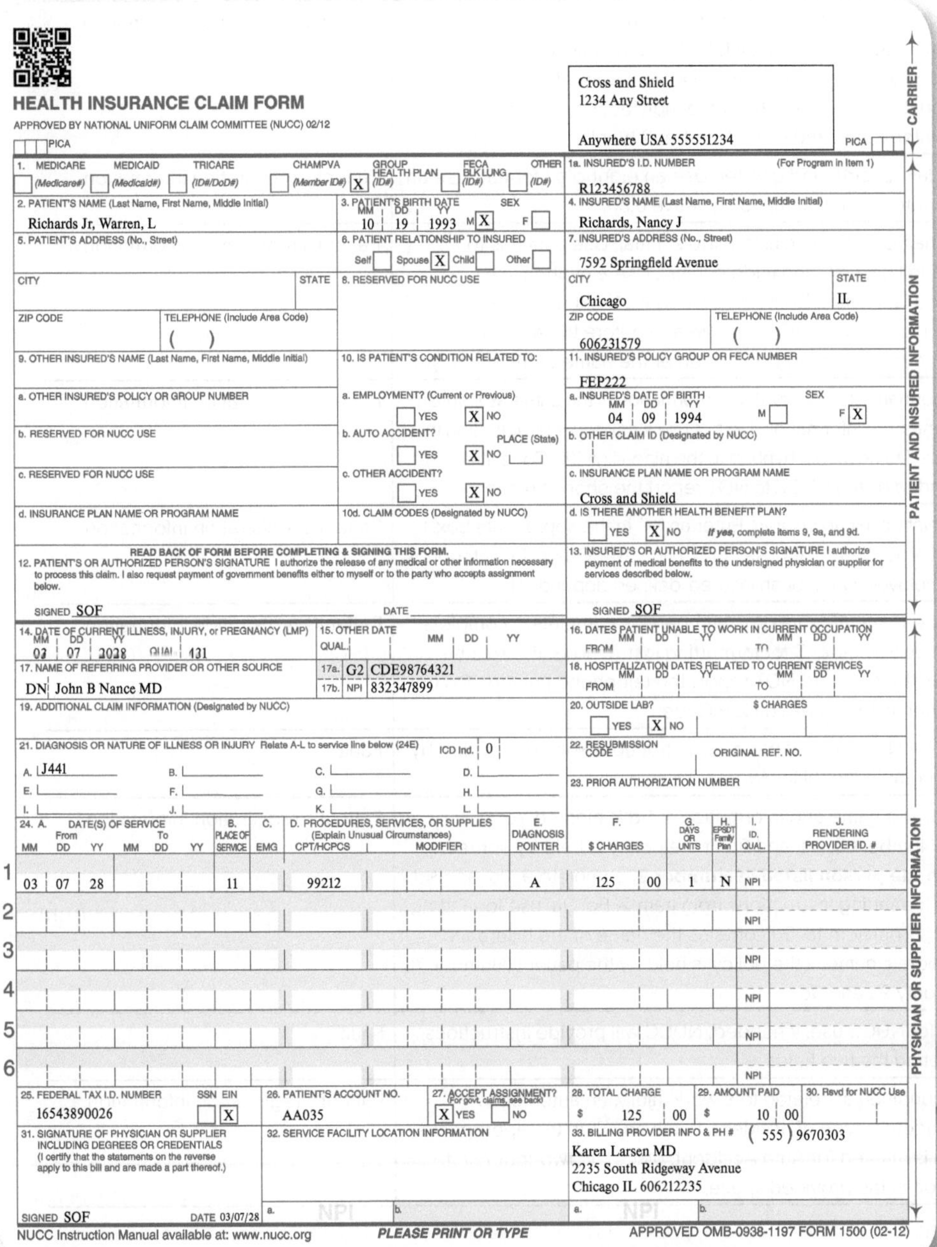

HEALTH INSURANCE CLAIM FORM
APPROVED BY NATIONAL UNIFORM CLAIM COMMITTEE (NUCC) 02/12

Cross and Shield
1234 Any Street
Anywhere USA 555551234

PICA — CARRIER

1. MEDICARE (Medicare#) MEDICAID (Medicaid#) TRICARE (ID#/DoD#) CHAMPVA (Member ID#) GROUP HEALTH PLAN (ID#) [X] FECA BLK LUNG (ID#) OTHER (ID#)
1a. INSURED'S I.D. NUMBER (For Program in Item 1): R123456788
2. PATIENT'S NAME (Last Name, First Name, Middle Initial): Richards Jr, Warren, L
3. PATIENT'S BIRTH DATE MM DD YY: 10 19 1993 SEX M [X] F
4. INSURED'S NAME (Last Name, First Name, Middle Initial): Richards, Nancy J
5. PATIENT'S ADDRESS (No., Street)
6. PATIENT RELATIONSHIP TO INSURED: Self Spouse [X] Child Other
7. INSURED'S ADDRESS (No., Street): 7592 Springfield Avenue
CITY STATE
8. RESERVED FOR NUCC USE
CITY: Chicago STATE: IL
ZIP CODE TELEPHONE (Include Area Code) ( )
ZIP CODE: 606231579 TELEPHONE (Include Area Code) ( )
9. OTHER INSURED'S NAME (Last Name, First Name, Middle Initial)
10. IS PATIENT'S CONDITION RELATED TO:
11. INSURED'S POLICY GROUP OR FECA NUMBER: FEP222
a. OTHER INSURED'S POLICY OR GROUP NUMBER
a. EMPLOYMENT? (Current or Previous) YES NO [X]
a. INSURED'S DATE OF BIRTH MM DD YY: 04 09 1994 SEX M F [X]
b. RESERVED FOR NUCC USE
b. AUTO ACCIDENT? YES NO [X] PLACE (State)
b. OTHER CLAIM ID (Designated by NUCC)
c. RESERVED FOR NUCC USE
c. OTHER ACCIDENT? YES NO [X]
c. INSURANCE PLAN NAME OR PROGRAM NAME: Cross and Shield
d. INSURANCE PLAN NAME OR PROGRAM NAME
10d. CLAIM CODES (Designated by NUCC)
d. IS THERE ANOTHER HEALTH BENEFIT PLAN? YES NO [X] *If yes*, complete items 9, 9a, and 9d.
READ BACK OF FORM BEFORE COMPLETING & SIGNING THIS FORM.
12. PATIENT'S OR AUTHORIZED PERSON'S SIGNATURE I authorize the release of any medical or other information necessary to process this claim. I also request payment of government benefits either to myself or to the party who accepts assignment below.
SIGNED SOF DATE
13. INSURED'S OR AUTHORIZED PERSON'S SIGNATURE I authorize payment of medical benefits to the undersigned physician or supplier for services described below.
SIGNED SOF
PATIENT AND INSURED INFORMATION

14. DATE OF CURRENT ILLNESS, INJURY, or PREGNANCY (LMP) MM DD YY: 03 07 2028 QUAL 431
15. OTHER DATE QUAL. MM DD YY
16. DATES PATIENT UNABLE TO WORK IN CURRENT OCCUPATION FROM TO
17. NAME OF REFERRING PROVIDER OR OTHER SOURCE: DN John B Nance MD
17a. G2 CDE98764321
17b. NPI 832347899
18. HOSPITALIZATION DATES RELATED TO CURRENT SERVICES FROM TO
19. ADDITIONAL CLAIM INFORMATION (Designated by NUCC)
20. OUTSIDE LAB? YES NO [X] $ CHARGES
21. DIAGNOSIS OR NATURE OF ILLNESS OR INJURY Relate A-L to service line below (24E) ICD Ind. 0
A. J441 B. C. D. E. F. G. H. I. J. K. L.
22. RESUBMISSION CODE ORIGINAL REF. NO.
23. PRIOR AUTHORIZATION NUMBER

	24. A. DATE(S) OF SERVICE From MM DD YY	To MM DD YY	B. PLACE OF SERVICE	C. EMG	D. PROCEDURES, SERVICES, OR SUPPLIES (Explain Unusual Circumstances) CPT/HCPCS MODIFIER	E. DIAGNOSIS POINTER	F. $ CHARGES	G. DAYS OR UNITS	H. EPSDT Family Plan	I. ID. QUAL.	J. RENDERING PROVIDER ID. #
1	03 07 28		11		99212	A	125 00	1	N	NPI	
2										NPI	
3										NPI	
4										NPI	
5										NPI	
6										NPI	

25. FEDERAL TAX I.D. NUMBER: 16543890026 SSN EIN [X]
26. PATIENT'S ACCOUNT NO.: AA035
27. ACCEPT ASSIGNMENT? (For govt. claims, see back) [X] YES NO
28. TOTAL CHARGE: $ 125 00
29. AMOUNT PAID: $ 10 00
30. Rsvd for NUCC Use
31. SIGNATURE OF PHYSICIAN OR SUPPLIER INCLUDING DEGREES OR CREDENTIALS (I certify that the statements on the reverse apply to this bill and are made a part thereof.)
SIGNED SOF DATE 03/07/28
32. SERVICE FACILITY LOCATION INFORMATION
a. NPI b.
33. BILLING PROVIDER INFO & PH # (555) 9670303
Karen Larsen MD
2235 South Ridgeway Avenue
Chicago IL 606212235
a. NPI b.
PHYSICIAN OR SUPPLIER INFORMATION
NUCC Instruction Manual available at: www.nucc.org PLEASE PRINT OR TYPE APPROVED OMB-0938-1197 FORM 1500 (02-12)

Figure 8.6

Completed CMS-1500 Form Source: National Uniform Claim Committee

Table 8.1 CMS-1500 Completion Guideline Chart*

ITEM NO.	DESCRIPTION	RESOURCE
Carrier block	Enter the name and address of the insurance payer in the upper right margin of the form. Use the following format: Line 1—Name Line 2—First line of address Line 3—Second line of address or leave blank Line 4—City, state (two digits) and nine-digit ZIP Code without punctuation Do not use punctuation in Lines 1 through 4.	ID Card
1	Type of insurance. Use an "X" to indicate the correct carrier. Do not mark more than one carrier.	Chart, patient's registration information
1A	Insured's ID number. Do not use spaces.	Patient's registration information
2	Patient's name. Enter last, first, middle initial. Use commas to separate the last, first, and middle initial. Use a hyphen in a hyphenated last name. Do not use periods. If the patient and the insured are the same individual, only report the insured's information and leave Number 2 blank.	Patient's registration information
3	Patient's date of birth and gender. Use an eight-digit format. Use an "X" to indicate gender. If unknown, leave blank.	Patient's registration information
4	Insured's name. Enter last, first, middle initial. Use commas to separate the last, first, and middle initial. Use a hyphen in a hyphenated last name. Do not use periods. A last name suffix should be placed after the last name and before the first name. For workers' compensation claims, enter the name of the employer.	Patient's registration information
5	Patient's permanent address. If the information is the same as insured, do not reenter the information. Do not use symbols or punctuation in the address. Do not use a hyphen in the nine-digit ZIP Code. It is recommended by the NUCC to NOT report the phone number.	Patient's registration information
6	Patient's relationship to insured. Enter an "X" in the appropriate box. If the patient is not "Self," "Spouse," or "Child," use "Other" for categories such as employee, ward, or an insured-defined dependent.	Patient's registration information
7	Insured's permanent address. If Number 4 is completed, complete Number 7. See Number 5 for formatting instructions. It is recommended by the NUCC to NOT report the telephone number. Do not use a hyphen in the nine-digit ZIP Code.	Patient's registration information
8	Reserved for NUCC use. If needed, instructions will be provided by NUCC for completing this field.	Fault
9, 9a, and 9d	Other insured's name and information. If 11d is marked Yes, complete Numbers 9, 9a, and 9d. If the policy is held **by someone other than the person listed in Number 2,** complete 9, 9a, and 9d. For 9, use formatting instructions from Item 2. For 9a, use formatting instructions from Item 1a. 9d contains the name of the insurance plan or program name. If the policy is held by the patient (Number 2), complete only 9a and 9d.	Patient's registration information
9b and 9c	Reserved for NUCC use. If needed, NUCC will provide instructions for completing the two fields.	Fault
10a, 10b, and 10c	Patient's condition as related to a work injury, an automobile accident, or other type of accident. Place an "X" in the appropriate box. If Yes is marked for Auto Accident, place the two letter state abbreviation in the provided space.	Patient's registration information

*Guidelines as of July 2020

Table 8.1 CMS-1500 Completion Guideline Chart—_continued_

ITEM NO.	DESCRIPTION	RESOURCE
10d	Claim Codes (designated by NUCC). If a payer requires the use of Condition codes, enter it in this field. Approved NUCC Condition Codes are available at http://NUCC.org under Code Sets.	Payer and NUCC website
11	Insured's policy, group, or FECA number. Do not use spaces or hyphens.	Patient's registration information
11a	Insured's date of birth and gender. Use an eight-digit format. Use an "X" to indicate gender. If unknown, leave blank.	Patient's registration information
11b	Other claim ID (designated by NUCC). Y4 Property Casualty Claim Number is to be used for Property Casualty claims. If required, enter the qualifier (Y4) to the left of the dotted, vertical line and the identifier number to the right of the dotted, vertical line. Enter the payor-assigned number to the right of the dotted line. Completion of 11b is required for workers' compensation or property and casualty claims, if the number is known.	Patient's medical claim information
11c	Insurance plan name or program name.	Patient's registration information
11d	Is there another health plan? Use an "X" to mark the appropriate box. If marked yes, complete 9, 9a, and 9d.	Patient's registration information
12	Patient's or authorized person's signature. Enter signature on file, SOF, or the patient's legal signature. If using a legal signature, enter the date either in six- or eight-digit format.	Patient's and/or insured's legal signature or the referenced signature on file in the patient's record
13	Insured's or authorized person's signature. Enter signature on file, SOF, or the insured's legal signature. If no signature on file exists, either leave Number 13 blank or enter No Signature on File.	Insured's legal signature or the referenced signature on file in the patient's record
14	Date of current illness, injury, pregnancy (LMP). Use either six- or eight-digit format. The applicable qualifier should be used to identify which date is reported on the claim form: qualifier 431 Onset of Current Symptoms or Illness or qualifier 484 Last Menstrual Period. Enter the qualifier on the right side of the dotted, vertical column.	Patient's record
15	Other date. Use six- or eight-digit format to enter any other date that is related to the patient's treatment or condition. If unknown, leave blank. A previous pregnancy is not considered a similar illness. Choose from the following qualifiers: 454 Initial Treatment 444 First Visit or Consultation 304 Latest Visit or Consultation 453 Acute Manifestation of a Chronic Condition 439 Accident 455 Last X-ray 471 Prescription 090 Report Start 091 Report End	Patient's record
16	Dates patient is unable to work in current occupation. Use six- or eight-digit format to indicate the "from" and "to" dates the patient is not able to work in his or her current occupation.	Patient's record
17	Referring doctor or other source. Enter the name and credentials of the referring, ordering, or supervising healthcare professional. Do not use periods or commas. Use a hyphen in a hyphenated last name. If more than one physician meets the criteria for Number 17, list only one physician using this hierarchy: referring, ordering, supervising physician. Select one of the three approved qualifiers and enter it to the left of the dotted, vertical line: DN Referring Provider DK Ordering Provider DQ Supervising Provider	Patient's record, physician's information, and NUCC website

continued

Table 8.1 CMS-1500 Completion Guideline Chart—*continued*

ITEM NO.	DESCRIPTION	RESOURCE
17a	Referring, ordering, or supervising physician's non-NPI number. Enter the NUCC qualifier to the left of the solid, vertical line. The following qualifiers are approved by NUCC: 0B State License Number 1G Provider UPIN Number G2 Provider Commercial Number LU Location Number Enter the number to the right of the solid, vertical line.	Patient's record, physician's information, and NUCC website
17b	Referring, ordering, or supervising physician's NPI number.	Patient's record, physician's information, and insurance manual
18	Hospitalization dates. Enter in six- or eight-digit format the admission and, if known, the discharge date for the inpatient hospitalization.	Patient's record
19	Additional claim information (designated by NUCC). Consult with insurance payer for completion instructions. Do not use a hyphen, space, or other type of separator between the qualifier and the number. A complete listing of approved NUCC qualifiers can be found at the NUCC website.	Insurance manual, NUCC website
20	Usage of outside lab services. Use an "X" to mark Yes or No. If no outside lab services were used (purchased), mark No. If outside lab services were purchased by the provider, such as processing blood or lab work, mark Yes and enter the amount paid for the services. Enter the amount right-justified in the $ CHARGES portion of the field using dollars and cents format (i.e., 1100 00). Do not use a dollar sign, commas, or periods. Enter the service information and service charge in line item 32.	Patient's record, patient's ledger
21	Diagnosis or nature of illness or injury. Using 9 for *ICD-9-CM* or 0 for *ICD-10-CM,* enter to the left of the dotted, vertical line which version of *ICD* codes are being used on the claim form. Enter the diagnostic code(s) related to the current visit on lines A–L. Do not use a decimal point in the appropriate place within the code.	Patient's record, coding manual
22	Resubmission code and reference number. To the left of the solid, vertical line, enter either 7 for replacement of a prior claim or 8 to void or cancel a prior claim. Contact the insurance payer for further instructions.	Insurance manual
23	Prior authorization code. If a prior authorization and/or a precertification code is required by the payer, enter the number with no spaces or hyphens.	Contact pay
24a	NOTE: For 24a–24h, use the bottom, unshaded portion of the field. Specific information for completing the shaded, upper portion of the field can be found at http://NUCC.org. Dates of service. Using a six-digit format, enter the dates of service for the procedure listed on the line. Only one service per line may be listed. For services rendered on one day, enter only the From date. If required by the payer, the same date may be listed in the To column.	Patient's record, patient's ledger
24b	POS code. Enter the two-digit place of service code. Place of service codes may be found at www.cms.gov/Medicare/Coding/place-of-service-codes/Place_of_service_code_Set.html.	Patient's record, patient's ledger
24c	Emergency. If required by the payer, enter "Y" for Yes or leave blank for No. If required, the definition of "emergency" must meet the criteria of the insured's insurance provider.	Patient's record

Table 8.1 CMS-1500 Completion Guideline Chart—*continued*

ITEM NO.	DESCRIPTION	RESOURCE
24d	Procedures, services, or supplies. Using the *CPT* or *HCPCS* code set for the year in which services or supplies were rendered, enter the appropriate code. Up to four two-digit modifiers may be entered in the Modifier column. If more than four modifiers are needed, check with the insurance provider on the appropriate use of -99 modifier.	Patient's record, coding manual
24e	Diagnostic pointer. Enter the line letter from Number 21 that relates to the service stated on the current line in Number 24. Use only the line letter, such as A or D, not the diagnostic code. If more than one diagnostic code relates to the rendered service, list the primary diagnostic line letter first. Diagnostic line letters should be left-justified with no commas or spaces, such as ABDF.	Patient's record
24f	Charges. Enter the charge related to the service listed in 24d. Enter the amount in dollars and cents format (24 00), right-justified with no commas or periods. If there is no charge for the service, enter 0 00 in 24f.	Patient's record, patient's ledger
24g	Days or units. Enter the number of days/units associated with the service listed on line 24. The number should be left-justified with no leading zeros. Fractions should be shown by using a decimal point. Examples would be .5, 1, and 1.5. When reporting anesthesia services, report the time in minutes.	Patient's record, patient's ledger
24h	Early and periodic screening and diagnostic testing. Enter a "Y" or "N" if a reason code is NOT required (such as a state requirement). If there is a reason code requirement, such as a state requirement, refer to the NUCC website for the correct code. If reporting family planning services is required, enter a "Y"; if there is not a requirement to report family planning services, enter an "N."	Patient's record, patient's ledger, NUCC website, or payer's manual
24i	ID qualifier. Enter the qualifier, found at http://NUCC.org, identifying the non-NPI identifier type of the providing physician in the shaded area.	Physician's information
24j	Rendering provider's ID. Enter the non-NPI number in the shaded, upper portion of 24j and the NPI number in the unshaded, lower portion of the field, only when the provider of the service is different from the provider listed in 33a and 33b.	Physician's information
25	Federal tax ID number. Enter the Employer Identification Number (EIN) or the Social Security Number of the billing provider listed in Number 33. Enter an "X" to mark the appropriate box for either EIN or SSN. Numbers should be left-justified without hyphens.	Physician's information
26	Patient's account number. Enter the patient's account number assigned by the provider. The number should be left-justified without hyphens.	Patient's record, patient's ledger
27	Accept assignment? Use an "X" to indicate Yes or No for all payers. Accepting assignment means the physician agrees to accept payment based on the payer's fee schedule.	Physician's information, insurance manual
28	Total charge. Enter the total amount for all charges on the current claim form. The amount should be in dollars and cents format and right-justified without periods or commas. Use "00" for whole dollar amounts (125 00).	Patient's record, patient's ledger
29	Amount paid. Enter the amount the patient or another payer paid on covered services listed on the current claim form. Enter the total amount paid in dollar and cents format and right-justified without periods or commas. Use "00" for whole dollar amounts.	Patient's record, patient's ledger

continued

Table 8.1 CMS-1500 Completion Guideline Chart—*continued*

ITEM NO.	DESCRIPTION	RESOURCE
30	Reserved for NUCC use. If needed, instructions will be provided by NUCC for completing this field.	Fault
31	Signature of physician or supplier including degrees or credentials. Enter the legal signature, signature on file, or SOF, along with the date the form was signed. Use either six- or eight-digit format or use alphanumeric format, such as January 13, 2028.	Physician's information
32, 32a, and 32b	Service facility location information. If laboratory or services were purchased by the providing physician, as indicated by a "Y" in Number 20, list the complete address of the provider from whom services were purchased. Enter the address in three-line format: (1) name, (2) street address, (3) city, state, and ZIP Code. Enter the address with no punctuation or symbols, including no hyphen in the nine-digit ZIP Code. Enter the NPI number of the facility in 32a and the qualifier and non-NPI number in 32b. Qualifiers are located at the NUCC website. Do not enter a space between the qualifier and the non-NPI number in 32b (GS12345678). Complete field 32 only if the service provider is different from the billing provider (field 33).	Patient's record, patient's ledger, NUCC website, or payer's manual
33, 33a, and 33b	Billing provider's information and phone number. Enter the name, address, and phone number of the billing provider. Enter the address in three-line format: (1) name, (2) street address, (3) city, state, and ZIP Code. Enter the address with no punctuation or symbols including no hyphen in the nine-digit ZIP Code or no separators in the telephone number. Enter the NPI number of the billing provider in 32a and the qualifier and non-NPI number in 32b. Qualifiers are located at the NUCC website. Do not enter a space between the qualifier and the non-NPI number in 33b (G212345678).	Physician's information, NUCC website

COMPLIANCE *TIP*

Updated guidelines for completing claim forms are found at the National Uniform Claim Committee's website at http://NUCC.org. Guidelines are updated yearly—usually in July.

CMS-1500 forms for specific completion instructions. It is beneficial to keep a log with an example of a properly completed claim form for each insurance carrier. The log can be easily referenced when completing future claims. CMS-1500 forms are purchased from vendors and are printed in red. Black ink should be used to complete the paper form.

After a claim has been completed and sent to the insurance company, make a notation in the patient ledger by entering the date and the phrase "Submitted to insurance" after the last entry. When insurance claims are submitted using an electronic submission program, the program places the submission date in the patient's electronic ledger account. An updated patient statement is then sent to the patient for billing purposes on the next billing date. The patient or another designated person is still responsible for the complete charge, even if insurance is involved. However, the medical provider must be careful to adhere to guidelines of the insurance carrier regarding when a patient is to be billed.

Using Computer Billing Programs. Generating claim forms (whether paper or electronic) on the computer is one of the major uses of computer technology in the medical office today. The computer automatically processes the information required to create a completed claim by transferring the patient's and the insured's information, the charges, the procedure and diagnostic codes, billing/rendering/referring provider information, and so forth from the various databases set up in the computer onto the insurance claim form.

The computer stores facts about the medical practice in the practice database; information about the carriers that most patients use in the insurance carrier database; information about payments made by patients, as well as benefits received from insurance companies, in the transaction database; and information about each patient—personal as well as clinical data—in the patient database. Careful attention must be given when keying information and updating system data. Errors in keying will be transferred to the claim form.

When all new data and transaction information have been entered and checked regarding a patient's visit to the physician, the administrative medical assistant creates the electronic claim. The format for the claim—either the CMS-1500, HIPAA 837P/5010 version, or a specialized claim form—is also designated. The software program then organizes the necessary databases and selects the data from each one as needed to produce a completed claim form. When this is completed, the administrative medical assistant will electronically transmit the claim to the insurance carrier for processing.

Electronic Claims Versus Paper Claims. The main difference between electronic claims and paper claims is the means by which they are transmitted to the insurance carrier. The use of electronic claims not only speeds up transmission and payments but also ensures a greater degree of accuracy and costs less.

Paper claims, whether printed from a computer billing program or typed, are usually transmitted to insurance carriers through the mail. When they reach the insurance carrier, the information on the form must be keyed into the insurance company's computer by data entry personnel. Alternatively, the information may be scanned using an optical character reader (OCR). In either case, a certain percentage of error is introduced.

The following are tips for preparing claims that will be scanned:

1. Use an eight-digit format for dates (01/02/2028) unless instructions are given to use a six-digit format for dates.
2. Send reports and other supporting documentation unattached from the claim form.
3. Start over when a mistake is made on claim forms prepared by hand, and correct individual errors when prepared on the computer. Refrain from erasing, striking out errors, or applying white-out products.
4. Read and input *ICD-10-CM, CPT,* and *HCPCS* codes carefully. *ICD-10-CM* has digits and letters that look similar. Be careful to avoid interchanging the digit *0* and the alphabetic letter *O*. Other combinations not to read or input incorrectly are the digit *5* and alphabetic letter *S,* and the combination of the digit *1* and the alphabetic letter *l*.

Electronic claims, on the other hand, are transmitted from one computer to another over the telephone, Internet, or other electronic transmission method. Because claim information is entered once, not twice, chances of error or omission are greatly reduced. It also costs less to file claims electronically; fewer personnel are involved and paper forms, envelopes, and postage are not required.

An advantage to transmitting claims electronically is that the medical office receives immediate feedback whenever claims are transmitted. Medical offices generally transmit claims in batches, grouped by insurer. Tracking numbers are used to follow the progress of claims. When an insurance carrier receives electronic claims, it sends a transmittal report back to the sender, acknowledging receipt of the claims. The administrative medical assistant should compare the acknowledgment of claims against the reports of sent claims. If a claim is not listed on the transmittal receipt, the claim should be retransmitted.

Each office has its own schedule for sending claims. The usual practice is to transmit claims every day or every other day. Larger practices may transmit claims multiple times a day, such as late morning and afternoon. Individual carriers will have time guidelines for providers to submit claims. Guidelines may be as little as 30 days from the date of service or as long as December 31 of the year after the year in which the service was provided. For example, a patient had a colonoscopy performed on March 18, 2023. Under the latter guidelines, the last date to submit this claim to the carrier would be December 31, 2024. Provider schedules for submitting claims to carriers should be based on the carrier's guidelines and any negotiated contract time guidelines.

When claims are transmitted electronically, the medical office receives a file acknowledgment—immediate feedback that tells the medical office the file has arrived at the insurance carrier's claims department. If the file is missing details (for example, if a required field is left blank) or if the claim form contains incorrect information, such as an invalid patient identification number, the computer will immediately notify the sender that the file has been rejected. The medical office that sent the claim can then fix the error and resubmit the claim.

Whether the claim is paper or electronic, it is often the overlooked, seemingly simple errors that prevent the provider from producing a **clean claim**—a claim that is accepted by the insurance payer for adjudication. The following are some common errors:

- Service facility names and associated information, such as address or phone number, are missing, incomplete, or incorrect.
- Referring provider information is missing.
- Patient birth date is invalid.
- Procedure and diagnostic codes are not current or are invalid.
- There are typographical errors and transpositions of numbers.

Clean claims are processed in a more timely manner; and, in turn, benefit payments are received faster by the provider. Software programs, known as **scrubber programs,** are used to check for errors on insurance claim forms before they are submitted.

Using Clearinghouses. A **clearinghouse** is a service bureau that collects electronic claims from many different medical practices and forwards the claims to the appropriate insurance carriers. Some insurance carriers who receive insurance claims electronically require information to be formatted in a particular way. Part of the service a clearinghouse provides is to translate electronic claim data to fit the setup of each carrier's claims processing department. Because of this factor, many medical practices choose to use a clearinghouse instead of transmitting claims directly to insurance carriers themselves. Usually, a fee is negotiated with the clearinghouse for its services. With or without the use of a clearinghouse, electronic claims reach the insurance carrier almost immediately compared with paper claims.

Following Up on Claims

When an EOB or ERA from a third-party payer arrives, the assistant checks that

- all the procedures listed on the claim also appear on the EOB/ERA.
- any unpaid charges are explained.
- the codes on the EOB/ERA match those on the claim.
- the payment listed for each procedure is correct.

The assistant must routinely follow up on all submitted claims. Many medical offices use the Internet to contact carriers to check claim status. For claims submitted using HIPAA transactions, HIPAA 276 and 277 are used to ask payers about the status of a claim. The number 276 refers to the provider's inquiry, and 277 refers to the payer's response. The timeline for the follow-up varies according to the insurance carrier, the insurance program, and if participating, their written contract. Most medical offices follow up on claim status 7 to 14 days after the claims are submitted. Experience with insurance will enable you to know when follow-up on a claim is necessary.

Some physicians automatically rebill in 30 days if they have not heard from an insurance company. This may produce a duplicate claim and result in a delay of payment of the original claim. Most medical offices, however, send a tracer as the first contact about overdue claims. A tracer, whether sent in print or by e-mail, contains the basic billing information and asks the carrier about its status. Using an electronic program, an aging report can be produced and used to determine how long a claim has been submitted yet not paid or denied. Outstanding claims are aged (how long the claim has been submitted), usually by a certain number of days, such as 1–30 days or 31–60 days.

In addition to regular claim follow-up, the administrative medical assistant will need to follow up claims that have been denied for unclear reasons or are late because of special situations. Examples include the following:

- An unclear denial of payment or an incorrect payment is received on an EOB or ERA; follow-up should be done to determine the cause of the problem and to rectify it.
- The carrier asks for more information to process the claim—namely, a report on a new procedure for which there is no *CPT* specific code and an unspecified code was used; the assistant should follow up with a report from the physician, describing the procedure and the situation in which it was used.
- The carrier notifies the medical office that a claim is being investigated with regard to a possible elective condition; after a period of 30 days from receiving such a notice, if nothing further has been received, follow-up should be done.

In some situations, the administrative medical assistant will need to submit a new claim. Examples include the following:

- A mistake has been made in billing: The physician forgot to check off a procedure on the patient encounter form.
- A claim was overlooked by the physician's office: A patient had a series of visits for allergy injections, and one of the visits was not included.

Similarly, there are situations in which the insurance carrier rejects a claim and asks for resubmission:

- The wrong diagnosis or procedure codes are submitted.
- Information is incomplete or missing (for example, no accident date is given).
- The charges, units, and costs do not total properly.

In short, the administrative medical assistant should study the ERA/EOB carefully to understand any noncovered benefits, deductibles, copayment responsibilities, and other reasons for any noncoverage in the claim. If any of the explanations on a claim seem unfair or unclear, the insurance carrier should be contacted for help. Most insurance carriers have staff members whose primary job is to answer questions about claims. If necessary, an appeal should be initiated by the medical office. It is the responsibility of the assistant to take the time and care necessary to process and complete clean insurance claims accurately and to follow up in whatever way is required, so that prompt and precise compensation is received.

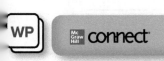

GO TO PROJECT 8.2 AND PROJECT 8.3
AT THE END OF THIS CHAPTER

Just as it is important for the medical office's cash flow to have claims approved and paid promptly by insurance carriers, it is also important to help ensure prompt payments from patients. The administrative medical assistant can facilitate the prompt receipt of payments from patients by keeping all transactions in each patient's account current and by being alert to the status of each account, such as 30 days past due.

The method of payment is arranged at the time of the patient's first visit. In most offices, a combination of methods is used and may include the following:

- Patients pay at the time of the visit by cash, check, debit card, credit card, or other electronic payment method. This type of collection is referred to as **collection at the time of service.** Copayments, as required by HMOs and other managed care plans, are always collected at the time of service.
- Bills are mailed to patients as designated by office policy, such as weekly or monthly or at the end of a procedure or hospital stay.
- Patients pay a fixed amount weekly or monthly until the bill is paid in full.
- Bills are sent to health insurance carriers.
- Some physicians work on a cash-only basis.
- A patient with a poor credit rating or whose checks have been returned for nonsufficient funds may be on a cash-only basis.

Methods of Payment

The assistant must be careful to enter each payment in the patient's ledger and in the daily summary record. The patient's name, the services rendered, the charges, the payment received on the account, and any balances should be included.

Payments should be given to the administrative medical assistant, not the physician. A receipt must be given to the patient who pays cash. An example of a receipt is shown in Figure 8.7. Copies of receipts are kept as permanent records. The patient should be advised to keep the receipt and a copy of the patient encounter form for income tax purposes in claiming medical deductions. If the patient pays by check, the canceled check is the receipt. Credit, debit card, and other forms of electronic payments appear on the patient's statement from his or her financial institution. Patients also receive a copy of the authorization. For smaller amounts (for example, $25 or less), patients may not need to sign an authorization form.

Certain rules must be observed to safeguard money received. Cash, checks, and money orders should be kept in a secure location, such as a locked drawer. Currency should be separated by denomination. Checks should be immediately stamped on the

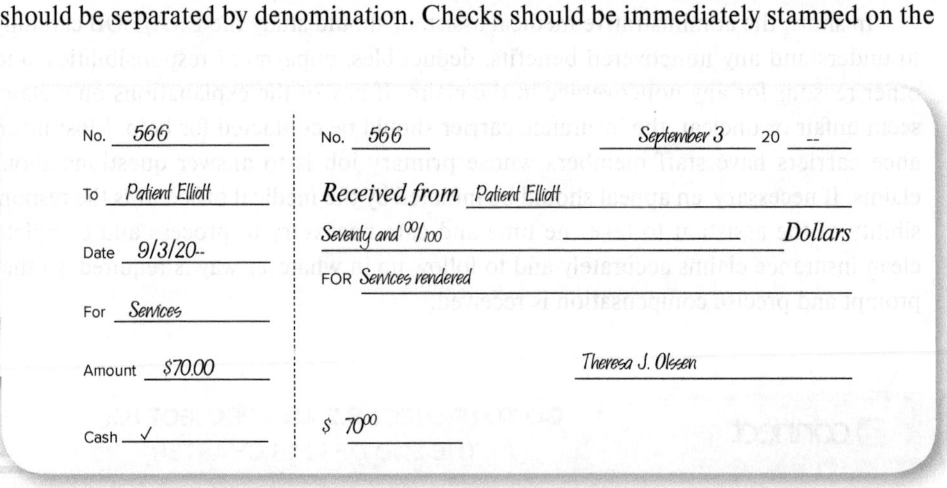

Figure 8.7

Completed Receipt

No. 566	No. 566 September 3 20 --
To Patient Elliott	*Received from* Patient Elliott
Date 9/3/20--	Seventy and 00/100 _____ *Dollars*
	FOR Services rendered
For Services	
Amount $70.00	Theresa J. Olssen
Cash ✓	$ 70 00

back with a restrictive endorsement, which specifies "Pay to the order of . . . " or "For deposit only." To minimize the danger of theft, money should be deposited in the bank daily.

Sending Statements

Although most bills are sent out once a month, a statement may be sent at the end of a procedure or episode of care, or upon discharge from the hospital. Practices decide to do either monthly billing or cycle billing. With **monthly billing,** bills are sent out once a month and are timed to reach the patient no later than the last day of the month, but preferably by the 25th of each month. Such a billing schedule enables patients to pay physicians' bills along with other monthly bills.

Traditionally, medical offices have used monthly billing. However, another system of billing, called **cycle billing,** is becoming more popular with medical offices. Cycle billing is designed to avoid once-a-month peak workloads and to stabilize the cash flow. It has been used by credit companies, utility companies, and other large businesses for some time. With cycle billing, all accounts are divided into fairly equal groups, the number of groups depending on how many times you wish to do billing during a month. If you decide to do billing four times a month (once a week), for example, you would divide the accounts into four groups, usually alphabetically, with each group billed on a different date. If cycle billing is used, the patient should be informed on the first visit approximately when the bill will be mailed.

There are two advantages of using cycle billing: (1) The workload is apportioned throughout the entire month and (2) a consistent monetary flow occurs throughout the month versus an influx of payments during only a specific period during the month. Billing is a major task for the administrative medical assistant. If bills are prepared once a month, entire days are usually sacrificed from other routine duties during that period in order to get statements in the mail. Cycle billing allows the assistant to factor in billing as part of a daily or weekly routine. An additional benefit is that the possibility of error is reduced, because more time and consideration can be given to each account.

Payment Plans

For the patient who is unable to pay a medical bill in one lump sum, a schedule of payments, or contract, can be agreed upon. The agreement should be in writing, and a copy of the plan should be given to the patient as a reminder of the commitment to pay the physician. The amount to be paid weekly or monthly is stated in the agreement, and it is used as a reference when corresponding with the patient about unpaid bills. Details of the contractual agreement should be documented in the patient's hardcopy or electronic record.

If the practice meets all four of the following criteria, a Truth-in-Lending Agreement must be completed and given to the patient to sign:

1. Credit is offered to patients.
2. Credit is offered on a regular basis, more than 25 times per year.
3. Finance charges are applied.
4. More than four payment installments.

Many practices have partnered with financial lending institutions to assist patients with paying medical debits.

Fee Adjustment

Should the need arise, the physician can adjust the cost of any procedure; the physician will then inform the administrative medical assistant of the **fee adjustment.** Fees should not be reduced as a way to receive payment quickly and avoid collection procedures.

One type of fee adjustment a medical office makes regularly with certain health plans is called a **write-off.** As explained elsewhere in the textbook, according to the rules of many insurance plans—for example, with most HMOs—when the physician's fee for a given service is higher than the insurance company's allowed fee for that service, a participating (PAR) provider is not permitted to bill the patient for the unclaimed portion of the fee. Instead, the physician must write off this amount by subtracting it from the patient's bill and accept the payment from the insurance company and the patient as payment in full—up to the allowable charge—for the procedure. Write-offs are entered into the patient ledger as fee adjustments. A nonparticipating (nonPAR) physician who does not accept the allowable charge may be permitted to bill the patient up to the physician's normal fee and not write off the difference. As discussed earlier, this is called balance billing.

If a physician chooses to reduce or cancel a fee, the decision must be in writing for the protection of the physician, since it is possible for such a reduction or canceling of a fee to be misinterpreted and even lead to a discrimination suit. For the same reasons, in computerized billing programs, it is important not to delete any transactions. Most electronic programs do not allow deletion of financial transactions. Rather, corrections, changes, and write-offs are made with adjustments to the existing transactions. Most billing programs contain a column in the patient ledger that displays such entries. The adjusting entries give both the medical office and the patient a history of events in case there is a billing inquiry or an audit.

In cases that involve a considerable sum, the patient may not be able to pay the fee and may have to seek financial assistance. The assistant should be acquainted with the local agencies to which a patient can be referred when financial assistance is needed. It is common for providers to have an established business relationship with lenders, thereby enabling patients to apply for credit in the medical office.

In the past, physicians have chosen to waive—not collect—charges for services rendered to other medical personnel, such as another physician or nurse, and their family members. However, many federal and state laws now prohibit the practice of professional courtesy. Filing an insurance claim and collecting benefits while waiving deductibles and other required payments are unlawful and violate Anti-Kickback laws.

At times, it may be in the best interest of the practice to render services for lesser or no fees. Patients are asked to sign and date documentation of the financial agreement, known as a hardship agreement, which becomes a permanent part of the medical record. Patients requesting a hardship agreement will be asked to provide supporting financial documentation of hardship and income.

Health Insurance

Many patients carry health insurance that provides payment for a portion of their medical expenses. Depending on whether or not the physician accepts the health insurance the patient has, the payment arrangement varies. Essentially, there are two options: (1) Patients are billed at the time of service or (2) they are billed after the insurance claim has been processed.

After an office visit, the new charges are entered into the patient's account. If the physician has not accepted assignment, patients are usually required to pay in full at the end of the visit. The administrative assistant gives the patient a receipt for the payment. In some cases, patients in this situation arrange to be billed later for payments due, depending on the office's policy. A written agreement containing the payment amount, the due date, and other pertinent payment information should be signed by the patient, and he or she should be given a copy of the contract. As a courtesy, the provider may file an insurance claim for the patient, even though for nonPARs this is not a requirement.

In contrast, when the physician accepts assignment and is going to file a claim, the patient usually pays only the required deductible and any coshare (required percentage or stated dollar amount) at the time of service. The amount of the patient's coshare payment is entered and subtracted from the balance due. Then the insurance claim for the service is created and transmitted to the insurance carrier. When the insurance payment is received, it is entered in the patient's account. Ideally, the total paid by the patient and all carriers should equal the allowable amount for the service(s) provided.

If there are procedures for which the insurance company did not pay or paid less than expected, the administrative medical assistant must sort out the various charges and benefits. The assistant determines which charges the patient should be billed for, if any are to be written off by the medical office, and which, if any, should be resubmitted— or even appealed—by studying the EOB or ERA. The patient's account is then updated accordingly, and a patient statement is sent on the appropriate billing date.

Third-Party Liability

Sometimes a person other than the patient assumes liability, or responsibility, for the charges. Such responsibility is called **third-party liability.** The assistant must contact this third party for verification of financial obligation. Relatives, particularly children of aged parents, may say they will be responsible for payment of the bill, but this promise must be in writing. Oral promises are not legally binding. A third party is not obligated by law unless he or she has signed an agreement to pay the charges. Therefore, a signed promise obtained prior to treatment will greatly reduce the credit risk. Other examples of third-party liability are workers' compensation claims and auto accidents. Claim numbers are needed to submit claims, and prior authorization, in most cases, is needed before treatment is rendered.

By contrast, a **guarantor** is an individual who is financially responsible for the account. Often, it is the policyholder of the insurance plan that covers the patient. The bottom line is that the individual who signed the registration form is financially responsible for payment of the account charges. For example, a parent who is a policyholder may be the guarantor for his or her **dependent** children. To be certain of the legal interpretation of guarantor, it is always a good idea to reference state laws for the particular state in which medical services were rendered. As part of the Health Care Reform Legislation of 2010 and effective September 23, 2010, adult children covered under a parent's insurance policy may continue being covered under the parent's medical insurance policy up to the age of 26, regardless of whether the adult child is a student or married.

connect   **GO TO PROJECT 8.4 AT THE END OF THIS CHAPTER**

8.4 DELINQUENT ACCOUNTS

A medical practice, like any business, has outstanding accounts. It is regrettable that patients are often slow and even delinquent in paying physicians. There are various reasons a patient may not pay a bill. For example, the patient may unintentionally or intentionally ignore the bill, the patient may not have the money to pay the bill, or the patient may be unwilling to pay the bill for a reason such as disagreeing with the amount of the bill. Examples of other reasons for nonpayment of medical bills include a patient's excessive debt, unemployment, illness, disability, family problems, and marital problems. The administrative medical assistant must know how to handle patients' accounts properly to reduce the physician's losses from unpaid bills.

Communicating with Patients

In a sense, the collection process actually begins with effective communications with patients about their responsibility to pay for services. When patients understand the charges and agree to pay them in advance, collecting the payments is not usually a problem. Most patients pay their bills on time. However, every practice has some patients who do not pay their bills when they receive their monthly statements.

One way to minimize problems with payments is to notify patients in advance of the probable cost of procedures that are not going to be covered by their plan. For example, many plans do not provide coverage for experimental or elective treatments or cosmetic procedures without medical necessity. Many patients, however, consider the services as good and necessary and are willing to pay for them. For these noncovered services, patients should be asked in writing to agree to pay. An agreement signed by the patient prior to service should also specify why the service will not be covered and the cost of the procedure. As mentioned previously, for Medicare patients, this form is called an Advance Beneficiary Notice (ABN) for noncovered services, a form that providers should have patients sign. It explains the service, the reason it will not be covered by Medicare, and the estimated charge. This form is also used when Medicare declares a service not reasonable and necessary and, therefore, does not cover it. Patients are asked to sign the ABN in advance of services being rendered.

A patient should also be informed about fees before a complicated set of procedures begins. A physician–in particular, a nonPAR physician–may need to clarify the payment arrangements with a patient before services are performed.

Guidelines for Payment

Management or the accounting department in every office must determine the **collection ratio** (total collections divided by net charges of the practice). The percentage will show the effectiveness of the collections (the higher the percentage, the more effective the collections). Management would then set the guidelines for payments–how much is to be collected daily, how much should be collected on each account, and so forth. As a general rule, at least one-third of the outstanding accounts should be collected each day.

Using the following figures, calculate the collection ratio and whether or not the collection methods are effective based on the guideline just stated.

	Total Collections	Net Charges	Collection Ratio	Effective Y/N
Day 1	$2,450.25	$6,320.00	_____	_____
Day 2	$1,425.50	$5,226.75	_____	_____

Collection methods are considered effective for Day 1–the collection ratio is 38.77 percent. However, the collection strategies for Day 2 are not effective. The collection ratio for Day 2 is only 27.27 percent.

HIPAA TIPS

Members of the healthcare team are prevented from leaving messages with live parties or on voice mail when those messages may violate patient confidentiality due to HIPAA regulations. Never mention a past due balance in a message. Simply leave a message to return your call. It is then important to document all calls in the patient's financial ledger.

Why should you not mention a past due balance during a message?

The Office Collection Policy

It is often the duty of the administrative medical assistant to collect payments on overdue accounts. Each month delinquent accounts (any unpaid accounts with a balance that is 30 days past due) should be aged to show their status in the collection process (that is, 30, 60, or 90 days past due). If a computerized billing program is used, a patient aging report is generated to show which patients' payments are due or overdue. For this reason, payments must always be entered promptly, so that at billing time there is no question about any balance due. For example, if payments received by the office totaled $5,000 for the month of January and the net outstanding accounts (accounts receivable) was $25,000, the collection ratio is 20 percent ($5,000 divided by $25,000).

Every office needs to establish a written course of action to be taken on overdue accounts. The physician will need to establish the office collection policy regarding collection procedures, including when to send statements, reminders, and letters and when to take final action. Usually, an automatic reminder notice and a second statement are mailed when a bill has not been paid 30 days after it was issued. Some medical offices phone a patient with a 30-day overdue account. If the bill is not then paid, a series of collection letters is generated at intervals, each more stringent in its tone and more direct in its approach. Collections letters should be sent using Certified Mail. Some medical offices use an outside collection agency to pursue large unpaid bills. Federal laws regulate credit and collections for businesses. Also, individual states may have laws that guide the collection process. Usually, as a last resort, payment for outstanding accounts may be pursued in small claims or civil claims court. The material in this chapter discusses basic collection procedures.

Laws Governing Collections

Collections from payers are considered business collections. Collections from patients, however, are consumer collections and are regulated by federal and state law. The Fair Debt Collection Practices Act of 1977 and the Telephone Consumer Protection Act of 1991 regulate debt collections, forbidding unfair practices, such as making threats, and the use of any form of deception or violence to collect a debt.

The Fair Debt Collection Practices Act (FDCPA) is enforced by the Federal Trade Commission (FTC) and regulates collection agencies and attorneys. Original creditors, such as a medical practice, are governed by state laws, which closely follow the FDCPA regulations. Medical practices should refer to state laws governing collection practices.

Under the FDCPA, debt collectors may contact a person by mail, telephone, e-mail, text, or fax. If a patient contacts the practice in writing to request that collection attempts stop, the practice may not contact the patient again for collection purposes except to notify the patient there will be no further contact or if the practice intends to take specific action, such as a lawsuit. Other guidelines under the FDCPA are as follows:

1. If an attorney is used by the patient, the practice may only contact the attorney. Other individuals may be contacted to find out where the patient lives and/or works. Most states prohibit contacting third parties for location information more than once. Financial issues may only be discussed with the attorney.
2. If the patient is contacted, within 5 days after the patient is first contacted, a written notice—called a validation notice—must be sent to the patient stating the amount and to whom the money is owed and what action the patient may take if he or she does not believe the money is owed. It is recommended to send the letter via Certified Mail, Return Receipt requested.
3. If the patient sends the practice a letter within 30 days after receiving the validation notice stating the money is not owed by them, the practice should not contact the patient again about the debt; however, the patient may be contacted again to send written verification of the medical debt, such as a copy of the bill or insurance EOB/ERA.

Certain actions are legally off limits. Harassing a patient or making false statements are illegal. Additionally, medical practices cannot threaten to arrest a patient for non-payment of a debt or garnish wages; collect interest, fees, or other charges in addition to the amount owed unless an original written/signed agreement allows such charges; or contact the patient using a postcard.

Collection by Telephone

A common method of collection is to phone the patient personally. The Telephone Consumer Protection Act of 1991 (TCPA), with revisions, provides laws governing tele-marketing and collection telephone calls. A phone call can be effective in reminding a person who has unintentionally forgotten to pay. Tact and experience are necessary in order to be effective in phone collections.

The following are some techniques of phone collection:

- Be sure you are talking to the person who is responsible for payment of the account. Avoid disclosure of PHI by following HIPAA regulations.
- Identify yourself, the practice, and the purpose of the call.
- Make the collection call in the evening, especially if the person who is responsible for payment is out during the day, but no later than 9 P.M. Collection calls may be placed after 8 A.M. but no later than 9 P.M. (local time of the called party) and not on Sunday or another day the patient recognizes as a Sabbath day.
- Never call a patient at a place of employment to inquire about an unpaid bill if the patient has requested not to be called at their workplace.
- Always use a pleasant manner and positive wording (such as "May I process your payment today using your credit or debit card?"). In other words, speak with an expectation of payment to reflect your confidence that the problem can be resolved.
- Ask to discuss the bill to determine whether the patient has any questions. This query should elicit some response, which is your cue to continue the rest of the conversation.
- Listen carefully and take accurate notes of the conversation.
- Do not show irritation in your voice or appear to be scolding the patient.
- Inform the person that you need to know why the bill has not been paid or why inquiries about the unpaid bill have not been answered.
- If the patient promises to pay, ask when you can expect a payment, the method of payment (cash, debit card, etc.), and the amount. Then make a note about the conversation, saying, for example, "I am making a note in your account file that you promised to pay $100 on September 10. Is that correct?"
- If the patient would prefer that you call his or her attorney, do not contact the patient directly again, unless asked to do so by the attorney. If the patient requests that no more calls be made to him or her concerning the debt, continue correspondence through the mail, with thorough documentation and evidence of delivery.

When collecting by phone, always keep complete, accurate records of who said what, who promised to pay, how much was promised, and when the payment was promised. Note any unusual circumstances. Ask the person responsible for the bill to write down the arrangement. An effective collection tool is to mail a confirmation of the phone details to the patient.

An important revision to the TCPA was implemented in 2014 in reference to using automated (autodialed) calls containing any telemarketing information to patients. The revision references telemarketing calls but states that collections calls that contain any telemarketing content do fall under the requirements of the revision. Under the 2014 revision, autodialed calls (collection calls) that do not contain any telemarketing content can be made to wireline (landline) phones without patient expressed consent. However, before automated calls can be made to a patient's wireless number, regardless of the presence or absence of telemarketing content, the patient must have given expressed oral or written consent that his or her wireless (cell) number may be used by the medical office. It is strongly recommended that written consent be obtained from the patient. The revision applies to autodialed calls and does not apply to calls that are manually dialed and that do not contain any type of prerecorded message.

Collection by Letter

The longer a bill remains unpaid, the less likelihood there is of collecting it. A bill should be followed up most vigorously after being overdue for 3 months. An effective method of collection at this point is to write a letter to the patient. Writing collection letters that bring results is a skill. Collection letters should be personal letters, not form letters. The letter should show that you are sincerely interested in the patient's problem and want to work out a solution. Collection letters should be brief, with short sentences. The letters should appeal to the patient's sense of pride and fair play, as well as a desire for a good credit rating. The amount that is due should be stated clearly in each collection letter, and the patient should be asked to call the assistant to discuss the situation by a stated date. Figure 8.8 shows an example of an effective first collection letter.

It is common practice to send no more than three collection letters, each letter using a more assertive tone. The second letter should refer to the first sent letter, and the third letter often attempts to stress the importance of payment before the account is submitted to a collection agency.

KAREN LARSEN, MD
2235 South Ridgeway Avenue   312-555-6022
Chicago, IL 60623-2240   Fax: 312-555-0025

July 1, 20--

Ms. Clair Munson
3492 Green Avenue South
Chicago, IL 60624–3422

Dear Ms. Munson:

In reviewing our accounts, I find that you have an overdue balance of $162.

As you are aware, all bills are due within 30 days of service. Is there some reason we have not heard from you?

Please send us your check for $162 or contact our office by July 10, 20--, to clear your account.

Sincerely,

Theresa J. Olssen

Theresa J. Olssen
Medical Administrative Assistant

Figure 8.8

Collection Letter

Terminated Accounts

The physician-patient relationship may be terminated for many reasons, but all reasons must be well documented to avoid the possible appearance of medical abandonment. The physician may close the medical practice, move to a different area, leave the patient's insurance network, or feel the patient needs care from a specialist. Patient behavior, or lack of medically compliant behavior, may also result in termination of the physician-patient relationship, such as the patient not adhering to the treatment plan. A physician who finds it impossible to extract payment from a patient may decide to terminate the physician-patient relationship. The account is then referred to as a **terminated account.**

If a patient is dismissed, careful and thorough documentation should be made. A letter documenting the dismissal should be sent to the patient by Certified Mail, Return Receipt requested. An offer to continue providing care on a cash-only basis for a stated period of time is offered to the patient so the patient's current status of health is not endangered. It will also provide evidence that the physician has neither medically abandoned nor refused care to the patient during the time when the patient is seeking another medical provider. Additionally, the physician may provide referrals and copies of the patient's records to other physicians for continuity of care. If a patient comes to the office requesting medical care after an account has been terminated, the physician should be consulted and may decide to see the patient on a cash-only basis.

Collection by Agency

If the patient has not paid the bill after a reasonable time and routine collection procedures have failed, the physician has two ways of attempting collection. The physician can sue the patient and go to court, which is a time-consuming and costly procedure. The other method is to turn the account over to a **collection agency.** Once an account has been turned over for collection, the office will have no further contact with the patient concerning billing.

The use of a collection agency is not a desirable option for collecting lower monetary unpaid bills, as most agencies work on a contingency basis. Approximately 20 to 50 percent of the amount due is lost when the account is turned over to an agency, and the longer the bill goes unpaid, the less money the physician will receive when the account is finally settled.

There are various types of collection agencies, and a physician will want to investigate an agency thoroughly to determine its reputation.

Statute of Limitations

If the physician fails to collect a fee within a certain period of time, the collection becomes illegal under the statute of limitations and no further claim on the debt is possible. Each state sets its own time limitation, which varies from 3 to 15 years. The physician should obtain legal counsel for advice concerning these statutes.

Credit Arrangements and the Truth in Lending Act

For large bills or special situations, some practices may elect to extend credit to patients. When credit agreements are made, patients and the practice agree to divide the bill into smaller payments over a period of months. If no finance charges are applied to unpaid balances, this type of arrangement is between the practice and the patient, and no legal regulations apply. High-deductible health plans and greater out-of-pocket expense for patients is contributing to the increase in credit arrangements for healthcare.

If, however, the practice adds finance or late charges, routinely offers credit arrangements (25 or more times per year), or the number of payments is more than four installments, the arrangement is governed by the federal Truth in Lending Act, which became law on July 1, 1968, and is part of the Consumer Credit Card Protection Act. Regulation Z requires that a disclosure form be completed and signed. The disclosure form notifies the patient in writing about the total amount, the finance charges (stated as a percentage), when each payment is due and the amounts, and the date the last payment is due. The disclosure form must be in clear, understandable language and signed by both the practice manager and the patient.

If a physician extends credit to one patient, under the Federal Equal Credit Opportunity Act (1975), the physician must extend the opportunity for credit arrangement to all patients who request it. Refusal can only be made based on ability or inability to pay; and if credit is refused, the physician must notify the patient of the refusal and reason for refusal. The patient has up to 60 days to request the reason for denial in writing.

Writing Off Uncollectible Accounts

If no payment has been made after the collection process, the administrative medical assistant follows the office policy on bills it does not expect to collect. Usually, if all collection attempts have been exhausted and it would cost more to continue than the amount to be collected, the process is ended. In this case, the amount is called an uncollectible account or bad debt and is written off from the expected revenues. Future services for patients who are responsible for uncollectible accounts are usually on a cash-only basis.

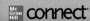 **GO TO PROJECT 8.5 AT THE END OF THIS CHAPTER**

8.1 Recognize and calculate charges for medical services, and process patient statements based on the patient encounter forms and the physician's fee schedule.	• The administrative medical assistant handles patient transactions, including entering charges for medical services rendered and payments received from patients and third-party payers. • The assistant enters transactions in the appropriate patient's account by referring to information on the patient's encounter form for the visit and the physician's fee schedule. Other charges, such as hospital charges, should be entered from course documents, such as a hospital rounds report. • Determine any charges that are the patient's responsibility, such as an office visit copayment. • Update the patient's account.

8.2 Compare and contrast the process of completing and transmitting insurance claims using both hardcopy and electronic methods.	• Complete the insurance claim form, either electronic or paper. The most commonly used claim form format is the CMS-1500 claim format.
	• Verify patient demographic, encounter, and insurance information.
	• Transmit, electronically or by Postal Service, the claim form to the insurance company, which decides to pay the fee, deny the claim, or pay a certain portion of the claim.
	• Verify the accuracy of the payment, and post any payments received from the insurance company to the patient's account.
	• Bill patient for coshares.
	• Both paper and electronic claims
	  — use patient information collected during the registration.
	  — use diagnostic and procedural information from the patient's encounter.
	  — gather needed information from either electronic or hardcopy records.
	• Electronic claims are entered only once, creating fewer opportunities for errors, whereas paper claims—even if produced electronically—may be scanned by the payer or physically reentered, creating greater opportunities for errors.
	• Payments resulting from electronic claims submission are faster and, most commonly, are electronic funds transfers. Payments from paper claims may be electronically deposited but may also be sent to the provider via a hardcopy check through the Postal Service, creating a much slower process.

8.3 Describe the different types of billing options used by medical practices for billing patients.	• The administrative medical assistant is responsible for receiving prompt payments from patients. The method of payment is arranged during the patient's first visit and may include a combination of the following: — Patients pay at the time of the visit by cash, check, or debit/credit card (coshares are always collected at this time). — Bills are mailed to patients monthly or at the end of a procedure or hospital stay, using either monthly or cycle billing. — Patients may pay, if necessary, according to an agreed-upon payment plan. — Bills are sent to health insurance carriers, and after payment is received, depending on the terms of the plan, the patient is billed for any balance due. — Patients pay for all charges when physicians work on a cash-only basis. • The physician can adjust the cost of any procedure, should the need arise. However, the decision must be documented, in writing, to protect against a malpractice suit if the adjustment is ever misinterpreted. • Adjusting entries are used to make corrections to patient accounts within a computerized billing system. Transactions are never deleted—they are adjusted.
8.4 Paraphrase the procedures and options available for collecting delinquent accounts.	• Guidelines are determined by each office in regard to payment—how much is to be collected daily, how much should be collected on each account, and so on. • Communications with patients from the start about what is expected from them in terms of payment are the beginning of the collection process. • Patients should be notified in advance of all procedures that are not covered by insurance. • Policies and procedures for handling overdue accounts are determined by each office in conjunction with state and federal laws. • Collection processes may be ended and the amount written off as a bad debt when the amount to be collected is less than the cost of collecting the debt. • State statutes are used to determine the legal period of time to continue the collection of a debt.

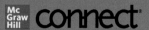

Chapter Projects

Project 8.1   **(LO 8.1) Updating Patient Statements**

 If you are instructed to complete this project using EHRclinic, your instructor will assign you the project as part of a Connect assignment.

WP Dr. Larsen asks you to update the billing. The established patients' statements are stored as files with the student materials on the EHRclinic® site at www.mhhe.com/EHRclinic, labeled according to the patients' last names. Save the statements onto your own external storage device. These are the billing statements that you will work from. Use Dr. Larsen's fee schedule—Working Paper 50 (WP 50)—and the following information to update the patients' statements. After updating the statements, print all of them for your file.

October 11, 20–:

- David Kramer*   NP preventive checkup,   Diagnostic code: ZØØ.129
                         age 5; UA (81001);
                         HGB (85018)

- Erin Mitchell*   99202; UA (81001);   Diagnostic code: N39.Ø
  *David Kramer, Erin   UC (87088)
  Mitchell, Donald
  Mitchell are on one
  account. The guarantor
  is Alan Mitchell.

- Gary Robertson   99212; UA(81001); UC (87088) Diagnostic code: N39.Ø
- Laura Lund   99213; Pap smear   Diagnostic code: N94.6
- Jeffrey Kramer   99212   Diagnostic code: H66.9Ø
- Joseph Castro   99212   Diagnostic code: T15.82XA

October 12, 20–:

- Todd Grant   99212; ECG   Diagnostic code: RØØ.Ø
- Thomas Baab   EP preventive, age 54;   Diagnostic code: ZØØ.ØØ
                         UA(81001); CBC; SMA-8;
                         PSA; fasting lipid panel
- Ardis Matthews   99212   Diagnostic code: AØ8.4
- Marc Phan   99212   Diagnostic code: J4Ø

Project 8.2   **(LO 8.2) Internet Research: Comparing Appeal Processes**

Every third-party payer has its own appeal process. Using your favorite search engine, visit the website of your health plan, a friend's plan, or a major plan you know about, and research the plan's appeal process. Then go to the Medicare website at www.medicare.gov and read about how to appeal a Medicare claim. How do the processes compare? Which process is more complicated? Why do you think this is the case? Answer these questions, and be prepared to discuss your findings.

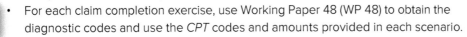

Project 8.3 **(LO 8.2) Completing Claim Forms**

Using the information listed here and NUCC instructions in Table 8.1, go to your assignment in Connect and use the online, electronic claim form in the chapter project "Completing Claim Forms" to complete the following five insurance claims:

- The place of service is Code 11 (24B).
- The physician is Jack E. Smith, MD, Suite 101, 400 E. Elm Street, Anytown, USA 12345-6789. His EIN IS 07071023. Phone 312-555-0874. NPI# is 6374322.
- The patients all live in Anytown, USA.
- For each claim completion exercise, use Working Paper 48 (WP 48) to obtain the diagnostic codes and use the *CPT* codes and amounts provided in each scenario.

A. **Edward Walker, 432 East High Street 12345-0432**
Date of Birth: 3/18/31
Patient is insured person, Medicare PLUS, 1601 Sunny Street,
Someplace, USA 66778-1601
Signature on file
Medicare Beneficiary Identifier: 1FG4TF6NJ28
Patient Phone Number: 555-555-5555
Patient Account Number: WALKEED0
Abdominal pain and non-insulin-dependent diabetes mellitus, Type 2
Seen in office

4/20/2028	Office visit, intermediate, 99213	$30.00
	Test feces for blood, 82270	$15.00
	Automated hemogram, 85027	$20.00
	Phlebotomy, 99195	$15.00

B. **Amber Shemwell, 3456 Sweetberry Lane 12345-3456**
Date of Birth: 11/27/82
Patient is insured person, Travelers Insurance Company, 1822 West Street
Someplace, USA 66778-1822. Insurance is through her employer.
Group Number GF061010.
Not related to employment or accident
Signature on file
Insured's ID Number: 98765A
Patient Phone Number: 555-444-4444
Patient Account Number: SHEMWAM0
Arthritis, acute low back pain
Seen in office

4/21/2028	Office visit, intermediate, 99213	$30.00
	X-ray lumbar spine, AP & lateral, 72100	$129.00
	Phlebotomy, 99195	$15.00
	Automated hemogram, 85027	$20.00
	X-ray lumbar spine, AP & lateral, 72100	$129.00

C. **Sherry Johnson, daughter, 2350 West Schaffer Road, 12345-2350**
Date of Birth: 11/25/99
Insured: Jeffrey Johnson Date of Birth: 9/5/1974. Address is the same as patient.
Self-employed
BCBS Insurance, 5501 Linn Road, Someplace, USA 66772-5501
Signature on file
Insured's ID Number: 99999D
Patient Phone Number: 312-555-4563
Patient Account Number: JOHNSSH0
Acute sinusitis
Seen in office

04/24/2028	Office visit, limited, 99212	$25.00

D. **Melissa Jones, wife, 286 South Roberts Road, 12345-0286**
Date of Birth: 12/3/73
Self-employed
Metropolitan Insurance, 5712 Long Avenue, Suite 309, Someplace, USA 66772-5712
Insured: Brad Jones Date of Birth: 10/15/68
Signature on file
Insured's ID Number: 112222
Patient Phone Number: 312-555-4845
Patient Account Number: JONESME0
Acute edema, proteinuria, acute vaginitis
Seen in office

04/25/2028	Office visit, extended, 99204	$45.00
	Catheterization, urethra, 51701	$30.00
	Endometrial biopsy, 58100	$130.00
	Urinalysis, 81001	$20.00

E. **Adam Westerfield, 2584 Bradford Road, 12345-2584**
Date of Birth: 8/13/45
Medicare, 1801 Sunny Street, Someplace, USA 66778-1081
(This is the patient's primary insurance)
Aetna, 626 Short Boulevard, Anywhere, USA 52407
(This is the patient's secondary insurance)
Signature on file
Insured's ID Number: 2BB3NT2RR34 (Medicare Beneficiary Identifier) 57893321 (Aetna)
Patient Phone Number: 312-555-3635
Patient Account Number: WESTEAD0
Insulin-dependent diabetes mellitus, Type 1
Seen in office

4/24/2028	Office visit, intermediate, 99213	$30.00
	Assay blood fluid, glucose, 82947	$30.00
	Phlebotomy, 99195	$15.00

(LO 8.3) Posting Payments

If you are instructed to complete this project using EHRclinic, your instructor will assign you the project as part of a Connect assignment.

One insurance payment is received and two patients stop in the office on October 12 with checks to update their accounts.

- Insurance payment of $35.20, check number 1816, is received for Florence Sherman's 10-05-28 office visit.
- Theresa Dayton pays $33.60, check number 4211.
- Thomas Baab pays $82.20, check number 1160.

Post the payments to their statements. Reprint these statements.

Project 8.5 **(LO 8.4) Preparing an Effective Collection Letter**

After updating the statements, you notice that Suzanne Roberts has not made a payment for 3 months. There are collection notations on her statement: September 27, reminder sent; October 7, a follow-up phone call. Compose a letter to Ms. Roberts, requesting payment. Date the letter October 17. This document should be typed and submitted to your instructor. Remember to update the patient's account ledger.

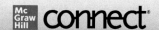
Listening Skills (LO 8.4)

Is listening the same as hearing? The answer is no. Hearing is a physical ability and listening is a skill. The ability to listen helps us make sense of what another person is saying. It greatly enhances our understanding and may even open doors that may not otherwise be open. If you are a good listener, you will be more productive in your career, and more opportunities will come your way. You should find it easy to establish positive working relationships with physicians, office managers, patients, and colleagues. Good listeners are well respected. As a healthcare professional, you will need to not only speak but also listen to the individuals you deal with on a daily basis. **Describe a situation in the collection process that will require you to both listen and speak. What could occur if communication fails during this situation?**

Respond to Facts, Not Feelings (LO 8.2)

As a part of your responsibilities, you are answering the phones for the day. An angry patient calls and begins yelling at you about an EOB that she has received that denied her claim as being "not medically necessary." It will be important that you attempt to listen to the facts the patient is giving. **How would you handle this situation?**

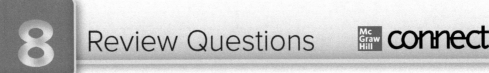
USING TERMINOLOGY

Match the term or phrase on the left with the correct answer on the right.

_____ 1. [LO 8.2] Electronic claim

_____ 2. [LO 8.2] CMS-1500 form

_____ 3. [LO 8.3] Cycle billing

_____ 4. [LO 8.4] Collection agency

_____ 5. [LO 8.1] Fee schedule

_____ 6. [LO 8.4] Collection ratio

_____ 7. [LO 8.3] Write-off

_____ 8. [LO 8.2] Clearinghouse

_____ 9. [LO 8.2] ERA

_____ 10. [LO 8.1] Patient statement

a. An accounting of patient services, charges, payments/adjustments, and balance

b. Payment determination report sent by insurance carrier

c. Percentage that shows the effectiveness of collection methods

d. Insurance claim prepared on and transmitted by computer

e. Service used to pursue payment for services

f. Listing of medical procedures/services and usual charges

g. Universal claim form

h. Billing method used to provide consistent cash flow

i. Service that collects, corrects, and transmits insurance claims

j. Financial adjustment for PAR providers of the difference between submitted and allowable charges

CHECKING YOUR UNDERSTANDING

Select the most correct answer.

1. [LO 8.1] Dr. Alonzo has rendered a noncovered procedure to Mrs. Shepherd, who is covered by Medicare. She was not advised before the procedure that it is not covered. The medical office should

    a. charge Mrs. Shepherd for the procedure.
    b. obtain Mrs. Shepherd's signature on an ABN.
    c. adjust the procedure charge off Mrs. Shepherd's account.
    d. charge Mrs. Shepherd the Medicare allowable amount for the service.

2. [LO 8.1] An appointment was scheduled for a new patient, who asked how much the fee would be for the visit. The administrative medical assistant should

    a. quote the highest new patient exam fee to the patient.
    b. transfer the call to the office manager.
    c. quote the midlevel new patient exam fee to the patient.
    d. provide an estimate of the exam but explain that the estimate is prior to other services, such as blood work.

3. [LO 8.2] Hardcopy insurance claim forms will produce which of the following?

    a. ERA

    b. EHR

    c. PAR

    d. EOB

4. [LO 8.2] Which of the following is not necessary information on an insurance claim form?

    a. Patient's gender

    b. Patient's sexual orientation

    c. Insured's employment data

    d. Procedure codes

5. [LO 8.2] To complete the insurance form, the medical biller/coder needs the dates when Juan Gomez was unable to work. To find this information, the coder would refer to the

    a. patient's chart.

    b. patient registration form.

    c. lab report.

    d. patient's ledger.

6. [LO 8.2] Before mailing patient statements, which of the following reports should be reviewed for delinquent accounts?

    a. ERA

    b. Aging report

    c. Daily report

    d. EOB

7. [LO 8.3] For her office visit, Katie was asked to pay $20, which is her cost for today's office visit through her managed care health plan. The $20 represents Katie's

    a. prior account balance.

    b. copayment/coshare.

    c. payment toward a scheduled procedure.

    d. monthly payment amount.

8. [LO 8.3] Listed on an account are the father, the mother, and two minor children. One insurance policy, held by the mother, covers all four family members. Who is the guarantor of the account?

    a. Mother

    b. Father

    c. Insurance carrier

    d. Mother and father

9. [LO 8.4] The administrative medical assistant must call patients whose accounts are 30 to 60 days past due. All of the following are recommended phone strategies *except*

    a. call during evening hours prior to 9 P.M.

    b. ask why the bill has not been paid.

    c. discuss results of lab tests and/or procedures.

    d. use effective listening techniques.

10. **[LO 8.4]** Statutes of limitations for collecting debt

    a. are mandated by the federal government.

    b. may exceed 15 years.

    c. are set state to state and may vary.

    d. are not relevant to the office collection policy.

THINKING IT THROUGH

These questions cover important points in this chapter. Using your critical-thinking skills, play the role of an administrative medical assistant as you answer each question. Be prepared to discuss your responses.

1. **[LO 8.2]** Wayne Elliot asks you why he was charged for two office visits when his daughters, Emily and Rose, were seen at the same time in the same room for the same problem—an earache. Explain the reasoning behind the charges.

2. **[LO 8.3]** You receive an EOB for a patient who is covered by an HMO. The HMO did not pay for services received on May 5, which is when the patient visited Dr. Larsen for her annual PET scan. You check your records and find that the same insurance carrier paid for previous PET scans for the same patient in past years. What should you do?

3. **[LO 8.4]** You receive an ERA from Blue Cross Blue Shield for a Medicare patient. The amount received for the claim is $60, which is $20 less than the provider's usual fee of $80. Since the doctor you work for accepts assignment for Medicare patients, the medical practice will need to write off this amount. You decide to delete the initial fee of $80 in the computerized patient ledger and key in $60, so that the account balances. Why is this a mistake?

4. **[LO 8.3]** You notice that an elderly patient is scheduled for a minor surgical procedure that will remove unsightly dark patches of skin, a procedure that is considered cosmetic by most insurance companies. Why is it a good idea to point this out to the patient before the procedure?

Practice Finances

LEARNING OUTCOMES

After studying this chapter, you will be able to

9.1 explain, using accounting terminology, the procedures for maintaining two essential financial records.

9.2 summarize the main focus of the Red Flag Requirements as they relate to the medical office as a business.

9.3 list three banking duties of the administrative medical assistant.

9.4 explain how an employee's net salary is determined.

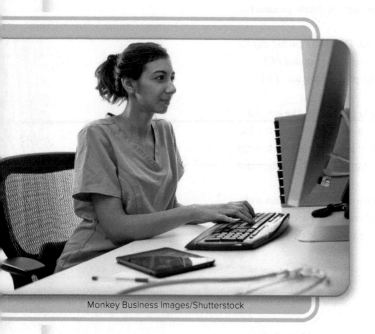

Monkey Business Images/Shutterstock

KEY TERMS

Study these important words, which are defined in this chapter, to build your professional vocabulary:

absolute accuracy	blank endorsement	Employer Identification Number (EIN)	interest
accounting	bookkeeping	e-signature	monthly summary
accounts payable (A/P)	cash basis	FICA (Federal Insurance Contributions Act)	patient ledger cards
accounts receivable (A/R)	charge/receipt slips		payroll
accrual method	daily journal	full endorsement	petty cash fund
aging reports	deductions	FUTA (Federal Unemployment Tax Act)	posting
annual summary	deposits		practice analysis report
audit	direct earnings	income statement	procedure day sheet
balance sheet	EFT (electronic funds transfer)	indirect earnings	Red Flag Requirements
bank reconciliation			restrictive endorsement

ABHES

4.e. Perform risk management procedures.

5.c. Assist the patient in navigating issues and concerns that may arise (i.e., insurance policy information, medical bills, and physician/provider orders).

7.a. Gather and process documents.

7.b. Navigate electronic health records systems and practice management systems.

7.c. Perform billing and collection procedures.

10.b. Demonstrate professional behavior.

www.abhes.org/accreditationmanual

The ABHES standards appear with permission of The Accrediting Bureau of Health Education Schools

CAAHEP

V.P.4.a. Coach patients regarding office policies.

V.P.6. Demonstrate professional telephone techniques.

VII.C.1.a. Define the following bookkeeping term: *charges*.

VII.C.1.b. Define the following bookkeeping term: *payments*.

VII.C.1.c. Define the following bookkeeping term: *accounts receivable*.

VII.C.1.d. Define the following bookkeeping term: *accounts payable*.

VII.C.1.e. Define the following bookkeeping term: *adjustments*.

VII.C.3.a. Identify precautions for accepting the following type of payments: cash.

VII.C.3.b. Identify precautions for accepting the following type of payments: check.

VII.C.3.c. Identify precautions for accepting the following type of payments: credit card.

VII.C.3.d. Identify precautions for accepting the following types of payments: debit card

VII.C.4.a. Describe types of adjustments made to patient accounts, including non-sufficient funds (NSF) checks.

VII.C.5. Identify types of information contained in the patient's billing record.

VII.P.1.a. Perform accounts receivable procedures to patient accounts, including posting charges.

VII.P.1.b. Perform accounts receivable procedures to patient accounts, including posting payments.

VII.P.1.c. Perform accounts receivable procedures to patient accounts, including posting adjustments.

VII.P.2. Prepare a bank deposit.

2015 Standards and Guidelines for the Accreditation of Educational Programs in Medical Assisting, Appendix B, Core Curriculum for Medical Assistants, Medical Assisting Education Review Board (MAERB), 2015.

INTRODUCTION

The physician's time and medical expertise are perhaps the most valuable assets in a medical practice. Because the practice is a business as well as a service, it is required to produce a profit. The administrative medical assistant protects and enhances the assets of the practice by handling many financial responsibilities on the business side. When assistants are working with patients' financial information, standards should be in place to protect patients from identity theft. Governmental Red Flag Requirements are federal standards that medical practices should follow.

9.1 ESSENTIAL FINANCIAL RECORDS

Administrative medical assistants help with **accounting**—the methodical recording, classifying, and summarizing of business transactions—in the medical office. The physician must have a record of all transactions and must be able to prepare tax records. Either an accountant employed by the practice or the Internal Revenue Service (IRS) may wish to perform an **audit,** or review of all financial data, in order to ensure the accuracy and completeness of the data. The assistant also makes all records available to the IRS and keeps all source documents for tax purposes. These tasks require a working knowledge of tax regulations and of the accounting process. The part of the process that is the accurate recording of transactions is called **bookkeeping.**

Accounting for the practice may be done in one of two ways: on a cash basis or on an accrual basis. If the practice operates on a **cash basis,** charges for services are not recorded as income to the practice until payment is received and expenses are not recorded until they are paid. With the **accrual method,** income is recorded as soon as it is earned, whether or not the payment is received, and expenses are recorded when they are incurred. Whichever way the practice decides to keep its accounts, there are certain essential records that must be carefully kept and maintained. The assistant's task is to enter data accurately the first time and to perform the task of **posting** to records, or transferring amounts from one record to another.

The financial records that are used daily in the practice include the following:

- *The daily journal:* The **daily journal** is a record of services rendered, daily fees charged, payments received, and adjustments. It is also called a *general journal, day sheet,* or *daily earnings record.* Most medical providers now use computerized daily journals (day sheets), commonly referred to as a *procedure* day sheet (which will be discussed later in this chapter).
- *Charge/receipt slips:* **Charge/receipt slips** provide a record of the physician's services and the charges for these. These slips are also called *patient encounter forms* (discussed earlier in the text).
- *Ledgers:* **Patient ledger cards** contain a patient's name, services rendered, charge, payment, and balance. Computerized patient ledgers are referred to as simply "patients' accounts." **Accounts payable (A/P)** ledgers record expense amounts owed to a supplier or creditor. Examples of accounts payable are rent, equipment rental, and office supplies. **Accounts receivable (A/R)** ledgers record the balance of payments due from patients or others (third-party payers) on current accounts.
- *Summaries:* The **monthly summary** shows the daily charges and payments for an entire month. The **annual summary** provides the monthly charges and payments for an entire year. In some practices, quarterly summaries are prepared (a *quarter* is a 3-month period).

Each of these records may be maintained electronically, and most offices, even if they have not fully implemented EHRs, maintain their financial records with electronic software.

The assistant is responsible for accurately entering the data and keeping these essential records current. Data input errors have a ripple effect. When a mistake is made on financial data, other financial areas are also affected. For example, a patient was evaluated at a 99213 level, but the code 99214 was entered. The error affects not only the patient's account but also the daily accountability of how many procedures of each type have been rendered and their daily, weekly, and monthly totals. Accurate data input is a key skill for medical office personnel.

Financial records are the basis for ongoing decisions about collections and disbursements, and they provide a picture of the financial health of the practice. In all businesses, the managers speak of the importance of the **balance sheet,** the financial statement for a particular date that indicates the total assets (possessions of value, such as equipment), liabilities (debts), and capital (available dollars). Summaries are an important part of the balance sheet.

Another important financial document of the practice is the **income statement,** which shows profit and loss for a stated period of time, such as a quarter or year. All income is categorized and reported as gross income (income prior to deductions). Expenses are also categorized and totals are listed. Taxes are included as a business expense. A net total (income after expenses are deducted) is calculated. Income statements are a critical analysis tool for determining the financial health of a business.

Accounting Software

Most practices use an accounting software package to perform all necessary accounting functions. Several software applications have been customized with vocabulary and features specific to medical practices. Software programs require some effort to learn and manipulate. However, they save time by automatically performing routine tasks and most mathematical calculations.

Daily Journal

The daily journal, manual and electronic, is used to record daily fees charged and payments received. It is, then, the financial source document (journal) used for accounts receivable (fees charged) and cash receipts (payments received). Fees charged, payments received, and adjustments must be recorded promptly in the daily journal.

It is necessary to have an accurate balance of accounts. The manual daily journal, used with older manual systems, in Figure 9.1, shows typical entries and balances entered onto a manual daily journal. There is a section, usually in the lower left corner of the page, labeled "Proof of Posting." In this case, *proof* does not mean that the correct amounts were charged. *Proof* means only that the columns balance. Accuracy is obtained by using the section at the bottom of the journal page, in the center, labeled "Accounts Receivable Control." *Accounts Receivable* in the label refers to the balance due from patients on current accounts. By maintaining this section of the daily journal, the practice keeps a "control" on the amount of money it is owed. Every day, the charges are added and the payments are subtracted from the previous day's balance. The result is the current day's accounts receivable balance.

The section labeled "Daily Cash" in the lower right corner is used to account for the daily cash flow, or the amount of cash received that day, normally from patients

Figure 9.1

Manual Daily Journal

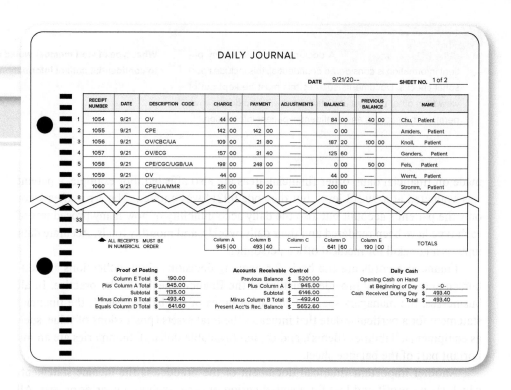

DAILY JOURNAL

DATE 9/21/20--   SHEET NO. 1 of 2

RECEIPT NUMBER	DATE	DESCRIPTION CODE	CHARGE	PAYMENT	ADJUSTMENTS	BALANCE	PREVIOUS BALANCE	NAME
1	1054	9/21	OV	44 00	—	—	84 00	40 00	Chu, Patient
2	1055	9/21	CPE	142 00	142 00	—	0 00	—	Amders, Patient
3	1056	9/21	OV/CBC/UA	109 00	21 80	—	187 20	100 00	Knoll, Patient
4	1057	9/21	OV/ECG	157 00	31 40	—	125 60	—	Ganders, Patient
5	1058	9/21	CPE/CGC/UGB/UA	198 00	248 00	—	0 00	50 00	Fels, Patient
6	1059	9/21	OV	44 00	—	—	44 00	—	Wernt, Patient
7	1060	9/21	CPE/UA/MMR	251 00	50 20	—	200 80	—	Stromm, Patient
8									
33									
34									
	ALL RECEIPTS MUST BE IN NUMERICAL ORDER			Column A 945 00	Column B 493 40	Column C —	Column D 641 60	Column E 190 00	TOTALS

Proof of Posting		Accounts Receivable Control		Daily Cash	
Column E Total	$ 190.00	Previous Balance	$ 5201.00	Opening Cash on Hand at Beginning of Day	$ -0-
Plus Column A Total	$ 945.00	Plus Column A	$ 945.00	Cash Received During Day	$ 493.40
Subtotal	$ 1135.00	Subtotal	$ 6146.00	Total	$ 493.40
Minus Column B Total	$ −493.40	Minus Column B Total	$ −493.40		
Equals Column D Total	$ 641.60	Present Acc'ts Rec. Balance	$ 5652.60		

making payments using cash. Petty cash, mentioned later in this chapter, is used not to receive cash payments but to pay for small cash items.

In the figure, the following events are recorded for Patient Chu. All transaction data was recorded on Receipt #1054 dated 9/21/20–.

1. Tamara's encounter was for an office visit (OV).
2. Her charge for today's OV was $44 (Column A).
3. She did not make a payment today (Column B).
4. No adjustment was made to today's charge (Column C).
5. The total balance on her account is $84 (Column D).
6. Tamara had a previous account balance of $40. Therefore, adding the previous balance (Column E) to today's charge (Column A) and subtracting any payments and/or adjustments (Columns B and C) results in Tamara's account balance (Column D): $40 + $44 − $0 = $84.

Computerized Daily Journal. Medical management software provides electronic daily journal forms. The example shown in Figure 9.2 is a Procedure Day Sheet. The **procedure day sheet** lists numerically all procedures performed on a given day. It also provides patient names, document numbers, places of service (POS), and debits and credits.

Methods of Bookkeeping

There are two main methods of bookkeeping: single-entry method and double-entry method. A third and older method, which is a manual accounting system referred to as a *pegboard system,* was used extensively by medical practices in the past, but most medical offices have transferred accounting functions to computerized systems. Debits and credits summarized in columns at the bottom of the day sheet are used to balance the manual day sheets.

• *Single-entry method:* This system requires only one entry for each transaction and is the oldest system. It is, however, a challenging system to use because it is not a self-balancing method; therefore, users find it hard to recognize errors.

Entry	Date	Chart	Name	Document	POS	Debits	Credits
80048							
146	9/21/2028	Clarence R: AA0039	Rogers, Clarence	0309240000		51.00	
		Total of 80048			Quantity: 1	$51.00	$0.00
81001							
89	9/21/2028	Theresa D: AA012	Dayton, Theresa	0309240000		24.00	
117	9/21/2028	Ardis M: AA022	Matthews, Ardis	0309240000		24.00	
		Total of 81001			Quantity: 2	$48.00	$0.00
85025							
88	9/21/2028	Theresa D: AA012	Dayton, Theresa	0309240000	11	25.00	
116	9/21/2028	Ardis M: AA022	Matthews, Ardis	0309240000	11	25.00	
		Total of 85025			Quantity: 2	$50.00	$0.00
87088							
118	9/21/2028	Ardis M: AA022	Matthews, Ardis	0309240000		35.00	
		Total of 87088			Quantity: 1	$35.00	$0.00
88150							
87	9/21/2028	Theresa D: AA012	Dayton, Theresa	0309240000		33.00	
125	9/21/2028	Ana M: AA024	Mendez, Ana	0309240000		33.00	
		Total of 88150			Quantity: 2	$66.00	$0.00
93000							
145	9/21/2028	Clarence R: AA0039	Rogers, Clarence	0309240000		70.00	
		Total of 93000			Quantity: 1	$70.00	$0.00

Figure 9.2

Procedure Day Sheet

- *Double-entry method:* This system requires more knowledge of accounting principles than the single-entry method does. It is a method based on the accounting equation: assets equal liabilities plus owner equity. In businesses where this method is used, one account must be debited and another account credited after each transaction. Thus, the system takes more time to use.

Summaries

In many practices, the physician will want to analyze charges, cash receipts, and disbursements at the end of the month, at the end of each quarter, and at the end of the year. The purpose of analyzing summaries is to compare the present financial performance of the practice with its performance last year, last quarter, or last month. The physician, and in some cases an accountant, will look at cash receipts from certain kinds of services (such as EP Level III E/M codes), the expenses involved in running the office, and other categories. The analysis will help the physician plan for the future of the practice by cutting back on expenses, for example, or by investing in equipment that will enable the practice to offer more patients a particularly profitable service.

Computer Summaries. The use of a software program to provide summaries is an efficient way to assemble information. The database can be manipulated to provide a summary by procedure code or by the number of procedures within a certain time frame. It also can provide a comparative summary over time of payments used to make a deposit. Such software solutions are available in specialized medical accounting software programs.

In some electronic record systems, for example, a **practice analysis report** may be generated monthly or for another specified period of time. The purpose of the report is, as its name shows, to analyze the revenue of the practice for a specified period of time. In the report, the description of and revenue for each procedure are shown first, as in Figure 9.3a. A summary page at the end of the report then shows the total charges, patient payments, copayments, adjustments, and so on. The summary page is shown in Figure 9.3b. This report may also be used to generate financial statements for the practice.

Karen Larsen MD
Practice Analysis
Show all data where the Date From is between 9/1/2028, 9/30/2028

Code	Description	Amount	Units	Average	Cost	Net
80048	SMA-8 Basic metabolic panel	51.00	1	51.00	0.00	51.00
81001	UA with microscopy	48.00	2	24.00	0.00	48.00
85025	Hemogram (CBC) with differential	50.00	2	25.00	0.00	50.00
87088	UC	35.00	1	35.00	0.00	35.00
88150	Pap	66.00	2	33.00	0.00	66.00
93000	Electrocardiogram (ECG)	70.00	1	70.00	0.00	70.00
99212	OV, EP, Focused	44.00	1	44.00	0.00	44.00
99213	OV, EP, Expanded	60.00	1	60.00	0.00	60.00
99395	Preventive, EP, 18-39 yrs.	272.00	2	136.00	0.00	272.00
INSPAY	Insurance payment	-917.15	22	-41.69	0.00	-917.15
PATPAY	Patient payment - check	-411.60	7	-58.80	0.00	-411.60

(a)

Karen Larsen MD
Practice Analysis
Show all data where the Date From is between 9/1/2028, 9/30/2028

Code	Description	Amount	Units	Average	Cost	Net
		Total Procedure Charges				$696.00
		Total Global Surgical Procedures				$0.00
		Total Product Charges				$0.00
		Total Inside Lab Charges				$0.00
		Total Outside Lab Charges				$0.00
		Total Billing Charges				$0.00
		Total Charges				$696.00
		Total Insurance Payments				-$917.15 *
		Total Cash Copayments				$0.00
		Total Check Copayments				$0.00
		Total Credit Card Copayments				$0.00
		Total Patient Cash Payments				$0.00
		Total Patient Check Payments				-$411.60
		Total Credit Card Payments				$0.00
		Total Receipts				-$1,328.75
		Total Debit Adjustments				$0.00
		Total Credit Adjustments				$0.00
		Total Insurance Debit Adjustments				$0.00
		Total Insurance Credit Adjustments				$0.00
		Total Insurance Withholds				$0.00
		Total Adjustments				$0.00
		Net Effect on Accounts Receivable				-$632.75
		*Total Insurance Payments Include Insurance Takebacks of				$0.00

Practice Totals

Total # Procedures	53
Total Charges	$3,000.00
Total Payments	-$1,814.55**
Total Adjustments	
Accounts Receivable	$1,185.45

**Total Payments include Insurance Takeback Adjustments of $0.00

(b)

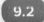

Karen Larsen MD
Patient Aging by Date of Service
As of October 7, 2028
Show all data where the Date From is on or before 10/7/2028

Chart	Name		Current 0 - 30	Past 31 - 60	Past 61 - 90	Past 91 ---->	Total Balance
AA012	Theresa Dayton		33.60				33.60
Last Pmt: -20.00	On:9/30/2028	(312)555-2231					
AA037	Suzanne Roberts				156.00		156.00
Last Pmt: -50.00	On:7/22/2028	(312)555-2267					
AA039	Clarence Rogers		86.20				86.20
Last Pmt: -100.00	On:9/30/2028	(312)555-5297					
AA040	Florence Sherman		35.20				35.20
Last Pmt: -8.80	On:10/5/2028	(312)555-1217					
	Report Aging Totals		$155.00	$0.00	$156.00	$0.00	$311.00
	Percent of Aging Total		38.5 %	0.0 %	50.2 %	0.0 %	100.0 %

Figure 9.4

Aging Report

In addition, many electronic medical record systems provide other useful summaries, such as **aging reports.** This analysis lists the amounts of money owed to the practice, and the report is organized according to the number of days due. In such a report, the aging begins on the date of the transaction and will report those debts that are current—or 0 to 30 days—and several other time frames of past due debts. See the example of an aging report in Figure 9.4.

Software spreadsheet capabilities also enhance the physician's ability to analyze the performance of the practice. These spreadsheets may be designed to provide profit and loss reports, expense reports, and budget planning documents. To create a program to serve your practice, the designer customizes the spreadsheet by specifying the format and creating formulas that will provide the desired calculations.

WP

Mc Graw Hill connect

IF ASSIGNED, GO TO OPTIONAL PROJECT 9.1 AT THE END OF THIS CHAPTER

9.2 IDENTITY THEFT IN THE MEDICAL OFFICE

Medical identity theft is a fast-growing area of criminal activity. Thieves steal an individual's personal information—such as a patient's name, Medicare or other provider identification number, and other identifying information—for purposes of securing healthcare, obtaining drugs, submitting fraudulent claims to gain illegal monetary benefits, or other illegal activity. This type of illegal activity can be conducted by medical personnel who know the workings of the medical insurance system. Computer hackers also attempt to gain access to a patient's personal information for purposes of medical identity theft. The thief who commits the crime can also be someone the patient knows and trusts. The medical office assistant must pay close attention to ERAs/EOBs and verify that their actual patient did receive the service listed.

Just as HIPAA regulations were implemented to protect patients' nonpublic health information, regulations known as **Red Flag Requirements** focus on identifying and verifying individuals in relation to information presented to the practice. In other words, the medical practice must make sure that persons presenting for services are who they say they are. Using the criminal act of identity theft to acquire medical and other types of services illegally is a growing challenge for society.

The following are some examples of possible identity theft:

- Checks with a different name than the patient's
- Patient complaints about bills for services they did not receive
- Medical records showing treatment that is inconsistent with the physical exam and/or history as reported by the patient

Who Must Comply

Financial institutions (that is, banks, credit unions, and other lending institutions) and other creditors must comply with federal Red Flag Requirements. Whether a medical practice is considered a "creditor" has been the topic of much debate. In 2010, the Red Flag Program Clarification Act amended the original definition of a *creditor*. Three requirements were defined in the act. If an entity, including a physician's office, uses any of the three criteria in the course of normal business, it would need to develop and implement an identity theft program utilizing the Red Flag Requirements. The three *creditor* criteria are

1. The practice obtains or uses consumer reports, either directly or indirectly, in connection with credit transactions.
2. The practice furnishes information to a consumer reporting agency in connection with credit transactions.
3. The practice advances funds to, or on behalf of, a patient based on an obligation of the patient to repay the funds.

EXAMPLE: RED FLAG REQUIREMENT CREDITOR

Dr. Larsen's office collects patients' payment histories on a quarterly basis and reports this information to a credit bureau. Based on Criterion 2, Dr. Larsen's medical practice is defined as a *creditor* and would need to develop and implement an identity theft program.

An individual may obtain medical services by using another person's identity, creating risk that the victim's medical records will be intermixed with the criminal's records. This may lead to serious consequences when the victim seeks medical treatment. Therefore, medical practices must know with a reasonable amount of certainty that persons seeking and receiving treatment are who they say they are. Even if a medical practice does not meet the criteria of a creditor, developing and implementing an identity theft program will help medical practices verify a patient's identity and protect patient information.

Covered Accounts

Covered accounts that must be protected are any personal accounts that allow multiple payments or transactions. This qualifies medical patients' accounts, as they usually are the primary source of financial transaction documents for a patient. Also, if there is a reasonable and predictable risk to the patient/customer or to the safety of the creditor, the account is considered a covered account because it is a transaction account. A transaction account is any account from which or into which the owner (patient) makes payments and/or transfers. If covered accounts are part of the medical practice, an identity theft program must be followed.

Red Flag Implementation

Each company/organization that fits the definition of a creditor with covered accounts (covered entity) must follow the Red Flag Requirements, also known as the *Red Flag Rules*. If a medical practice does not meet the criteria of a "covered entity," it is still a good financial practice to develop and implement an identity theft policy based on the Red Flag Requirements. The following are the parts of the Red Flag Requirements:

1. *Recognize and list red flags (warning signs) pertinent to your practice.* Each practice should study and identify triggers that suggest identity fraud. Make a comprehensive list. Alerts and updates from a consumer reporting guide may be used to list red flags. Other red flags may be in the form of suspicious documents, a change in PHI (such as an address change), and unusual account activity.

2. *Describe how your practice will discover/detect each red flag.*
   a. Put steps in place to obtain identifying information and to verify the identity of an individual who is seeking services.
   b. Implement effective methods of authenticating the identity of the patient requesting service or other transactions. Traditionally, a photo ID, such as a driver's license, was sufficient. However, more stringent methods may need to be used. Primary and secondary identifiers should be listed as acceptable forms of identification. Primary identifiers may include a valid driver's license or state ID card, valid passport, U.S. alien registration card, and military ID. Fingerprint readers may be used to authenticate identity. Examples of secondary identifiers may include Social Security cards, firearm licenses, insurance cards, and voter registration cards. Patients should present either two primary identifiers or one primary and one secondary identifier—the policy of identifiers should be established, in writing, by the practice.
   c. Monitor the activity of your patients' accounts.
   d. Verify the authenticity of a change of address. Identity thieves will change the legitimate address on the account, so that all fraudulent activity is sent to the changed address.

3. *Prevent and diminish identity theft with appropriate responses.* The medical office should respond to identity theft triggers to an appropriate degree. For example, an account may only need to be monitored for identity abuse, or it may need to be closed.

4. *Update the Red Flag Requirements plan.* The effectiveness of policies and procedures needs to be evaluated to ensure that they cover the current red flags.

A Red Flag Requirements plan should be overseen by individuals who are senior in the practice, such as the physician, office manager, and head nurse. Also, the plan must include steps for training medical team members in identity theft triggers and detection. Using guidelines from the federal government, medical offices should design and implement a plan that is appropriate for the size and nature of the practice. Many helpful websites contain information and suggestions for developing a Red Flag Requirements plan, including the Federal Trade Commission website at ftc.gov.

9.3 BANKING

It is clear that handling the banking functions of the practice accurately and promptly contributes to the financial health of the practice. The administrative medical assistant is responsible for many of these banking duties, including preparing deposits and reconciling bank statements. Banking tasks require **absolute accuracy,** correctness that is 100 percent, because the assistant acts as the physician's agent in these matters.

Checks and Checking Accounts

An order (written or electronic) to a bank to pay a specific amount of money to another party is referred to as a *check*. The practice may have at least two types of checking accounts—one regular business checking account and an account that pays interest. There may also be a savings account in the name of the practice. Money for taxes or expenses that are not immediate will be kept in a checking or savings account where it will earn **interest,** or money paid by the bank to depositors in return for the bank's use of the depositor's money. You will use the regular business account most frequently: to deposit patient payments and to draw checks for the payment of office expenses. Although this account may not pay interest, it allows for availability and flexibility.

Negotiable Checks. A check is an order to a bank to pay a specific amount of money. In order for the check to be negotiable—that is, to allow the legal transfer of money, it must meet several requirements. It is important for you to know what these are; you should examine all checks given to you before accepting them. To be negotiable, a check must

- state the specific amount to be paid. The amount should be printed in figures and in dollars and cents. The amount should also be stated in words. For example, the figure amount of $125.00 would also be written as "one hundred twenty-five dollars and 00/100." It is recommended the wording be printed, not written in cursive. If the figure amount and the printed wording amount are different, the wording amount is considered the legal amount of the check.
- be made out (made payable) to the payee. The payee may be the title of the practice rather than the physician's name, depending on the title of the account.
- carry the name of the bank that is making the payment.
- specify the date on which payment is to be made.
- be signed by the payer, the person who writes the check and is promising to pay the money.
- make a note in the memo line, if desired, about the purpose of the check. For example, this line could include the patient's chart/account number. However, whether or not the memo line contains information will not affect the validity of the check.

Be sure that you understand and follow office policies about accepting checks. For example, a patient visiting the office for the first time may be required to present identification before the check is accepted.

The following kinds of checks are usually not acceptable:

- *Postdated checks:* The mindset of "A check dated in the future (postdated) cannot be cashed until that future date" is incorrect. A postdated check can be presented to the bank for cash or deposit when the check is written! If a postdated check is accepted, ask for a explanation why the check is postdated. If the patient does not have funds in the account when the check is written but will have funds on the check's post date, it may be in the best interest of the medical practice to wait until the date of the check to deposit the check. Fees and penalties may be incurred by the practice if the check is presented to the bank and funds are not in the account.
- *Predated checks:* A check dated in the past should only be accepted based on the medical practice's financial policy. Financial institutions should be consulted for acceptance of predated checks. Predated checks may be expired and nonnegotiable.
- *Third-party checks:* In this case, *third party* refers not to an insurer but to anyone other than the patient. A third party check is a check written to the patient by a person unknown to the practice.
- *Checks annotated "Paid in Full":* When the amount of the check does not correspond to the total or full amount due for the services rendered, the office should

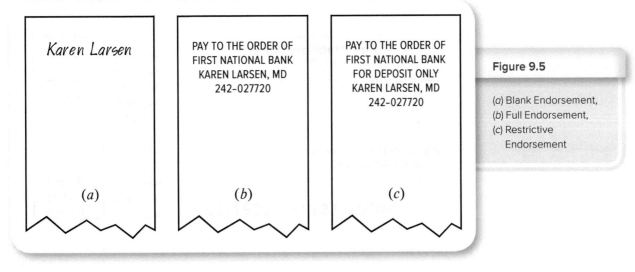

Figure 9.5

(a) Blank Endorsement,
(b) Full Endorsement,
(c) Restrictive Endorsement

not accept a check marked "Paid in Full." Accepting a check with the notation "Paid in Full," "PIF," or "PFIC" and consequently presenting it to the bank for deposit or cash means the practice agrees with the amount on the check and accepts it as a full settlement of the patient's account.

Check Endorsements. All checks received should be endorsed as soon as they are accepted. This lessens the chance that they will be lost, stolen, or forgotten. Three types of endorsements may be used (Figure 9.5):

- *Blank endorsement:* In a **blank endorsement,** (Figure 9.5a), the signature of the person to whom the check is payable (the payee) is placed on the back of the check. Once a check is endorsed this way, the check may be cashed by anyone. Blank endorsements are not used in business.
- *Full endorsement:* A **full endorsement** (Figure 9.5b), indicates the person, company, account number, or bank to which the check is being transferred, followed by the payee's name.
- *Restrictive endorsement:* A **restrictive endorsement** (Figure 9.5c) is the safest and most commonly used endorsement in business. The check is restricted by being marked "For Deposit Only." The use of the check is thus limited because the party to whom the money should be paid and the purpose have been stated. The restrictive endorsement is convenient for business use. The assistant may use a "For Deposit Only" rubber stamp and may deposit the check without obtaining the physician's signature.

Deposits. The checks and cash placed into the account belonging to the practice are called **deposits.** Once the daily monetary intake from endorsed checks and cash has been verified using the procedure day sheet, a deposit slip is prepared. For a sizable practice, depositing checks daily is important because it improves the cash flow and ensures that checks sent by the practice will not bounce. If the practice is specialized or very small, deposits may be made less often during the week. The bank where the checking account is maintained provides deposit slips. These are preprinted with the title of the account and the account number. A sample deposit slip is shown in Figure 9.6. On the first line, marked "Cash," the amount of currency—bills and coins—is entered. Some deposit slips list "Cash" and "Coins" on separate lines. Beneath this entry, each check is listed separately. Some banks prefer to have the check identified by the signature name on the check, the check number, or the bank name. If needed, some deposit slips may allow for additional deposit information to be recorded on the back of the form.

Figure 9.6

Deposit Slip

DEPOSITED IN

First National Bank

Chicago, IL 60623-2791

THIS DEPOSIT ACCEPTED UNDER AND SUBJECT TO THE PROVISIONS
OF THE UNIFORM COMMERCIAL CODE.

DATE _9/21/20--_

Karen Larsen, MD
2235 South Ridgeway Avenue
Chicago, IL 60623-2240

⑆07015550⑆ 2242027720 ⑈

	DOLLARS	CENTS
Cash	53	20
Checks list separately		
Ambers, Patient	142	00
Feis, Patient	248	00
Stromn, Patient	50	20
Total from Other Side	0	00
Subtotal	493	40
Less Cash Received	0	00
TOTAL	493	40

Transfer the total from the back to the front of the deposit slip. Subtotal the front and back amounts. When money is to be given to the depositor from the deposit, place the amount to be withheld from the deposit on the front of the slip. This is called "Less Cash Received." Subtract the Less Cash Received amount from the subtotal to calculate the total amount of the deposit. The amount of the deposit is then entered on the first unused checkbook stub or in the check register. When manually preparing any banking document, only blue or black ink should be used. Other colors are difficult for electronic scanning equipment to read.

It is important to obtain a deposit receipt from the bank. All deposit slips, receipts, the checkbooks, and the check register should be kept in a secure and locked place in the office.

Returned Checks. The bank may return a check that has not been completed properly: The check may be missing a date or signature. The check will also be returned if there is not enough money in the account to cover the amount shown on the check. In this case, the check is stamped, or identified "NSF," or "non-sufficient funds." The bank may charge a fee for returned checks, and in turn the practice will charge the patient a fee for the returned check. After the returned check has been received, make a debit entry in the patient's account, recharging for the amount of the check. Include the returned check fee on the account. Notify the patient of the returned check and related fees. Usually, payment from the patient should be a cash or debit/credit card payment. Be sure to inform the patient of the due date and to document information discussed with the patient (if not in letter format).

The Banking Policy of the Practice

The physician must indicate the persons in the practice authorized to sign all checks. One person may be authorized to write checks, and another may be authorized to sign. This is a good internal system to avoid mistakes and misappropriations. The physician may require two signatures for each check or may set limits on the amounts of money for which anyone other than the physician may write checks.

Bank Reconciliation

Each month the bank mails or sends an electronic statement of the checking account, such as the one shown in Figure 9.7. The monthly statement shows the beginning balance, total credits (deposits added to the account during the month), total debits (checks paid out of the account during the month), any service charges that apply, and the resulting new balance.

First National Bank
Chicago, IL 60623-2791

STATEMENT OF
ACCOUNT NUMBER
242 027720

CLOSING DATE	ITEMS
6/30/20--	12

Figure 9.7

Bank Statement

KAREN LARSEN, MD
2235 SOUTH RIDGEWAY AVENUE
CHICAGO, IL 60623-2240

CHECKING ACCOUNT STATEMENT

BEGINNING BALANCE	(+) TOTAL CREDITS	(−) TOTAL DEBITS	(−) SERVICE CHARGE	(=) NEW BALANCE
2,592.74	1,030.00	919.06		2,703.68

CHECKS & OTHER DEBITS	DEPOSITS & OTHER CREDITS	DATE	BALANCE
1622 − 2.54	165.00	6/2	2,755.20
	100.00	6/3	2,855.20
1623 − 97.00		6/6	2,758.20
1625 − 450.00		6/7	2,308.20
	120.00	6/9	2,428.20
1627 − 29.37		6/13	
1628 − 13.00			2,385.83
	85.00	6/14	2,470.83
1629 − 7.00	210.00	6/15	2,673.83
1630 − 15.62		6/20	2,658.21
	90.00	6/22	2,748.21
1631 − 37.98	185.00	6/23	
1633 − 65.12			2,830.11
1634 − 145.00		6/28	
1635 − 15.00			2,670.11
1636 − 41.43	75.00	6/29	2,703.68

SYMBOLS

C = CORRECTION	DM = DEBIT MEMO	RI = RETURN ITEM	ST = SAVINGS TRANSFER
CM = CREDIT MEMO	OD = OVERDRAFT	SC = SERVICE CHARGE	

The new balance on the statement must be compared with the checkbook balance to determine whether there is a difference between the amounts. This process is known as reconciling the bank statement, or **bank reconciliation.** Many banks provide a reconciliation form, such as the one shown in Figure 9.8, on one of the pages of the monthly statement.

You should take the following steps in the reconciliation process:

1. Compare the canceled (processed) checks returned by the bank with the items listed on the bank statement. When banks do not provide the actual canceled checks, miniaturized copied images of the checks are usually provided, or processed checks can be checked at the practice's online banking site. These, in addition to the listing of the checks on the statement, may be used for reference.

2. Compare the checks listed on the bank statement with the checkbook stubs to verify that check numbers and amounts agree. Deductions, such as service charges, are explained on the bank statement. These must be recorded in the checkbook. Checks that were written during the last month but have not yet been paid by the bank are not included with the statement. These are called "outstanding checks" and should be listed on the reconciliation form as shown in Figure 9.8.

Figure 9.8

Reconciliation Section of a
Bank Statement

CHANGE OF ADDRESS ORDER

TO CHANGE YOUR ADDRESS, PLEASE COMPLETE THIS FORM;
THEN CUT ALONG DOTTED LINE, AND MAIL OR BRING TO THE BANK.

NEW ADDRESS
_____

NUMBER AND STREET
_____

CITY   STATE AND ZIP CODE   NEW PHONE NUMBER
_____

DATE   CUSTOMER'S SIGNATURE
_____

- -

OUTSTANDING CHECKS	
NUMBER	AMOUNT
1602	125 00
1624	18 65
1626	22 19
1632	48 90
TOTAL	214 74

TO RECONCILE YOUR STATEMENT AND CHECKBOOK

1. DEDUCT FROM YOUR CHECK-BOOK BALANCE ANY SERVICE OR OTHER CHARGE ORIGINATED BY THE BANK. THESE CHARGES WILL BE IDENTIFIED BY SYMBOLS AS SHOWN ON FRONT.

2. ARRANGE ENDORSED CHECKS BY DATE OR NUMBER AND CHECK THEM OFF AGAINST THE STUBS IN YOUR CHECKBOOK.

3. LIST IN THE OUTSTANDING CHECKS SECTION AT THE LEFT ANY CHECKS ISSUED BY YOU AND NOT YET PAID BY US.

TO RECONCILE YOUR STATEMENT AND CHECKBOOK		
LAST BALANCE SHOWN ON STATEMENT	2,703	68
PLUS: DEPOSITS AND CREDITS MADE AFTER DATE OF LAST ENTRY ON STATEMENT	130	00
SUBTOTAL	2,833	68
MINUS: OUTSTANDING CHECKS	214	74
BALANCE: WHICH SHOULD AGREE WITH YOUR CHECKBOOK	2,618	94

3. Compare the deposits recorded in the checkbook with the credits listed on the bank statement. A deposit listed in the checkbook but not recorded by the bank at the time the statement was issued is called a "deposit in transit."

4. If the checking account earns interest, record the interest as a credit, similar to a deposit, in the checkbook.

5. Complete the reconciliation form following the directions.

If the final amount on the reconciliation form does not agree with the amount in the checkbook, compare the monthly statement with the checkbook again.

- Recheck the deposits entered on the bank statement against those you have entered in the checkbook.

- Confirm that all service charges shown on the statement are entered in the checkbook and have been properly deducted.

- Make sure no check has been drawn that has not been recorded in the checkbook. Compare all checks with the stubs to make sure the amounts agree.
- Review the list of outstanding checks to see whether an old check is still outstanding.
- Recheck all addition and subtraction.

When the checkbook is reconciled, make a notation to that effect in the checkbook on the last-used stub or register line.

Mc Graw Hill connect | **GO TO PROJECT 9.2 AT THE END OF THIS CHAPTER**

Banking Electronically

Banking electronically can contribute to both efficiency and accuracy. The tasks that you have when banking electronically are the same as those you perform when using paper procedures. You are still responsible for recording and physically depositing checks (unless the check was electronically deposited or paid). You still need to reconcile statements but do not need to wait for a hardcopy statement to be mailed. Online banking is typically in real time and is up to date. However, the software makes all the calculations automatically. This not only saves time but also reduces the chances for error. You no longer need to worry about a secure storage place for the checkbook and deposit slips. The password you use to access the bank account is the only item you must protect.

Banks' software systems allow you to

- check account balances.
- receive electronic deposits.
- find out which checks have cleared.
- transfer money from one account to another.
- pay certain bills.

Menus in banking software are user friendly. Main menus present broad topics, such as "Pay Bills," "Payment Center," and "Transfers." Reconciling monthly statements may also be done electronically with a computerized version of the reconciliation form. Technical support is available with most online banking software 24 hours a day, 7 days a week. The software is updated and maintained periodically, however, and during that time online banking transactions cannot be processed.

In June 2000, federal legislation (ESIGN) was signed that granted electronic signatures, or e-signatures, the same legal standing as printed signatures. An **e-signature** is a unique identifier, or "signature," created for each person through computer code. It can be a computer image of a person's handwritten signature or other digital marker (such as a code of numbers). Verifying the identities of those doing business in cyberspace is still an issue to be resolved. Many medical providers and other businesses are becoming technologically equipped to use e-signatures for processing financial and other documents. This practice will continue to grow as the technology becomes more efficient and economical.

The practice may also authorize a payer to transfer funds electronically. That is, a third-party payer, such as the federal government or an insurance company, deposits payments to the practice electronically directly into the practice's account.

Petty Cash

A **petty cash fund** contains small amounts of cash (such as $40–$100) to be used for small expenses. These expenses are usually so small that checks would not be written to pay for them: cab fares, postage stamps, payments to messengers, and delivery charges.

Each time you make a payment from the petty cash fund, make an entry in the petty cash register, or complete a voucher if this is the system used in your office. The register or voucher provides a record of these small expenses and ensures that only authorized payments are made from this fund. Receipts for expenditures from petty cash should be placed with the petty cash register/voucher.

To obtain money for the petty cash fund, the minor expenses for the month are estimated. A check for the estimated amount is drawn, payable to "Cash" or "Petty Cash." The check is endorsed and cashed in an assortment of small bills and change. The money is kept in a secure place, such as a locked metal cashbox in a drawer.

At the end of the month or when the amount of cash has been depleted to a predetermined amount, such as $25, the fund is replenished. First, from the record in the petty cash register and receipts, determine the total amount of disbursements made. Count the remaining cash in the fund. Be sure the two amounts add up to the original amount of the check that was last cashed. This procedure is called "proving the petty cash fund." A new check is then drawn to bring the fund back to its original amount.

EXAMPLE: PETTY CASH

The original amount of the petty cash fund was $100. According to the petty cash register, expenses added up to $89.75. Thus, there should be $10.25 in cash and $89.75 in receipts remaining in the fund. Count the cash to verify that the correct amount remains. Draw a check for $89.75 to bring the amount of petty cash back to $100 once the check has been cashed.

The petty cash expenditures should be recorded in the correct columns on the monthly summary sheet. They may be entered as petty cash.

Mc Graw Hill connect **GO TO PROJECT 9.3 AT THE END OF THIS CHAPTER**

9.4 PAYROLL

The total earnings of all the employees in the practice is called the **payroll.** Services, such as ADP (Automatic Data Processing, Inc. at adp.com), will process payroll for companies. However, if you are responsible for handling the payroll in your office, you will be completing the following tasks:

- Calculating the earnings of employees
- Subtracting the correct amounts of taxes and other **deductions,** or amounts of money withheld from earnings
- Creating employee payroll records
- Preparing salary checks
- Submitting payroll taxes
- Keeping current with IRS formulas and regulations that affect payroll; many tax tables and other information can be found on the IRS website (www.irs.gov)

Creating Employee Payroll Records

Because accurate records are required and because the process is complex, you will want to create a payroll information record for each person employed in the practice. For each employee, list the following information:

- Name, address, Social Security Number, marital status, and the number of dependents (W-4 form)
- Pay schedule; show how often the employee is paid—weekly or biweekly, for example
- Type of payment; show whether the employee is paid a straight salary or an hourly wage, bonuses, overtime, holiday, vacation, etc.
- Employee-requested deductions; an employee may have payments to an employer-sponsored insurance plan, a flexible healthcare spending account, contributions to a savings plan sponsored by the practice, or additional tax contributions withheld

If any employees are not citizens of the United States, they must be authorized to work in the United States. A completed Employment Eligibility Verification Form (Form I-9) must be filed with the federal government within 3 business days of the date when employment begins, and a copy of the I-9 form, along with supporting identification documents, should be kept with the payroll records. This document verifies that the person is a legally admitted alien or a person authorized to work in this country.

Employer and Employee Identification Numbers

All employers, whatever the size of the business, are required to have a tax identification number. This **Employer Identification Number (EIN)** enables the IRS to track the financial activity of employers in meeting payroll and tax obligations. An example of an EIN is 12-3456789. The nine-digit number is obtained by requesting Form SS-4 from the IRS. Employees are required to be identified by Social Security Numbers.

Taxes Deducted from Earnings

Direct earnings are salaries (fixed amounts paid regardless of hours worked) or wages (pay based on an hourly or daily specific rate) paid to employees. **Indirect earnings** are specific employer-paid benefit programs, such as paid leave, housing allowance, and health insurance.

When employees are first hired, they must complete the Employee's Withholding Allowance Certificate (Form W-4), on which they state the number of allowances or exemptions to be used when the employer is calculating how much money to withhold from their salaries as deductions. Employers should verify annually that the information on file is still current. A new W-4 should be completed when major life changes (marriage, divorce, births, or deaths) occur. Name changes should be made only when the change is verified by a new Social Security card. The amounts to be withheld from an employee's salary for federal and state taxes are determined from wage-bracket tables supplied by the IRS. The amount withheld depends on the amount of money earned, the number of exemptions claimed, and the current tax rate. The IRS also supplies wage-bracket tables that apply to various payroll cycles: daily, weekly, semimonthly, and monthly. Refer to the state and local tax tables to determine the additional amounts of money to be withheld.

FICA Tax

A law known as **FICA (Federal Insurance Contributions Act)** governs the Social Security system. This law requires that a certain amount of money be withheld for Social Security. The employee pays half the required contribution, and the employer pays the other half. This amount is deducted in two separate payroll taxes: One helps finance

Medicare, and the other helps fund Social Security pension benefits. These amounts, dictated by the IRS, are a percentage of the employee's taxable earnings, considering payroll periods and allowances claimed. Because Congress can change this amount yearly, you must obtain information from the IRS or from the physician's accountant.

Calculating Payroll

Spreadsheet programs perform these complex calculations very quickly. It is important for you to understand the formulas used and the process involved. Websites such as www.adp.com offer the opportunity to use free online payroll calculators.

- *Gross earnings:* Calculate gross earnings. For an employee on salary, the salary amount for the period is the employee's gross earnings, regardless of whether or not the employee worked more than 35 or 40 hours. For an hourly wage worker, the hourly rate multiplied by the number of hours worked yields the employee's gross earnings. If an hourly wage employee works overtime hours, the hourly wage is typically paid at the rate of 150 percent of the base pay. This is commonly referred to as "time and a half." For example, if an employee is paid $12 per hour base wage, the overtime hourly wage would be $18 ($12 × 150%).
- *Exemptions; state and local tax deductions:* Find the number of exemptions the employee claimed on Form W-4. Refer to the IRS tax table (Circular E) for the amount to be deducted, based on the gross earnings and the exemptions. State and local taxes are often at a set rate—for example, 5 percent of gross earnings. Subtract this amount from gross earnings.
- *FICA taxes:* Withhold, and deduct, half the amount due for the pay period from the employee's gross earnings. The other half is paid by the practice. There is one rate for the Social Security deduction and another for the Medicare deduction. Verify the current withholding rate prior to calculating the amounts.
- *Voluntary deductions:* Deduct any amounts the employee has requested for insurance, a savings plan, additional tax withholding, and so on. Deductions are either pretax deductions (deducted from the employee's pay prior to calculating the taxable amount of income) or posttax deductions (deducted after the employee's taxable amount of income has been calculated). An example of a pretax deduction includes contributions made to retirement accounts. An example of a posttax deduction would be a contribution to a charitable organization.
- *Employer's obligation:* Post the employer's FUTA (see next section), FICA contribution, and taxes due to federal and state unemployment funds to the physician's account.
- *Net earnings:* When total deductions are taken from gross earnings, the result is the employee's net earnings.
- *Net pay statement:* Prepare an itemized statement, either hardcopy or electronic, of gross pay, deductions, and net pay, and include it with the employee's pay.

Employers' Tax Responsibilities

Employers are required to help fund the **FUTA (Federal Unemployment Tax Act)** account, which is used to help those who have been without work for a specified time as they seek new employment. This dollar amount is a percentage of each employee's gross earnings but is not to be deducted from the employee's earnings. Usually, payments into a state and federal unemployment fund are applied as credit against the amount of FUTA tax.

FUTA requires only the employer to contribute to the unemployment insurance fund. An employer is required to pay FUTA if $1,500 or more has been paid to an employee in any calendar quarter in the current or previous year.

Employers' Deposit and Tax Return Obligations. The practice must make federal tax withholding payments and FICA payments to a federal deposit account in a federal reserve bank or in another authorized bank. The money must be deposited at least monthly. The IRS imposes a severe penalty for the failure to make these deposits.

The employer is required to file a quarterly tax return, Form 941, to report federal income and FICA taxes withheld from employee paychecks.

Employees' W-2, I-9, and 1095 Forms. Employees need payroll information from the previous year to file their taxes with the federal and state governments. Employers prepare a W-2 showing wages and deductions for each employee who received earnings during the previous year. Employer identification information is also listed on the W-2.

Employers are also required by federal law to verify the identity and employment eligibility of each employee. A properly completed Form I-9 must be completed for each hired employee.

Additionally, employers who offer health insurance coverage to employees are required by federal law to provided Form 1095-B or 1095-C for each employee. Basically, Form 1095 is used to show if an employee had medical insurance coverage during the calendar year, who (dependents) was covered, and if any gaps in coverage occurred. Form 1095-B is used by employers with 50 or fewer full-time employees. Form 1095-C is used by employers offering medical insurance coverage with 50 or more full-time employees or the equivalent of 50 full-time employees.

Other forms may be required by state and/or federal laws; therefore, the employers should always be current with the requirements.

Payroll Records: Contents and Retention

The practice is required by law to retain payroll data for a minimum of 3 years. However, a longer retention period may be required to prove income and deductions. A typical format for this record is shown in Figure 9.9.

Each employee's earnings record must contain the employee's name; Social Security Number; address; number of exemptions claimed; gross salary earned; net

INDIVIDUAL EMPLOYEE'S EARNINGS RECORD

Name: Molly Benson
Address: 5985 West Park Ave.
City: Chicago, IL 60650
Telephone: 555-4251

Social Security No.: 555-55-5555
Marital Status: Single
No. of Allowances: 1
Birthdate: 5/29/1978

Position: AMA (part-time)
Monthly Rate:
Weekly Rate: $528
Overtime Rate: $25/hour

| Period Ending 20-- | Hours Worked | Gross Earnings | | | Deductions | | | | | | | | Net Pay | | Accumulated Earnings (Gross) | |
		Regular	Overtime	Total	FICA	Federal Withholding	State Withholding	City Withholding	Insurance	Other	Total				
6-13	24	528 00		528 00	40 40	63 19	15 84				119 43	408 57	12,672 00	
6-20	24	528 00		528 00	40 40	63 19	15 84				119 43	408 57	13,200 00	
6-27	24	528 00		528 00	40 40	63 19	15 84				119 43	408 57	13,728 00	
7-4	24	528 00		528 00	40 40	63 19	15 84				119 43	408 57	14,256 00	
7-11	24	528 00		528 00	40 40	63 19	15 84				119 43	408 57	14,784 00	
7-18	24	528 00		528 00	40 40	63 19	15 84				119 43	408 57	15,312 00	
7-25	24	528 00		528 00	40 40	63 19	15 84				119 43	408 57	15,840 00	
8-8	24	528 00		528 00	40 40	63 19	15 84				119 43	408 57	16,368 00	
8-15	24	528 00		528 00	40 40	63 19	15 84				119 43	408 57	16,896 00	

Figure 9.9

Individual Employee's Earnings Record

salary paid; income taxes withheld; and FICA, state, and local taxes deducted. The column labeled "Other" is used to record certain other deductions required by law or voluntary deductions made under an agreement with the employer. For example, many employers deduct, at the employee's request, amounts for savings bonds, insurance, or union dues. All amounts deducted by the employer are held in trust. The employer must remit the monies to the proper authority in a timely manner.

Electronic Payroll: Direct Deposit

Through direct deposit, the employee's net pay is automatically withdrawn from the practice's account and deposited into the employee's account. The physician must contract with the bank for this procedure, known as **EFT (electronic funds transfer),** and employees must give employers their account numbers (bank routing number and employee's account number). The employee receives a deposit stub showing the gross pay, net pay, and specific deductions. This aspect of electronic banking has many advantages for both employers and employees:

1. The loss or theft of paychecks is eliminated. When an employee is on vacation or absent, the check is deposited.
2. Productivity and cost savings are increased. Time and expense are saved because no paychecks need to be written.
3. Employees have the convenience of eliminating a trip to the bank to deposit a paycheck, and the money is available on the day of deposit.

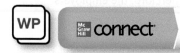

GO TO PROJECTS 9.4, 9.5, and 9.6 AT THE END OF THIS CHAPTER

9.1 Explain, using accounting terminology, the procedures for maintaining two essential financial records.	• Five accounting terms related to the assistant's responsibilities are
	— *accounts payable*—expense amounts owed to the supplier or creditors.
	— *accounts receivable*—balance of payments due from patients or others on current accounts.
	— *bookkeeping*—the part of accounting that is the accurate recording of transactions.
	— *daily journal*—the record of services rendered, daily fees, charges, payments received, and adjustments.
	— *audit*—an IRS review of all financial data to ensure the accuracy and completeness of the data.
	• The procedures for maintaining two essential financial records (electronic or manual) follow:
	— Daily journal:
	  • Daily, record the fees charged.
	  • Daily, record the payments received.
	  • Accurately maintain the Accounts Receivable Control section with the record of payments received from patients.
	  • Daily, balance the columns for Proof of Posting.
	  • Accurately record the amount of cash received during the day in the Daily Cash section to account for cash flow.
	— Monthly summary:
	  • Accurately summarize the daily charges and payments on a monthly basis.

9.2 Summarize the main focus of the Red Flag Requirements as they relate to the medical office as a business.	• Medical practices must protect not only patients' protected health information under HIPAA but also patients' financial information. Identity thieves have increasingly used criminal activities to gain medical services and benefits, such as insurance payments. • Medical practices must establish policies and procedures that enable them to form a reasonable belief that the individual requesting services is actually that person.

	• Policies and procedures should identify — the primary and secondary types of identification required from patients. — account red flags. — the courses of action to take when fraudulent activity is suspected.
9.3 List three banking duties of the administrative medical assistant.	• Three banking duties performed by the assistant are — accepting valid checks in payment for services rendered. — depositing cash, checks, and other forms of payment into the practice's account(s). — reconciling bank statements.
9.4 Explain how an employee's net salary is determined.	• The assistant's duties related to the payroll process are — calculating gross earnings—determining the salary amount, or multiplying the number of hours worked by the hourly wage amount. — determining the proper exemptions, and state and local tax deductions—subtracting these from the gross earnings. — subtracting FICA tax—withholding half the specified amount from the employee's paycheck; the employer pays the other half. — subtracting voluntary deductions—if the employee has asked that amounts be withheld for insurance, savings, and so on, deducting these amounts. — subtracting the total deductions from the gross earnings—the result is the employee's net salary. — posting the taxes that are the physician's obligation to the practice account.

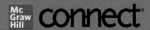

Chapter Projects

Project 9.1   (LO 9.1) Updating Daily Journals (Optional)

Complete the daily journals started for October 17 (WP 51) and October 18 (WP 52).

Note that the patients have been listed for you. Use patient statements to verify each previous balance. Post each day's transactions onto both the daily journal and the patient statement, computing the current balance. Information for charges has been obtained from each patient's encounter form or from payments received on account.

Total Columns A, B, C, D, and E. Complete the Proof of Posting, Accounts Receivable Control, and Daily Cash sections. Post the daily ending accounts receivable balance onto the next daily journal.

Note that no deposits were yet made.

Project 9.2   (LO 9.3) Reconciling a Bank Statement

Using the following information from the bank's monthly statement and the physician's checkbook information, reconcile the bank statement with the physician's balance. What is the missing "Deposit Not on Bank Statement" amount? Be prepared to show and justify your work.

INFORMATION ON BANK STATEMENT

Beginning Balance	$ 10,142.10
Total Debits/Checks	$ 8,090.54
Total Credits/Deposits	$ 17,983.18
New Balance	$20,034.74

INFORMATION FROM PHYSICIAN'S CHECKING ACCOUNT

Balance	$19,307.63
Outstanding Checks	$ 982.16
	$ 823.30
Deposit Not on Bank Statement	$ _____

Project 9.3   (LO 9.3) Reconciling Petty Cash

Each month, $150 is available in petty cash funds for small office expenditures. Expenses paid from petty cash during the month are listed here.

Postage	$26.00
Office supplies	$46.25
Delivery charge	$ 9.50
Physician's parking fee	$ 12.00

1. What is the total for expenditures for the month from petty cash?
2. What is the balance, after expenditures, of petty cash?
3. How much is needed to replenish petty cash for the next month?

Be prepared to show your work and justify your totals.

Project 9.4 — (LO 9.4) Internet Research: Using the IRS as a Resource

Using a favorite search engine, key in "Internal Revenue Service." Go to the site for the IRS, and examine the information available. Look especially at the tax forms, the help for small businesses, and the section on payroll tax rules. Determine why this site is helpful to a medical practice. Be prepared to discuss the specific helpful information that you find.

Project 9.5 — (LO 9.3) Updating Payments and Deposits

The following payments were received, in the form of checks, on October 21:

Patient Name	Check Number	Amount
Joseph Castro	629	$ 44.00
Suzanne Roberts	857	$156.00
Gene Sinclair	1279	$ 44.00

 If you are instructed to complete this project using EHRclinic, your instructor will assign you the project as part of a Connect assignment.

If optional Project 9.1 was completed, then complete a daily journal (WP 53), and post transactions to patient statements for the three payments received from Castro, Roberts, and Sinclair on October 21. Complete one deposit slip (WP 54) to include payments received on October 17 (Armstrong and Villano), 18, and 21. Date the deposit slip October 21.

Project 9.6 — (LO 9.4) Calculating an Employee's Payroll

Complete the following table by calculating the number of hours each employee worked during the payroll period. Then calculate the employee's base pay by multiplying the number of hours worked in the payroll period by the employee's hourly wage. (For employees who worked more than 40 hours, only multiply their first 40 hours by their hourly wage.) Round to the nearest cent.

Employee	M	T	W	TH	F	Base Hours	Rate per Hour	Base Pay
Connie Bradley	10	11	11	Off	10		12.00	
Dara Cecil	8	7	8	7	Off		12.00	
Misty Dark	Off	11	10	11	10		12.25	
Jennifer Eckel	5	Off	8	8	8		12.25	
Thomas Free	8	8	Off	7	6		12.50	
Anthony Gregson	Off	6	7	Off	8		13.50	
Tara Hughes	8	11	8	11	8		13.50	
Michael Ikard	9	9	9	9	9		15.25	
Leighanne Jones	7	8	Off	8	8		15.75	
Amanda Kat	11	8	11	10	9		14.25	

The following employees worked overtime hours. Using their rate per hour provided in the previous chart, multiply that hourly rate by 150% (1.5). Next, multiply that amount by the employees' overtime hours. Add the employees' overtime earning to their base pay (calculated in the previous step) to determine their gross earnings. Round all money figures to the nearest cent.

Employee	Total Overtime Hours	Overtime Rate	Overtime Earnings	Gross Earnings
Michael Ikard	5			
Misty Dark	2			
Connie Bradley	2			
Amanda Kat	9			
Tara Hughes	6			

Soft Skills Success

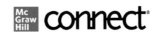

Integrity (LO 9.4)

As an administrative medical professional, it is your job to handle the payroll. You have worked with several of the employees for over 5 years, and you realize that a new hire is making more money hourly than the other employees in the same position. Somehow the employees have found out about this, and they ask you if it is true. **How should you handle this situation?**

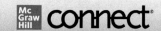
USING TERMINOLOGY

Match the term or phrase on the left with the correct answer on the right.

_____ 1. [LO 9.1] Procedure day sheet

_____ 2. [LO 9.1] Posting

_____ 3. [LO 9.3] Blank endorsement

_____ 4. [LO 9.4] Direct earnings

_____ 5. [LO 9.4] FICA

_____ 6. [LO 9.4] FUTA

_____ 7. [LO 9.1] Daily journal

_____ 8. [LO 9.3] Restrictive endorsement

_____ 9. [LO 9.2] Red Flag Requirements

_____ 10. [LO 9.1] Balance sheet

a. Record of provided services and their charges, payments received, and adjustments

b. Transferring accounts from one record to another

c. Period statement showing assets, liability, and capital

d. Numeric listing of all procedures and related information performed on a given day

e. Federal regulations requiring creditors to implement procedures to protect personal data pertaining to a covered account

f. Signature of the payee on the back of a check

g. States the payee and purpose of a check

h. Salaries/wages from an employer

i. Law requiring withholding from wages for Social Security

j. Law requiring employers to pay into an unemployment fund to be used by individuals unemployed for a specific amount of time but seeking new employment

CHECKING YOUR UNDERSTANDING

Select the most correct answer.

1. [LO 9.1] Dr. Conna is considering purchasing her own EKG equipment to perform the procedure at the office instead of renting the equipment from a DME (durable medical equipment) distributor. She asked Evan (her administrative medical assistant) to give her the total number of EKGs performed and the revenue generated for the month of September. Which of the following reports should Evan reference for the information?

   a. Aging report
   b. Procedure day sheet
   c. Practice analysis report
   d. Income statement

2. [LO 9.1] To prepare for sending out patient statements for Dr. Conna's practice, Evan needs to know which accounts are more than 30 days past due. Which of the following reports should he reference for the information?

   a. Aging report
   b. Procedure day sheet
   c. Practice analysis report
   d. Income statement

3. [LO 9.2] Since Dr. Conna is a cardiologist, she performs many high-cost procedures, which require her patients to establish a monthly payment schedule. Her office extends credit in accordance with the Truth in Lending Act. Based on extending credit, the practice may be considered a

   a. FICA employer.
   b. FUTA employer.
   c. red flag–covered account.
   d. red flag creditor.

4. [LO 9.2] Evan has been asked by Dr. Conna to establish policies and procedures to protect patients from identity theft. Which of the following is an identity theft alert?

   a. A patient requests a change of address.
   b. A patient is billed for a service she did not receive.
   c. The name on a check is different from the patient's name.
   d. All of these are identity theft alerts.

5. [LO 9.3] The monthly bank statement shows a balance of $5,060.13. Three checks in the amounts of $89.50, $310.92, and $25.00 are still outstanding. What is the actual available balance of the checking account?

   a. $5,485.55
   b. $5,060.13
   c. The available balance cannot be determined.
   d. $4,634.71

6. [LO 9.3] Using the same information from Question 5, calculate the monthly service charge of $10 into the actual available balance. What is the actual available balance after the service charge?

   a. $5,495.55
   b. $5,050.13
   c. The available balance still cannot be determined.
   d. $4,624.71

7. [LO 9.4] Evan's hourly wage is $18, and he works 7.5 hours per day, 5 days per week. Based on a tax withholding of 7.5 percent, how much should be withheld from his wages for taxes?

   a. $506.30
   b. $50.63
   c. $5.06
   d. $67.50

8. [LO 9.4] Using Evan's wage information from Question 7, if the state tax rate is 9 percent, what is his tax obligation?

   a. $6.08
   b. $607.50
   c. $60.75
   d. $61.00

9. [LO 9.3] Which of the following would *not* typically be paid from petty cash funds?

   a. Charges for COD delivery
   b. Cost of postage stamps
   c. Registration fee for a medical conference
   d. All of these would typically be paid from petty cash.

10. [LO 9.3] An endorsement on the back of a deposited check states the following:

    PAY TO THE ORDER OF FIRST ANYWHERE BANK AND TRUST
    FOR DEPOSIT ONLY
    ALIANNA WELLINS, MD
    123-99008876

    This is an example of which type of endorsement?

    a. Restrictive
    b. Blank
    c. Full
    d. Negotiable

THINKING IT THROUGH

These questions cover important points in this chapter. Using your critical-thinking skills, play the role of an administrative medical assistant as you answer each question. Be prepared to discuss your responses.

1. [LO 9.1] What are some of the major financial responsibilities that you have as an administrative medical assistant? What are the accounting terms used to describe these responsibilities?
2. [LO 9.1] You have been asked to help a colleague understand how to deal with the daily journal. How will you explain this?
3. [LO 9.3] Mr. Thompson is a patient whose insurance company has paid a portion of the fee for the physician's services; Mr. Thompson is responsible for the remaining amount. He is angry and determined to dispute the matter with the insurance company. For this reason, he has given you a postdated check for the amount owed to the doctor, $427.50. The check is dated 3 weeks from the current date. How will you handle this nonnegotiable check?
4. [LO 9.4] One of the staff members asks you to explain the difference between the terms *gross* and *net* on the paycheck. How do you respond?

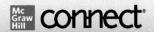

 If you are instructed to complete this project using EHRclinic, your instructor will assign you the project as part of a Connect assignment.

BEFORE YOU START

Today you will begin a second simulation in Dr. Larsen's office. The simulation dates are October 19, October 24, October 25, and October 26.

PROCEDURES

1. Check Simulation 1 and all patient-related projects for completion and accuracy prior to Simulation 2.
2. Review the section "Before You Start" in Simulation 1. Note that these procedures also apply to this simulation.
3. Review the "Procedures," because they apply to this simulation.
4. Pull the patients' charts following the appointment calendar, and put them in the appropriate day folder.
5. Prepare a separate deposit slip for each of the 4 days.
6. Prepare receipts for payments received in person.
7. Do not prepare receipts for payments received through the mail or electronically (WP 72, WP 77, and WP 85).

MATERIALS

You will need the following materials to complete Simulation 2. If these materials are not already in the proper folder, obtain them from the sources indicated. (*Note:* All WPs are located within Connect and in the Working Papers section of this textbook.)

Materials	Source
Appointment calendar	WPs 20–35
Diagnostic codes	WP 48
Fee schedule	WP 50
Deposit slips	WP 54
Patient Account/Chart Numbers	WP 87
Supplies folder	

To-Do Items

Day 1 folder:

Place patients' charts for October 19.

Telephone Log	WP 55
To-Do List	WP 56
Letter from Dr. Tai	WP 57
Receipts	WP 58
Patient encounter forms	WPs 59–63
Daily journal (Optional)	WP 64

Day 2 folder:

Place patients' charts for October 24.

Telephone Log	WP 65
To-Do List	WP 66
Patient encounter forms	WPs 67–71
Checks received	WP 72
Daily journal (Optional)	WP 73

Day 3 folder:

Place patients' charts for October 25.

Telephone Log	WPs 55, 65
To-Do List	WPs 56, 66
Patient encounter forms	WPs 74–76
Checks received	WP 77
Daily journal (Optional)	WP 78

Day 4 folder:

Place patients' charts for October 26.

Telephone Log	WPs 55, 65
To-Do List	WPs 56, 66
Patient encounter forms	WPs 79–84
Checks received	WP 85
Daily journal (Optional)	WP 86

Patients' folders:

The following items have been added to the patients' folders since Simulation 1.

Patient statements for all current patients	Project 8.1, 8.4

Simulation 2

MEDICAL VOCABULARY

Before working through this simulation's assignments, review the following terms to ensure that you are familiar with their spellings and meanings.

Ace wrap

bacitracin—anti-infective agent

chronicity—long duration of time

clindamycin—anti-infective agent

COPD—chronic obstructive pulmonary disease

DTP—diphtheria, tetanus, and pertussis vaccine

effusion—escape of fluid from blood vessels or lymphatics into tissues or a cavity

FSH—follicle-stimulating hormone

gravida—pregnant woman

HDL—high-density lipoprotein

hematuria—urine containing blood

hemoccult—test for hidden (occult) blood within stool

hidradenitis—inflammation of sweat glands

incontinence—inability to prevent discharge of excretions, such as urine or feces

IPV—inactivated polio vaccine

IVP—intravenous pyelogram

LDL—low-density lipoprotein

lymphadenitis—inflammation of lymph node or nodes

medial condyle—middle rounded prominence on a bone

MMR—measles-mumps-rubella vaccine

Naprosyn®—analgesic, antipyretic

OTC—over-the-counter

proximal—nearest

purulent—containing pus

pustular—marked by pustules (small skin elevations containing pus)

pyelonephritis—inflammation of renal pelvis and kidney

Robaxin®—skeletal muscle relaxant

suppurative—producing pus

tendonitis/tendinitis—inflammation of tendon

valgus—bent or twisted outward from midline of body

varus—bent or twisted inward toward the midline of body

Vicodin®—analgesic

Z-Pak®—antibiotic

PART 4

Preparing for Employment

CHAPTER 10
Preparing for Employment in the Medical Office

Part 4 discusses the importance of preparation as the administrative medical assistant begins and progresses through the path to a medical career. Presented are steps and strategies to make the career search as successful as possible.

CONSIDER THIS: Self-analysis can help the administrative medical assistant match skills and attributes to a career choice. *What are your top five skills and personal attributes and how can they be used in a medical environment?*

Chapter 10

Preparing for Employment in the Medical Office

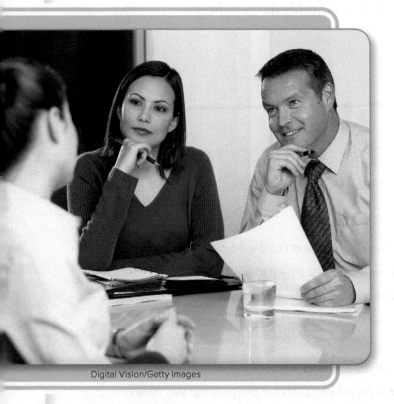

Digital Vision/Getty Images

LEARNING OUTCOMES

After studying this chapter, you will be able to

10.1 list and explore visible and hidden career/employment resources.

10.2 assimilate information and prepare an employment application.

10.3 compose a cover/application letter.

10.4 assimilate data and compose résumés using different format styles.

10.5 assemble personal and professional information and appropriate dress for the interview process and conduct a mock interview.

10.6 compose a follow-up thank-you letter.

KEY TERMS

Study these important words, which are defined in this chapter, to build your professional vocabulary:

chronological résumé

cover/application letter

e-portfolio

functional résumé

hidden job markets

key words

personal reference

plain-text résumé

power words

professional reference

scannable résumé

shoulder surfing

visible job markets

ABHES

1.a. Describe the current employment outlook for the medical assistant.

7.a. Gather and process documents.

10.a. Perform the essential requirements for employment such as résumé writing, effective interviewing, dressing professionally, time management, and following up appropriately.

10.b. Demonstrate professional behavior.

www.abhes.org/accreditationmanual

The ABHES standards appear with permission of The Accrediting Bureau of Health Education Schools

CAAHEP

V.C.7. Recognize elements of fundamental writing skills.

V.P.2. Respond to nonverbal communication.

V.P.8. Compose professional correspondence utilizing electronic technology.

X.C.9. List and discuss legal and illegal interview questions.

2015 Standards and Guidelines for the Accreditation of Educational Programs in Medical Assisting, Appendix B, Core Curriculum for Medical Assistants, Medical Assisting Education Review Board (MAERB), 2015.

INTRODUCTION

Just a short time ago, employment opportunities were mostly confined to a local, state, or national job market. Many employees worked at and retired from first jobs with very little mobility. Times have changed, and so have opportunities for employment. The workforce is very fluid and the Internet presents a global market.

Whether the job search is local or international, one key to being successful is being prepared. It begins with evaluating your skills and goals and matching them to various career opportunities. The search continues through exploring sources of career opportunities, composing a professional cover/application letter and accurately completing an application, preparing a résumé (or more than one), interviewing for a position, and conducting follow-up techniques.

 10.1 SEARCHING SOURCES OF EMPLOYMENT OPPORTUNITIES

Your Skills and Goals

As you begin your search for employment, first evaluate your skills (personal and professional) and your overall goal. Make a list of your personal traits and professional skills. Many individuals are not content in their current position for various reasons, one of which may be that their personal and professional skills are mismatched with their current job requirements. Following are some questions to ask yourself as you begin your list:

- Am I skilled in public communications?
- Do I enjoy searching for answers or solving problems (do I like word puzzles/word searches, etc.)?
- Am I more productive working on my own or as a member of a team?
- Do I organize my personal and professional lives?
- Have I held or do I hold positions of leadership, such as club officer?
- What are my technical skills?
- Do I pursue above and beyond what is required of me?

As you begin to evaluate yourself through these and other questions, match your answers to general job requirements or environments. For example, someone who enjoys and is proficient at solving word searches may be suited to finding errors in submitted insurance claim forms and submitting corrected claims to carriers. An individual who frequently holds an office, such as president or treasurer, within an organization may not be content in a professional position that does not provide an opportunity to grow professionally and assume more responsibility. Listing and objectively evaluating personal and professional skills is the first step in seeking employment.

Sources of Employment Opportunities

After you have compiled an evaluation of your skills and traits, the next step is to begin searching for employment opportunities. Some sources are more visible and traditional, while others fall within the hidden job market of opportunities. At times, employers want a large number of responses for available positions; however, some position vacancies are complicated by a vast number of applicants. Traditional job markets, or **visible job markets**, also referred to as published markets (job markets composed of resources that are traditional and the most obvious), produce a greater number of responses to positions, while nontraditional job markets, or **hidden job markets** (job markets that are less obvious and require more initiative by the job seekers to access) are more confined

Visible Resources. Many resources are available to job seekers through easily accessible venues. Following is a sampling of some visible job markets:

- *Internet.* Doing a topic search for job listings will produce a vast number of results. Several online employment services are available, such as www.Monster.com and www.linkedin.com. Some sites collect résumés, which they forward to employers, while some sites list complete position information, including the employer. One advantage of using Internet employment websites is the number of choices they provide. However, corporations listed on these sites may receive a great number of résumés per day. Résumés that are not prepared in a computer-friendly format (discussed later in this chapter) may not convey the intended information, and therefore may not be reviewed.

- *Social media.* Career opportunities can also be located through social media (Facebook, Twitter, Instagram, etc.). Many organizations maintain their own links through various social media venues. Also, personal contacts through social media sites may post employment opportunities, sometimes prior to the organization posting the vacant position.
- *Classified ads in national and local newspapers.* Ads may include desired information, such as the name and address of the organization, but many do not include specific data other than the position requirements. Résumés are frequently sent to a P.O. box, and no company or individual name is listed. Most newspaper classified ads can also be found on the newspaper's Web page.
- *Professional publications.* Journals published by professional organizations contain position opportunities. Student memberships are available through most professional organizations, usually at a discounted rate. National organizations typically have local chapters, which can supply information about local career opportunities.
- *Career/job fairs.* Most schools will host an event that brings together prospective employers and employees. Local communities may also host a career fair. When attending a fair, an applicant should be professionally dressed, have an application/cover letter (discussed later in this chapter), and have résumés in various formats (also discussed later in this chapter).
- *Job boards.* Schools and businesses post available positions on accessible traditional and/or electronic forums. For businesses, positions may first be posted to provide currently employed individuals the opportunity to apply first (known as in-house posting). Beginning and ending dates are listed on the vacancy notice. For example, a volunteer within a medical facility will know when positions have been internally posted and when external applicants may apply for the position. School career centers and/or placement offices also post the available positions that have been sent to them.
- *Temporary employment agencies.* Short-term exposure to various positions can be gained through local temporary job services. Job seekers who have little or no experience may find it beneficial to use these services to gain documentable experience. There may be a fee for the services. The temporary position may change to a permanent opportunity; however, the goal of a temporary employment agency is to provide short-term coverage of job responsibilities.
- *Employment services.* Companies may fill positions through local and governmental employment services. Companies that have a vacancy contact the employment service and ask to review the files of individuals who meet the job requirements. Those selected are interviewed by the service or by the company. Individuals should keep the file with the employment service up to date. Privately owned employment services may charge a fee for their services.

This list is not inclusive of all career resources but gives job seekers some avenues to pursue for employment.

Hidden Resources. Many times, less obvious job markets are overlooked and opportunities are lost. Job seekers must have the initiative to seek out these markets and opportunities. Following are examples of hidden markets:

- *Face-to-face networking.* Everyone has a network of individuals, which frequently is overlooked in the job-seeking process (Figure 10.1). People in your network can

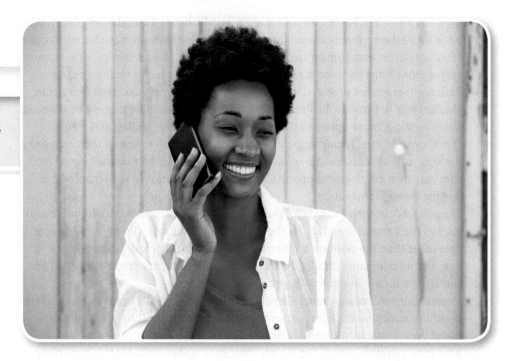

Figure 10.1

Practicing Networking
Skills mimagephotography/
Shutterstock

provide up-to-date information on industry trends and changes, as well as current and upcoming vacancies. Teachers and classmates typically have the same or similar interests and goals. Relatives and friends, fellow club or organization members, and acquaintances from the community frequently know about upcoming vacancies before the positions are posted. If someone with whom you work is leaving, an opportunity could be provided for you to apply for the vacancy. A network also includes people from sporting events, health clubs, workout classes, and physicians' offices. The list continues to include many, varied places where other individuals can be encountered.

- *Electronic networks.* These kinds of networks also are a vast source of employment opportunities. However, you should be careful of seeking information electronically if you are currently employed and have not submitted a letter of resignation. Also, refrain from posting negative comments about your current employment and colleagues. Electronic information, once posted, spreads quickly.
- *Telephone directories.* Yellow pages, traditional or electronic, are a valuable source of employers in a specific area. It is easy to locate all the physicians in a given specialty by using yellow pages.
- *Chamber of commerce.* The chamber of commerce in an area can provide a list of local businesses and organizations.
- *Direct contact with companies.* Information about available positions can be obtained from personally visiting a business. Keep in mind, however, that this is a "fact-gathering" visit. From the visit, a position-related cover/application letter and résumé can be prepared. An applicant should take a generic application letter and résumé, in case there is an opportunity to speak with a manager. A clean, neat, professional appearance will make a favorable impression.

McGraw Hill connect

**GO TO PROJECTS 10.1 AND 10.2
AT THE END OF THIS CHAPTER**

10.2 COMPLETING AN ONLINE AND A TRADITIONAL APPLICATION

It is common for prospective employers to ask candidates to fill out an application prior to interviewing. Information requested on an application frequently is more complete than information provided on a résumé. A complete educational and work history, such as exact dates of employment, complete company addresses, supervisors' names and contact information, and salary or wage amounts, is commonly requested. This information is typically summarized on a résumé. Applications serve as a snapshot of the applicant, which helps employers choose interview candidates. Additionally, applicants must attest to the completeness and truthfulness of the presented application data by signing a statement of authenticity on the application. Individuals have been hired for a position and later fired because they provided false information on an application and/or a résumé.

Online applications are an effective and efficient method of submitting data. An advantage of submitting electronically is the opportunity to correct data. When preparing an application traditionally, applicants must either key the information in on a computer or fill it in by hand. Read through the entire application before inserting information. By doing this, the applicant will have a a better idea of where to place information, thereby avoiding possible mistakes. If a computer is used to fill out an application and print it, errors can be easily corrected; however, applications prepared by hand require more effort to submit correctly. Correction fluid may be used to correct the occasional error on a handwritten application; but unless the applicant is skilled with using correction fluid, the correction will be obvious. The company may require the correction to be initialed by the applicant. It is best to redo the application. For this reason, when an applicant knows the application will be prepared by hand, additional copies of the application should be available. Blue or black ink should be used to complete an application. Be sure to look for specific instructions on the application concerning ink color. Data on a handwritten application should be printed and neat.

Whether the application is filed electronically or traditionally, several tips apply:

- Determine the information you will need and have it accessible. Samples of information include the following:
  - *Personal information:* In addition to complete name and address, an applicant's Social Security Number may be requested (used to do a background check of the applicant), but date of birth is not. Daytime and evening contact landline telephone numbers and cell phone number are requested. E-mail addresses may also be requested.
  - *Name of position desired:* State the name of the position or positions to which the application applies; whether full-time, part-time, seasonal, or shift work is desired; the date you are available to begin work; and the desired salary. So that you do not eliminate yourself from possible employment because of a stated salary requirement, it is best to answer by giving a range, such as $25,000–$30,000, or using the words "Open" or "Negotiable" to the desired salary. While it is easiest to state "Open" or "Negotiable," you should research similar positions in the geographic region and have an idea of the salary requirements, to help you avoid under- or overpricing yourself for the available position. However, if you require a certain amount and will consider nothing less, then state your desired amount.
  - *Work history information:* Your work history is your employers' names and complete addresses, your supervisors' names and contact information, your

dates of employment, beginning and ending salary or wage information, your responsibilities, your titles, and your reasons for leaving (if separated from employment). If you were fired or laid off, it is best not to place blame when stating the reason for leaving. Statements such as "My professional goal became different from the company's goal" or "The organization went through realignment" show a positive attitude.

Address any gaps in your work history. Individuals have a variety of reasons for not being in the workforce. Reasons should be very brief statements, such as attending school, caring for aging parents, and the like. Be prepared to address reasons for frequent changes in jobs. Reasons such as seasonal work or temporary positions should be listed. If you have more work history than there is room for on the application, the short statement "Additional work experience is available upon request" may be used on the application. Most applications ask for work experience in reverse chronological order.

— *Criminal history:* Honesty is the best policy. State the facts—what happened and how you have changed from the experience.

— *Military history:* Be prepared to record dates, ranks, awards, and commendations.

— *Education:* Have available postsecondary education information. Applications usually ask for the names and addresses of institutions, dates attended, degrees/ credentials earned, hours completed, and grade point average (GPA) or ranking in class. Some employers also request high school information, including the name and address of the high school, diploma or GED, and class ranking or GPA. Any specialized training, awards, or honors may also be requested. Some employers will require an official transcript to prove educational accomplishments.

— *References:* Stating "References are available upon request" is not a best practice for completing an application. A minimum of three references is typically requested. After asking permission, list three (or the requested number) individuals who know your work ethic, skills, and personal aptitudes. Relatives or clergy should not be listed as references. Fellow workers and committee members with whom you have served are good candidates for references. Sometimes an applicant has been out of the workforce, training for a new career. In this case, a fellow long-term classmate or an instructor may be used as a reference. Whomever you use, be sure of what they will say! Provide each person's name, title, address, e-mail, and phone number. State how long you and the reference have known each other, as well as any company information for professional references.

- Spell every word correctly, apply correct punctuation, and use proper grammar.
- Fill in every question. If the question does not apply, then mark "Not Applicable" or "N/A" in the blank.
- Follow all directions on the application.
- Use only positive wording. Also, use wording on the application that reflects desired requirements of the position, such as Web design training and electronic health records experience. This is discussed in more detail later in the chapter.
- Describe your skills using action verbs and concrete nouns. Consider using "keys at 70 words per minute with no errors" instead of "good keyboarding skills" or "interpersonal verbal and communication skills" instead of "good with people."
- Refrain from using acronyms. Spell them out completely.
- Sign and date the application.

Continue the same style of wording when preparing all employment documents— applications, cover letters, résumés, and follow-up letters.

The purpose of a **cover/application letter** is to personalize the application process by introducing the applicant to the employer and to gain an interview. It can be referred to as either a *cover letter* or an *application letter*. The letter places a name and snapshot of relevant information in front of the reader and should entice the prospective employer to schedule an interview. An application may or may not accompany the cover letter.

Prior to writing a cover/application letter, do research to gather data about the company and the position(s). Learn specific job requirements, and try to locate the name of the person to whom you will address your letter. The more you know about a company, the better prepared you will be to write a cover/application letter and to link your skills or traits to specific position requirements. Information can be obtained through the Internet, local business chambers of commerce, libraries, and newspapers, as well as the human resources departments of organizations. If it is a small company and the position has been advertised, information can be obtained through an office manager. However, if the position has not yet been advertised, obtain information and submit an application on the first day that applications are being accepted.

Although there are variations of cover/application letters, correct format, grammar, spelling, and punctuation are essential. The format style should be consistent in the cover/application letter, résumé, and follow-up letter. Left-justified letters and résumés are standard. However, a modified-block-style letter may also be used with a modified-block-style résumé and follow-up letter. When preparing the three employment documents, print them on the same color of high-quality paper. Bright colors (pink, purple, orange) should not be used. Neutral pastel colors, such as beige, wheat, or gray, are easier to read.

The parts of a cover/application letter are the letterhead or return address, inside address, salutation, typical three-paragraph body, and closing.

- *Letterhead or return address:* Many cover/application letters contain personally created letterheads with the applicant's name, address, phone number, and e-mail address. The format should be professional and not distract from the body of the letter. E-mail addresses should always be professional and not offensive. For example, the e-mail address hotmom@hotmail.com or ivoryqueen@gmail.com should not be used as professional contact information. If sending a cover/application letter by e-mail, include the return address contact information at the end of the e-mail after the name.
- *Date:* If the date that you composed the letter is different from the date that you are sending it, use the date you send the letter.
- *Inside address:* This is the name and address of the organization to which you are applying. Through prior research, you should know the name of the person to whom you will address the cover/application letter.
- *Salutation:* Correctly spell the name of the individual and use *Mr., Mrs., Ms., Dr.,* and so on with the name. Since this is a professional business letter, a colon (:) should follow the salutation. It is not professionally appropriate to use "To Whom It May Concern:" or "Dear Human Resources:." This sets a negative tone—one of not caring enough to find out the receiver's name. Sometimes, after extensively researching but not finding a name, the writer may use "Dear Members of the Search Committee:" or address the letter to the manager of a specific department, such as "Dear Coding Department Manager:."
- *Three-paragraph body:* Extensive work experience or education may necessitate a four-paragraph format, although it is usually possible to use concise wording and maintain a three-paragraph format. Prepare the body of the letter in the "you" approach, and refrain from the "I" approach. In other words, state how the organization will benefit from your skills and traits.

— Paragraph 1 is the most important position of the letter. The opening sentence should be professional yet grab the reader's attention. State the position for which you are applying and how, where, and when you learned of the position; also, refer to the position title and how your qualifications match those of the position. Also state if someone has referred you for the position.

- Ineffective example: "I heard about your administrative medical assistant position and would like to apply for the job." This example is missing how, where, and when the applicant learned of the position and is written in the "I" approach.

- Instead use: "Your advertisement in the October 23, 2028, *Washington Central Post* seeks an administrative medical assistant, and the 11 years that I have worked in a progressive medical environment will be an asset to your established office. Please consider this letter as application for your administrative medical assistant position."

— Use paragraph 2 to sell your skills and qualities to the employer. Three main topics are addressed: work experience/traits/skills, education, and résumé. Each of the topics should be related to the job requirements, placing first the category that most closely relates to the position. Use concrete nouns and action verbs to create a specific verbal portrait.

- Ineffective example: "I am creative and able to multitask." The example uses the "I" approach.

- Instead use: "During a rapid patient-growth period, I redesigned limited office space to maximize office workflow. This was accomplished while also implementing a new electronic health records system."

- Avoid repeating information that will be contained in the résumé.

Compare the following two second-paragraph examples for their overall effectiveness.

EXAMPLE ONE (INEFFECTIVE)

"I have had 11 years of medical office experience, where I was able to work with people, function as a team member, and learn new duties. I received an associate degree in office systems with an emphasis in medical coding and billing. My résumé is enclosed."

EXAMPLE TWO (EFFECTIVE)

"Serving as a liaison between patients and insurance carriers enabled me to enhance my analytical and problem-solving skills. The result was an overall yearly increase in collectible accounts of 43 percent. During a 5-year period, my democratic leadership style led the office team in developing requirements for and implementing an electronic health records system. Computer technology, medical office, and coding skills acquired through my associate degree training have been and will continue to be an asset in technological environments, such as Anywhere Medical Center. You may further review my relevant work experience and education on the enclosed résumé."

— Paragraph 3 is the "action" paragraph. The primary focus of paragraph 3 is a polite request for an interview. Provide contact times and phone numbers through which the employer may contact you. If the greeting on your contact phone is not professional, change it to a more appropriate greeting. A statement of appreciative anticipation of the next step or of further discussion about the position can be

1234 Any Street
Somewhere, USA 12345-5555
October 23, 2024

Dr. Mike Doe
5555 St. Christopher's Street
Somewhere, USA 12345-5555

Dear Dr. Doe:

During our October monthly medical coders' meeting, Nancy Smith referred me to your office vacancy for a medical insurance specialist.
After discussing the position requirements with Nancy, I am confident
that the skills and experience I possess would match those required in
the position, and I am, therefore, applying for the position of medical
insurance specialist.

Your position requires a certified coder. Since graduating from
Anywhere Community and Technical College with an associate degree in
health information technology, I have attained two national credentials
(Certified Professional Coder [CPC] and Chart Auditing) and have worked
with local physicians to implement policies and procedures that proac-
tively detect auditing errors. This has resulted in an 80 percent reduction in rejected claims and a 75 percent increase in revenue. During
the same 10-year period, I worked with the medical office team to develop patient satisfaction surveys, analyze results, and incorporate
changes into the office environment. The enclosed résumé lists further
work and educational achievement.

During an interview we can further discuss how to put these and other
qualifications to work for your orthopedic practice. Please contact me
at 555-555-5555 or at nennabayes@anyspace.com Monday through Saturday
prior to 9 P.M. to arrange a time for an interview.

Sincerely,

Nenna Bayes
Nenna Bayes

Enclosure

added to the third paragraph. Following is an example of a correctly worded third paragraph.

- "Putting my skills to work in a highly reputable medical office such as yours is an opportunity that I have been seeking. May I discuss my qualifications with you further during an interview? Please use the phone number in the letterhead to contact me Monday through Saturday prior to 10 P.M. to schedule a time for us to meet."

- *Closing:* Many acceptable closings may be used in a cover/application letter, including "Yours sincerely," "Sincerely," and "Respectfully." Follow the closing with a comma and leave room for the signature. How much room is left depends on the software being used. No less than three spaces should be left. If the letter is being submitted electronically, attach the electronic signature to the letter. Be sure to include the "Enclosure" notation under the name for the enclosed résumé. The following is an example of a proper closing.

Sincerely,

Nenna Bayes

Enclosure

Figure 10.2 provides an example of a cover/application letter of an applicant who is applying for the position of medical insurance specialist in an orthopedic surgeon's office.

McGraw Hill **connect** **GO TO PROJECT 10.3 AT THE END OF THIS CHAPTER**

Investing time and energy into preparing a professional résumé pertinent to your career goal(s) is time and energy well spent. The primary goal of a résumé is not to obtain a position but to gain an interview with the employer and to convey what you can do for the employer. Employers may have numerous résumés to review and only a few seconds to spend on each one. Résumés should be brief, easy to read and/or scan for relevant information, and well written. Just one typographical or grammatical error could land the résumé in "File 13"–the trash can. Investing time to learn about the company and the available position and developing a résumé are the first steps to passing through the initial sorting process.

Various formats, which will be discussed later in this section, are used to present résumé data. Whichever format is chosen, there are basic dos and don'ts for résumé preparation.

Do

- Use **power words,** action verbs, to showcase skills–"increased accounts receivable revenue by 23 percent in a 6-month period." Power words are verbs that emphasize actions within a job position and should follow bullets (use professional bullets, not cute bullets) within the résumé–for example:
  - Billed and collected $15,000 from previously uncollectible accounts receivable
  - Developed history and physical and other patient documentation forms for newly implemented electronic health records system
- Use correct tense. For activities that are still being performed, use present tense. For completed activities, use past tense.
- List military service, collegiate sports, leadership roles, and volunteer work. Military candidates are often viewed as responsible and reliable, with very good work ethics. Involvement in collegiate sports demonstrates teamwork and willingness to follow instructions. The ability to assume responsibility is evident through leadership positions and volunteer projects.
- Supply complete employment information, including company names, company locations (addresses, including phone numbers), and dates employed.
- Maintain a consistent, uncluttered format.
- Use left justification, not right justification.
- Use high-quality résumé paper. If you prepare a cover/application letter, use the same high-quality résumé paper for both the letter and the résumé.
- Prepare different résumés tailored to various career opportunities; rearrange bulleted items to fit the available position's requirements and skills. Have a traditional résumé even if you also have a scannable/electronic résumé.
- Include professional recognitions and awards; educational honors and a grade point average of 3.0 or higher may be listed.
- Limit the use of bold and other functional fonts to highlight data and a font size no larger than 13.
- Confine résumé data, if possible, to one page–use no more than two pages. Administrative positions, such as office manager, may require more pages.
- Ask a qualified individual to proofread the résumé for format, grammar, and content.
- Review social network sites for any comments, postings, photographs, statuses, and so on that may reflect badly on your image. What may have seemed funny at the time may suggest a lack of good judgment or immaturity to a prospective employer.

Don't

- Don't handwrite a résumé!
- Don't use complete sentences or add unnecessary wording. This is referred to as "fluff."

- Don't go back too far for work experience. The rule of thumb is approximately 10 years unless the last position is the only position listed.
- Don't lie about or overstate résumé data. This can lead to dismissal.
- Don't provide personal information such as age (including birth year), marital status, race, religion, physical data (weight/height, etc.), family, sexual orientation, or Social Security Number (unless necessary to perform mandatory background check).
- Don't break up words with hyphens. Press Enter and move the complete word to the next line.
- Don't use first-person pronouns.
- Don't use a work e-mail or professionally distasteful e-mail address, such as singlegal@yahoo.com or loserboy@hotmail.com.
- Don't list numerous classes on the résumé—have a transcript available, if applicable.
- Don't list references but prepare a list in case an employer requests one.
- Don't list salary data on the résumé.
- Don't supply reasons for leaving previous positions, but be prepared to discuss these issues. Also, be prepared to discuss gaps in employment history.

Résumé Formats

After investing time in researching the company and available career opportunities, the next step is to match your employment, education, and other relevant history to the position requirements. Compile the information, and decide which résumé format is best suited to display the information. Basically, there are two categories—chronological and functional. A third format option is a scannable/electronic résumé, which is prepared in either chronological or functional format (or a combination of both) and formatted for optical character reading (OCR). The most widely used file format for submitting résumés over the Internet is the plain-text format.

Chronological Format. The traditional and most common résumé style is the **chronological résumé.** One advantage of this style is that employers can quickly view educational and employment-related information. However, gaps in these areas are also evident. Another advantage of this format is that it is relatively easy to compose. The following sections are included in a chronological format: a heading, a career objective, a summary of qualifications (a recent addition to résumé formats), education, work history, and optional components.

- *Heading:* This section contains identifying and contact information. State your name, address, phone numbers, and e-mail address. List your complete name, including your middle initial. Use a slightly larger font for the name. An address should include the street address, P.O. box number, city, state, and ZIP Code. List the phone number(s) to be used when more information is needed or to arrange for an interview. Include area codes with the phone numbers. As stated previously, e-mail addresses should be professional and not distasteful. Do not include a work e-mail on the résumé.
- *Career objective:* Opinions are divided as to whether a career objective should be included. If you choose to include a career objective, it should be specific to the position and written from the employer's perspective. A concisely written objective should be limited to no more than three lines. Consider the following examples.
  — Instead of "To obtain an administrative medical assistant position in a progressive medical office where I can use my training and skills"
  — Consider "Seeking an administrative medical assistant position where my training in medical front office and clinical skills can contribute to the efficient team dynamics of patient care"
- *Résumé profile:* As with the career objective, this is also an optional section. However, the inclusion of a well-written profile can entice the employer to read further.

Evaluate your experience (work, education, awards, accomplishments, technical and soft skills, etc.), and write a summary that targets the position's qualifications. A rule of thumb is to limit the number of bulleted items to five or six. **Key words,** words used throughout the résumé that directly relate to the position's requirements, should be used in this section. If a position requirement is "use of EHR clinic® software," consider using "Trained using EHR clinic® software" instead of "Medical office software training." Key words are especially important when résumés will be scanned. A résumé profile is also referred to as a *career summary, summary of qualifications, résumé summary,* or *profile statement.*

- *Education:* List your education in reverse chronological order (the most current first)—for many, this is collegiate information. List the school name and complete address as well as your major and minor. Grade point averages (GPAs) may be listed if they are at least 3.0 or higher. Academic awards and recognitions may be listed in this section or in a separate, later section. Only list classes that directly relate to the position, and the list should be concise. A transcript of classes should be made available for review. If college information is listed, it is not necessary to include high school information. If no college information is listed, supply the same data for high school education. If you obtained a GED, list the date on the GED.

- *Work history:* List employment in reverse chronological order. If work experience is most relevant to the available position, place it before the education section. List work experience and/or transfer skills, such as electronic health records experience, that demonstrate qualification for the position. For each position, list (1) employer's name and complete address; (2) dates of employment; (3) your most significant job title; and (4) significant duties, accomplishments, and promotions. An employment application may require complete work history, but a résumé can be selective. If selective employment is listed, be prepared to explain the gaps in employment. A statement such as "Other employment experience is available upon request" may be added to the bottom portion of this section. If this statement is added, have the additional listing prepared using the same format and style as the résumé. Use power words and action verbs to describe job responsibilities. Do not list every responsibility, only those that relate to the position you are seeking. Avoid using personal pronouns and complete sentences.

- *Optional components:* Special skills and capabilities, community service, professional affiliations and/or activities, military service, awards/honors/achievements, and references are examples of optional sections within a chronological résumé. Employers seek individuals who not only are qualified for the position but also demonstrate a sense of community interest and self-enhancement. Many employers require community service as part of employment. Volunteering for community service demonstrates caring for other individuals and community needs and/or goals. Opportunities for community service are varied—a few examples include community cleanup, food drives, and national organization functions, such as walking to raise money for Alzheimer's disease. Opinions are divided on whether or not to include the notation "References available upon request." Whether you place such a notation on the résumé or not, a reference page should be prepared and available for the employer—keep a hardcopy of the reference listing with you and available for a prospective employer. Prior to placing anyone on a reference list, always ask that person's permission, and be sure the individual will give a positive recommendation. List three to five references on a separate sheet prepared in the same format and on the same high-quality paper as the résumé. Most, if not all, of the references should be **professional references,** individuals who know your work skills. If necessary, a **personal reference,** someone who knows your ethics, honesty, and trustworthiness, may be used. For each reference, include
  — the reference's name, with a courtesy title, such as Mr., Mrs., or Ms. (many names can be either male or female).

- the reference's position title, if applicable.
- the name and complete address of the company.
- the reference's phone number(s) with area code(s).
- the reference's e-mail address, if given to you by the reference.

Figure 10.3 provides a sample of a chronological résumé, and Figure 10.4 shows a reference list.

NENNA L. BAYES

1234 Any Street
Somewhere, USA 12345-5555

Cell Phone: 555-555-5555
E-mail: nennabayes@anyspace.com

Figure 10.3

Chronological Résumé

OBJECTIVE

A position in a medical facility in which medical billing and coding experience can be used to sustain and increase revenue from accounts receivable and increase positive patient satisfaction

RÉSUMÉ PROFILE

- Nationally certified professional coder (CPC)
- Nationally certified chart auditor (CCA)
- Developed, implemented, and analyzed patient satisfaction policies and procedures
- Implemented revenue-collection strategies that increased revenue by 23 percent in a 6-month period

EDUCATION

2021–Present, Pursuing Bachelor of Science in Health Information Technology, Anywhere University, Somewhere, USA 12345-5555

- Anticipated graduation date of 2024
- Presidential Scholarship for Academic Achievement
- 112 of 128 hours completed

2019–2021, Associate of Applied Science degree awarded May 2019, Anywhere Community and Technology College, Somewhere, USA 12345-5555

- National Collegiate Honor Society
- GPA 3.98 on a 4.0 scale

Technical skills include the following:

- Microsoft Office Suite Certification (Word, Excel, Access, Outlook, and PowerPoint)
- Proficient in medical office practice management and electronic health records software (EHR clinic®)
- Input technology—keyboarding skills of 85 corrected words per minute, voice-recognition software, and various scanning devices
- Records and database management

EXPERIENCE

May 2019–Present

- Medical Insurance Specialist and Administrative Coordinator for Physicians Center of Somewhere, 8888 Center Street, Somewhere, USA 12345-8888
  - Created and implemented revenue-intensive procedures that reduced uncollectible debt by 23 percent
  - Conducted certified continuing education workshops for physicians and staff
  - Streamlined staff workload to increase staff and patient satisfaction
  - Updated all coding reference and course materials quarterly and annually

COMMUNITY SERVICE

- Chairperson for SkillsUSA
- Organized Zumba Community Fitness Fair
- Conducted update training for Somewhere area medical coders
- Volunteer for Humane Society

PROFESSIONAL AFFILIATION

- American Academy of Professional Coders
- American Federation of Office Administrators

Figure 10.4

NENNA L. BAYES

1234 Any Street
Somewhere, USA 12345-5555

Cell Phone: 555-555-5555
E-mail: nennabayes@anyspace.com

PROFESSIONAL REFERENCES

- Mr. Mark Someone, Office Manager
  Physicians Center of Somewhere
  8888 Center Street
  Somewhere, USA 12345-5555
  555-555-5555
  e-mail—marksomeone@pcos.com

- Ms. Susie Sunshine, Medical Assistant
  Physicians Center of Somewhere
  8888 Center Street
  Somewhere, USA 12345-5555
  555-555-5555
  e-mail—susiesunshine@pcos.com

- Mr. Allan Anyone, Regional President
  AAPC Organization
  9999 Local Avenue
  My Town, USA 55555-4444
  444-444-4444
  e-mail—anyone@aapcky.org

- Mrs. Annie Okley, Vice Chair
  Medical Assistants Foundation
  7777 National Boulevard
  Professionals, USA 44444-3333
  333-333-3333
  e-mail—aokley@maf.edu

Functional Format. **Functional résumés** organize skills and accomplishments into data groups that directly support the position goal, such as management, patient care, or software implementation. Being able to group skills together is one advantage of a functional résumé; however, it takes a little more thought and time to compose this style of résumé. It can best serve individuals who are changing fields and/or have gaps in their employment history. The typical organization of a functional résumé includes the following sections:

- Heading
- Summary of qualifications/skills (optional)
- Skills heading (use bulleted skills)
- Work experience with contact information; since skills will be listed in the previous section, only list the company name, dates of employment, and title
- Education—if education is most relevant to the position, list it prior to the work experience or skills section
- Optional sections

Figure 10.5 shows an example of a functional résumé. The same information was used to prepare both the chronological résumé (Figure 10.3) and the functional résumé samples. Notice the different placement of the information, such as the education section, in each résumé.

Figure 10.5

Functional Résumé

NENNA L. BAYES

1234 Any Street
Somewhere, USA 12345-5555

Cell Phone: 555-555-5555
E-mail: nennabayes@anyspace.com

OBJECTIVE

A position in a medical facility in which medical billing and coding experience can be used to sustain and increase revenue from accounts receivable and increase positive patient satisfaction

RÉSUMÉ PROFILE

- Nationally certified professional coder (CPC)
- Nationally certified chart auditor (CCA)
- Developed, implemented, and analyzed patient satisfaction policies and procedures
- Implemented revenue-collection strategies that increased revenue by 23 percent in a 6-month period

ACHIEVEMENTS

- Billing and Coding Skills
  - Created and implemented revenue-intensive procedures that reduced uncollectible debt by 23 percent
  - Conducted certified continuing education workshops for physicians and staff
  - Streamlined staff workload to increase staff and patient satisfaction
  - Updated all coding reference and course materials quarterly and annually
- Administrative Skills
  - Supervised nine employees within the medical billing and coding department
  - Resolved patient complaints by taking direct, proactive action and conducted follow-up to resolution
  - Established work team and developed patient satisfaction survey—used results to implement patient satisfaction policies and procedures
  - Reorganized workflow within department, resulting in 45 percent, measurable increased productivity
- Technical Skills
  - Microsoft Office Suite Certification (Word, Excel, Access, Outlook, and PowerPoint)
  - Proficient in medical office practice management and electronic health records software (EHR clinic®)
  - Input technology—keyboarding skills of 85 corrected words per minute, voice-recognition software, and various scanning devices
  - Records and database management

EXPERIENCE

May 2019–Present
- Medical Insurance Specialist and Administrative Coordinator for Physicians Center of Somewhere, 8888 Center Street, Somewhere, USA 12345-8888

EDUCATION

2021–Present, Pursuing Bachelor of Science in Health Information Technology, Anywhere University, Somewhere, USA 12345-5555
- Anticipated graduation date of 2024
- Presidential Scholarship for Academic Achievement
- 112 of 128 hours completed

2019–2021, Associate of Applied Science degree awarded May 2019, Anywhere Community and Technology College, Somewhere, USA 12345-5555
- National Collegiate Honor Society
- GPA 3.98 on a 4.0 scale

continued

Figure 10.5

continued

COMMUNITY SERVICE
- Chairperson for SkillsUSA
- Organized Zumba Community Fitness Fair
- Conducted update training for Somewhere area medical coders
- Volunteer for Humane Society

PROFESSIONAL AFFILIATION
- American Academy of Professional Coders
- American Federation of Office Administrators

There may be a situation in which the best style to use is a combination of chronological and functional formats. If you choose to combine formats, be sure to use the proper format for each section but format the entire résumé in a consistent style, such as underlining all side headings.

Scannable and Plain-Text Résumés. In today's technological workplace, résumés frequently are scanned into a database and referenced for interviews. An applicant should be prepared to submit two, differently formatted résumés: (1) a traditionally formatted chronological, functional, or combined chronological/functional résumé; and (2) a scannable résumé. When preparing a **scannable résumé** for electronic (OCR) scanning, all of the formatting elements should be removed. Use only white paper and do not fold or attach anything to it. A folded résumé can lead to misreads by the OCR. Use black ink and a high-quality laser or ink-jet printer. Following are more tips for preparing a scannable résumé:

- Use an OCR-friendly font such as Times New Roman, Courier, Helvetica, or Arial.
- Use 10- to 14-point type font.
- Avoid using italics, underlining, shading, and other unusual elements. Some OCRs can read solid bullets, asterisks, and bold, but use them sparingly. It is best to remember that, when the OCR's capabilities are unknown, omit the "extras." "When in doubt, leave them out!"
- Place phone numbers on separate lines—the OCR may read numbers on the same line as one number.
- Use plenty of white space.
- Refrain from using columns.
- Limit the résumé to one page, if possible.
- Use key words listed in the job description. Electronic resumes are typically reviewed by a scanning program that looks for key words listed in the job description.

A **plain-text résumé,** a résumé with simplified formatting and electronically saved as a .txt file, can be e-mailed or cut and pasted into an online résumé drop box. A résumé prepared using guidelines for scannable formatting but not saved as a plain-text file may transmit misinformation. When preparing a résumé to be sent as a plain-text file, use the same simplified formatting features used to prepare a scannable résumé and save the file as a plain-text file (save the résumé using a .txt file). Plain text is the most widely used file format for submitting résumés via the Internet. When submitting through an e-mail, be sure the subject specifically states the purpose of the message. Use all the previously mentioned tips for a scannable résumé, but also

- use shorter lines.
- format all text to the left.

- remove all tabs. If indentations are desired, use the space bar.
- save the résumé as "Plain Text" or "Text Only."
- correct any errors (after saving in previous step) and resave the résumé.

Figure 10.6 shows an example of the previous résumé saved in plain-text format.

Figure 10.6

Plain-Text Résumé

NENNA L. BAYES

```
1234 Any Street
Somewhere, USA 12345-5555
Cell Phone: 555-555-5555
E-mail: nennabayes@anyspace.com
```

OBJECTIVE
```
A position in a medical facility in which medical billing and coding
experience can be used to sustain and increase revenue from accounts
receivable and increase positive patient satisfaction
```

RÉSUMÉ PROFILE
```
· Nationally certified professional coder (CPC)
· Nationally certified chart auditor
· Developed, implemented, and analyzed patient satisfaction policies
  and procedures
· Implemented revenue-collection strategies that increased revenue by
  23 percent in a 6-month period
```

EDUCATION
```
2021-Present, Pursuing Bachelor of Science in Health Information
Technology, Anywhere University, Somewhere, USA 12345-5555
· Anticipated graduation date of 2024
· Presidential Scholarship for Academic Achievement
· 112 of 128 hours completed
```
```
2019-2021, Associate of Applied Science degree awarded May 2019,
Anywhere Community and Technology College, Somewhere, USA 12345-5555
· National Collegiate Honor Society
· GPA 3.98 on a 4.0 scale
```
```
Technical skills include the following:
· Microsoft Office Suite Certification (Word, Excel, Access, Outlook,
  and PowerPoint)
· Proficient in medical office practice management and electronic
  health records software (EHR Clinic®)
· Input technology: keyboarding skills of 85 corrected words per
  minute, voice-recognition software, and various scanning devices
· Records and database management
```

EXPERIENCE
```
May 2019-Present
· Medical Insurance Specialist and Administrative Coordinator for
  Physicians Center of Somewhere, 8888 Center Street, Somewhere,
  USA 12345-8888
  · Created and implemented revenue-intensive procedures that reduced
    uncollectible debt by 23 percent
  · Conducted certified continuing education workshops for
    physicians and staff
  · Streamlined staff workload to increase staff and patient satisfaction
  · Updated all coding reference and course materials quarterly and
    annually
```

Figure 10.6

continued

COMMUNITY SERVICE

- Chairperson for SkillsUSA
- Organized Zumba Community Fitness Fair
- Conducted update training for Somewhere area medical coders
- Volunteer for Humane Society

PROFESSIONAL AFFILIATION

- American Academy of Professional Coders
- American Federation of Office Administrators

Employment E-Portfolios. In today's electronic age, employers expect their employees to be trained in the use of technology. Websites and links are provided for applicants to upload employment credentials directly or indirectly to the employer. Scanners are used to search for key words within applications and résumés, such as the name of software programs or applicants' certification(s). Another source of technology usage in the employment process is e-portfolios. An employment **e-portfolio** is an electronic collection of data that showcases the applicant's accomplishments, skills, and qualifications. Essentially, it is an expansion of a résumé.

Instead of producing paper or hardcopy employment documents, each document is placed in an electronic file. Similar to applications, the contents of an e-portfolio are varied but have basic elements that should be included.

The difference between a regular paper/hardcopy résumé and an e-portfolio is the expansion of the résumé elements. For example, a paper résumé has a Community Service section that gives short examples of volunteer service, such as "Volunteer for Humane Society." In an e-portfolio, an applicant has the opportunity to expand on the type of service provided by the applicant and to include a letter of recommendation from a supervisor at the Humane Society. Pictures depicting the applicant working with animals could also be included. Following is a list of basic components that may be included in an e-portfolio:

- A copy of the résumé
- Letters of recommendation
- Listing of references
- Projects and/or presentations prepared by the applicant
- Expansion of résumé components. Examples could include scanned copies of educational transcripts, industry-related certifications, thank-you letters relating to community service, awards, and military service documents. Also include an expanded list of accomplishments, skills, and qualifications.
- Examples of work. For new graduates, include examples of classwork. Examples can include software-related work, class-related certificates (e.g., medical terminology certificate), written work, composed documents such as brochures and newsletters, screenshots of EHR software usage, and other applicant-produced class work examples. For an applicant who is changing from one position to another, the same examples would be appropriate; however, all examples should be void of any identifying information. All patient data should be removed.

This list is not inclusive of all possible e-portfolio components. Résumés and e-portfolios should be tailored to fit the employment opportunity. For quick and easy reference, include labels for each electronic file. E-portfolio files should follow the layout of the résumé (which should be the first item in the e-portfolio). Examples of file labels are résumé PROFILE and CODING CERTIFICATIONS.

Store an e-portfolio on an external device that can be transported and left at the end of the interview. Although the interviewer may not keep the external device, it is a good idea to be prepared to leave it with the interviewer. Additionally, an applicant can also take a hardcopy of the e-portfolio to leave with the interviewer(s).

Mc Graw Hill connect

GO TO PROJECTS 10.4 AND 10.5 AT THE END OF THIS CHAPTER

10.5 THE INTERVIEW

An interview may be one of the most stressful steps of the employment process if the applicant has not prepared. Even with preparation, will the applicant be nervous? Yes! Will the interviewer know the applicant is nervous? Yes! However, there is a way to make the interview less stressful and as successful as possible, and that is to do the "3 Ps"—prepare, prepare, and prepare.

Do the Research

It is more efficient to match skills to job requirements if the job seeker knows something about the company or office. Doing research will enable the applicant to learn more about the company's philosophy, profitability, stability, community service, and reputation. Also, knowing information about the organization will enable the applicant to formulate answers to anticipated interview questions and to ask questions during the interview. Several sources of company information are available.

Network Individuals. Person-to-person information is a valuable resource. Former and current employees of a company are important sources of firsthand information. However, listen carefully to distinguish between facts about the company and individuals' feelings. College placement offices and former students who are employed in your field of interest can also supply up-to-date information. As mentioned earlier, local chapters of professional organizations can provide information about local employers.

The Internet. Searching the Internet can yield a wealth of information. If the company has social media sites, blogs, and/or message boards, read through the postings, and remember to look for facts. If negative statements are posted, gather information from other sources, such as newspaper articles, to determine if the postings are valid. If you decide to post, only post professional questions about company facts—steer clear of any negative postings.

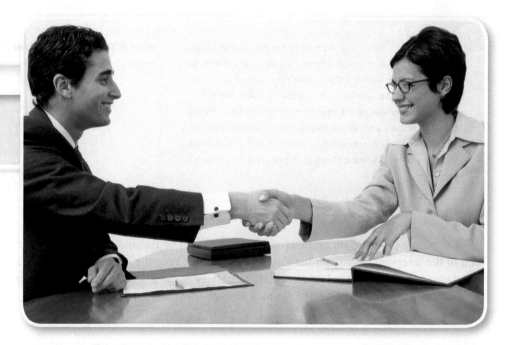

Figure 10.7

The Interview
Latin Stock/Image Source/
Alamy Stock Photo

Company Printed Resources. Most larger companies make available published literature, such as mission statements/philosophies and community involvement activities. These may also be published on their websites. Financial statements, organizational structures, and position descriptions also provide company details.

Preparing for the Interview

Remember the "3 Ps"—prepare, prepare, and prepare. After researching the company, it is time to start preparing physically and mentally for the interview. Before the day of the interview, call the company for directions and make a trial run. As you travel to the interview site, note how long it takes to arrive. On the way, observe any detour or construction signs, school buses, or other factors that require more travel time. Look for parking areas, observing the availability of spaces and cost. Plan to arrive at least 10 minutes prior to the scheduled interview time and add those 10 minutes into the travel time. Also, if taking a bus or subway, add wait time. When traveling the route, look for alternative ways to the company—plan for the unexpected!

Gather Materials. If necessary, purchase a folder to use for interview materials. In it, place *copies* (not originals) of your résumé, your reference listing, recommendation letters, a list of additional work experience, your transcript, and examples of your work. De-identify any medical examples (Figure 10.7). These items may also be placed into a portfolio binder. If everything is equal between two competing applicants, the applicant who has expended the time and effort to assemble information into a portfolio may have the advantage. Take a pen or pencil and a notepad to the interview. The interviewer may ask for additional documents or information, which you should note. In today's technological age, it is also acceptable to take notes on a small, handheld device, such as a smart device. Ask permission of the interviewer to take notes. Place the device in Silent mode. An applicant who is prepared to take notes appears organized. If using a cell phone to take notes, be sure to turn the ringer off.

Dress Appropriately. Clean and pressed—this should be the interviewee's overall physical presentation (Figure 10.8). The person's attire should reflect what he or she would

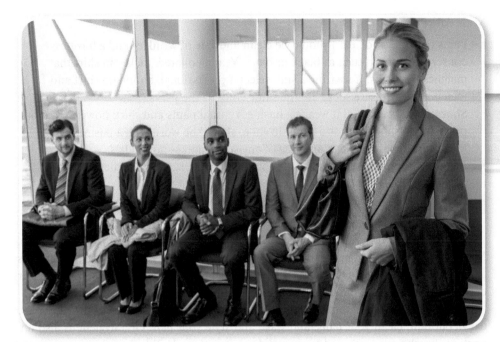

Figure 10.8

Dressing for the Interview
Fredrick Kippe/Alamy Stock Photo

wear if employed in the position. However, there are some exceptions. When interviewing for a position that requires a uniform (such as scrubs), professional office dress, not the uniform (scrubs), is appropriate. If you are unsure about how to dress, it is best to be conservative. In other words, when in doubt, don't! Here are some basic guidelines for female and male interview attire.

Female Attire

- Business dress should have a modest length and neckline. Select a color that is not too flashy. Red and pink are examples of less favorable colors for an interview. Business pants or a skirt and blouse/top are also appropriate.
- Stockings (hose) should be worn with a dress or skirt. Wear closed-toed shoes with a modest heel—no sandals. Be sure shoes are clean and free of scuff marks.
- Nails should be clean, trimmed, and a modest length. If wearing nail polish, use clear or neutral colors.
- Rings and other jewelry should be limited. Many companies have a policy concerning the type and amount of jewelry to be worn. Check prior to the interview and follow any company policy. If one does not exist, follow these suggestions: no more than one ring per hand—engagement and wedding band are considered one ring; one bracelet (which does not make noise); a watch, if desired; no more than two modest earrings in each earlobe; and a conservative necklace. Tattoos should be covered for the interview—the applicant should investigate the company's policy on body art. Also, nose rings, tongue rings, or other body piercings (excluding earrings) should be removed for the interview; again, the company policy on body piercings should be known prior to the interview. What is trendy in one social circle may not be considered professional dress.
- Perfume and/or scented lotions should be a very light scent or not worn at all to the interview. The interviewer may be allergic to the scent.
- Undergarments should be worn but should never be visible through clothing.
- Hair should be clean and conservatively styled. Keep hair away from the face and out of the eyes.

Male Attire

- Pants (cotton, wool, etc.) should be clean and free of wrinkles and a business-conservative color, such as black or blue. Wear a collared, tucked-in shirt that matches the pants. If wearing a suit, select a professional, button-up shirt and matching tie. Be sure socks are the same color as the pants.
- Shoes should be casual if wearing business casual pants and shirt; however, a more professional shoe, such as a wing tip shoe, should be worn with a business suit. Make sure shoes are clean and free of any scuff marks—no sandals.
- Fingernails, piercings, and tattoos should follow the same guidelines as those previously listed for females.
- Hair should be clean and well styled. Keep hair out of the face and eyes. Trim facial hair according to company policy.

Purchasing appropriate clothing for the interview does not have to be expensive. Many thrift and secondhand consignment shops offer a wide variety of business clothes at a fraction of new-store prices. Determine a budget and stick to it. Be a better consumer by using store advertisements and coupons.

Be aware of your personal hygiene. Take a shower or bath the day of the interview, use deodorant, clean your nails, and wash and style your hair. Oral hygiene is also important—brush your teeth and tongue and use mouthwash. Take breath mints and use them just before the interview. When nervous, some individuals have sweaty palms—take tissues to absorb the moisture. To help you feel alert, get at least 8 hours of productive sleep the night before. It is best not to smoke prior to the interview; smoke smell tends to attach to clothing and hair. Check documents, such as résumés, to be sure they are free of smoke smell.

Prepare for Interview Questions. Another way to prepare for an interview is by anticipating the questions the interviewer may ask and developing appropriate responses ahead of time. Employers want to know about the applicant's skills, training, experience, availability, and future plans. Although not every question can be anticipated, the following are some common, general interview questions and statements:

- Tell me about yourself.
- Why should we hire you?
- What is your strongest asset?
- Tell me what experience you have that relates to this position.
- Why do you want to work for our company?
- Can you travel?
- Are you willing to relocate?
- What do you see as your greatest weakness, and what have you done or are planning to do to overcome this?
- Do you work better individually or as part of a team?
- Why are you looking for a position?
- What have you learned from past mistakes?
- Professionally, where do you see yourself in 5 years?
- Do you plan to continue your education?
- Do you view yourself as a leader or as a follower?
- Have you ever been fired from a position? (Be honest and tactful when you answer this question. Placing blame on another individual may give the impression that you cannot take responsibility. State the reason for the separation and what you have learned from the experience.)
- What are the two most important accomplishments in your life so far?
- How would another person describe you?

Practice answering these and other interview questions several times before the actual interview. Even though the wording may be different, the intended content will probably be the same. For many interview questions, there is no right or wrong answer. Most questions are subjective, allowing interviewees to display their work ethics and character through their answers.

In an interview, it is illegal to ask questions about certain areas of an applicant's life. Under Title VII of the 1964 Civil Rights Act and subsequent amendments, it is illegal to discriminate against an employee or job applicant based on several factors: race, color, national origin, sex, gender identity, sexual orientation, religion, age, disability, family status, or political views. Basically, an interviewer is prohibited from asking any question(s) of the applicant that could or may lead to bias. If such a question is asked, the interviewee has three options: (1) Let the situation go and answer the question; (2) mention that the question is illegal, and choose either to answer or not to answer the question; or (3) file a complaint. The choice is up to the interviewee.

Sometimes the wording of the question itself, not the intention, makes it illegal. Such questions are legal only if their content directly relates to a position's requirements. Illegal questions can be grouped into the following categories:

- Affiliations
  - *Not Allowed:* "To which organizations do you belong?"
  - *Allowed:* "Do you belong to any professional organizations that you feel are relevant to this position?"

- Age
  - *Not Allowed:* "How old are you?" "Are you a Baby Boomer?" "When did you graduate from high school?"
  - *Allowed:* "Are you over the age of 18?"

- Arrest Record
  - *Not Allowed:* "Have you ever been arrested?"
  - *Allowed:* "Have you ever been convicted of one of the following crimes?" (The crime must be related to the position, such as a drug conviction relating to a position in a medical office.)

- Citizenship
  - *Not Allowed:* "Are you a U.S. citizen?"
  - *Allowed:* "Do you have the proper paperwork to work in the United States?"

- Health and/or Disabilities
  - *Not Allowed:* "Do you have any disabilities?" "Have you been hospitalized for any major illness in the last 3 years?" "Are you under the care of a mental health professional or have you ever been treated for any type of mental illness?"
  - *Allowed:* Upon completion of the interview and after receiving a thorough description of the job's duties, the applicant may be asked if he or she can perform the essential functions of the position. Many employers require a medical examination after the applicant has been hired. There are also stipulations regarding the release of the information obtained from these exams.

- Gender
  - *Not Allowed:* "Do you have any problem with having a male/female supervisor?" "What is your opinion of office romances?"
  - *Allowed:* "Please tell me about any previous supervising experience."

- Height/Weight
  - *Not Allowed:* "How tall are you?" "How much do you weigh?"

- *Allowed:* "Are you able to lift a 100-pound patient from the examination table back into a wheelchair?" (Questions concerning height and weight are allowed only if they relate to minimum position requirements.)

- Marital and/or Family Status
  - *Not Allowed:* "Are you married?" "Are you single?" "How many children do you have?" "Do you plan to have children or more children?"
  - *Allowed:* "Are you willing to work overtime as needed?" "Can you travel?" (If asked of one candidate, these questions must be asked of each candidate applying for the position.)

- Military
  - *Not Allowed:* "Did you receive an honorable or a dishonorable discharge from your military service?"
  - *Allowed:* "What type of training did you receive while in the service?"

- National Origin or Race
  - *Not Allowed:* "Where are you from?" "Were you born in the United States?" "Your name is unusual—what is the origin of your name?"
  - *Allowed:* "Have you ever worked under a different name?"

- Religion
  - *Not Allowed:* "Where do you go to church?" "Which religious holidays do you celebrate?"
  - *Allowed:* "Are you a member of any organizations that you feel are relevant to and would enhance your performance in this position?"

Keep in mind that this list is not inclusive of all illegal questions and legal wordings, but it is meant to be a guide. Positions such as those in security or medical facilities do require the interviewer(s) to extract the candidate's position-related knowledge and qualifications in some of these areas, but the questions must be directly related to the position requirements. Credit history and background checks are commonly performed on applicants in certain areas.

Requests for Private Social Media Data

Social networks are considered a source of public information and are being referenced by employers to access public information posted by applicants. However, some job applicants are being asked to give login information to employers or to log in accounts from the employer's computer network so that nonpublic information, protected by privacy settings, may be viewed. This practice is called **shoulder surfing.** Shoulder surfing is a direct violation of social media networks' privacy policies, which state that users are to protect login information and forbid anyone from soliciting the login data or accessing another individual's account. Maryland is the first state to pass legislation banning employers from asking for social media passwords of job applicants and company employees. Several other states have laws prohibiting employers from accessing social networking accounts. An interviewer may not ask for login information but may, instead, ask the interviewee to log into the social media site or to "friend" certain company individuals, such as the human resource director or a department director. Both of these actions are considered shoulder surfing.

What do you do if you are asked for your social media login information during an interview? Ultimately, the decision of whether to reveal login data is up to the interviewee. Before making the decision to reveal login information, consider how it could be perceived. If an applicant is willing to divulge protected information during an interview, this same person, if hired, may be willing to divulge protected health information or company information in other situations. Following are examples of how to decline the request for login information, logging into an account, or "friending" a company official.

1. "I take my privacy agreements seriously, and it is against my user agreement to share login information with anyone else. I must respectfully decline your request."

2. "Privacy is a matter that I take seriously. Should I be employed with ABC Healthcare Systems, I would honor all patient protected health information and all company information just as I am now honoring my own privacy, even if this means losing this great employment opportunity with your organization. If presented with a similar situation, I would not jeopardize patient or company information. Therefore, I would prefer to keep my social media profile private."

Currently, there are a few exceptions to shoulder surfing requests, one being candidates for law enforcement positions. However, this, too, is being legally challenged.

As mentioned earlier in this chapter, an applicant's social media comments, photos, blogs, and so on may be used to evaluate a potential employee. Items that are protected through an applicant's privacy settings but are shared by our social media friend may create a possible opportunity for employers to view an applicant's social media information. It is wise for job applicants to remove potentially offensive postings from their social presence before applying for a position. Following are some tips for maintaining an online presence:

1. Search yourself electronically. Because of cookies, caches, etc., on an individual's computer, use a different computer to search for yourself.

2. Update, if needed, privacy settings.

3. Search for individuals having the same name. This could create a mix-up of social information.

4. Review photos and comments that are public.

Conducting the Interview

During the interview is when the applicant presents his or her skills, training, and experience to the employer. The employer will determine the applicant's suitability for the position through a series of questions and observations. It is basically a question-and-answer session. Most of the work has already been completed—the applicant has gathered information, compiled the necessary documents, practiced questions and answers, and made physical preparations (e.g., dress, rest). The old saying "You never get a second chance to make a first impression" is extremely important during the interview process. The interviewer will be assessing not only the applicant's verbal communication skills but also his or her nonverbal communication. The interviewer will evaluate the applicant's confidence, respect, and attentiveness through various ordinary actions, such as a handshake. When you are asked to enter the interview area, wait until a hand is offered before shaking hands. It is a sign of respect to wait for the interviewer to first extend a handshake. Use a firm, but not crushingly firm, handshake. Shake using the whole hand and avoid the "finger" shake (only touching the tips of another individual's fingers).

Be aware of nervous habits or the perception of nervous habits. Consider the following real-life example. During an interview, an applicant was asked if she was a nervous individual. She responded that normally she was not but that today she was. The applicant inquired of the interviewer why the question was asked. The interviewer answered that he had noticed the applicant's very short fingernails and had thought them to be a sign of chronic nervousness. The applicant then explained that she played the piano and needed her nails to be short, a sign of practicality that had been misinterpreted as a sign of nervousness.

Address the interviewer using a courtesy title, such as Mr., Ms., or Dr., and allow the interviewer to be seated and to extend an invitation to be seated before sitting down. This is another sign of respect and courtesy. The following are some more guidelines for being successful in an interview:

- Be on time. Arrive approximately 10 minutes early—and alone. Don't take a friend into the interview venue.
- Refrain from chewing gum, eating candy, or drinking a beverage. However, it is acceptable to take a bottle of water into the interview. Remember to take it with you when the interview is over.
- Maintain consistent eye contact with the interviewer.
- Maintain good posture, both when standing and when sitting. Sit up straight and do not lean. Place your feet flat on the floor or crossed at the ankle. Crossing the legs may be interpreted as too relaxed, and for females wearing a skirt or dress, modesty may be jeopardized. Keep your hands still and comfortably folded in your lap or placed at your side.
- Smile! Smile sincerely and frequently during the interview. Fake smiles are noticeable.
- Listen attentively to the interviewer. Active listening will help you formulate questions for the interviewer.
- Use concrete nouns and action verbs when discussing your experience, your training, and other related position information.
- Avoid saying "um" and "like" when answering questions.
- Turn off your cell phone. Even when a cell phone is placed on vibrate or silent mode, the incoming call or message may still be a distraction. As mentioned earlier, if you use the phone to take notes, turn off the ringer and ask permission of the interviewer and let the interviewer know you are taking notes on the phone.
- Ask questions of the interviewer at the point, usually near the end of the interview, when you are asked if you have any questions. Never say no. This conveys disinterest in the position. Instead, ask questions that will help you gain more knowledge of the position and its requirements. Questions concerning job duties, workload, schedule, evaluation strategies, company structure, and immediate supervisor are all applicable. Salary and benefits questions are best left for the next level—the job offer. Sample questions include the following:
  — Will my duties also include taking patient histories?
  — Are periodic meetings conducted for clinical and administrative medical staff?
  — Should I supply my own blood pressure cuff and stethoscope?
  — Does the practice have a mentor assigned to new employees?

An applicant may be presented with different types of interviews. Panel interviews (a group of interviewers) will ask the applicant interview questions. Some panels are set up to ask questions in a predetermined sequence, while other panels are designed for members to randomly ask questions. You should greet each panel member with a smile and direct eye contact. Shake hands with each panel member. Prepare for a panel interview in the same manner as you would prepare for a one-on-one interview: Use good posture, take notes, answer questions fully, be prepared to ask questions of the panel, and so on. Look at each panel member; do not focus on just one or a few members.

Phone interviews are becoming more common in today's global and fast-paced society. Mentally and physically prepare for a phone interview just as you would for a face-to-face meeting. Prior to the phone interview, confirm the interview time—be sure to consider differences in time zones. Locate a quiet place where you can fully concentrate on the interview without interruptions. Assemble all your employment credentials (e.g., résumé, transcript, and samples of work). Be sure to have a pen and paper to take notes and a glass of water to clear your throat. Dress professionally for the phone interview—no jeans or sweatpants.

During a phone interview, follow these tips:

- Disable the call-waiting feature.
- Do not use speakerphone.
- Listen for and eliminate any background noises, such as a fan, prior to the phone interview.
- Smile and use good posture. This will give you a feeling of physically presenting yourself to the interviewer in a positive nonverbal manner. If you prefer, stand.
- Concentrate totally on the phone interview—do not try to multitask.
- Listen attentively to questions, and ask for clarification if you did not understand.
- Speak at a slightly slower pace than normal.
- Refrain from chewing or eating during the phone interview.
- Keep your answers to less than 2 minutes in length. It is easier to continue talking on the phone than in person.
- Apologize if you accidentally interrupt, and allow the interviewer to finish.

Prior to the interview, an applicant should ask if any testing will be conducted either prior to or during the interview. In the medical setting, it is common practice for an applicant to be tested on his or her knowledge of medical terminology. If applying for a medical coding position, medical coding scenarios will be given for the applicant to code. Keyboarding or computer skills evaluations are common employment tests. "What ifs" scenarios, known as situational interview questions, are used to evaluate an applicant's soft-skill level, such as problem-solving and critical thinking. To reduce the stress level and increase the opportunity for successful testing, the applicant should remember the "3 Ps"—prepare, prepare, and prepare.

Ending the Interview

After all questions have been asked and answered, it is time to conclude the interview. The interviewer normally will nonverbally signal the end by standing or by verbally thanking the applicant. This is a good time, if not answered earlier, to ask what action is next and the anticipated time frame. It is also an opportune time for the applicant to reiterate his or her desire and qualifications for the position. When offered, shake the interviewer's hand and thank the interviewer by name. Also, thank others who were involved, such as an administrative assistant or a receptionist, when leaving the interview.

10.6 THE FOLLOW-UP CONTACT LETTER

After leaving an interview, you should immediately make notes of what happened during the interview, the information you gave and received, the names of people you met, and other details. Write a thank-you letter to the interviewer within a time frame of no more than 2 days. A thank-you letter serves two purposes. It (1) expresses gratitude to

Figure 10.9

Follow-Up Contact Letter

```
1234 Any Street
Somewhere, USA 12345-5555
October 30, 2024

Dr. Mike Doe
5555 St. Christopher's Street
Somewhere, USA 12345-5555

Dear Dr. Doe:

Talking with you on Wednesday, October 30, about the medical insurance
specialist position was informative and interesting. Your medical
facility is progressive, and interviewing with you confirmed my belief
that our professional goals are the same. Thank you for describing
details of the position.

Your recent implementation of electronic health records at Advanced
Treatment Center utilizes a software program with which I have previ-
ously worked and updated. Designing the history and physical interface
was both challenging and rewarding and was an experience that your
facility can utilize to increase physician/patient productivity and
satisfaction. Our discussion on accounts receivable reinforced my
interest in becoming an integral part of your medical office team.
Since the interview, I have considered different options for conducting
internal documentation auditing on a consistent basis and am anxious
to discuss the two different plans with you.

It is exciting to be considered for the medical insurance specialist
position with Advanced Treatment Center, and I look forward to joining
your staff. If you have additional questions or would like to discuss
the position further with me, please contact me at 555-555-5555 or at
nennabayes@anyspace.com.

Sincerely,

Nenna Bayes
Nenna Bayes
```

the interviewer and (2) places the applicant's name and qualifications in front of the interviewer one more time.

Prepare the follow-up contact letter using the same format and paper quality as you used for your cover/application letter and résumé. Use very few, if any, first-person pronouns at the beginnings of sentences. Like the cover/application letter, the thank-you follow-up letter should have three paragraphs:

- Paragraph 1 expresses gratitude for the interview opportunity.
- Paragraph 2 emphasizes the applicant's qualifications and any information you may have forgotten during the interview. Refer to specific topics discussed in the interview.
- Paragraph 3 is forward looking in content. Show enthusiasm and eagerness to join the office team.

Figure 10.9 shows a sample follow-up letter.

It is easy to become discouraged during an employment search. Rejection is inherently part of the process; however, view rejection as an opportunity to learn, to improve, and to move forward. Rejection may have nothing to do with your level of skill or education but with timing, and a rejection becomes an opportunity to seek other career possibilities.

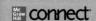

**GO TO PROJECT 10.6
AT THE END OF THIS CHAPTER**

10.1 List and explore visible and hidden career/employment resources.	• Many rich sources of employment opportunities are available for job seekers. Examples of visible/traditional markets include classified advertisements, professional journals, career job fairs, job boards, the Internet, temporary employment agencies, and employment services. • Less common markets for career opportunities include telephone directories, chambers of commerce, company websites, and social/professional networks.

10.2 Assimilate information and prepare an employment application	• Complete and accurate information is needed when completing an employment application:
	  — Personal information
	  — Employment information—including dates of employment and addresses
	  — Educational information
	  — Reference information
	• Complete all blanks.
	• Print legibly using blue or black ink.
	• Be truthful.
	• Sign and date the application.

10.3 Compose a cover/application letter.	• The first impression of a potential employee is frequently made through an application letter.
	• Use a properly formatted letter containing correct grammar and punctuation. Block-style format is common.
	• Prepare the letter using a suggested three-paragraph format:
	  — Paragraph 1 informs the reader from whom, where, and when the applicant heard of the position—the company may have more than one position to fill; actually state which position you are applying for.
	  — Paragraph 2 presents your qualifications (experience/education), linked to the available position. Refer to the enclosed résumé. If electronic, refer to the résumé attachment.
	  — In paragraph 3—an action paragraph—request an interview and provide contact data for the reader.
	• Use high-quality paper.
	• Proofread, proofread, and proofread!
	• Sign the letter using blue or black ink. If electronic, use an electronic signature.

10.4 Assimilate data and compose résumés using different format styles.	• The main purpose of a résumé is to secure an interview.
	• Data compiled for an application, such as personal information, addresses and dates of employment, and education information, may be used to compose a résumé.
	• Résumés take the "snapshot picture" provided on the application or within the application letter to the next level by providing more detail.
	• Formats are chronological and functional. Sometimes a combination of chronological and functional formats is used.
	  — Chronological format supplies data within categories (e.g., education) in reverse chronological order (the most current is placed first).
	  — Functional format supplies data in related skills and experience categories, such as management or administration.
	• Plain-text format résumés should be prepared for electronic or electronically read submission.
	• Categories commonly included in résumés are heading, objective, summary of qualifications, work experience, education, and optional categories (such as awards and community service).
	  — References should be listed on a separate reference page containing three to five professional references. The reference page should be available when requested.
	• Electronically collect employment credentials, samples of work, and other employment documents, and compile them in an e-portfolio. Label each electronic file, and arrange them in a format that reflects the format of the résumé.

10.5 Assemble personal and professional information and appropriate dress for the interview process and conduct a mock interview.	• Gather all requested and/or anticipated interview materials, and assemble them for review into a hardcopy or electronic portfolio. In addition to a cover/application letter and résumé, supply examples of professional work and educational documentation (transcript). Be prepared to leave information with the interviewer—take copies, not originals (unless an original transcript or other documentation is requested).

	• Dress should be professional and conservative. Check company policy on dress and accessories, such as rings, earrings and other piercings, and tattoos. • Use good personal hygiene—bathe/shower and use deodorant, brush teeth and use mouthwash, clean hair and nails, and refrain from using strong colognes and/or scented lotions. • Assemble a list of anticipated interview questions and questions to ask the interviewer. • Practice shaking hands, sitting, and standing.
10.6 Compose a follow-up thank-you letter.	• Within 24 hours—no more than 2 days—after the interview, compose and send a thank-you letter to the interviewer. The letter serves two purposes: — Expression of gratitude — Reminder of your qualifications • Use the same format for the follow-up letter as you used for the cover/application letter. If you used block style for the cover/application letter, use block style for the follow-up letter. • Prepare the follow-up letter using the same high-quality paper you used for the cover/application letter and résumé. • Construct the letter using a three-paragraph format: — In paragraph 1, express gratitude for the interview. — In paragraph 2, remind the reader of your qualifications. — In paragraph 3, express your anticipation of employment with the company.

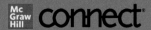
Project 10.1 — (LO 10.1) Preparing Interview Questions

Imagine that you have the opportunity to interview a number of administrative medical assistants about their jobs. What information would you like to learn from them? With a partner, brainstorm a list of questions to ask the administrative medical assistants. Divide your list of questions into three categories: tasks, skills, and personal attributes. Be prepared to discuss your questions and/or submit your project findings to your instructor.

Project 10.2 — (LO 10.1) Locating Positions

Research various sources of available administrative medical assistant positions and select a position. Research and collect data about the position and the company. You will use this information to compose employment credentials. If possible, locate job opportunities in your geographic area by visiting the websites of your state's department of labor and of local newspapers.

Project 10.3 — (LO 10.3) Preparing a Cover/Application Letter

Using the data you collected in Project 10.2, compose a cover/application letter for the position of administrative medical assistant.

Use block-style formatting for the letter. Prepare it in the three-paragraph format discussed in this chapter.

Project 10.4 — (LO 10.4) Preparing a Résumé

Prepare a résumé to accompany the cover/application letter you prepared in Project 10.3. Select the style (chronological or functional) that best suits your qualifications. After preparing the résumé, save it and reopen it. Save a copy of the résumé as plain text.

Project 10.5 — (LO 10.4) Compiling an E-Portfolio

Begin collecting documents for your e-portfolio. The application letter and résumé prepared in Projects 10.3 and 10.4 are a good beginning. Refer to the e-portfolio section within this chapter, and compile electronic data to be used in your e-portfolio. You may need to scan documents into an electronic file. After you have gathered all documents to be included in your e-portfolio, electronically arrange the documents in a format that is the same as the format of your résumé. Label each electronic file to reflect categories on your résumé and the additional documents. Examples of labels are EDUCATION and TRANSCRIPTS. Save the e-portfolio, and be prepared to submit it to your instructor.

Project 10.6 — (LO 10.6) Composing a Follow-Up Letter

You have just completed an interview for the position in Project 10.3. Prepare a follow-up thank-you letter addressed to your interviewer, using that person's name. If you were not able to obtain an individual's name, address the letter to Dr. Karen Larsen, 2235 South Ridgeway Avenue, Chicago, IL 60623-2240.

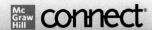
Interpersonal Skills (LO 10.5)

Interpersonal skills are all the behaviors and feelings that exist within all of us that influence our interactions with others. These skills are also referred to as communication skills, people skills, and/or soft skills. We learn them by watching our parents, the television, and our peers. Healthy interpersonal skills reduce stress, reduce conflict, improve communication, increase understanding, and promote joy. Improving these skills builds confidence and enhances our relationships with others. **How can interpersonal skills improve your chances when applying for a job? Can interpersonal skills make or break your interview?**

Positive Attitude (LO 10.5)

A positive attitude helps you cope more easily with daily life and helps you avoid worry. A positive attitude makes you happier and more successful. With a positive attitude, you see the bright side of life and expect the best. If your attitude is positive enough, it becomes contagious. Choose to be happy. Find reasons to smile more often, and associate with happy people. **Why is surrounding yourself with positive people so important?**

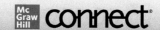
USING TERMINOLOGY

Match the term or phrase on the left with the correct answer on the right.

_____ 1. [LO 10.1] Hidden job market

_____ 2. [LO 10.3] Cover/application letter

_____ 3. [LO 10.4] Chronological résumé

_____ 4. [LO 10.4] Professional reference

_____ 5. [LO 10.4] Functional résumé

_____ 6. [LO 10.4] Key words

_____ 7. [LO 10.5] Shoulder surfing

a. Document that concisely presents an applicant's specific traits that match a career opportunity

b. Career opportunity resources that are less visible

c. Words that are directly related to a position

d. Data presented in categories, with the most recent listed first

e. Individual who can attest to an applicant's work ethic

f. Data organized by categories that directly support a position goal

g. Employers asking for access to private social media data

CHECKING YOUR UNDERSTANDING

Select the most correct answer.

1. [LO 10.1] Latisha recently graduated from a medical office program. While attending school, she worked part-time during evenings in the records department at a local hospital. She is now ready to seek full-time employment in her field of study. Where could she go to begin compiling employment possibilities?

   a. Friends and social networks
   b. Website for the hospital where she works
   c. School career center
   d. All of these are correct.

2. [LO 10.2] When filling out an employment application, periods of unemployment should be

   a. left off the application.
   b. placed on the application with a short explanation, such as "attending college."
   c. placed on the application and left blank.
   d. placed on the application and highlighted, so that it can be discussed during the interview.

3. [LO 10.2] Which of the following would not be considered an appropriate reference for an application or a résumé?

   a. Work colleague of the applicant
   b. Applicant's instructor during recent training
   c. Applicant's clergy
   d. Fellow committee member

4. [LO 10.3] Which of the following is an example of a sentence composed using the "you" approach?

a. "Training during the past 2 years in the medical office program at Anywhere Community and Technical College has provided me with skills that can be used to complement your HIT department."

b. "I have attended school during the past 2 years at Anywhere Community and Technical College."

c. "My skills and training in the medical office program during the past 2 years can be used by your HIT Department."

d. "I recently became certified in medical records and would like to use my skills in your HIT department."

5. [LO 10.3] As Latisha composes a cover/application letter, she is unsure of where to mention her résumé. In which paragraph should she place a reference to her enclosed résumé?

a. First

b. Second

c. Third

d. Second and third

6. [LO 10.4] During her search for employment opportunities, Latisha found an open HIT position with a multi-physician clinic. The résumé is to be submitted online. Which format should she use to submit her online résumé?

a. Functional, because she likes it better and already has a résumé prepared using this format

b. Chronological with bold side headings

c. Chronological, because her recent educational training and certification directly relate to the position requirements

d. Chronological/plain-text format, because her recent educational training and certification directly relate to the position requirements

7. [LO 10.4] Which of the following statements is composed using the most effective power wording?

a. "Implemented revenue collection strategies that increased the collection ratio from 22 percent to 62 percent during a 9-month period."

b. "Assisted in increasing the collection ratio from 22 percent to 62 percent."

c. "Increased the collection ratio from 22 percent to 62 percent."

d. "Worked with the office team to increase the collection ratio rate."

8. [LO 10.5] During an interview for a medical coding position, which requires AHIMA or AAPC coding certification, which of the following questions may legally be asked of the interviewee?

a. "To which organizations do you belong?"

b. "Are you a certified coder through AHIMA or AAPC?"

c. "Do you hold membership in organizations?"

d. "May I see a list of all the organizations to which you belong?"

9. [LO 10.5] Which of the following questions should not be asked by the applicant during the first interview?

   a. "How many patients does the practice see during a normal working day?"
   b. "Will I be cross trained with other members of the medical office team?"
   c. "Do you prefer I wear scrubs or other office dress?"
   d. "Will I receive a yearly cost-of-living salary increase?"

10. [LO 10.6] Which of the following salutations should be used for a follow-up thank-you letter?

    a. Dear Human Resource Director:
    b. To Whom It May Concern:
    c. Dear Mr. Sanders:
    d. Dear Allen,

THINKING IT THROUGH

These questions cover important points in this chapter. Using your critical-thinking skills, play the role of an administrative medical assistant as you answer each question. Be prepared to discuss your responses.

1. [LO 10.5] Donna Smith is an administrative medical assisting student who is currently finishing her education and preparing to seek employment in the healthcare field. Donna does not have transportation, so she has to rely on others for transportation or uses public transportation.

   As a result of this issue, she has arrived late to several interviews.

   Now, it is your turn to think it through!
   a. Should Donna discuss her lack of transportation during the interview? Why or why not?
   b. If Donna has a problem with transportation, should she be seeking employment?
   c. Due to Donna's transportation issue, she was repeatedly tardy for her last job. Should this information be shared during the interview process? Why or why not?

2. [LO 10.5] Nathan was granted an interview for an administrative medical assistant position. During the interview, the employer asked Nathan how the medical office's mission statement (displayed in the waiting area and on the facility's website) aligned with Nathan's professional goal(s). Also, Nathan's résumé, which was referred to during his interview, contained the old name of the medical practice. Nathan was not offered the position. Why do you think Nathan was not offered the position? Why is it important to learn about a potential employer before attending a job interview?

3. [LO 10.5] Addison was nervous during her interview and consistently looked from the floor to a picture located to the right of the interviewer, Ms. Jackson. Ms. Jackson asked Addison if something was bothering her, since she seemed to be distracted. Why is good eye contact important when meeting and speaking with potential employers?

4. [LO 10.2] "Getting a job is a full-time job in itself." Do you agree with this statement? Why or why not?

5. [LO 10.5] Why is being late for an interview one of the most serious mistakes a job applicant can make?

AAMA (American Association of Medical Assistants) A national association providing continuing education, professional networking opportunities, and certification examinations to its members.

absolute accuracy Correctness that is 100 percent; correctness without error, required for handling financial transactions.

accepting assignment The agreement by a healthcare provider who participates in an insurance plan to accept the allowed charge as payment in full for services.

accession book A book containing a list of consecutive numbers used to assign each patient a number in practices where a numeric filing system is used; see also *numeric filing*.

accounting A system used to classify, record, and summarize financial transactions.

accounts payable (A/P) The unpaid amounts of money owed by the practice to creditors and/or suppliers.

accounts receivable (A/R) The unpaid amounts of money owed to the medical practice by patients and third-party payers.

accrual method The accounting method whereby income is recorded as soon as it is earned, whether or not payment is received; expenses are recorded when they are incurred.

accuracy Correctness, including attention to detail; the trait often ranked most important in assistants by physicians.

ACO (accountable care organization) A network of providers who share in the medical and financial responsibility of patient care.

active files Those records belonging to patients currently seeing the physician.

administrative medical assistant (AMA) The title given to medical office professionals who perform administrative tasks in a wide variety of settings.

Advance Directives Legal documents stating the patient's wishes for medical care should the patient not be able to make medical decisions. Examples include living wills, DNRs, and medical durable powers of attorney.

agenda An outline of a meeting, specifying location, time, date, and major topics to be discussed.

aging reports Reports that show the passage of time between the issuing of a request for payment (invoice) and the receipt of payment; used to determine late payments and collect them.

AHDI (Association for Healthcare Documentation Integrity) A national organization that promotes professional standards and growth for the field of medical transcription.

AHIMA (American Health Information Management Association) A national organization that serves health information management professionals, keeps professionals current with legislation, and provides consumers of health services with topics of interest to them.

allowed charge The maximum amount that an insurer will pay for a service or procedure; also called *allowable* or *maximum*.

alphabetic filing A system of filing whereby documents are kept according to names, titles, or classifications in alphabetical order.

AMT (American Medical Technologists) A national organization that promotes professional standards and growth; certification available through the association's examination.

annotate The act of making notes that are either helpful or necessary in the margins of communications before forwarding them to the physician.

annual summary A report providing the monthly charges and payments for an entire year.

application software Computer programs that apply the computer's capabilities to specific uses, such as word processing, graphics, database management, and spreadsheets.

arbitration The process whereby a neutral third party judges the merits of a complaint by one party against another, with the consent of the parties; serves as an alternative to trial, and the judgment is binding.

ARMA (Association of Records Managers and Administrators) An international association that includes among its members information managers, archivists, librarians, and educators; sets standards for filing, record retention, and other aspects of records management.

assault The clear threat of injury to another.

assertiveness The ability to step forward to make a point in a confident, positive manner.

assessment The physician's interpretation of subjective and objective findings as contained in the SOAP record; also called *diagnosis* or *impression*.

assignment of benefits The permission given by a policyholder that allows a third-party payer to pay benefits directly to the healthcare provider.

audit A review of all financial data by an independent party outside the practice—the IRS or an accountant—to ensure the accuracy and completeness of all financial transactions.

authoritarian/autocratic A leadership style that provides clear and definitive expectations to team members.

authorization Expressed (stated) permission given by the patient and required to convey information about a patient to anyone (including the patient).

balance billing Collecting payment from the insured patient of the difference between a provider's usual fee and a payer's lower allowed charge.

balance sheet A report for a stated period indicating the practice's complete assets, liabilities, and capital.

bank reconciliation The process of comparing the balance on the monthly bank statement with the checkbook balance to determine whether there is agreement or a difference in the amounts.

battery Any bodily contact without permission; in medicine, interpreted to include procedures performed without the patient's consent or those that go beyond the degree of consent given.

bibliography A list of all references used by an author in the preparation of a manuscript; listed in a separate section at the end of the text.

bioethics The branch of ethics that deals specifically with medical treatment, technology, and procedure; see also *ethics*.

birthday rule A guideline for determining which of two parents with medical coverage has the primary insurance for a child; states that the policy held by the insured with the earliest birthday in the calendar year is the primary policy.

blank endorsement The presence of only a signature to enable a check to be cashed or deposited; the most common form of endorsement.

block-style letter Arrangement of a letter so that all lines, including those beginning new paragraphs, begin at the left margin.

Blue Cross Blue Shield Association (BCBSA) One of the largest private-sector insurers in the United States; offers both indemnity and managed care plans with many variations.

bookkeeping The accurate recording of financial transactions.

capitation A form of payment made by the insurance company in advance of medical services received; the prepayment by the insurance carrier of a fixed amount to a physician to cover services for a member of a particular plan.

carrier An insurance company; also known as a *third-party payer*.

cash basis The system of accounting whereby charges for services are not recorded as income to the practice until payment is received and expenses are not recorded until they are paid.

CDHP (consumer-driven health plan) An insurance plan that combines a high-deductible, low-premium insurance plan with a medical services payment account.

Centers for Medicare & Medicaid Services (CMS) The federal agency responsible for setting up the terms of Medicare and reviewing managed care plans that want to become Medicare-covered providers; part of the Department of Health and Human Services, CMS was called the Health Care Financing Administration (HCFA) before 2001.

Certificate of Mailing A receipt purchased at the time of mailing that documents the date the material was presented for mailing to the U.S. Postal Service.

certification An essential minimum standard of competence in a particular medical specialty achieved through training and successful completion of a comprehensive examination.

Certified Mail A service offered by the U.S. Postal Service whereby the Postal Service keeps a record of delivery and the sender receives a mailing receipt.

CHAMPVA (Civilian Health and Medical Program of the Veterans Administration) The government health insurance program that covers the medical expenses of families of veterans with total, permanent, service-connected disabilities; covers spouses and dependents of veterans who die as a result of injuries sustained in the line of duty.

channel The chosen method of transmitting a message.

charge/receipt slips Records of the doctor's services to each patient and the charges, combined with a tear-off receipt for the patient.

CHEDDAR A system of documenting medical data in a patient's chart using seven sequential categories: chief complaint, history, exam, details of problem/complaint, drug data, assessment, and return visit or referral.

chief complaint (CC) The reason for the patient's visit to seek the physician's advice.

chronological résumé The traditional and most common résumé style, which lists information in reverse chronological order.

clean claim A medical insurance claim that is free of errors and that can be adjudicated.

clearinghouse A service bureau that collects electronic claims from many different medical practices and forwards the claims to the appropriate insurance carriers.

closed files The records of those patients who have moved away from the area, died, or terminated their relationship with the physician.

cloud computing Performing computerized tasks such as processing, storing, backing up, and synchronizing electronic data over the Internet instead of using a local network.

cluster scheduling A method that brings several patients in at the same time, such as on the hour, to be seen by the provider; also known as *wave scheduling*.

CMS-1500 claim form A paper claim for physician services.

code linkage The connection between the diagnostic and procedural information, examined by insurance carriers to evaluate the medical necessity of the reported charges.

coding (1) *Physical* placement of number, letter, color, or underscore beneath a word to indicate where a document should be filed; (2) the process of assigning codes to diagnoses and treatments based on standard code sets.

coinsurance The percentage of each claim that the insured person must pay; the percentage to be paid by the carrier is usually stated first, as in "a rate of 80-20."

Collect on Delivery (COD) The U.S. Postal Service delivery service that collects postal and other fees from the recipient when the postal material is delivered.

collection agency A business whose purpose is to collect unpaid debts for the creditor; usually used after other methods of securing payment have failed.

collection at the time of service The payment for services by patients at the time of the visit, by cash, check, or credit card where acceptable; the payment method required for insurance copayments.

collection ratio A percentage used to show the effectiveness of collection practices; the higher the collection ratio, the better the collection practices.

color-coding The organization of files according to a system of colored file folders.

compliance The act of adhering to legal rules and regulations as well as high ethical standards through practices and procedures within the medical practice, in all aspects of medical care.

confidentiality The legal requirement that a patient's medical information be kept secret except in certain clearly defined instances.

contributory negligence The failure of a patient to follow the advice and/or instructions of the physician, thus contributing to neglect or an outcome that may not be satisfactory.

coordination of benefits (COB) The clause in insurance policies that states that the insured who has two insurance policies may have only a maximum of 100 percent of the health costs.

copayment (copay) The set charge, required by HMOs and some other insurers, to be paid by patients every time they visit the physician's office.

cover/application letter A letter that introduces the applicant to the employer by supplying relevant information about the applicant as it relates to the available position.

CPT (Current Procedural Terminology) A book published by the American Medical Association and updated annually; contains the most commonly used system of procedure codes.

cross-reference sheet The indication, made on a sheet of paper or card, of other files where a copy of a particular document may be found.

customary fee A physician's charge for a procedure or service determined by what physicians with similar training and experience in a certain geographic area typically charge.

cycle billing A method of billing patients designed to stabilize cash flow and workload; involves dividing patients into groups of a size roughly equal to the number of times billing will take place during the month.

daily journal A record of services rendered by the physician, daily fees charged, and payments received; also called *general journal* or *daily earnings record*.

database The complete history of a patient as contained in a problem-oriented medical record (POMR): includes the problem; medical, social, and family histories; a review of systems, and the physician's conclusions; also, any collection of related data, sets, or subsets of information.

dead storage An area reserved for records that have been closed or that must be stored permanently; usually physically separate from where active files are kept.

decoding The application of meaning by the receiver of a transmitted message.

deductible A certain amount of medical expense the insured must incur before the insurance carrier will begin paying benefits.

deductions The amounts of money withheld from earnings to cover required taxes, insurance, and so on.

Defense Enrollment Eligibility Reporting System (DEERS) The system used to list individuals covered through TRICARE.

defensive medicine Those practices of the physician designed to help him or her avoid incurring lawsuits, such as ordering tests and/or additional tests to confirm a diagnosis, as well as follow-up visits.

delegative/laissez-faire A leadership style that uses a "hands-off" policy and tends to allow other office team members to make their own decisions.

Delivery Confirmation The U.S. Postal Service delivery service that provides the date and time of delivery or attempted delivery.

dependability The ability to complete work on schedule, do required tasks without complaint, and always communicate willingness to help; closely related to accuracy and thoroughness.

dependent A person related to a policyholder, such as a spouse or child.

deposition A sworn statement to the court before any trial begins and usually made outside of court.

deposits Checks or cash put into a bank account.

diagnosis (Dx) A term used interchangeably with *assessment* or *impression*; gives a name to the condition from which the patient is suffering.

diagnosis-related groups (DRGs) A system used by Medicare to establish payment for hospital stays; based on groupings of diagnostic codes that show the relative value of medical resources used throughout the nation for patients with similar conditions.

direct earnings Salaries paid to employees; see also *indirect earnings*.

double-booking appointments The practice used, when the schedule is full, of entering overflow patient appointments in a second column beside regular appointments; in some cases, triple columns are used.

durable power of attorney A legal document giving a stated person the legal right to make decisions for another. This can be for medical decisions, financial decisions, or both.

e-mail A telecommunications system for exchanging written messages through a computer network; also known as *electronic mail*.

e-portfolio An electronic collection of employment credentials and samples of work designed to showcase an applicant's qualifications.

e-signature A unique identifier created for each person through computer code; has the same legal standing as a printed signature.

editing The assessment of a document to determine its clarity, consistency, and overall effectiveness.

efficiency The ability to use time and other resources to avoid waste and unnecessary effort.

EFT (electronic funds transfer) The automatic withdrawal of employees' net pay from the practice account and the deposit to each employee's account; arranged for with the bank by the physician.

electronic claims Claims that are completed and transmitted to insurance companies by computer, with the assembling of data and completion of claims done using medical billing software.

electronic health records (EHRs) Healthcare databases compiled over the course of different patient encounters.

electronic remittance advice (ERA) The report sent to the patient and healthcare provider by the insurance carrier informing them of the final reimbursement determination, and containing the same additional information as the EOB; used for electronic claims.

emancipated minor A minor who has achieved independence through circumstances or by court order from his or her parents or legal guardians.

emergency Acute symptoms of sufficient severity that the delay of medical attention would result in serious jeopardy to an individual or unborn child, serious impairment of body functions, or dysfunction of a body organ or part.

empathy Sensitivity to the feelings and situations of others that allows one to mentally put oneself in the other person's situation.

Employer Identification Number (EIN) A tax identification number that employers are required to have by the Internal Revenue Service (IRS).

encoding Using words and gestures to convey a message.

endnotes References that the author may have used as background or relevant information, placed on a separate page following the text of the manuscript.

ergonomics The science of designing the work environment to meet the needs of the human body, while reducing the risks of injury or hazards without decreasing output.

established patient (EP) A patient who has seen the physician or a physician of the same specialty within the same practice in the last 3 years.

ethics The standards of conduct that grow out of one's understanding of right and wrong.

ethnocentrism The tendency to believe that one's own race or ethnic group is the most important and that some or all aspects of its culture are superior to those of other groups.

etiquette Those behaviors and customs that are standards for what is considered good manners.

explanation of benefits (EOB) The report sent to the patient and the healthcare provider by the insurance carrier informing them of the final reimbursement determination, explaining the decision, and appending reimbursement due the provider; used for paper claims.

express consent The patient's approval, which may be given either orally or in writing; required for procedures that are not part of routine care.

family history (FH) Facts about the health of the patient's parents, siblings, and other blood relatives that may be significant to the patient's condition.

fee adjustment The reduction of a fee based on the physician's decision of the patient's need; see also *write-off*.

fee schedule A list maintained by each physician or medical practice of the usual procedures the office performs and the corresponding charges.

fee-for-service A payment method through an insurance carrier whereby the patient (policyholder) pays for medical services at the time of receiving them and is reimbursed by the insurance company once it has reviewed and approved a claim describing the services; alternately, the policyholder's directive that the carrier pay the service provider directly once services are received.

feedback A receiver's response(s) to a message.

FICA (Federal Insurance Contributions Act) The law that governs the Social Security system and requires that a certain amount of money be withheld for Social Security benefits; employer pays half the amount withdrawn and employee pays the other half.

file server A central computer within a computer network, used to store the computer programs and data that must be shared by all the computers in the network; also called, simply, a *server*.

first draft The first complete keying of a manuscript.

first-class mail The classification of mail weighing 13 ounces or less, which includes all correspondence, whether handwritten or typewritten, such as bills and statements of account, and is sealed against postal inspection.

fixed office hours Designated hours during which the physician is available for scheduled appointments. Each patient is given a set appointment time.

flexibility Adaptability to new or changing requirements.

folders Containers used to hold those items that are to be filed; frequently made of a sturdy material to withstand handling.

footnotes Notes, usually at the bottom of a page, used to cite sources of information or quotations used in the text.

fraud An intentionally dishonest practice that deprives others of their rights, such as falsifying credentials or submitting false or duplicate insurance claims.

full endorsement The signature on a check indicating the person, account number, or bank to which the check is being transferred, and the payee's name.

functional résumé The résumé format in which skills and accomplishments are organized into data groups that directly support the position goal.

FUTA (Federal Unemployment Tax Act) The federal law that requires employers to pay a percentage of each employee's salary; the amount paid provides a fund for employees once they are unemployed and seeking new jobs.

gender rule An older method of determining a dependent's primary insurance coverage when both parents have coverage. The father's insurance would be primary.

good judgment The ability to use knowledge, experience, and logic to assess all aspects of a situation in order to reach a sound decision.

Good Samaritan Act A law designed to protect trained medical personnel who provide emergency care from liabilities for civil damages that may arise from the circumstances.

graphics application A software program that allows the user to manipulate images and to create original images electronically.

guarantor The insurance policyholder for a patient.

guide A rigid divider placed at the end of a section of files to indicate where a new section or category of files begins.

HCPCS Pronounced "hic-pics"; stands for *Healthcare Common Procedure Coding System,* for use in coding services for Medicare patients.

Health Insurance Portability and Accountability Act (HIPAA) The federal law that protects the security and privacy of health information by regulating how electronic patient information is stored and shared.

hidden job markets Employment markets that are less obvious and require more initiative by job seekers to access.

history of present illness (HPI) Information taken from the patient about symptoms: when they began, what factors affect them, what the patient thinks is the cause, remedies tried, and any past treatment for the symptoms.

HMO (health maintenance organization) The oldest form of managed care; a medical center or designated group of physicians provides medical services to insured persons for a monthly or annual premium.

honesty Truth telling, expressed in words and actions; a quality that enables the person to be trusted at all times and in all situations.

IAAP (International Association of Administrative Professionals) A worldwide organization that sponsors continuing education and a certification examination with the successful completion earning the designation of Certified Administrative Professional (CAP); also works with employers to promote excellence; formerly known as Professional Secretaries International (PSI).

ICD-10-CM *(International Classification of Diseases, 10th edition, Clinical Modification)* A list of alphanumeric codes required by the federal government and used by physicians and other healthcare providers in the outpatient setting to classify and code diseases and conditions.

ICD-10-PCS *(International Classification of Diseases, 10th edition, Procedure Coding System)* A list of alphanumeric codes required by the federal government and used by inpatient facilities to classify and code procedures.

implied consent The patient's agreement that is not stated outright but is shown by the patient's having gone to the doctor's office for treatment.

impression A term used interchangeably with *assessment* or *diagnosis*; gives a name to the condition from which the patient is suffering.

inactive files The records of those patients who have not seen the doctor for a stated period of time as defined by the practice.

income statement A financial statement showing profit and loss for a stated period of time, such as a quarter or a year.

indemnity plan An insurance plan that provides a percentage of payment to the physician on a fee-for-service basis; the patient assumes responsibility for the remaining portion of the cost.

indexing The process of *mentally* selecting the name, title, or classification under which a document or an item will be filed.

indirect earnings Amounts of money other than salary supplied to the employee, such as paid leave; also benefits such as employer-paid benefit programs that are worth amounts of money.

informed consent The ability of the patient to make a sound decision to agree because the problem has been explained in clear language and the physician has given treatment options and a prognosis.

initiative The exercise of one's power to act independently.

inspecting documents The act of checking each item received for filing to be sure that the information is complete and that the item is in good physical condition.

insured May be the person who takes out an insurance policy and is responsible for the payments; may also refer to anyone, such as a spouse or dependent, covered by an insurance policy.

Insured Mail Articles sent through the U.S. Postal Service or other carriers that are covered against loss or damage through the purchase or provision of insurance.

interest Money paid by the bank to depositors in return for the use of the depositor's money.

Internet A vast, worldwide computer network that links millions of computers; enables almost instantaneous sharing of information in various digital forms—text, graphics, sound, video, and so on.

itinerary A daily schedule of events for a traveler, containing such information as flight numbers and times and hotel and car arrangements.

key words Words used throughout the résumé that directly relate to the position requirements.

label An oblong piece of paper, frequently adhesive, used to identify a file by title or subject.

laptop A portable computer, designed to fit into a briefcase; able to run on either plug-in current or batteries.

lateral files Drawers or shelves that open horizontally where files are arranged sideways from left to right instead of from front to back.

liability Legal responsibility.

licensure The act of the state whereby healthcare providers, and those in other professions, are granted licenses to practice under certain conditions, including meeting the requirements of education and training.

litigation The bringing of lawsuits against an individual or other entity.

living will A written document providing directions for medical care to be given if a competent adult becomes incapacitated or otherwise unable to make decisions personally; see also *Advance Directives.*

mainframe A computer designed to store massive databases that many users may all access at the same time.

malpractice An act that a reasonable and prudent physician would not do, or the failure to do some act that such a physician would do.

managed care A system that combines the financing and delivery of healthcare services to members.

management qualifications Usually regarded for the administrative medical assistant as the ability to be a team player, the ability to do strategic planning, and the ability to increase productivity.

mature minor An unemancipated minor who has demonstrated through a set of consistent standards that he or she possesses the maturity to understand and comprehend the nature, risk, and consequences of medical treatment.

maturity Emotional and psychological integrity composed of many qualities and skills.

Meaningful Use Set of standards defined by CMS that specify how EHRs are to be used and allow eligible providers to earn financial incentives for the use of certified EHRs by meeting stated objectives.

Medicaid A health benefit program, jointly funded by federal and state governments, designed for people with low incomes who cannot afford medical care.

medical abandonment The physician's failure to furnish care for a particular illness for as long as it is required unless the patient has been discharged in an appropriate manner.

Medical Practice acts The laws of each state governing who must be licensed to give care, the rules for obtaining licensure, the grounds for revoking licenses, and the reports required by state law.

Medicare The federal health plan that provides insurance to citizens and permanent U.S. residents 65 years and older, people with disabilities (including kidney failure), and dependent widows; divided into Part A, hospitalization insurance; Part B, outpatient insurance; Part C, Medicare Choice; and Part D, prescription coverage.

medicolegal A type of document that provides evidence of patient care and is considered a legal document in a court of law.

meeting minutes Official record of a meeting, including the major pieces of business conducted; the names and contributions of any attendees who spoke; the date, place, and time of the meeting; those present and absent; and the duration of the meeting.

message Ideas formulated by the sender to be received by the recipient.

microcomputer A computer designed for one user; may reside on a desktop or may be portable, and may be called a PC, laptop, or microcomputer.

micrographics The process of storing records in miniaturized images, usually in a microfiche sheet or ultrafiche format, viewed on readers that enlarge the images.

minicomputer A computer having less power than a mainframe; may operate for a single user or along with many terminals.

mixed/standard punctuation The placing of a colon after the salutation of a letter and the placing of a comma after the complimentary closing.

mobile-aisle files Open-shelf files that are moved manually or by motor.

modified-block-style letter The arrangement of a letter whereby the dateline, complimentary closing, and signature all begin at the center of the page and all other lines begin at the left margin.

monthly billing The system of sending each patient an updated statement of payments made and charges owed to the physician once per month; these are all sent from the office at the same time every month.

monthly summary The report that shows the daily charges and payments for the entire month.

networking A means of communicating, exchanging information, and pooling resources among a group of electronically locally linked computers.

new patient (NP) A patient who has not seen the physician or a physician of the same specialty within the same practice group for 3 or more years.

no-show A patient who, without notifying the physician's office, fails to show up for an appointment.

noise Internal and external interference with the communication process.

numeric filing A system of document storage in which each patient is assigned a number; see also *accession book.*

objective The physician's examination of the patient contained in the SOAP record; results of the examination may be shown under the heading "Physical Examination (PE)."

online Connected to a computer network for purposes of communicating, gathering, or exchanging information.

open and fixed office hours A method of scheduling patients that combines times during which patients are seen *without* prearranged appointment times (open scheduling) and *with* scheduled appointment times (fixed scheduling).

open office hours A method of seeing patients during hours when the physician is available and no appointment is made, such as from 10 A.M. to noon; patients are seen on a first-come-first-seen basis.

open punctuation No punctuation used outside the body of a letter unless the line ends with an abbreviation.

open-shelf files Shelves that hold files, may be adjustable or fixed, and may extend from floor to ceiling; shelves accept files placed sideways with identifying tabs protruding.

operating system The internal programming that tells the computer how to use its own components by controlling the basic functions of the computer and directing the computer to interact with the user and with input and output devices.

optical character reader (OCR) Equipment used to scan materials for data, such as a ZIP Code.

out guide A card placed as a substitute for a file folder; indicates that a file has been removed.

output device A device used to display electronic data.

outside services file A list of professional and other resources kept in either paper or electronic format.

participating (PAR) provider A physician who joins an insurance plan and agrees to provide services according to the rules and payment schedules of the insurance plan.

participative/democratic A leadership style in which the leader not only offers advice but also participates in the team dynamics and seeks input from other team members.

password A code assigned to a computer user as a security measure; limits access to computer files and safeguards information.

past medical history (PMH) A listing of any illnesses the patient has had in the past; includes treatments and procedures performed.

patient education materials Printed materials provided to patients to give information on caring for their health, lists of resources, descriptions of frequently requested tests and procedures, and the like.

patient encounter form The list made of procedures, diagnoses, and charges during any particular patient visit.

patient information brochure A booklet that provides vital information about the practice, such as services offered, qualifications of the physicians, instructions for making appointments, and ordering refills of prescriptions.

patient information form A form used to collect a patient's personal and insurance information; usually updated at least every 12 months.

patient ledger cards A record that contains a patient's name, services rendered, charge, payment, and balance.

patient statement The copy provided to the patient of all charges incurred by the patient and all payments made by the patient or the patient's insurance company; also called the *patient bill.*

payroll The total earnings of all the employees in the practice.

perfectionism Unrealistic expectations and goals and being dissatisfied with anything less.

personal computer A computer designed for one user; may reside on a desktop or may be portable, as laptop and notebook computers are; referred to as a *PC* or as a *microcomputer.*

personal reference An individual who knows a job seeker's personal ethics, honesty, and trustworthiness.

petty cash fund A fund containing small amounts of cash used for expenses so minor that checks would not be written to pay them: postage stamps, cab fares, and the like.

physical exam (PE) A complete examination of the patient in which findings for each of the major areas of the body are stated or an examination that covers only the body systems pertinent to that particular visit.

plain-text résumé A résumé with simplified formatting; used to submit an online résumé.

plan The treatment, as stated in the SOAP record, listing prescribed medication, instructions given to the patient, and recommendation for surgery or hospitalization.

policies and procedures manual An employee handbook that contains job descriptions, job responsibilities, instructions for completing routine tasks, personnel policies, and so on.

POLST (Physician Orders for Life-Sustaining Treatment) A transportable medical document completed and kept by the patient that states the type of life-sustaining treatment(s) he or she may or may not want. It is signed by both the patient and the patient's physician.

POS (point of service) A managed care option that combines features of a traditional HMO and a PPO allowing patients to use out-of-network providers while still using a PCP.

posting The activity of transferring an amount from one record to another.

POSTNET A bar code interpretation of the ZIP Code or the ZIP+4 consisting of a series of long and short vertical lines, which is placed on the lower portion of the mailing address.

power words Action verbs used to showcase your skills.

PPO (preferred provider organization) A popular type of managed care plan that contracts to perform services for members at specified rates, usually lower than fees charged to regular patients; also provides members with a list of healthcare providers from which to receive services at lower rates.

practice analysis report The report used to analyze the revenue of the practice during any specified length of time; contains lab charges, patient payments, copayments, adjustments, and so on.

preauthorization The requirement by HMOs and some other insurance plans that the physician obtain permission from the insurance plan before delivering certain types of services.

premium The rate charged to a person who holds an insurance policy; usually paid on a regular basis, monthly or quarterly.

primary care provider (PCP) The physician who coordinates the patient's overall care and ensures that various medical services are necessary; described as a "gatekeeper" and often an internist or a general practitioner.

Priority Express Mail Service offered by the U.S. Postal Service that provides next-day delivery of items.

Priority Mail A service offered by the U.S. Postal Service; 2-day delivery service to most domestic destinations.

problem-oriented medical record (POMR) A patient record organized around a list of the patient's complaints or problems; contains a database of the patient's history, initial plan, and problem list.

problem-solving The ability to find solutions through flexibility, advice seeking, information gathering, and good judgment.

procedure day sheet A numeric listing of all the procedures performed on a given day; includes patient names, document numbers, and places of service; may be a computerized journal form.

professional image The appearance, manner, and bearing that reflect health, cleanliness, and wholesomeness; shown by evidence of healthful habits, good grooming, and appropriate dress.

professional reference An individual who knows a job seeker's work ethics and skills.

proofreading The careful reading and examination of a document for the sole purpose of finding and correcting errors.

provider A physician or other healthcare professional.

punctuality The ability to be on time.

Real ID Act Federal law that established minimal standards for verifying an individual's identification.

reasonable fee A charge for the physician's service that is a usual and stated charge and/or the charge by physicians in the geographic area with similar experience.

records management The systematic control of the steps in the life of a record, from its creation through its maintenance to its disposition.

Red Flag Requirements Mandated federal regulations that must be implemented by creditors to protect covered financial accounts from identity theft.

referral The recommendation from the primary care provider (PCP) that the patient use a specialist for a specific service; in the referral document, the PCP names the provider and states the service.

Registered Mail Items sent through the U.S. Postal Service for which a delivery record is maintained at the mailing Post Office; a receipt is given to the sender at the time of mailing.

registration A permit granted to a physician for prescribing and dispensing pharmaceutical medications.

relative value scale (RVS) The assignment of values to medical services based on an analysis of the skill and time required to provide them; values are multiplied by a dollar conversion factor to calculate fees.

release mark An indication by initial or by some other agreed-upon mark that a document has been inspected and acted upon and is ready for filing.

release of information (ROI) Written permission signed by the patient, authorizing the proper transfer of information to those who have made a legitimate request or have a legitimate need; often called simply a "release."

reprints Copies of an already published article; available from the publisher for a small fee or free when the physician is the author.

resource-based relative value scale (RBRVS) The payment system used by Medicare; establishes relative value units for services based on what each service costs to provide.

respondeat superior A common-law legal doctrine that makes employers liable for the actions of employees when those actions are performed within the scope of their employment.

Restricted Delivery Direct delivery through the U.S. Postal Service; item delivered only to the addressee or addressee's authorized agent.

restrictive endorsement Signing, or endorsing, of a check by writing or stamping "For Deposit Only," the account number to which the check should be deposited, and the signature.

Retail Ground The classification of mail for items 70 pounds or less and no more than 130 inches in length and girth; mailing fee is based on weight, distance to travel, and shape.

retention The length of time that records are kept; regulated in many cases by state law; also regulated by Medicare.

Return Receipt A piece of paper provided by the U.S. Postal Service to give the sender proof of delivery.

review of systems (ROS) The physician's specific questions to the patient about each of the body's systems.

rule out (R/O) A possible diagnosis that must be proved or "ruled out" by further tests. In the outpatient setting, a rule out diagnosis cannot be submitted to an insurance carrier—only confirmed signs and symptoms can be submitted.

scannable résumé A format style used for résumés read by optical character readers.

screening calls The practice of evaluating calls to decide on appropriate appointment action.

scribe An unlicensed assistant who accompanies the physician and enters medical data into an electronic health record or chart at the direction of the physician.

scrubber program Software used to detect and correct medical insurance claims prior to being submitted to the insurance carrier.

self-motivation The quality expressed by willingness to contribute without being asked or required to undertake a task.

settlement An agreement by parties on opposing sides; may be the result of a court decision or an agreement arrived at without trial; may involve compensation to the complaining party.

shared medical appointments A method of scheduling patients with the same condition in a group setting and at the same time.

shoulder surfing The practice of employers requesting access to an employee's and/or interviewee's private social media information.

Signature Confirmation U.S. Postal Service delivery service that provides the date, ZIP, time of delivery (or attempt), and signature of the person who accepted the delivery.

SOAP An acronym used to refer to the most common system for outlining and structuring notes on a patient's chart; the acronym stands for the headings used: Subjective, Objective, Assessment, and Plan.

social history (SH) Information that may be pertinent to treatment regarding the patient's marital history; occupation; interests; and eating, drinking, and smoking habits.

sorting The arrangement of documents in the order in which they will be filed.

Special Handling A U.S. Postal Service for-a-fee service to be used when sending items that are fragile and require extra care. The package should be marked "FRAGILE."

sponsor The TRICARE and CHAMPVA term for enlisted military personnel through whom medical coverage is provided.

spreadsheet programs Software used for financial planning and budgeting.

statute of limitations A law made by each state government setting a time limit beyond which the collection of a debt, or the prosecution of many kinds of crimes, is not subject to legal action; varies from 3 to 8 years.

storing The placement of an item in its correct place in a file; also called *filing*.

stress Emotional and/or physiological reactions to external motivators.

subject filing A system of document storing whereby the placement of related material is alphabetic by subject categories.

subjective The patient's description of the problem or complaint, including symptoms, when symptoms began, associated factors, remedies tried, and past medical history.

subpoena A legal document ordering that all materials related to a lawsuit be delivered to court; also, a legal document requiring people to appear in court and to divulge information.

subpoena duces tecum A legal order for a person to appear, testify, and present specified documents.

summons A written notice to the person being sued (defendant), ordering the person to answer charges presented in the document.

supercomputers The most powerful computers available.

tab A projection that extends beyond the rest of the file folder so that the folder may be labeled and easily viewed.

tab cut Position of tab on file folder.

tact The ability to speak and act considerately, especially in difficult situations.

team player One who is generous with his or her time, helping other staff members when necessary; who observes both the written and unwritten rules of the office; and who practices professional and personal courtesy.

telephone etiquette A set of skills and attitudes used when answering the phone that allows the assistant to sound alert, interested, and concerned.

template A standard electronic version of a frequently used document; may be altered slightly from one use to the next; saves user time in keying and formatting commonly used documents and forms.

terminated account The account of a patient from whom it has not been possible to extract payment; also the status of accounts at the end of the patient-physician relationship for other reasons.

third-party liability The assumption of responsibility for charges related to a patient by someone other than the patient—for example, a patient's insurance carrier would have financial third-party liability.

third-party payer An insurance company that agrees to carry the risk of paying for medical services for the insured.

thoroughness The ability to perform tasks with attention to completeness, correctness, and detail.

title page The first manuscript page, which contains the title of the manuscript and the author's name, degree and/or title, and affiliation.

transcription A method of recording data whereby the medical provider dictates data into a recording device and an individual trained in medical keyboarding skills keys the information into documentation format.

travel agent A professional, often certified by the travel industry, who may work independently or within a travel company; handles all aspects of travel arrangements at no charge to the customer.

triage The determination of how soon a patient needs to be seen by the physician based on whether the patient's condition requires immediate attention.

TRICARE The Department of Defense health insurance plan for military personnel and their families; coverage extends to active or retired members of the U.S. Army, Navy, Marines, Air Force, Coast Guard, Public Health Service, and National Oceanic and Atmospheric Administration, and dependents of military personnel killed on active duty; formerly called *CHAMPUS*.

urgent A condition that requires immediate medical attention as a result of an unforeseen illness, injury, or condition but is not defined as an emergency.

usual fee A healthcare provider's average charge for a certain procedure or service, usually shown on the physician's fee schedule.

vertical carousel file system A file storage container that uses a motorized carousel-like motion to bring selected drawers/files to a desired location for retrieval.

vertical files Drawer files, contained in cabinets of various sizes; files are arranged from front to back.

virus (computer) A malicious computer program written with the intent of harming other data, software, and/or computers.

visible job markets Employment markets composed of resources that are traditional and most obvious.

visionary A management style that focuses on the overall goals and mission of the medical environment and encourages team members to move together in the same positive direction.

voice-recognition technology A program used along with a word processing application to transcribe spoken words into text without the use of a keyboard.

wave scheduling Groups of patients are scheduled and arrive for appointments at the same stated time, such as on the hour (e.g., 1 P.M.). Another group (or wave) of patients will arrive at the next schedule time (e.g., 2 P.M.).

wireless communication The use of radio waves rather than wires or cables to transmit data through a computer network.

word processing program Software used to enter, edit, format, and print documents.

work ethic The collective habits and skills that help the worker deal effectively with work tasks and with people.

workers' compensation State law and insurance plan requiring employers to obtain insurance in case of employee accident or injury.

write-off The subtraction of an amount from a patient's bill; entered into the patient ledger as an adjustment.

ZIP Abbreviation for Zone Improvement Plan, which is a system of the U.S. Postal Service of designating delivery of mail based on numerical codes.

ZIP+4 An extension of the postal ZIP system that adds an additional four codes, which represent a geographic segment such as a building number to the original ZIP Code.

Bibliography

1500 Claim Form Reference Instruction Manual. National Uniform Claim Committee, July 2020. Accessed November 20, 2020. www.nucc.org/index.php/1500-claim-form-mainmenu-35/1500-instructions-mainmenu-42. *(Ch. 8)*

AHIMA. "Retention and Destruction of Health Information." Updated October 2013. Accessed October 10, 2019. http://library.ahima.org/doc?oid=300217#.XZ9yVyV7m1s *(Ch. 5)*

AHIMA. "Using Medical Scribes in a Physician Practice." *Journal of AHIMA* 83, no. 11 (November 2012): 64–69. Accessed October 1, 2019. http://library.ahima.org/doc?oid=106220#.WNFzgXQrJPN *(Ch. 5)*

American Association of Medical Assistants. *AAMA Code of Ethics.* 2018-2019. Accessed July 10, 2019. www.aama-ntl.org/docs/default-source/members-only/aama-bylaws.pdf. *(Ch. 2)*

American Board of Medical Specialties. "Specialties and Subspecialties." 2019. Accessed July 10, 2019. https://www.abms.org/member-boards/specialty-subspecialty-certificates/ *(Ch. 1)*

"Are Checks with "Payment in Full" in the Memo Line Legally Binding?". LevelSet. October 28, 2019. Accessed December 18, 2019. https://www.levelset.com/blog/beware-checks-payment-in-full-memo-mechanics-lien-rights/. *(Ch. 9)*

Arkovich, Christie D. "Debt Collectors Calling Your Cell Phone: TCPA Protection You Should Not Overlook." December 2, 2019. www.christiearkovich.com/debt-collectors-calling-your-cell-phone-tcpa-protections-you-sho.html. *(Ch. 8)*

"Best Practices for Mail Screening and Handling Processes: A Guide for the Public and Private Sectors." Interagency Security Committee, U.S. Department of Homeland Security, September 27, 2012. Accessed September 12, 2019. www.dhs.gov/sites/default/files/publications/Mail_Handling_Document_NonFOUO%209-27-2012.pdf. *(Ch. 4)*

"Bipartisan Budget Act of 2018: Fraud Penalties Up, Stark Law Clarified." *Bloomberg Law Health Law and Business News* (June 4, 2018). Accessed July 10, 2019. https://news.bloomberglaw.com/health-law-and-business/bipartisan-budget-act-of-2018-fraud-penalties-up-stark-law-clarified *(Ch. 2)*

Blackett, Karine B. *Career Achievement: Growing Your Goals.* New York: McGraw-Hill, 2011. *(Ch. 1 and 10)*

Bohm, Allie. "Maryland Legislature to Employers: Hands Off Facebook Passwords." ACLU.org, April 9, 2012. Accessed December 17, 2019. www.aclu.org/blog/maryland-legislature-employers-hands-facebook-passwords. *(Ch. 10)*

Centers for Medicare & Medicaid Services. "2016 Program Requirements." February 14, 2017. Accessed March 21, 2017. www.cms.gov/Regulations-and-Guidance/Legislation/EHRIncentivePrograms/2016ProgramRequirements.html. *(Ch. 2)*

Centers for Medicare & Medicaid Services. "Are You a Covered Entity?" (August 2, 2020). Accessed February 1, 2021. https://www.cms.gov/regulations-and-guidance/administrative-simplification/hipaa-aca/areyouacoveredentity.html *(Ch. 2)*

Christie, Les. "The New American Household: 3 Generations, 1 Roof" (April 3, 2012). *CNN Money* (April 3, 2012). Accessed October 15, 1019. https://www.cnn.com/2012/04/03/us/the-new-american-household-3-generations-1-roof/index.html *(Ch. 6)*

"CMA (AAMA) Occupational Analysis." American Association of Medical Assistants, *CMA (AAMA)* (November 2017). Accessed July 10, 2019. https://www.aama-ntl.org/medical-assisting/occupational-analysis *(Ch. 1)*

Cohn, D'Vera, and Jeffrey S. Passell. "A Record 64 Million Americans Live in Multigenerational Households." *Fact Tank, Pew Research* (April 5, 2018). Accessed October 15, 2019. https://www.pewresearch.org/fact-tank/2018/04/05/a-record-64-million-americans-live-in-multigenerational-households/ *(Ch. 6)*

"Consumer Driven Care Fact Sheet." *Consumer Driven Care* (February 13, 2017). www.consumerdrivencare.com/factsheet. *(Ch. 7)*

CPT Professional Edition, 2021. American Medical Association. 2021. *(Ch. 7)*

"Cultural Clues: Communicating with Your Deaf Patient" (January 2012). University of Washington Medical Center, January 2012. Accessed July 10, 2019. http://depts.washington.edu/pfes/PDFs/DeafCultureClue.pdf. *(Ch. 1)*

"Debt Collection." Federal Trade Commission, Consumer Information, March 2018. Accessed December 2, 2019. www.consumer.ftc.gov/articles/0149-debt-collection. *(Ch. 8)*

Department of Homeland Security. "REAL ID Frequently Asked Questions for the Public." Last published October 2, 2019. Accessed October 15, 2019. Available at www.dhs.gov/real-id-public-faqs. *(Ch. 6)*

"Disclosures for Emergency Preparedness—A Decision Tool: Authorization." U.S. Department of Health and Human Services, July 26, 2013. Accessed December 10, 2019. https://www.hhs.gov/hipaa/for-professionals/special-topics/emergency-preparedness/authorization/index.html *(Ch. 2)*

"The Different Types of Health Insurance Plans." *eHealth* (September 22, 2016). Accessed October 5, 2016. https://resources.ehealthinsurance.com/individual-and-family/different-types-health-insurance-plans. *(Ch. 7)*

The Douglas Whaley Blog. "The Payment-in-Full Check: A Powerful Legal Maneuver," blog entry by Douglas Whaley, April 11, 2011. Accessed December 18, 2019. http://douglaswhaley.blogspot.com/2011/04/payment-in-full-check-powerful-legal.html *(Ch. 9)*

Doyle, Allison. "Hard Skills vs. Soft Skills: What's the Difference?" *The Balance Careers* (February 4, 2019). Accessed September 4, 2019. https://www.thebalancecareers.com/hard-skills-vs-soft-skills-2063780 *(Ch. 1)*

Doyle, Allison. "How to Write a Job Application Letter." *The Balance Careers* (July 30, 2019). Accessed December 17, 2019. https://www.thebalancecareers.com/how-to-write-a-job-application-letter-2061569 *(Ch. 10)*

Eischen, Clifford, and Lynn Eischen. *Résumés, Cover Letters, Networking, and Interviewing,* 3rd ed. Mason: South-Western Cengage Learning, 2010. *(Ch. 10)*

"Emancipation Law and Legal Definition." *USLegal* (2012). Accessed July 10, 2019. http://definitions.uslegal.com/e/emancipation. *(Ch. 2)*

Ericson, Brad. (2019). "Easy Tips for Writing a Professional Email." *Healthcare Business Monthly* 6(9), 54–57. *(Ch. 7)*

"Essential Health Benefits." HealthCare.gov. Accessed December 10, 2019. www.healthcare.gov/glossary/essential-health-benefits. *(Ch. 7)*

"Expected HIPAA Updates and HIPAA Changes in 2019." *HIPAA Journal* (January 31, 2019). Accessed July 12, 2019. https://www.hipaajournal.com/hipaa-updates-hipaa-changes/ *(Ch. 2)*

"Facts About the Official 'Do Not Use' List of Abbreviations." The Joint Commission, June 28, 2019. Accessed October 1, 2019. www.jointcommission.org/facts_about_do_not_use_list. *(Ch. 5)*

"FECC Approves New TCPA Rules—Telephone Consumer Protection Act." *The National Law Review* (June 18, 2015). Accessed December 2, 2019. www.natlawreview.com/article/fcc-approves-new-tcpa-rules-telephone-consumer-protection-act. *(Ch. 8)*

Feldman, Paige Miles. "The Choice Is Not Always Yours: A Minor's Right to Make Medical Decisions." *Campbell Law Observer* (February 5, 2015). Accessed July 10, 2019. http://campbelllawobserver.com/the-choice-is-not-always-yours-a-minors-right-to-make-medical-decisions. *(Ch. 2)*

Gambel, Molly. "FTC Releases New Guidance for Red Flags Rule." Becker's Healthcare, *Becker's Hospital Review* (June 14, 2013). Accessed December 18, 2019. www.beckershospitalreview.com/legal-regulatory-issues/ftc-releases-new-guidance-for-red-flags-rule.html. *(Ch. 9)*

Griffith, Eric. "What is Cloud Computing?" *PCMag* (May 3, 2016). Accessed October 10, 2019. www.pcmag.com/article2/0,2817,2372163,00.asp. *(Ch. 5)*

HCPCS Level II Expert, 2021. American Academy of Professional Coders, 2021. *(Ch. 7)*

Heathfield, Susan M. "Payroll File Contents." *The Balance* (March 14, 2019). Accessed December 18, 2019. www.thebalance.com/payroll-file-contents-1918224. *(Ch. 9)*

Hicks, Joy. "OSHA Employee Safety Precautions for the Medical Office." *VeryWellHealth* (May 18, 2019). Accessed October 15, 2019. https://www.verywellhealth.com/osha-employee-precautions-2317277. *(Ch. 3)*

HIPAA Basics for Providers: Privacy, Security, and Breach Notification Rules. Department of Health and Human Services, Centers for Medicare & Medicaid Services, September 2018. Accessed December 10, 2019. www.cms.gov/Outreach-and-Education/Medicare-Learning-Network-MLN/MLNProducts/Downloads/HIPAAPrivacyandSecurity.pdf. *(Ch. 2)*

ICD-10-CM Expert for Physicians and Hospitals, 2021. American Academy of Professional Coders, 2021. *(Ch. 7)*

"Illegal Interview Questions." Better Team. July 30, 2019. Accessed December 17, 2019. https://www.betterteam.com/illegal-interview-questions *(Ch. 10)*

"Informed Consent." American Cancer Society, July 2014. Accessed July 10, 2019. https://www.cancer.org/treatment/finding-and-paying-for-treatment/understanding-financial-and-legal-matters/informed-consent/what-is-informed-consent.html *(Ch. 2)*

"Insurance and Extra Services." U.S. Postal Service, 2019. Accessed September 13, 2019. www.usps.com/ship/insurance-extra-services.htm. *(Ch. 4)*

Internal Revenue Service. "Recordkeeping." IRS, updated April 26, 2019. Accessed December 18, 2019. www.irs.gov/businesses/small-businesses-self-employed/recordkeeping. *(Ch. 9)*

"Job Seekers Getting Asked for Facebook Passwords." *USA Today* (March 21, 2012). Accessed December 17, 2019. http://usatoday30.usatoday.com/tech/news/story/2012-03-20/job-applicants-facebook/53665606/1. *(Ch. 10)*

Lindberg, Sara, and Legg, Timothy. "Eustress: The Good Stress." *Healthline* (January 3, 2019). Accessed October 15, 2019. https://www.healthline.com/health/eustress. *(Ch. 6)*

Lofquist, Daphne A. "Multigenerational Households: 2009–2011." United States Census Bureau, *American Community Survey Briefs* (October 2012). Accessed October 15, 2019. https://www2.census.gov/library/publications/2012/acs/acsbr11-03.pdf. *(Ch. 6)*

Magloff, Lisa. "Types of Management Leadership Styles." *Chron: Small Business* (2017). Accessed October 15, 2019. http://smallbusiness.chron.com/types-management-leadership-styles-10024.html. *(Ch. 6)*

"Mail and Shipping Services." U.S. Postal Service, 2019. Accessed September 13, 2019. www.usps.com/ship/mail-shipping-services.htm. *(Ch. 4)*

Marques-Lopez, Dalizza D. "Not So Gray Anymore: A Mature Minor's Capacity to Consent to Medical Treatment." University of Houston Law Center, October 2006. Accessed July 10, 2019. www.law.uh.edu/healthlaw/perspectives/2006/(DM)MatureMinor.pdf. *(Ch. 2)*

"Meaningful Use Program Renamed; Stage 3 Requirements Revised." AAP News. June 13, 2019. Accessed October 1, 2019. https://www.aappublications.org/news/2019/06/13/hit061319 *(Ch. 5)*

Medical Identity Theft and Medicare Fraud, Brochure. Department of Health and Human Services, Office of Inspector General. Accessed December 14, 2019. https://oig.hhs.gov/fraud/medical-id-theft/OIG_Medical_Identity_Theft_Brochure.pdf. *(Ch. 9)*

"Medical Records Collection, Retention, and Access." Health Information and the Law Project, 2012. Accessed October 10, 2019. www.healthinfolaw.org/topics/60. *(Ch. 5)*

Medicare Managed Care Manual, Chapter 4. Centers for Medicare & Medicaid Services, April 22, 2016. Accessed December 10, 2019. www.cms.gov/Regulations-and-Guidance/Guidance/Manuals/downloads/mc86c04.pdf. *(Ch. 7)*

"Multigenerational Households on Rise in U.S." NBCNews.com, October 25, 2012. Accessed October 15, 2019. http://economywatch.nbcnews.com/_news/2012/10/25/14669859-multigenerational-households-on-rise-in-us?lite. *(Ch. 6)*

Niemeyer, Brooke. "What Are Debt Collection Laws? For Instance, Can a Debt Collector Call You at Work?" *Credit.com* (March 25, 2019). Accessed December 2, 2019. https://www.credit.com/debt/top-10-debt-collection-rights/ *(Ch. 8)*

"NHA Certifications." National Healthcareer Association. Accessed September 4, 2019. www.nhanow.com. *(Ch. 1)*

Occupational Outlook Handbook, 2018–2019 Edition. Bureau of Labor Statistics, U.S. Department of Labor. Accessed July 3, 2019. www.bls.gov/ooh/healthcare/medical-assistants.htm. *(Ch. 1)*

"Office-Based Physician Electronic Health Record Adoption." Health IT Quick-Stat #50. The Office of the National Coordinator for Health Information Technology, January 2019. Accessed October 1, 2019. dashboard.healthit.gov/quickstats/pages/physician-ehr-adoption-trends.php. *(Ch. 5)*

Patel, Sonal. "New Anti-Kickback Provisions Affect Labs and Physicians." *Healthcare Business Monthly* (April 2019). American Academy of Professional Coders. *(Ch. 2)*

"Patient's Bill of Right—What Is the Patient's Bills of Rights?" Health Source Global. Accessed July 10, 2019. www.healthsourceglobal.com/docs/Patient%20Bill%20of%20Rights_merged.pdf. *(Ch. 2)*

Peterson, Thad. "100 Top Job Interview Questions—Be Prepared for the Interview." *Monster* (2019). Accessed December 17, 2019. https://www.monster.com/career-advice/article/100-potential-interview-questions *(Ch. 10)*

"Postal Explorer." U.S. Postal Service. 2019. Accessed September 12, 2019, pe.usps.com. *(Ch. 4)*

Prichard, Justin. "How to Write a Check: A Step-by-Step Guide." *The Balance* (November 20, 2019). Accessed December 11, 2019. https://www.thebalance.com/how-to-write-a-check-4019395 *(Ch. 9)*

Prichard, Justin. Writing and Cashing Postdated Checks *The Balance* (July 29, 2019). Accessed December 11, 2019. www.thebalance.com/postdated-checks-315335. *(Ch. 9)*

"Priority Mail." U.S. Postal Service, 2019. Accessed September 13, 2019. www.usps.com/ship/priority-mail.htm?gclid=CPDNtti4xs4CFZM2aQodlmwJMA. *(Ch. 4)*

"Priority Mail Express." U.S. Postal Service, 2019. Accessed September 13, 2019. www.usps.com/ship/priority-mail-express.htm. *(Ch. 4)*

Procedural Coding Expert, 2021. American Academy of Professional Coders, 2021. *(Ch. 7)*

"Protect Your Patients, Protect Your Practice: What You Need to Know About the Red Flag Rules." Practice Management Center. American Medical Association, 2011. Accessed December 11, 2019. https://www.cms.org/uploads/red-flags-rule-edu.pdf. *(Ch. 9)*

Purcell, Glynnis. "The Top 7 Management Styles: Which Ones Are Most Effective?" *Workzone* (August 27, 2019). Accessed October 15, 2019. https://www.workzone.com/blog/management-styles/ *(Ch. 6)*

"REAL ID Flying with REAL ID." Transportation Security Administration, Department of Homeland Security. Accessed October 15, 2019. https://www.tsa.gov/real-id. *(Ch. 6)*

"REAL ID Frequently Asked Questions for the Public." Department of Homeland Security. October 2, 2019. Accessed October 15, 2019. https://www.dhs.gov/real-id-public-faqs. *(Ch. 6)*

"Record Retention Guideline." MedPro Group, 2017. Accessed October 10, 2019. https://www.medpro.com/documents/10502/359074/Record+Retention+Guideline2017.pdf *(Ch. 5)*

"Removing a Patient from Your Practice: A Physician's Legal and Ethical Responsibilities." Modern Medicine Network, March 16, 2015. Accessed July 10, 2019. https://www.medicaleconomics. com/health-law-policy/removing-patient-your-practice-physicians-legal-and-ethical-responsibilities *(Ch. 2)*

Rodriquez, Christy. "REAL ID: Everything You Need to Know." *Upgraded Points* (October 5, 2019). Accessed October 15, 2019. https://upgradedpoints.com/real-id-act. *(Ch. 6)*

Stein, Loren. "Glossary of Common Medical Specialties." Sentry Drug, March 11, 2013. Accessed September 4, 2019. www. sentrydrug.com/main/patient-resources/library_modal/646265/ glossary-of-common-medical-specialties. *(Ch. 1)*

Sullivan, Thomas. "New Laws to Be Implemented Regarding Kickbacks and Opioid Treatment." *Policy & Medicine, A Rockpointe Publication* (December 30, 2018). Accessed July 10, 2019. https://www.policymed.com/2019/01/new-laws-to-be-implemented-regarding-kickbacks-and-opioid-treatment.html *(Ch. 2)*

"Summary of the HIPAA Security Rule." Health Information Privacy, HHS.gov, last reviewed July 13, 2013. Accessed December 10, 2019. https://www.hhs.gov/hipaa/for-professionals/security/ index.html *(Ch. 2)*

Taylor, Nicole Fallon. "Are You Asking Candidates These Illegal Job Interview Questions?" *Business News Daily* (July 6, 2018). Accessed December 18, 2019. www.businessnewsdaily. com/4037-illegal-interview-questions.html. *(Ch. 10)*

Toporoff, Steven. "Red Flag Rules: What Providers Need to Know." Pedorthic Footcare Association, 2019. Accessed December 11, 2019. https://www.pedorthics.org/page/ RFRWHCPNTK/Red-Flag-Rules-What-Healthcare-Providers-Need-to-Know.htm *(Ch. 9)*

Torrey, Trisha. "Doctors Firing or Dismissing Patients." Updated July 29, 2019. Accessed September 12, 2019. https://www. verywellhealth.com/can-my-doctor-fire-or-dismiss-me-as-a-patient-2615017. *(Ch. 2)*

Torrey, Trisha. "How to Get Copies of Your Medical Records." Updated September 19, 2019. Accessed October 10, 2019. https://www.verywellhealth.com/how-to-get-copies-of-your-medical-records-2615505. *(Ch. 2)*

"Travel." Transportation Security Administration, Department of Homeland Security. Accessed October 15, 2019. www.tsa.gov/ traveler-information. *(Ch. 6)*

"The Patient Bill of Rights: Your Right to Respect and Good Care." *HCA Healthcare* (July 20, 2016). Accessed July 10, 2019. https://hcahealthcare.com/hl/?/134184/The-Patient-Bill-of-Rights–Your-Right-to-Respect-and-Good-Care *(Ch. 2)*

"Triage: A Guide to Urgency for Non-Clinical Staff in General Practice for Telephone and Walk In Presentations." Rural Health West, 2014. Accessed December 10, 2019. http://www. practiceassist.com.au/PracticeAssist/media/ResourceLibrary/ General%20Practice%20Accreditation/ACCREDITATION_ POSTER_Front_Desk_Triage_V1.pdf *(Ch. 4)*

"Triage Protocol for Non-Clinical Staff." Medical Protection Society, October 2014. Accessed September 11, 2019. https://www.medicalprotection.org/ireland/practice-matters/ may-2014/example-triage-protocol-for-non-clinical-staff *(Ch. 4)*

Waldman, Joshua. "What to Do If a Company Asks for Your Facebook Password in a Job Interview." *Ladders* (July 31, 2014). Accessed December 30, 2019. www.theladders.com/p/1467/ what-to-do-if-company-asks-for-facebook-password-in-job-interview. *(Ch. 10)*

Westgate, Aubrey. "To Reduce Medical Practice Risks, Implement a Compliance Plan." *Physicians Practice* (October 10, 2013). Accessed December 17, 2019. www.physicianspractice. com/mgma13/reduce-medical-practice-risks-implement-compliance-program. *(Ch. 2)*

"What Is Considered Protected Health Information Under HIPAA?" *HIPAA Journal* (April 2, 2018). Accessed July 12, 2019. https://www.hipaajournal.com/what-is-considered-protected-health-information-under-hipaa/ *(Ch. 2)*

"Who's Answering the Phone? Why Telephone Policies Are Important." Medical Protective. Accessed December 2, 2019. www.server5.medpro.com/documents/11006/16730/Who_Is_ Answering_the_Phone.pdf. *(Ch. 8)*

"Your ePortfolio: An Essential Job Marketing Tool." *Getting Hired* (September 15, 2016). Accessed December 17, 2019. https://www.gettinghired.com/en/blog/2016/9/your-eportfolio-essential-job-marketing-tool *(Ch. 10)*

Working Papers

WORKING PAPERS

Working Papers are also included in Connect

PERSONAL ATTRIBUTES, WORK ETHIC AND PROFESSIONALISM, AND INTERPERSONAL RELATIONSHIPS

Directions: Match the term in Column 2 with its definition in Column 1.

Column 1

_____ 1. On time and ready to work

_____ 2. Inspired to increase knowledge and to advance

_____ 3. Able to produce work with few or no errors

_____ 4. Able to understand how a patient feels

_____ 5. Careful to pay attention to detail

_____ 6. Truthful; trustworthy

_____ 7. Privacy for all patient information

_____ 8. Ability to take independent action

_____ 9. The correct appearance for the job

_____10. Able to present ideas and information without offending

_____11. A person who works well with associates and pitches in when needed

_____12. Able to make good use of time and materials and to be organized

_____13. Able to present ideas to others with confidence

_____14. Pleasant and friendly

_____15. Able to adapt to new conditions; willing to try new ideas

Column 2

a. accurate

b. assertive

c. cheerful

d. confidentiality

e. efficient

f. empathetic

g. flexible

h. honest

i. initiative

j. professional image

k. punctual

l. self-motivated

m. tactful

n. team player

o. thorough

PHYSICIAN'S OBLIGATIONS AND MEDICAL LAW

Directions: The following items refer to the obligations of the physician and/or medical law. Mark each statement with either "T" for *true* or "F" for *false*. Be prepared to discuss your answers.

_____ 1. The Principles of Medical Ethics state that the physician may refuse to accept a new patient.

_____ 2. A license to practice is good for the life of the physician.

_____ 3. A physician must obtain an annual permit for narcotic registration.

_____ 4. The physician is legally obligated to inform a patient of all possible reactions to a medication.

_____ 5. A physician must obtain a written consent before seeing a new patient.

_____ 6. A physician is legally obligated to seek a referral if the conditions are beyond the physician's scope of knowledge.

_____ 7. A physician's license to practice medicine is valid in all 50 states.

_____ 8. Medical practice acts, established by law, govern the practice of medicine.

_____ 9. The physician cannot refuse to perform a procedure on a patient because of that physician's moral beliefs.

_____ 10. The Drug Education Administration issues narcotic registration and renewals.

_____ 11. When a patient visits a physician for an appointment, he or she is establishing implied consent.

_____ 12. A physician must obtain the maximum amount of education in a particular medical specialty before becoming certified in that specialty.

_____ 13. The adult age as defined by law is known as *majority*.

_____ 14. Express consent is not required in an emergency situation.

_____ 15. A physician must sign a consent form before performing any procedure.

MEDICAL LIABILITY AND COMMUNICATIONS

Directions: The following items refer to medical liability and communications. Mark each statement with either "T" for *true* or "F" for *false*. Be prepared to discuss your answers.

_____ 1. The charge of battery exists when there is a clear threat of injury to another.

_____ 2. A subpoena orders the defendant to answer the stated charges.

_____ 3. Contributory negligence may exist if the patient has failed to follow the physician's advice and treatment.

_____ 4. Access to health records is the form that contains written permission to release patient information.

_____ 5. Defensive medicine means the physician is dissolving legal responsibility.

_____ 6. An authorization for release of information does not have the physician's signature.

_____ 7. A statute of limitations controls the time limit for starting a lawsuit.

_____ 8. Using e-mail to transmit medical documents is preferred over faxing documents.

_____ 9. In a lawsuit, the burden of proof that malpractice exists rests on the patient.

_____10. The physician may be charged with medical abandonment if the physician discontinues care without sending proper notification to the patient.

_____11. Statutory reports require that the patient's condition be reported to the patient's insurance.

_____12. Operating beyond the patient's expressed consent may establish a charge of battery.

_____13. A deposition is sent to the defendant requiring the defendant's appearance in court.

_____14. The Good Samaritan Act states that a patient may start a lawsuit upon reaching majority.

_____15. HIPAA is a federal law that protects the security and privacy of a patient's electronic health information.

LEGAL TERMS

Directions: Match the term in Column 2 with its definition in Column 1.

Column 1

_____ 1. Standards of right and wrong conduct

_____ 2. Adherence to rules and regulations

_____ 3. Patient's permission for treatment when he or she enters a doctor's office

_____ 4. Legal responsibility

_____ 5. Testimony under oath, usually outside of court

_____ 6. Behavior and customs that are considered good manners

_____ 7. Time limit for a lawsuit to start

_____ 8. Physician's leaving a case before the patient is recovered or transferred

_____ 9. State law that governs the state's practice of medicine

_____ 10. Patient's written agreement to have a procedure performed

_____ 11. Clear threat of injury

_____ 12. Depriving others of their rights by dishonest means

_____ 13. A lawsuit

_____ 14. Legal document ordering all relevant documents to be submitted to the court

_____ 15. Authorization to send the patient's information to another physician

_____ 16. Operating beyond the patient's given consent

_____ 17. Written notice sent to the defendant asking for an answer to the charges

_____ 18. Resolution of a case brought about by an unbiased third party

_____ 19. Protection for the physician from liability of civil damages in emergency care

_____ 20. Confidential information that must be submitted to the state department

Column 2

a. abandonment

b. arbitration

c. assault

d. battery

e. compliance

f. deposition

g. ethics

h. etiquette

i. express consent

j. fraud

k. Good Samaritan Act

l. implied consent

m. liability

n. litigation

o. Medical Practice Act

p. release of information

q. statute of limitations

r. statutory report

s. subpoena

t. summons

OUTSIDE SERVICES

Hugh Arnold, MD 2785 South Ridgeway Avenue, Suite 440 Chicago, IL 60647-2700 312-555-6800 **Internist**	Martinez Transcription Service 2200 South Ridgeway Avenue Chicago, IL 60623-2000 312-555-2424 **Betze Martinez**
Jason Berger, MD 5000 North Oak Park Drive Chicago, IL 60634-0005 312-555-7050 **Personal friend**	Elizabeth Miller-Young, MD 2901 West Fifth Avenue, Suite 205 Chicago, IL 60612-9002 312-555-3500 **OB/GYN**
Consumer Pharmacy Pharmacists: Dale Geddal, MD 312-555-1252 Joy Rishard, MD **Pharmacy in medical center**	Mark Newman, MD 2785 South Ridgeway Avenue Chicago, IL 60647-2700 312-555-2700 **On-call doctor**
Lynn Corbett, MD Professional Building 8672 South Ridgeway Avenue, Suite 300 Chicago, IL 60623-2240 312-555-2300 **Cardiologist**	Margery Pierce, MD 6452 North Ridgeway Avenue, Suite 209 Chicago, IL 60626-5462 312-555-4880 **Pediatrician**
Richard Diangelis, MD 2785 South Ridgeway Avenue, Suite 280 Chicago, IL 60647-2700 312-555-1575 **Ophthalmologist**	Laura Sinn, MD 2901 West Fifth Avenue, Suite 100 Chicago, IL 60612-9002 312-555-7850 **Urologist**
Greg Koski, MD Professional Building 8672 South Ridgeway Avenue, Suite 350 Chicago, IL 60623-2240 312-555-4500 **Orthopedic surgeon**	Theresa Townsend, MD 500 South Dearborn Street Chicago, IL 60605-0005 **Chairperson** 312-555-2200 **Chicago Medical Society**
University Hospital 5500 North Ridgeway Avenue Chicago, IL 60625-1200 312-555-2500	**Education services:** Juanita Yates 312-555-2950 **Human resources:** 312-555-1200 **Resident services:** Lee Eaton 312-555-3043

CHART NOTE

Sherman, Florence
DOB: 05/22/19__
AA040

10/05/20__
CHIEF COMPLAINT: Trouble with vision.

SUBJECTIVE: Patient is a 65-year-old female who had two episodes during the last week of jagged lights occurring in central visual field. These lasted 15-20 minutes; no other symptoms. Patient has long history of migraines.

OBJECTIVE: Within normal limits; specifically, no evidence of tear or hole in the retina.

ASSESSMENT: Migraine equivalent vs. posterior vitreous detachment.

PLAN: 1. Discussed with ophthalmologist, Richard Diangelis, MD. Patient advised about signs and symptoms of detachment of the retina and told to seek immediate medical attention should any of these signs appear.
          2. Trial of Midrin for migraines.
          3. Recheck in 1 to 2 months.
          4. Patient requests referral to Dr. Diangelis.

Karen Larsen, MD/ls

PROOFING AND EDITING REPORTS

↓ 2 inches

Doublespace body.
Page numbers on upper
right starting on page 2.

↓ 2

RUBELLA (GERMAN MEASLES)

DEFINITION

Rubella (german measles) is a *highly* communicable viral disease characterized by diffuse, punctate, macular rash. Rubella is a relatively benign viral illness unless there is transplacental transmission. (Define the following terms: *communicable, diffuse, punctate, transplacental,* and *macular*.)

ETIOLOGY

Rubella is caused by rubella virus (*Rubivirus*) that is spread by air borne direct contact with nasopharyngeal secretions. This disease is communicable from one week before *the* rash appears to five days after the rash disappears. Rubella is most common in children but may also affect adults who were not infected during childhood. (Define the following terms: airborne, direct contact, and nasopharyngeal.)

INCIDENCE

Rubella occurs most often in the spring, but there are major epidemics occurring in 6 to 9 year cycles. (Investigate recent epidemics vs. the use of the vaccine.)

PATHOPHYSIOLOGY

The virus invades the nasopharynx and travels to the lymphglands, causing lymphadenopathy. Then in 5 to seven days it enters the blood stream stimulating an immune response causing the *skin* rash. This rash lasts about three days. (Define lymphadenopathy.)

CLINICAL SYSTEMS

The first Clinical symptoms of rubella include swollen gands, fever, sore throat, cough, and fatigue. The *often* pruritic rash generally starts in 1 to 5 days after the prodrome. The rash begins on the face and *the* trunk and spreads to the upper and lower extremities. Symptoms of headache and conjunctivitis may occur after the rash. (Define conjunctivitis, pruritic, and swollen glands.)

ADDITIONAL ASSIGNMENT:

Investigate what complications may occur to a fetus and a child with rubella, describing each complication plus its incidence.

Investigate what complications may occur in adults with rubella, describing each complication plus its incidence.

Investigate what diagnostic testing can be done for the occurrence *of* rubella.

Investigate treatment options.

MUMPS (INFECTIOUS PAROTITIS)

DEFINITION

Mumps is an ^acute^ viral disease that may include myalgia, anorexia, malaise, headache, low-grade fever, ^and^ parotid gland tenderness and unilateral or bilateral swelling, although many#other organs can be involved. (Define the following terms: *myalgia, anorexia,* and *malaise.*)

ETIOLOGY

Mumps is caused ^by^ paramyxovirus transmitted in saliva droplets or direct contact. The virus lives in the salvila six to (9) days before the parotid gland swelling. The highest communicable period is 48 hours before the on set of swelling but continues until swelling is decreased. Incubation period range^s^ from 14 to 25 days.

INCIDENCE

(Investigate the incidence in the past 10 years.)

PATHOPHYSIOLOGY

During the incubation period, the virus invades ^the^ salivary glands which causes tissue edema —and and infiltration of lymphocytes. Degeneration of cells in the glandular tissue produce^s^ necrotic debris that plugs the ducts.

CLINICAL SYMPTOMS

The prodrome ^of mumps^ generally begins with ~~generally begins~~ myalgia, anorexia, malaise, headache, and low-grade fever. Next the patient may have an ear ache aggravated by chewing, temperature of 101° to 104° F, and pain from chewing food or drinking acidic liquid. Both the parotid gland and other salivary glands ^may^ become swollen. (Define *prodrome.*)

ADDITIONAL ASSIGNMENT:

Investigate what complications may occur with mumps in ^both^ children and adults.

Summarize how mumps would be diagnosed.

Summarize outpatient and inpateint complications of treatment.

COMMUNICATIONS TERMS

Directions: Match the term in Column 2 with its definition in Column 1.

Column 1

_____ 1. The type of letter formatting that begins all parts of the letter at the left margin

_____ 2. Manuscript source at the bottom of the page on which the source is cited

_____ 3. Careful reading and examination of a document to find and correct errors

_____ 4. Style that has a colon after the salutation and a comma after the complimentary closing

_____ 5. To skim a document and write notes in the margin

_____ 6. Letter that begins the date line, complimentary closing, and signature line at the center point

_____ 7. Style without punctuation after the salutation and complimentary closing

_____ 8. Assessing a document to determine its clarity, consistency, and overall effectiveness

_____ 9. Manuscript sources placed on a separate page following the last page of text

Column 2

a. annotate

b. block-style letter

c. editing

d. endnotes

e. footnote

f. modified-block-style letter

g. open punctuation

h. proofreading

i. standard/mixed punctuation

MESSAGE FORMS

MESSAGE

TO _____

DATE _____ TIME _____

FROM _____

PHONE _____

☐ PLEASE CALL   ☐ RETURNED YOUR CALL   ☐ WILL CALL AGAIN

REGARDING _____

_____

_____

_____

_____

_____

TAKEN BY _____

MESSAGE

TO _____

DATE _____ TIME _____

FROM _____

PHONE _____

☐ PLEASE CALL   ☐ RETURNED YOUR CALL   ☐ WILL CALL AGAIN

REGARDING _____

_____

_____

_____

_____

_____

TAKEN BY _____

MESSAGE

TO _____

DATE _____ TIME _____

FROM _____

PHONE _____

☐ PLEASE CALL   ☐ RETURNED YOUR CALL   ☐ WILL CALL AGAIN

REGARDING _____

_____

_____

_____

_____

_____

TAKEN BY _____

MESSAGE

TO _____

DATE _____ TIME _____

FROM _____

PHONE _____

☐ PLEASE CALL   ☐ RETURNED YOUR CALL   ☐ WILL CALL AGAIN

REGARDING _____

_____

_____

_____

_____

_____

TAKEN BY _____

MESSAGE FORMS

MESSAGE

TO _____
FROM _____
PHONE _____
DATE _____ TIME _____
☐ PLEASE CALL   ☐ RETURNED YOUR CALL   ☐ WILL CALL AGAIN
REGARDING _____
_____
_____
_____
TAKEN BY _____

MESSAGE

TO _____
FROM _____
PHONE _____
DATE _____ TIME _____
☐ PLEASE CALL   ☐ RETURNED YOUR CALL   ☐ WILL CALL AGAIN
REGARDING _____
_____
_____
_____
TAKEN BY _____

MESSAGE

TO _____
FROM _____
PHONE _____
DATE _____ TIME _____
☐ PLEASE CALL   ☐ RETURNED YOUR CALL   ☐ WILL CALL AGAIN
REGARDING _____
_____
_____
_____
TAKEN BY _____

MESSAGE

TO _____
FROM _____
PHONE _____
DATE _____ TIME _____
☐ PLEASE CALL   ☐ RETURNED YOUR CALL   ☐ WILL CALL AGAIN
REGARDING _____
_____
_____
_____
TAKEN BY _____

MESSAGE FORMS

MESSAGE

TO _____ DATE _____ TIME _____

FROM _____

PHONE _____

☐ PLEASE CALL   ☐ RETURNED YOUR CALL   ☐ WILL CALL AGAIN

REGARDING _____

_____

_____

_____

TAKEN BY _____

MESSAGE

TO _____ DATE _____ TIME _____

FROM _____

PHONE _____

☐ PLEASE CALL   ☐ RETURNED YOUR CALL   ☐ WILL CALL AGAIN

REGARDING _____

_____

_____

_____

TAKEN BY _____

MESSAGE

TO _____ DATE _____ TIME _____

FROM _____

PHONE _____

☐ PLEASE CALL   ☐ RETURNED YOUR CALL   ☐ WILL CALL AGAIN

REGARDING _____

_____

_____

_____

TAKEN BY _____

MESSAGE

TO _____ DATE _____ TIME _____

FROM _____

PHONE _____

☐ PLEASE CALL   ☐ RETURNED YOUR CALL   ☐ WILL CALL AGAIN

REGARDING _____

_____

_____

_____

TAKEN BY _____

MESSAGE FORMS

MESSAGE

TO _____ DATE _____ TIME _____

FROM _____

PHONE _____

☐ PLEASE CALL   ☐ RETURNED YOUR CALL   ☐ WILL CALL AGAIN

REGARDING _____

_____

_____

_____

TAKEN BY _____

MESSAGE

TO _____ DATE _____ TIME _____

FROM _____

PHONE _____

☐ PLEASE CALL   ☐ RETURNED YOUR CALL   ☐ WILL CALL AGAIN

REGARDING _____

_____

_____

_____

TAKEN BY _____

MESSAGE

TO _____ DATE _____ TIME _____

FROM _____

PHONE _____

☐ PLEASE CALL   ☐ RETURNED YOUR CALL   ☐ WILL CALL AGAIN

REGARDING _____

_____

_____

_____

TAKEN BY _____

MESSAGE

TO _____ DATE _____ TIME _____

FROM _____

PHONE _____

☐ PLEASE CALL   ☐ RETURNED YOUR CALL   ☐ WILL CALL AGAIN

REGARDING _____

_____

_____

_____

TAKEN BY _____

MESSAGE FORMS

MESSAGE

DATE _____ TIME _____

TO _____

FROM _____

PHONE _____

☐ PLEASE CALL ☐ RETURNED YOUR CALL ☐ WILL CALL AGAIN

REGARDING _____

_____

_____

_____

TAKEN BY _____

MESSAGE

DATE _____ TIME _____

TO _____

FROM _____

PHONE _____

☐ PLEASE CALL ☐ RETURNED YOUR CALL ☐ WILL CALL AGAIN

REGARDING _____

_____

_____

_____

TAKEN BY _____

MESSAGE

DATE _____ TIME _____

TO _____

FROM _____

PHONE _____

☐ PLEASE CALL ☐ RETURNED YOUR CALL ☐ WILL CALL AGAIN

REGARDING _____

_____

_____

_____

TAKEN BY _____

MESSAGE

DATE _____ TIME _____

TO _____

FROM _____

PHONE _____

☐ PLEASE CALL ☐ RETURNED YOUR CALL ☐ WILL CALL AGAIN

REGARDING _____

_____

_____

_____

TAKEN BY _____

MESSAGE FORMS

MESSAGE

TO _____

FROM _____

PHONE _____

DATE _____ TIME _____

☐ PLEASE CALL ☐ RETURNED YOUR CALL ☐ WILL CALL AGAIN

REGARDING _____

_____

_____

_____

TAKEN BY _____

MESSAGE

TO _____

FROM _____

PHONE _____

DATE _____ TIME _____

☐ PLEASE CALL ☐ RETURNED YOUR CALL ☐ WILL CALL AGAIN

REGARDING _____

_____

_____

_____

TAKEN BY _____

MESSAGE

TO _____

FROM _____

PHONE _____

DATE _____ TIME _____

☐ PLEASE CALL ☐ RETURNED YOUR CALL ☐ WILL CALL AGAIN

REGARDING _____

_____

_____

_____

TAKEN BY _____

MESSAGE

TO _____

FROM _____

PHONE _____

DATE _____ TIME _____

☐ PLEASE CALL ☐ RETURNED YOUR CALL ☐ WILL CALL AGAIN

REGARDING _____

_____

_____

_____

TAKEN BY _____

MESSAGE FORMS

MESSAGE

TO _____

FROM _____

PHONE _____

☐ PLEASE CALL   ☐ RETURNED YOUR CALL   ☐ WILL CALL AGAIN

REGARDING _____

_____

_____

_____

DATE _____   TIME _____

TAKEN BY _____

MESSAGE

TO _____

FROM _____

PHONE _____

☐ PLEASE CALL   ☐ RETURNED YOUR CALL   ☐ WILL CALL AGAIN

REGARDING _____

_____

_____

_____

DATE _____   TIME _____

TAKEN BY _____

MESSAGE

TO _____

FROM _____

PHONE _____

☐ PLEASE CALL   ☐ RETURNED YOUR CALL   ☐ WILL CALL AGAIN

REGARDING _____

_____

_____

_____

DATE _____   TIME _____

TAKEN BY _____

MESSAGE

TO _____

FROM _____

PHONE _____

☐ PLEASE CALL   ☐ RETURNED YOUR CALL   ☐ WILL CALL AGAIN

REGARDING _____

_____

_____

_____

DATE _____   TIME _____

TAKEN BY _____

MESSAGE FORMS

MESSAGE

TO _____
DATE _____ TIME _____
FROM _____
PHONE _____
☐ PLEASE CALL   ☐ RETURNED YOUR CALL   ☐ WILL CALL AGAIN
REGARDING _____
_____
_____
_____
TAKEN BY _____

MESSAGE

TO _____
DATE _____ TIME _____
FROM _____
PHONE _____
☐ PLEASE CALL   ☐ RETURNED YOUR CALL   ☐ WILL CALL AGAIN
REGARDING _____
_____
_____
_____
TAKEN BY _____

MESSAGE

TO _____
DATE _____ TIME _____
FROM _____
PHONE _____
☐ PLEASE CALL   ☐ RETURNED YOUR CALL   ☐ WILL CALL AGAIN
REGARDING _____
_____
_____
_____
TAKEN BY _____

MESSAGE

TO _____
DATE _____ TIME _____
FROM _____
PHONE _____
☐ PLEASE CALL   ☐ RETURNED YOUR CALL   ☐ WILL CALL AGAIN
REGARDING _____
_____
_____
_____
TAKEN BY _____

SCHEDULING DECISION MAKING

Directions: The calls in Column 1 are for a family practice physician. The physician does see emergencies in the office. Choose the appropriate response from Column 2 to indicate when an appointment should be made for *STAT, Today, Tomorrow, Later,* or a message taken—*Take message.*

Column 1

_____ **1.** Loni Kayen desires weight control, 312-555-9834.

_____ **2.** North Lab's report on prothrombin time for Walter Boone; control was 11.6; patient, 18, 312-555-6757.

_____ **3.** Hank Holm at 312-555-4432 wants to talk to the doctor about his left leg cast; it seems too tight, feels numbness in his toes.

_____ **4.** Brian Verk at 312-555-2389 needs diabetes recheck.

_____ **5.** Kay Frank, bee sting, left face check, swelling and a hard spot in the middle; she has no allergies; 312-555-6734.

_____ **6.** Beth Cater has a urinary problem, hurts to urinate, no blood in urine, 312-555-9823.

_____ **7.** True Value Drug, 312-555-9877, prescription refill Diane Yvon, Coumadin 5 mg each a.m. before breakfast #30, last filled 2 months ago.

_____ **8.** Hu Grangdon, rash over abdomen times 2 days, itching, no new foods or meds, 312-555-3341.

_____ **9.** Ben Jones, BP recheck, 312-555-3478.

_____ **10.** Dana Lund, annual Pap smear, 312-555-0043.

_____ **11.** Donna Kelly, son Alex got hit in head with a bat, bleeding, swelling, 312-555-9822.

_____ **12.** North X-ray, 312-555-6757, chest x-ray on Ann Tyn is negative.

_____ **13.** Pamela Bond, 6-week checkup for baby Keith, 312-555-5636.

_____ **14.** Rein Los Ames, age 2 months, cranky, pulling right ear, slight temperature, 312-555-3223.

_____ **15.** Tom Urness, 312-555-5574, age 47, noticed blood in stools, very concerned, read about colon cancer in recent magazine.

_____ **16.** Karin Olsson, age 72, infected hangnail with green pus, hurts, swollen, 312-555-9966.

_____ **17.** Wendy Rinke, age 8, something in her eye, red, watering. Father was sanding where she was playing, 312-555-7845.

Column 2

a. STAT

b. Today

c. Tomorrow

d. Later

e. Take message

APPOINTMENT SCHEDULE INFORMATION

KAREN LARSEN, MD, OFFICE SCHEDULE
2235 South Ridgeway Avenue
Chicago, IL 60623-2240
312-555-6022
Fax: 312-555-0025

Monday, Tuesday, and Wednesday

Hospital rounds	8:00 A.M. – 10:00 A.M.
Travel time	10:00 A.M. – 10:30 A.M.
Patient appointments	10:30 A.M. – 12 noon
Lunch	12 noon – 1:00 P.M.
Teach and work at University Hospital	1:00 P.M. – 5:00 P.M.

Thursday

Patient appointments	8:00 A.M. – 5:00 P.M.

Friday

Hospital rounds	8:00 A.M. – 10:00 A.M.
Travel time	10:00 A.M. – 10:30 A.M.
Office for dictation, messages, writing, and course preparation	10:30 A.M. – 12 noon
Office closed	12 noon – 5:00 P.M.

Saturday

Patient appointments	8:00 A.M. – 12 noon

Length of Appointments

Complete physical examination	1 hour
All other appointments, unless designated	15 minutes

Appointment Abbreviations

abd	abdominal
BP	blood pressure
✓	checkup
Dx	diagnosis
ECG	electrocardiogram
F/U	follow-up visit
FX	fracture
GI	gastrointestinal
N & V	nausea and vomiting
NP	new patient
CPE, PE	physical examination
preop	preoperative
postop	postoperative

APPOINTMENT CALENDAR PAGES

| Monday, October 9 | Tuesday, October 10 | Wednesday, October 11 |

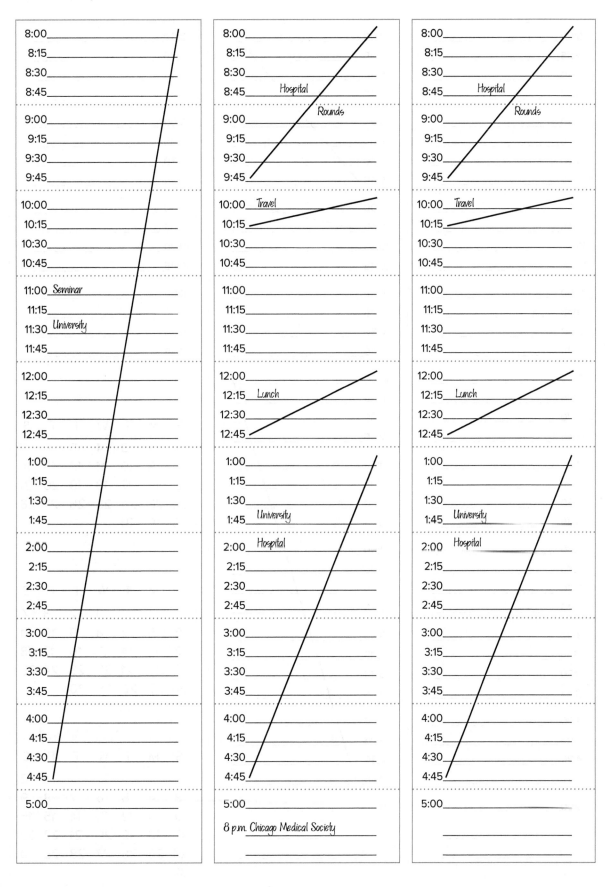

Monday, October 9

8:00
8:15
8:30
8:45

9:00
9:15
9:30
9:45

10:00
10:15
10:30
10:45

11:00 Seminar
11:15
11:30 University
11:45

12:00
12:15
12:30
12:45

1:00
1:15
1:30
1:45

2:00
2:15
2:30
2:45

3:00
3:15
3:30
3:45

4:00
4:15
4:30
4:45

5:00

Tuesday, October 10

8:00
8:15
8:30
8:45 Hospital

9:00 Rounds
9:15
9:30
9:45

10:00 Travel
10:15
10:30
10:45

11:00
11:15
11:30
11:45

12:00
12:15 Lunch
12:30
12:45

1:00
1:15
1:30
1:45 University

2:00 Hospital
2:15
2:30
2:45

3:00
3:15
3:30
3:45

4:00
4:15
4:30
4:45

5:00

8 p.m. Chicago Medical Society

Wednesday, October 11

8:00
8:15
8:30
8:45 Hospital

9:00 Rounds
9:15
9:30
9:45

10:00 Travel
10:15
10:30
10:45

11:00
11:15
11:30
11:45

12:00
12:15 Lunch
12:30
12:45

1:00
1:15
1:30
1:45 University

2:00 Hospital
2:15
2:30
2:45

3:00
3:15
3:30
3:45

4:00
4:15
4:30
4:45

5:00

APPOINTMENT CALENDAR PAGES

Thursday, October 12   Friday, October 13   Saturday, October 14

Thursday, October 12	Friday, October 13	Saturday, October 14
8:00	8:00	8:00
8:15	8:15	8:15
8:30	8:30	8:30
8:45	8:45 Hospital	8:45
9:00	9:00	9:00
9:15	9:15 Rounds	9:15
9:30	9:30	9:30
9:45	9:45	9:45
10:00	10:00 Travel	10:00
10:15	10:15	10:15
10:30	10:30	10:30
10:45	10:45	10:45
11:00	11:00	11:00
11:15	11:15	11:15
11:30	11:30	11:30
11:45	11:45	11:45
12:00	12:00	
12:15	12:15	
12:30	12:30	
12:45	12:45	
1:00	1:00 Office	
1:15	1:15	
1:30	1:30 Closed	
1:45	1:45	
2:00	2:00	
2:15	2:15	
2:30	2:30	
2:45	2:45	
3:00	3:00	
3:15	3:15	
3:30	3:30	
3:45	3:45	
4:00	4:00	
4:15	4:15	
4:30	4:30	
4:45	4:45	
5:00	5:00	

October

S	M	T	W	T	F	S
1	2	3	4	5	6	7
8	9	10	11	12	13	14
15	16	17	18	19	20	21
22	23	24	25	26	27	28
29	30	31				

November

S	M	T	W	T	F	S
			1	2	3	4
5	6	7	8	9	10	11
12	13	14	15	16	17	18
19	20	21	22	23	24	25
26	27	28	29	30		

December

S	M	T	W	T	F	S
					1	2
3	4	5	6	7	8	9
10	11	12	13	14	15	16
17	18	19	20	21	22	23
24	25	26	27	28	29	30
31						

APPOINTMENT CALENDAR PAGES

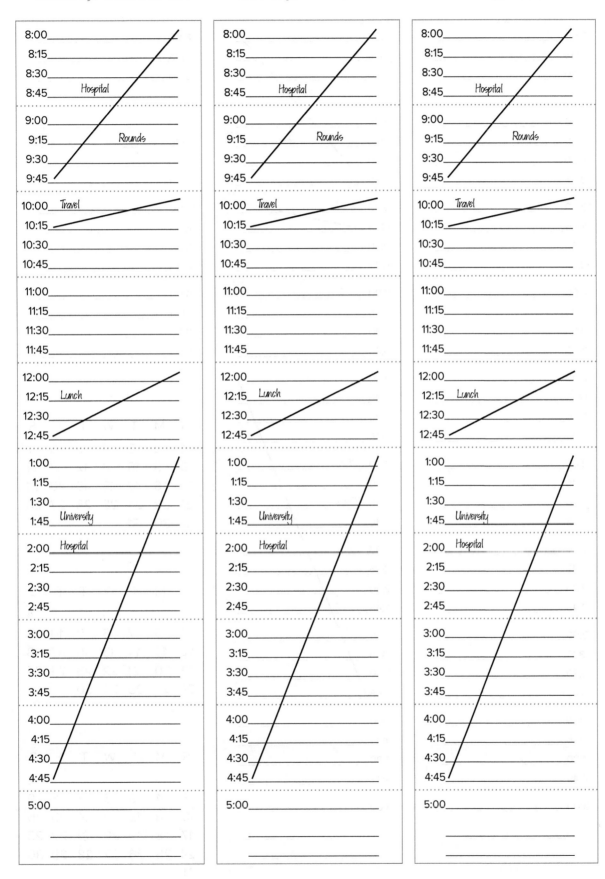

Monday, October 16	Tuesday, October 17	Wednesday, October 18

Monday, October 16

- 8:00
- 8:15
- 8:30
- 8:45 _Hospital_
- 9:00
- 9:15 _Rounds_
- 9:30
- 9:45
- 10:00 _Travel_
- 10:15
- 10:30
- 10:45
- 11:00
- 11:15
- 11:30
- 11:45
- 12:00
- 12:15 _Lunch_
- 12:30
- 12:45
- 1:00
- 1:15
- 1:30
- 1:45 _University_
- 2:00 _Hospital_
- 2:15
- 2:30
- 2:45
- 3:00
- 3:15
- 3:30
- 3:45
- 4:00
- 4:15
- 4:30
- 4:45
- 5:00

Tuesday, October 17

- 8:00
- 8:15
- 8:30
- 8:45 _Hospital_
- 9:00
- 9:15 _Rounds_
- 9:30
- 9:45
- 10:00 _Travel_
- 10:15
- 10:30
- 10:45
- 11:00
- 11:15
- 11:30
- 11:45
- 12:00
- 12:15 _Lunch_
- 12:30
- 12:45
- 1:00
- 1:15
- 1:30
- 1:45 _University_
- 2:00 _Hospital_
- 2:15
- 2:30
- 2:45
- 3:00
- 3:15
- 3:30
- 3:45
- 4:00
- 4:15
- 4:30
- 4:45
- 5:00

Wednesday, October 18

- 8:00
- 8:15
- 8:30
- 8:45 _Hospital_
- 9:00
- 9:15 _Rounds_
- 9:30
- 9:45
- 10:00 _Travel_
- 10:15
- 10:30
- 10:45
- 11:00
- 11:15
- 11:30
- 11:45
- 12:00
- 12:15 _Lunch_
- 12:30
- 12:45
- 1:00
- 1:15
- 1:30
- 1:45 _University_
- 2:00 _Hospital_
- 2:15
- 2:30
- 2:45
- 3:00
- 3:15
- 3:30
- 3:45
- 4:00
- 4:15
- 4:30
- 4:45
- 5:00

APPOINTMENT CALENDAR PAGES

Thursday, October 19   Friday, October 20   Saturday, October 21

Thursday, October 19

8:00
8:15
8:30
8:45

9:00
9:15
9:30
9:45

10:00
10:15
10:30
10:45

11:00
11:15
11:30
11:45

12:00
12:15
12:30
12:45

1:00
1:15
1:30
1:45

2:00
2:15
2:30
2:45

3:00
3:15
3:30
3:45

4:00
4:15
4:30
4:45

5:00

Friday, October 20

8:00
8:15
8:30
8:45   Hospital

9:00
9:15   Rounds
9:30
9:45

10:00   Travel
10:15
10:30
10:45

11:00
11:15
11:30
11:45

12:00
12:15
12:30
12:45

1:00   Office
1:15
1:30   Closed
1:45

2:00
2:15
2:30
2:45

3:00
3:15
3:30
3:45

4:00
4:15
4:30
4:45

5:00

Saturday, October 21

8:00
8:15
8:30
8:45

9:00
9:15
9:30
9:45

10:00
10:15
10:30
10:45

11:00
11:15
11:30
11:45

October

S	M	T	W	T	F	S
1	2	3	4	5	6	7
8	9	10	11	12	13	14
15	16	17	18	19	20	21
22	23	24	25	26	27	28
29	30	31				

November

S	M	T	W	T	F	S
			1	2	3	4
5	6	7	8	9	10	11
12	13	14	15	16	17	18
19	20	21	22	23	24	25
26	27	28	29	30		

December

S	M	T	W	T	F	S
					1	2
3	4	5	6	7	8	9
10	11	12	13	14	15	16
17	18	19	20	21	22	23
24	25	26	27	28	29	30
31						

APPOINTMENT CALENDAR PAGES

Monday, October 23   Tuesday, October 24   Wednesday, October 25

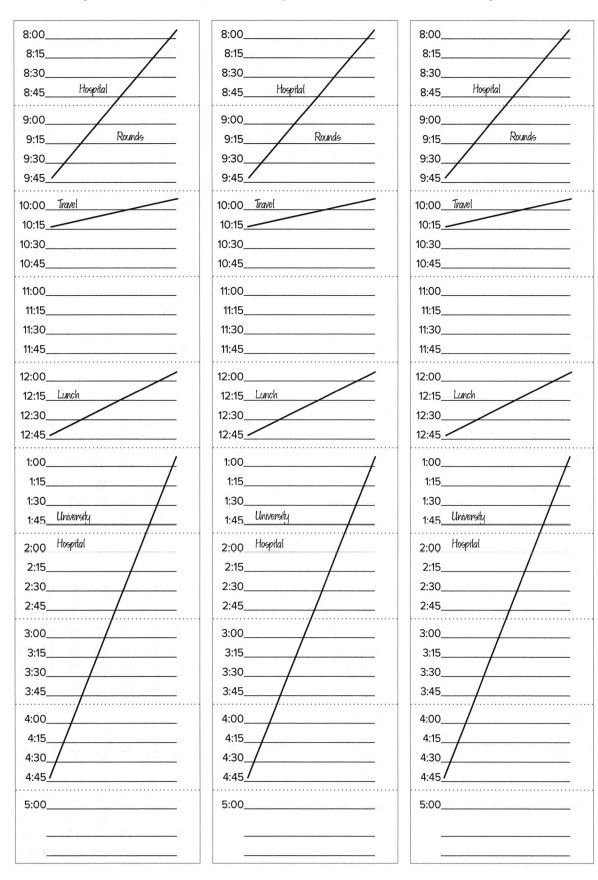

APPOINTMENT CALENDAR PAGES

Thursday, October 26   Friday, October 27   Saturday, October 28

Thursday, October 26	Friday, October 27	Saturday, October 28
8:00	8:00	8:00
8:15	8:15	8:15
8:30	8:30	8:30
8:45	8:45 *Hospital*	8:45
9:00	9:00	9:00
9:15	9:15 *Rounds*	9:15
9:30	9:30	9:30
9:45	9:45	9:45
10:00	10:00 *Travel*	10:00
10:15	10:15	10:15
10:30	10:30	10:30
10:45	10:45	10:45
11:00	11:00	11:00
11:15	11:15	11:15
11:30	11:30	11:30
11:45	11:45	11:45
12:00	12:00	
12:15	12:15	
12:30	12:30	
12:45	12:45	
1:00	1:00 *Office*	
1:15	1:15	
1:30	1:30 *Closed*	
1:45	1:45	
2:00	2:00	
2:15	2:15	
2:30	2:30	
2:45	2:45	
3:00	3:00	
3:15	3:15	
3:30	3:30	
3:45	3:45	
4:00	4:00	
4:15	4:15	
4:30	4:30	
4:45	4:45	
5:00	5:00	

October

S	M	T	W	T	F	S
1	2	3	4	5	6	7
8	9	10	11	12	13	14
15	16	17	18	19	20	21
22	23	24	25	26	27	28
29	30	31				

November

S	M	T	W	T	F	S
			1	2	3	4
5	6	7	8	9	10	11
12	13	14	15	16	17	18
19	20	21	22	23	24	25
26	27	28	29	30		

December

S	M	T	W	T	F	S
					1	2
3	4	5	6	7	8	9
10	11	12	13	14	15	16
17	18	19	20	21	22	23
24	25	26	27	28	29	30
31						

Working Papers

APPOINTMENT CALENDAR PAGES

Monday, October 30	Tuesday, October 31	Wednesday, November 1

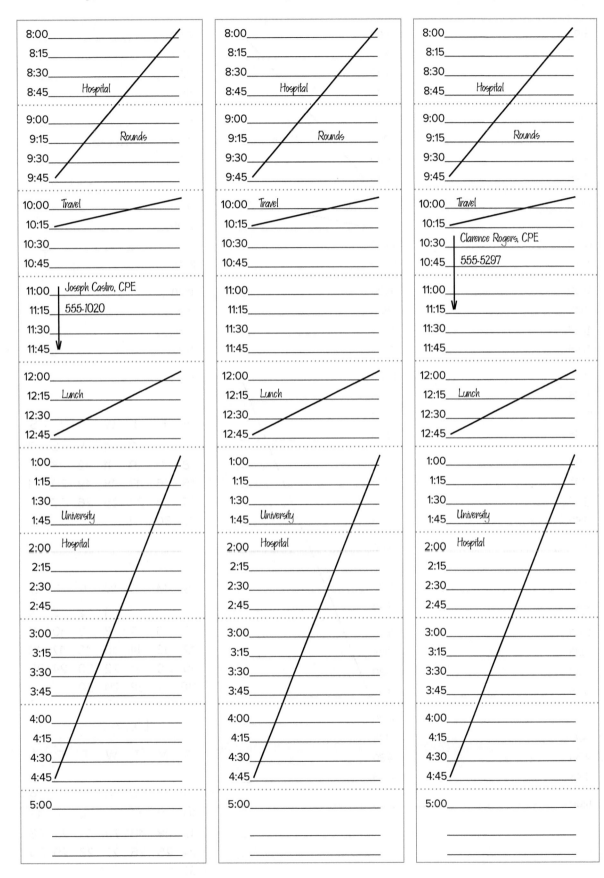

Monday, October 30

8:00
8:15
8:30
8:45 Hospital
9:00
9:15 Rounds
9:30
9:45
10:00 Travel
10:15
10:30
10:45
11:00 Joseph Castro, CPE
11:15 555-1020
11:30
11:45
12:00
12:15 Lunch
12:30
12:45
1:00
1:15
1:30
1:45 University
2:00 Hospital
2:15
2:30
2:45
3:00
3:15
3:30
3:45
4:00
4:15
4:30
4:45
5:00

Tuesday, October 31

8:00
8:15
8:30
8:45 Hospital
9:00
9:15 Rounds
9:30
9:45
10:00 Travel
10:15
10:30
10:45
11:00
11:15
11:30
11:45
12:00
12:15 Lunch
12:30
12:45
1:00
1:15
1:30
1:45 University
2:00 Hospital
2:15
2:30
2:45
3:00
3:15
3:30
3:45
4:00
4:15
4:30
4:45
5:00

Wednesday, November 1

8:00
8:15
8:30
8:45 Hospital
9:00
9:15 Rounds
9:30
9:45
10:00 Travel
10:15
10:30 Clarence Rogers, CPE
10:45 555-5297
11:00
11:15
11:30
11:45
12:00
12:15 Lunch
12:30
12:45
1:00
1:15
1:30
1:45 University
2:00 Hospital
2:15
2:30
2:45
3:00
3:15
3:30
3:45
4:00
4:15
4:30
4:45
5:00

APPOINTMENT CALENDAR PAGES

Thursday, November 2	Friday, November 3	Saturday, November 4

Thursday, November 2

8:00
8:15
8:30
8:45

9:00
9:15
9:30
9:45

10:00
10:15
10:30
10:45

11:00
11:15
11:30
11:45

12:00
12:15
12:30
12:45

1:00
1:15
1:30
1:45

2:00
2:15
2:30
2:45

3:00
3:15
3:30
3:45

4:00
4:15
4:30
4:45

5:00

Friday, November 3

8:00
8:15
8:30
8:45 Hospital

9:00
9:15 Rounds
9:30
9:45

10:00 Travel
10:15
10:30
10:45

11:00
11:15
11:30
11:45

12:00
12:15
12:30
12:45

1:00 Office
1:15
1:30 Closed
1:45

2:00
2:15
2:30
2:45

3:00
3:15
3:30
3:45

4:00
4:15
4:30
4:45

5:00

Saturday, November 4

8:00
8:15
8:30
8:45

9:00
9:15
9:30
9:45

10:00
10:15
10:30
10:45

11:00
11:15
11:30
11:45

October

S	M	T	W	T	F	S
1	2	3	4	5	6	7
8	9	10	11	12	13	14
15	16	17	18	19	20	21
22	23	24	25	26	27	28
29	30	31				

November

S	M	T	W	T	F	S
			1	2	3	4
5	6	7	8	9	10	11
12	13	14	15	16	17	18
19	20	21	22	23	24	25
26	27	28	29	30		

December

S	M	T	W	T	F	S
					1	2
3	4	5	6	7	8	9
10	11	12	13	14	15	16
17	18	19	20	21	22	23
24	25	26	27	28	29	30
31						

Working Papers

APPOINTMENT CALENDAR PAGES

Monday, November 6	Tuesday, November 7	Wednesday, November 8

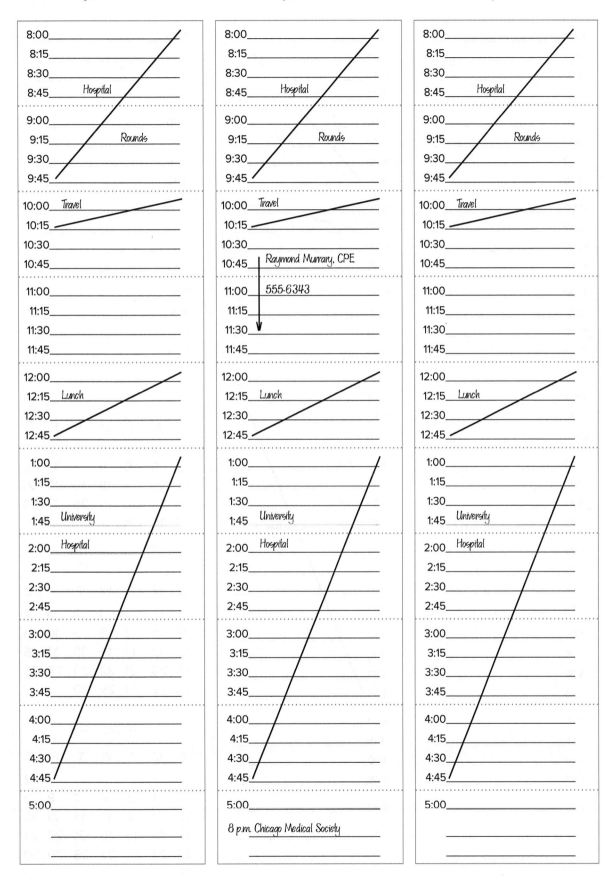

Monday, November 6

- 8:00
- 8:15
- 8:30
- 8:45 — Hospital
- 9:00
- 9:15 — Rounds
- 9:30
- 9:45
- 10:00 — Travel
- 10:15
- 10:30
- 10:45
- 11:00
- 11:15
- 11:30
- 11:45
- 12:00
- 12:15 — Lunch
- 12:30
- 12:45
- 1:00
- 1:15
- 1:30
- 1:45 — University
- 2:00 — Hospital
- 2:15
- 2:30
- 2:45
- 3:00
- 3:15
- 3:30
- 3:45
- 4:00
- 4:15
- 4:30
- 4:45
- 5:00

Tuesday, November 7

- 8:00
- 8:15
- 8:30
- 8:45 — Hospital
- 9:00
- 9:15 — Rounds
- 9:30
- 9:45
- 10:00 — Travel
- 10:15
- 10:30
- 10:45 — Raymond Murrary, CPE
- 11:00 — 555-6343
- 11:15
- 11:30
- 11:45
- 12:00
- 12:15 — Lunch
- 12:30
- 12:45
- 1:00
- 1:15
- 1:30
- 1:45 — University
- 2:00 — Hospital
- 2:15
- 2:30
- 2:45
- 3:00
- 3:15
- 3:30
- 3:45
- 4:00
- 4:15
- 4:30
- 4:45
- 5:00
- 8 p.m. Chicago Medical Society

Wednesday, November 8

- 8:00
- 8:15
- 8:30
- 8:45 — Hospital
- 9:00
- 9:15 — Rounds
- 9:30
- 9:45
- 10:00 — Travel
- 10:15
- 10:30
- 10:45
- 11:00
- 11:15
- 11:30
- 11:45
- 12:00
- 12:15 — Lunch
- 12:30
- 12:45
- 1:00
- 1:15
- 1:30
- 1:45 — University
- 2:00 — Hospital
- 2:15
- 2:30
- 2:45
- 3:00
- 3:15
- 3:30
- 3:45
- 4:00
- 4:15
- 4:30
- 4:45
- 5:00

APPOINTMENT CALENDAR PAGES

Thursday, November 9

8:00
8:15
8:30
8:45

9:00
9:15
9:30
9:45

10:00
10:15
10:30
10:45

11:00
11:15
11:30
11:45

12:00
12:15
12:30
12:45

1:00
1:15
1:30
1:45

2:00
2:15
2:30
2:45

3:00
3:15
3:30
3:45

4:00
4:15
4:30
4:45

5:00

Friday, November 10

8:00
8:15
8:30
8:45 _Hospital_

9:00
9:15 _Rounds_
9:30
9:45

10:00 _Travel_
10:15
10:30
10:45

11:00
11:15
11:30
11:45

12:00
12:15
12:30
12:45

1:00 _Office_
1:15
1:30 _Closed_
1:45

2:00
2:15
2:30
2:45

3:00
3:15
3:30
3:45

4:00
4:15
4:30
4:45

5:00

Saturday, November 11

8:00
8:15
8:30
8:45

9:00
9:15
9:30
9:45

10:00
10:15
10:30
10:45

11:00
11:15
11:30
11:45

October

S	M	T	W	T	F	S
1	2	3	4	5	6	7
8	9	10	11	12	13	14
15	16	17	18	19	20	21
22	23	24	25	26	27	28
29	30	31				

November

S	M	T	W	T	F	S
			1	2	3	4
5	6	7	8	9	10	11
12	13	14	15	16	17	18
19	20	21	22	23	24	25
26	27	28	29	30		

December

S	M	T	W	T	F	S
					1	2
3	4	5	6	7	8	9
10	11	12	13	14	15	16
17	18	19	20	21	22	23
24	25	26	27	28	29	30
31						

Working Papers

APPOINTMENT CALENDAR PAGES

Monday, November 13   Tuesday, November 14   Wednesday, November 15

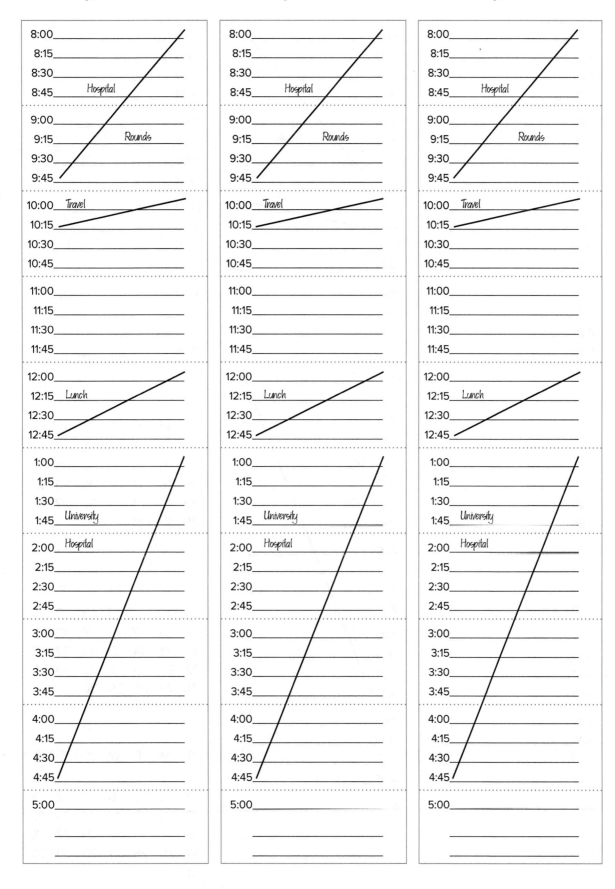

Monday, November 13	Tuesday, November 14	Wednesday, November 15
8:00	8:00	8:00
8:15	8:15	8:15
8:30	8:30	8:30
8:45 Hospital	8:45 Hospital	8:45 Hospital
9:00	9:00	9:00
9:15 Rounds	9:15 Rounds	9:15 Rounds
9:30	9:30	9:30
9:45	9:45	9:45
10:00 Travel	10:00 Travel	10:00 Travel
10:15	10:15	10:15
10:30	10:30	10:30
10:45	10:45	10:45
11:00	11:00	11:00
11:15	11:15	11:15
11:30	11:30	11:30
11:45	11:45	11:45
12:00	12:00	12:00
12:15 Lunch	12:15 Lunch	12:15 Lunch
12:30	12:30	12:30
12:45	12:45	12:45
1:00	1:00	1:00
1:15	1:15	1:15
1:30	1:30	1:30
1:45 University	1:45 University	1:45 University
2:00 Hospital	2:00 Hospital	2:00 Hospital
2:15	2:15	2:15
2:30	2:30	2:30
2:45	2:45	2:45
3:00	3:00	3:00
3:15	3:15	3:15
3:30	3:30	3:30
3:45	3:45	3:45
4:00	4:00	4:00
4:15	4:15	4:15
4:30	4:30	4:30
4:45	4:45	4:45
5:00	5:00	5:00

APPOINTMENT CALENDAR PAGES

Thursday, November 16	Friday, November 17	Saturday, November 18
8:00	8:00	8:00
8:15	8:15	8:15
8:30	8:30	8:30
8:45	8:45 *Hospital*	8:45
9:00	9:00	9:00
9:15	9:15 *Rounds*	9:15
9:30	9:30	9:30
9:45	9:45	9:45
10:00	10:00 *Travel*	10:00
10:15	10:15	10:15
10:30	10:30	10:30
10:45	10:45	10:45
11:00	11:00	11:00
11:15	11:15	11:15
11:30	11:30	11:30
11:45	11:45	11:45
12:00	12:00	
12:15	12:15	
12:30	12:30	
12:45	12:45	
1:00	1:00 *Office*	
1:15	1:15	
1:30	1:30 *Closed*	
1:45	1:45	
2:00	2:00	
2:15	2:15	
2:30	2:30	
2:45	2:45	
3:00	3:00	
3:15	3:15	
3:30	3:30	
3:45	3:45	
4:00	4:00	
4:15	4:15	
4:30	4:30	
4:45	4:45	
5:00	5:00	

October

S	M	T	W	T	F	S
1	2	3	4	5	6	7
8	9	10	11	12	13	14
15	16	17	18	19	20	21
22	23	24	25	26	27	28
29	30	31				

November

S	M	T	W	T	F	S
			1	2	3	4
5	6	7	8	9	10	11
12	13	14	15	16	17	18
19	20	21	22	23	24	25
26	27	28	29	30		

December

S	M	T	W	T	F	S
					1	2
3	4	5	6	7	8	9
10	11	12	13	14	15	16
17	18	19	20	21	22	23
24	25	26	27	28	29	30
31						

Working Papers

APPOINTMENT CALENDAR PAGES

Monday, November 20   Tuesday, November 21   Wednesday, November 22

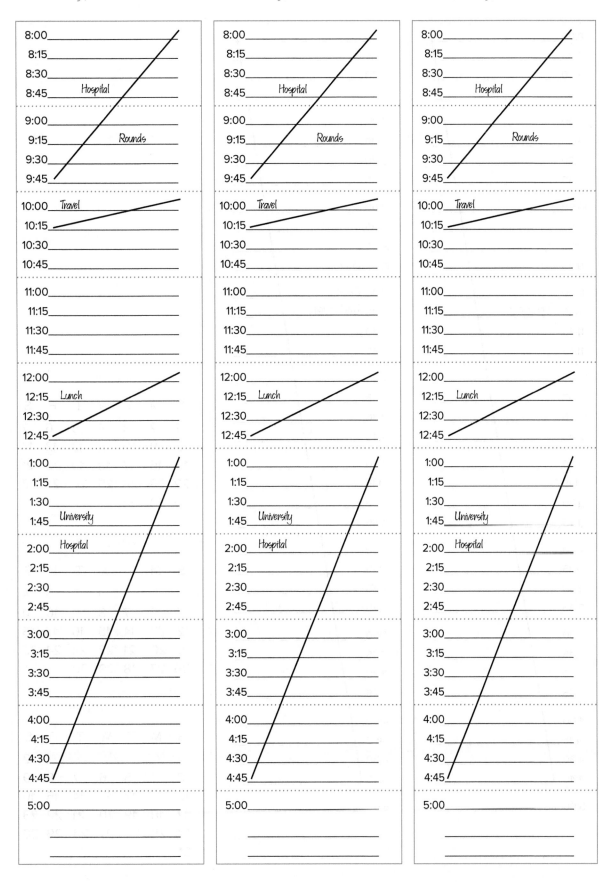

APPOINTMENT CALENDAR PAGES

Thursday, November 23   Friday, November 24

Thursday, November 23	Friday, November 24
8:00	8:00
8:15	8:15
8:30	8:30
8:45	8:45
9:00	9:00
9:15	9:15
9:30	9:30
9:45	9:45
10:00	10:00
10:15	10:15
10:30	10:30
10:45 Office	10:45 Office
11:00 Closed	11:00 Closed
11:15 Thanksgiving	11:15 Thanksgiving
11:30	11:30
11:45	11:45
12:00	12:00
12:15	12:15
12:30	12:30
12:45	12:45
1:00	1:00
1:15	1:15
1:30	1:30
1:45	1:45
2:00	2:00
2:15	2:15
2:30	2:30
2:45	2:45
3:00	3:00
3:15	3:15
3:30	3:30
3:45	3:45
4:00	4:00
4:15	4:15
4:30	4:30
4:45	4:45
5:00	5:00

October

S	M	T	W	T	F	S
1	2	3	4	5	6	7
8	9	10	11	12	13	14
15	16	17	18	19	20	21
22	23	24	25	26	27	28
29	30	31				

November

S	M	T	W	T	F	S
			1	2	3	4
5	6	7	8	9	10	11
12	13	14	15	16	17	18
19	20	21	22	23	24	25
26	27	28	29	30		

December

S	M	T	W	T	F	S
					1	2
3	4	5	6	7	8	9
10	11	12	13	14	15	16
17	18	19	20	21	22	23
24	25	26	27	28	29	30
31						

APPOINTMENT CALENDAR PAGES

Monday, November 27   Tuesday, November 28   Wednesday, November 29

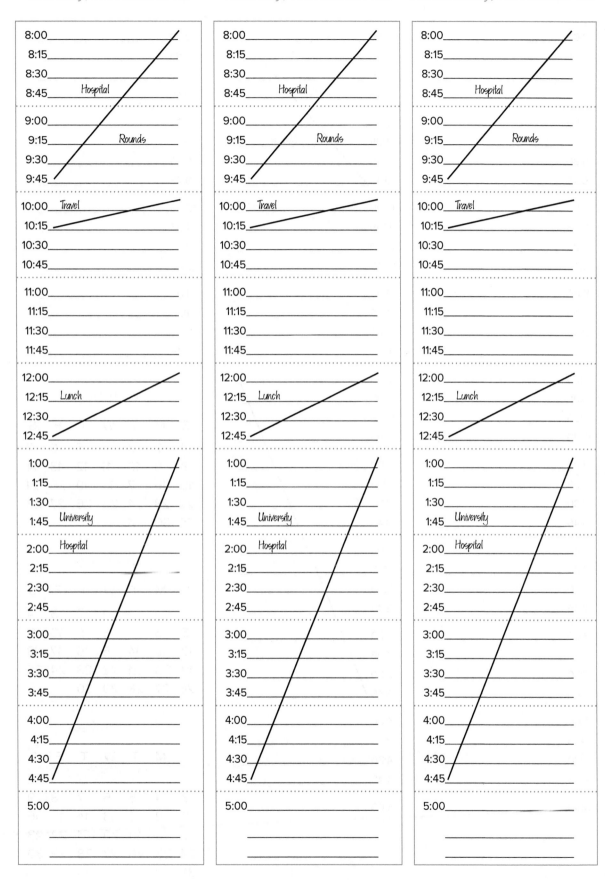

Monday, November 27	Tuesday, November 28	Wednesday, November 29
8:00	8:00	8:00
8:15	8:15	8:15
8:30	8:30	8:30
8:45 Hospital	8:45 Hospital	8:45 Hospital
9:00	9:00	9:00
9:15 Rounds	9:15 Rounds	9:15 Rounds
9:30	9:30	9:30
9:45	9:45	9:45
10:00 Travel	10:00 Travel	10:00 Travel
10:15	10:15	10:15
10:30	10:30	10:30
10:45	10:45	10:45
11:00	11:00	11:00
11:15	11:15	11:15
11:30	11:30	11:30
11:45	11:45	11:45
12:00	12:00	12:00
12:15 Lunch	12:15 Lunch	12:15 Lunch
12:30	12:30	12:30
12:45	12:45	12:45
1:00	1:00	1:00
1:15	1:15	1:15
1:30	1:30	1:30
1:45 University	1:45 University	1:45 University
2:00 Hospital	2:00 Hospital	2:00 Hospital
2:15	2:15	2:15
2:30	2:30	2:30
2:45	2:45	2:45
3:00	3:00	3:00
3:15	3:15	3:15
3:30	3:30	3:30
3:45	3:45	3:45
4:00	4:00	4:00
4:15	4:15	4:15
4:30	4:30	4:30
4:45	4:45	4:45
5:00	5:00	5:00

APPOINTMENT CALENDAR PAGES

Thursday, November 30   Friday, December 1   Saturday, December 2

Thursday, November 30	Friday, December 1	Saturday, December 2
8:00	8:00	8:00
8:15	8:15	8:15
8:30	8:30	8:30
8:45	8:45 Hospital	8:45
9:00	9:00	9:00
9:15	9:15 Rounds	9:15
9:30	9:30	9:30
9:45	9:45	9:45
10:00	10:00 Travel	10:00
10:15	10:15	10:15
10:30	10:30	10:30
10:45	10:45	10:45
11:00	11:00	11:00
11:15	11:15	11:15
11:30	11:30	11:30
11:45	11:45	11:45
12:00	12:00	
12:15	12:15	
12:30	12:30	
12:45	12:45	
1:00	1:00 Office	
1:15	1:15	
1:30	1:30 Closed	
1:45	1:45	
2:00	2:00	
2:15	2:15	
2:30	2:30	
2:45	2:45	
3:00	3:00	
3:15	3:15	
3:30	3:30	
3:45	3:45	
4:00	4:00	
4:15	4:15	
4:30	4:30	
4:45	4:45	
5:00	5:00	

October

S	M	T	W	T	F	S
1	2	3	4	5	6	7
8	9	10	11	12	13	14
15	16	17	18	19	20	21
22	23	24	25	26	27	28
29	30	31				

November

S	M	T	W	T	F	S
			1	2	3	4
5	6	7	8	9	10	11
12	13	14	15	16	17	18
19	20	21	22	23	24	25
26	27	28	29	30		

December

S	M	T	W	T	F	S
					1	2
3	4	5	6	7	8	9
10	11	12	13	14	15	16
17	18	19	20	21	22	23
24	25	26	27	28	29	30
31						

Working Papers

APPOINTMENT CARDS

YOUR APPOINTMENT IS:

AT

SPECIAL INSTRUCTIONS:

KAREN LARSEN, MD
2235 South Ridgeway Avenue
Chicago, IL 60623-2240
312-555-6022
PLEASE CALL IF YOU CANNOT KEEP THIS
APPOINTMENT.

YOUR APPOINTMENT IS:

AT

SPECIAL INSTRUCTIONS:

KAREN LARSEN, MD
2235 South Ridgeway Avenue
Chicago, IL 60623-2240
312-555-6022
PLEASE CALL IF YOU CANNOT KEEP THIS
APPOINTMENT.

YOUR APPOINTMENT IS:

AT

SPECIAL INSTRUCTIONS:

KAREN LARSEN, MD
2235 South Ridgeway Avenue
Chicago, IL 60623-2240
312-555-6022
PLEASE CALL IF YOU CANNOT KEEP THIS
APPOINTMENT.

YOUR APPOINTMENT IS:

AT

SPECIAL INSTRUCTIONS:

KAREN LARSEN, MD
2235 South Ridgeway Avenue
Chicago, IL 60623-2240
312-555-6022
PLEASE CALL IF YOU CANNOT KEEP THIS
APPOINTMENT.

YOUR APPOINTMENT IS:

AT

SPECIAL INSTRUCTIONS:

KAREN LARSEN, MD
2235 South Ridgeway Avenue
Chicago, IL 60623-2240
312-555-6022
PLEASE CALL IF YOU CANNOT KEEP THIS
APPOINTMENT.

YOUR APPOINTMENT IS:

AT

SPECIAL INSTRUCTIONS:

KAREN LARSEN, MD
2235 South Ridgeway Avenue
Chicago, IL 60623-2240
312-555-6022
PLEASE CALL IF YOU CANNOT KEEP THIS
APPOINTMENT.

YOUR APPOINTMENT IS:

AT

SPECIAL INSTRUCTIONS:

KAREN LARSEN, MD
2235 South Ridgeway Avenue
Chicago, IL 60623-2240
312-555-6022
PLEASE CALL IF YOU CANNOT KEEP THIS
APPOINTMENT.

YOUR APPOINTMENT IS:

AT

SPECIAL INSTRUCTIONS:

KAREN LARSEN, MD
2235 South Ridgeway Avenue
Chicago, IL 60623-2240
312-555-6022
PLEASE CALL IF YOU CANNOT KEEP THIS
APPOINTMENT.

YOUR APPOINTMENT IS:

AT

SPECIAL INSTRUCTIONS:

KAREN LARSEN, MD
2235 South Ridgeway Avenue
Chicago, IL 60623-2240
312-555-6022
PLEASE CALL IF YOU CANNOT KEEP THIS
APPOINTMENT.

YOUR APPOINTMENT IS:

AT

SPECIAL INSTRUCTIONS:

KAREN LARSEN, MD
2235 South Ridgeway Avenue
Chicago, IL 60623-2240
312-555-6022
PLEASE CALL IF YOU CANNOT KEEP THIS
APPOINTMENT.

YOUR APPOINTMENT IS:

AT

SPECIAL INSTRUCTIONS:

KAREN LARSEN, MD
2235 South Ridgeway Avenue
Chicago, IL 60623-2240
312-555-6022
PLEASE CALL IF YOU CANNOT KEEP THIS
APPOINTMENT.

YOUR APPOINTMENT IS:

AT

SPECIAL INSTRUCTIONS:

KAREN LARSEN, MD
2235 South Ridgeway Avenue
Chicago, IL 60623-2240
312-555-6022
PLEASE CALL IF YOU CANNOT KEEP THIS
APPOINTMENT.

YOUR APPOINTMENT IS:

AT

SPECIAL INSTRUCTIONS:

KAREN LARSEN, MD
2235 South Ridgeway Avenue
Chicago, IL 60623-2240
312-555-6022
PLEASE CALL IF YOU CANNOT KEEP THIS
APPOINTMENT.

YOUR APPOINTMENT IS:

AT

SPECIAL INSTRUCTIONS:

KAREN LARSEN, MD
2235 South Ridgeway Avenue
Chicago, IL 60623-2240
312-555-6022
PLEASE CALL IF YOU CANNOT KEEP THIS
APPOINTMENT.

YOUR APPOINTMENT IS:

AT

SPECIAL INSTRUCTIONS:

KAREN LARSEN, MD
2235 South Ridgeway Avenue
Chicago, IL 60623-2240
312-555-6022
PLEASE CALL IF YOU CANNOT KEEP THIS
APPOINTMENT.

OUT-OF-OFFICE SCHEDULING

Directions: You are working for several physicians: Dr. R. Gain, a cardiologist; Dr. J. Brent, a family practice physician; and Dr. E. Oren, a general surgeon. Determine what element is missing in the situations in Column 1. Choose the appropriate response from Column 2.

Column 1

_____ 1. Dr. Gain asks you to admit the patient, age 72, with a recent myocardial infarction to University Hospital today for controlled cardiovascular monitoring.

_____ 2. Dr. Oren asks you to schedule a gastrectomy for Les Weiner, age 65, at University Hospital next Monday or Tuesday morning.

_____ 3. Dr. Brent asks you to schedule Mary Maye for a bone marrow aspiration at University Hospital Lab because of her iron-deficiency anemia.

_____ 4. Peter Nu fractured his right wrist playing racquetball. Dr. Brent wants you to schedule an appointment with an orthopedic surgeon as soon as possible for possible surgery.

_____ 5. Dr. Brent asks you to refer a 4-year-old patient, Jan Davis, with acute lymphocytic leukemia to an oncologist next week to start a program of chemotherapy.

_____ 6. Dr. Oren wants you to schedule a short-stay surgery room at University Hospital for Tina Messer next Tuesday morning. Tina has a nodule in her right breast.

_____ 7. Dr. Gain wants you to admit Ian Wenth to University Hospital. Ian has pulmonary insufficiency caused by pneumonia and will need intensive oxygen therapy.

_____ 8. Patient Larry Phen has been diagnosed with emphysema. Dr. Gain now wants to refer Larry to a pulmonary specialist as soon as possible for therapeutic management.

_____ 9. Dr. Brent wants to refer this patient as soon as possible to Dr. Henri Wilson, a neurologist. The patient's migraines have increased in frequency and in severity; her therapeutic program needs to be reevaluated.

_____ 10. Dr. Oren wants you to admit Jane Hanson with appendicitis to University Hospital this morning.

Column 2

a. Specialist's name

b. Patient's name

c. Diagnosis or problem

d. When to be seen

e. Procedure to be performed

COMPUTER TERMS

Directions: Match the term in Column 2 with its definition in Column 1.

Column 1

_____ 1. Software that relates to specific tasks, such as word processing

_____ 2. Communications system for exchanging messages written on a computer over telephone lines

_____ 3. Portable, notebook-sized computers

_____ 4. The brain of a computer

_____ 5. Software that allows a person to edit a printed document

_____ 6. A display screen

_____ 7. Software that transcribes spoken words into text without using a keyboard

_____ 8. A system that allows a group of computers to communicate, exchange information, or pool resources

_____ 9. Software that allows the creation of images on the computer

_____10. A collection of related data

_____11. Temporary computer memory

_____12. Software that allows numeric data to be tabulated according to mathematical formulas

_____13. A device to input data

Column 2

a. application software

b. CPU

c. database

d. e-mail

e. graphics application

f. keyboard

g. monitor

h. networking

i. laptops

j. RAM

k. spreadsheet program

l. voice-recognition software

m. word processing program

COMPUTER TECHNOLOGY

Directions: The following items refer to computer technology. Mark each statement with either "T" for *true* or "F" for *false*. Be prepared to discuss your answers.

_____ 1. It is easier to locate open time slots for appointments on an electronic schedule than on a paper schedule.

_____ 2. Only one user at a time can access a file on a network.

_____ 3. A mainframe computer is necessary to operate any doctor's office.

_____ 4. A firewall prevents outside parties from having access to the office's particular files.

_____ 5. ROM is temporary; everything in ROM disappears when the computer is shut down.

_____ 6. When you are online, you are connected to a network.

_____ 7. An electronic medical record must be backed up with a paper medical record.

_____ 8. E-mail systems do not allow you to print messages.

_____ 9. A transaction database contains data on a specific patient's visit, including such items as services rendered during that visit, necessary diagnosis and procedure codes, and so forth.

_____ 10. The cost of filing an electronic insurance claim is higher than that of filing a paper copy.

_____ 11. A scanner allows you to enter information into the computer's memory without keying it.

_____ 12. Designing the work environment to conform to the physical needs of a user is ergonomics.

_____ 13. A firewall turns data into unrecognizable information during transmission.

_____ 14. Wireless communication transmits data through telephone wires.

_____ 15. The most powerful computer available is the supercomputer.

_____ 16. Virus checkers do not need to be updated.

_____ 17. A screen saver protects data from being seen by others.

_____ 18. Everyone in the medical office will be performing audit trails on computer usage.

_____ 19. Passwords are designed to limit access to computer files.

_____ 20. An office does not need a signed release-of-information form for use with electronic health records.

KNOWLEDGE OF THE EHR

Directions: The following items refer to electronic health records. Mark each statement with either "T" for *true* or "F" for *false*. Be prepared to discuss your answers.

_____ 1. The use of EHR has been an unnatural outgrowth of the widespread clinical use of computers in the healthcare industry.

_____ 2. For many facilities and private practices, the cost of EHR is prohibitive.

_____ 3. Frequent and ongoing training for medical team members is imperative to ensure the integrity of the input data and the security of the system.

_____ 4. Policies and procedures for updating personnel and evidence of the training should be placed in the personnel manual.

_____ 5. Implementation of electronic health records is mandated by the federal government.

_____ 6. Until electronic health records are fully implemented into the healthcare system, scanners will be provided by the federal government.

_____ 7. After all office medical documents have been scanned into the system, hardcopy lab reports, consultation letters, and so on will automatically be entered into the patient's electronic records and no scanning will ever be needed.

_____ 8. Converting paper-based records to electronic health records requires the scanning of paper records into the electronic database.

_____ 9. Errors will not occur in EHR, only in the paper-based record.

_____10. There is no need for proofreading electronic medical data.

_____11. An amendment can be used to make a correction in an electronic medical record.

_____12. An electronic signature or initials are not needed when correcting erroneous information in the EHR.

_____13. Completely removing electronic data is an acceptable practice when utilizing EHRs.

_____14. There are many advantages to converting from paper-based medical records to EHRs.

_____15. Initial cost and contract fees are relatively inexpensive for healthcare providers.

PATIENT INFORMATION FORM

Welcome	*Please complete this form using only ink. This information will remain confidential.*

PATIENT INFORMATION

Last name:	First name:	Initial:	Date of birth:	Home phone:

Address:	Marital status: (check appropriate box) S ☐ M ☐ D ☐ W ☐	Sex M F

City:	State:	ZIP:	Social Security Number:

Patient's employer: (If student, name of school.)	Employment address: Business phone:

Bill to:	Relationship:

Address:	City:	State:	ZIP:

NOTIFY IN CASE OF EMERGENCY

Name:	Relationship:

Address:	Phone:

City:	State:	ZIP:

INSURANCE INFORMATION

Primary insurance company:	Secondary insurance company:

Subscriber's name:	DOB:	Subscriber's name:	DOB:

Patient Insurance ID #:	Group #:	Patient Insurance ID #:	Group #:

OTHER INFORMATION

Reason for visit:	Name of referring physician:

Patient's signature/Parent or guardian's signature	Today's date

PATIENT INFORMATION FORM

Welcome	Please complete this form using only ink. This information will remain confidential.

PATIENT INFORMATION

Last name:	First name:	Initial:	Date of birth:	Home phone:

Address:	Marital status: (check appropriate box) S ☐ M ☐ D ☐ W ☐	Sex M F

City:	State:	ZIP:	Social Security Number:

Patient's employer: (If student, name of school.)	Employment address:
	Business phone:

Bill to:	Relationship:

Address:	City:	State:	ZIP:

NOTIFY IN CASE OF EMERGENCY

Name:	Relationship:

Address:	Phone:

City:	State:	ZIP:	

INSURANCE INFORMATION

Primary insurance company:	Secondary insurance company:

Subscriber's name:	DOB:	Subscriber's name:	DOB:

Patient Insurance ID #:	Group #:	Patient Insurance ID #:	Group #:

OTHER INFORMATION

Reason for visit:	Name of referring physician:

Patient's signature/Parent or guardian's signature	Today's date

RECORDS RELEASE

RECORDS RELEASE

TO: _____ Healthcare provider

_____ Address

_____ City, State, ZIP

I authorize the above-named healthcare provider to release the specified information listed below to the following physician:

Karen Larsen, MD   312-555-6022
2235 South Ridgeway Avenue   Fax: 312-555-0025
Chicago, IL 60623-2240

PATIENT: _____   DOB: _____

_____   Address

_____   City, State, ZIP

Please include _____   specific records

Signed _____   Date _____

RECORDS RELEASE

TO: _____ Healthcare provider

_____ Address

_____ City, State, ZIP

I authorize the above-named healthcare provider to release the specified information listed below to the following physician:

Karen Larsen, MD   312-555-6022
2235 South Ridgeway Avenue   Fax: 312-555-0025
Chicago, IL 60623-2240

PATIENT: _____   DOB: _____

_____   Address

_____   City, State, ZIP

Please include _____   specific records

Signed _____   Date _____

TELEPHONE LOG

TELEPHONE LOG

Date _____

TIME	CALLER	TELEPHONE NUMBER	REASON	DONE

TO-DO LIST

	TO-DO LIST	
		Date _____

RUSH	ITEMS TO DO	DONE

Working Papers

INSURANCE TERMINOLOGY

Directions: Match the term in Column 2 with its definition in Column 1.

Column 1

_____ 1. Insurance through employment, with all employees having one master policy

_____ 2. Person who is covered by an insurance policy

_____ 3. Insurance company that provides insurance benefits

_____ 4. Provides reimbursement for income lost because of insured's illness

_____ 5. Rate charged for policy

_____ 6. Healthcare professional who supplies the healthcare

_____ 7. Ensures that payment for medical expenses will not exceed 100 percent of the medical expenses

_____ 8. Generally covers hospitalization, lab tests, surgery, and x-rays

_____ 9. A term used to describe an insurance company in the context of the doctor's and patient's relationship

_____ 10. Covers medically necessary services while insured is an inpatient

_____ 11. Covers physician's services for office visits

_____ 12. Covers medical expenses in a catastrophic situation

_____ 13. In a family with two family insurance contracts, determines which policy will be the primary carrier for the children

_____ 14. Covers physician's fee for surgery

_____ 15. Person in whose name the policy is written

Column 2

a. basic insurance plan

b. birthday rule

c. carrier

d. COB

e. disability insurance

f. group insurance

g. hospital insurance

h. insured

i. major medical insurance

j. medical insurance

k. policyholder

l. premium

m. provider

n. surgical insurance

o. third-party payer

INSURANCE PLANS, PAYERS, AND PAYMENT METHODS

Directions: The following items refer to insurance plans and processing claims. Mark each statement with either "T" for *true* or "F" for *false*. Be prepared to discuss your answers.

_____ 1. Coinsurance is the amount of medical expense that the insured must pay before the insurance carrier begins paying benefits.

_____ 2. A government agency called the Centers for Medicare and Medicaid Services (CMS) administers the Medicare and Medicaid programs.

_____ 3. In an indemnity plan, patients receive medical services from a primary care physician who coordinates the patients' overall care.

_____ 4. Coinsurance is the percentage of each claim that the insured must pay, according to the terms of the insurance policy.

_____ 5. Everyone eligible for Medicare Part A (hospitalization insurance) automatically receives Medicare Part B (medical insurance).

_____ 6. *Balance billing* refers to billing the patient for any amount due on a provider's bill after the insurance company has taken care of its responsibility.

_____ 7. The allowable fee, in insurance terms, is the most the insurance company will allow any provider to collect for a covered procedure.

_____ 8. Every time HMO and PPO members visit their physician, they pay a set charge called a copayment.

_____ 9. A PAR provider who agrees to accept the allowed charge set forth by the insurance company as payment in full is accepting assignment.

_____ 10. In a capitated plan, a physician may receive $35 per month for each patient assigned to him or her, even if the patient receives no care during that month.

_____ 11. A Medicare participating provider decides whether to accept assignment on a claim-by-claim basis.

_____ 12. RBRVS is the payment system used by Medicare for determining how much it will pay for inpatient care.

_____ 13. When the amount the physician charges is more than the insurance company's allowed charge, the difference must be absorbed by the PAR provider.

ICD-10-CM DIAGNOSTIC CODES

Codes	Description	Codes	Description
N91.2	Amenorrhea, unspecified	K58.9	Irritable bowel syndrome w/o diarrhea
D64.9	Anemia	M25.50	Joint pain, unspecified
I20.9	Angina, pectoris, unspecified	I88.9	Lymphadenitis, nonspecific
I49.9	Arrhythmia, cardiac, unspecified	R59.1	Lymphadenopathy
M19.90	Arthritis, NOS/Osteoarthritis	N95.1	Menopausal disorder, symptomatic
M06.9	Arthritis, rheumatoid, unspecified	N93.9	Menstrual disorder, abnormal vaginal/uterine bleeding
J45.909	Asthma, unspecified, uncomplicated		
R82.71	Bacteruria	R11.0	Nausea
H01.009	Blepharitis, unspecified	E66.9	Obesity, unspecified
J20.9	Bronchitis, acute, unspecified	M81.0	Osteoporosis, age-related
J40	Bronchitis, not specified as acute or chronic	H60.399	Otitis externa, other, infective, unspecified ear
L03.90	Cellulitis/Abscess, unspecified	H66.90	Otitis media, unspecified, unspecified ear
I67.9	Cerebrovascular disease, unspecified		
R07.9	Chest pain, unspecified	R10.9	Pain, abdominal, unspecified
I50.9	CHF, unspecified	M54.5	Pain, back, low
K81.0	Cholecystitis, acute	M79.10	Pain, muscular
H10.9	Conjunctivitis, unspecified	R00.2	Palpitations
R05	Cough	R10.2	Pelvic and perineal pain
N30.00	Cystitis, acute, without hematuria	J02.9	Pharyngitis/Sore throat, unspecified
L30.9	Dermatitis, unspecified	J18.9	Pneumonia, unspecified organism
Z83.3	Diabetes family history	R63.1	Polydipsia
E10.9	Diabetes mellitus Type 1, without complications	R35.8	Polyuria
		Z32.01	Pregnancy test, positive results
E11.9	Diabetes mellitus Type 2, without complcations	Z01.818	Pre-op
		Z00.00	Preventive, adult
R19.7	Diarrhea, unspecified	Z01.419	Preventive including GYN exam, w/o abnormal findings
K57.32	Diverticulitis, large intestine, w/o bleeding, abscess, or perforation		
		Z00.129	Preventive, pediatric, w/o abnormal findings
R42	Dizziness/Lightheadedness		
N94.6	Dysmenorrhea, unspecified	Z02.0	Preventive, school admission
K30	Dyspepsia, functional	N40.0	Prostatic hypertrophy, benign,w/o lower urinary track symptoms
R30.0	Dysuria		
R60.9	Edema, unspecified	N41.9	Prostatitis
Z02.1	Employment exam	R80.9	Proteinuria, unspecified
R04.0	Epistaxis	R97.20	PSA, elevated
R53.83	Fatigue	R21	Rash/Skin eruption
T15.82XA	FB, left eye, external, multiple parts	R06.02	Shortness of breath
T15.81XA	FB, right eye, external, multiple parts	J01.90	Sinusitis, acute, unspecified
T15.80xA	FB, unspecified eye, external, multiple parts	R00.0	Tachycardia, unspecified
		R84.5	Throat culture, positive
R50.9	Fever, unspecified	H93.19	Tinnitus, unspecified ear
K29.70	Gastritis, unspecified, without bleeding	J03.90	Tonsillitis, acute, unspecified
K52.9	Gastroenteritis and colitis, noninfective, unspecified	K51.20	Ulcerative colitis/Proctitis
		J06.9	URI, unspecified
A08.4	Gastroenteritis, viral, unspecified	R35.0	Urinary frequency
K21.9	Gastroesophageal reflux	R32	Urinary incontinence, unspecified
R51.9	Headache, unspecified	N39.0	UTI
G43.909	Headache, migraine	N76.0	Vaginitis, acute
Z82.49	Heart disease, family history	B34.9	Viral infection, unspecifed
E78.00	Hypercholesterolemia	Z11.59	Viral screening, unspecified
E78.5	Hyperlipidemia, unspecified	R11.10	Vomiting, unspecified
I10	Hypertension, essential	D72.829	wbc high
J11.1	Influenza, with other respiratory manifestation	D72.819	wbc low
		R63.4	Weight loss, abnormal
G47.00	Insomnia, unspecified		**2021 edition**

JANET PROVOST'S PATIENT ENCOUNTER FORM

No.	Date	Description	Charge	Credit		Current Balance
				Payment	Adjustment	
	03/08/20--	Annual exam/CBC/UA	185.00	25.00	-------	160.00

Patient Information

7921 W. 42d Street
Address

Chicago, IL 60632-1426
City, State, ZIP

312-555-4279   312-555-6264
Home phone   **Work phone**

same   self
Responsible person   **Relationship**

Blue Cross/Blue Shield   PRO87265
Insurance   **Patient Insurance ID**

Patient _____ Provost, Janet _____

Date: 03/08/20--   **Chart #AA033**

Karen Larsen, MD
2235 S. Ridgeway Avenue
Chicago, IL 60623-2240

312-555-6022

Fax: 312-555-0025

Diagnoses:

1. ___ ZØØ.ØØ ___

2. _____

3. _____

4. _____

OFFICE VISITS

New Patient	Established Patient

Preventive Medicine

	_____ 99381	under 1 year	_____ 99391	
	_____ 99382	1–4	_____ 99392	_____ 99211
_____ 99202	_____ 99383	5–11	_____ 99393	_____ 99212
_____ 99203	_____ 99384	12–17	_____ 99394	_____ 99213
_____ 99204	_____ 99385	18–39	_136_ 99395	_____ 99214
_____ 99205	_____ 99386	40–64	_____ 99396	_____ 99215
	_____ 99387	65+	_____ 99397	

Hospital Visits
Initial:
_____ 99221
_____ 99222
_____ 99223
Subsequent:
_____ 99231
_____ 99232
_____ 99233
Discharge:
_____ 99238
_____ 99239
Nursing Facility
Initial:
_____ 99304
_____ 99305
_____ 99306

Other
_____
_____

Lab:
_____ 80048 Basic metabolic panel
_____ 87110 Chlamydia culture
_____ 85651 ESR; nonautomated
_____ 83001 FSH
_____ 82947 Glucose, blood
_25_ 85025 Hemogram (CBC) with differential
_____ 80076 Hepatic function panel
_____ 85018 HGB
_____ 86701 HIV-1
_____ 83002 LH
_____ 80061 Lipid panel
_____ 86617 Lyme antibody

_____ 86308 Monospot test
_____ 88150 Pap
_____ 85610 Prothrombin time
_____ 84152 PSA
_____ 86430 Rheumatoid factor
_____ 82270 Stool hemoccult x 3
_____ 87430 Strep screen
_____ 84478 Triglycerides
_____ 84443 TSH
_24_ 81001 UA with microscopy
_____ 87088 UC
_____ 84550 Uric acid, blood
_____ 81025 Urine pregnancy test
_____
_____

Injections:
_____ 90471 admin 1 vac
_____ 90472 each add'l vac
_____ 90716 Chickenpox
_____ 90702 DT
_____ 90700 DTaP
_____ 90657 Influenza 0.25mL
_____ 90658 Influenza 0.5mL
_____ 90710 MMRV, subcutaneous
_____ 90707 MMR
_____ 90649 4vHPV
_____ 90713 Polio vac inactivated (IPV)
_____ 90714 Td

ECG:
_____ 93000 ECG

Other
_____
_____

2021 Edition

FEE SCHEDULE

Fee Schedule—Karen Larsen, MD

New Patient	Established Patient

Preventive Medicine

New Patient		Preventive Medicine	Established Patient	
	139 99381	under 1 year	110 99391	
	145 99382	1–4	123 99392	
	142 99383	5–11	128 99393	29 99211
73 99202	177 99384	12–17	148 99394	44 99212
100 99203	165 99385	18–39	136 99395	60 99213
147 99204	178 99386	40–64	148 99396	87 99214
190 99205	199 99387	65+	119 99397	134 99215

Hospital Visits

Initial:

121 99221

172 99222

217 99223

Subsequent:

65 99231

90 99232

132 99233

Discharge:

100 99238

150 99239

Nursing Facility

Initial:

53 99304

77 99305

109 99306

Other

_____

_____

Lab:

51 80048 Basic metabolic panel

74 87110 Chlamydia culture

21 85651 ESR; nonautomated

97 83001 FSH

21 82947 Glucose, blood

25 85025 Hemogram (CBC) with differential

55 80076 Hepatic function panel

13 85018 HGB

77 86701 HIV-1

97 83002 LH

72 80061 Lipid panel

86 86617 Lyme antibody

33 86308 Monospot test

33 88150 Pap

23 85610 Prothrombin time

91 84152 PSA

30 86430 Rheumatoid factor

15 82270 Stool hemoccult x 3

39 87430 Strep screen

21 84478 Triglycerides

69 84443 TSH

24 81001 UA with microscopy

35 87088 UC

20 84550 Uric acid, blood

23 81025 Urine pregnancy test

_____

_____

_____

Injections:

10 90471 admin 1 vac

8 90472 each add'l vac

133 90716 Chickenpox

31 90702 DT

78 90700 DTaP

30 90657 Influenza 0.25mL

35 90658 Influenza 0.5mL

40 90710 MMRV, subcutaneous

104 90707 MMR

51 90649 4vHPV

52 90713 Polio vac inactivated (IPV)

26 90714 Td

ECG:

70 93000 ECG

Other

_____

_____

_____

2021 Edition

DAILY JOURNAL

DATE _____10/17/20--_____   SHEET NO. ____102____

	RECEIPT NUMBER	DATE	DESCRIPTION CODE	CHARGE	PAYMENT	ADJUSTMENTS	BALANCE	PREVIOUS BALANCE	NAME
1	1090	10/17	OV	44 00	---	---	44 00	---	Sherman, Florence
2	1091	10/17	OV/Strep screen	83 00	16 60	---	66 40	---	Villano, Juan
3	1092	10/17	OV	44 00	---	---	147 00	103 00	Robertson, Gary
4	1093	10/17	OV/LAB	241 00	48 20	---	192 80	---	Armstrong, Monica
5	1094	10/17	OV	44 00	---	---	44 00	---	Casagranda, George
6									
7									
32									
33									
34									
			TOTALS	Column A	Column B	Column C	Column D	Column E	TOTALS

◄ ALL RECEIPTS MUST BE
IN NUMERICAL ORDER

Proof of Posting

Column E Total $ _____
Plus Column A Total $ _____
Subtotal $ _____
Minus Column B Total $ _____
Equals Column D Total $ _____

Accounts Receivable Control

Previous Balance $ ____6260.40____
Plus Column A $ _____
Subtotal $ _____
Minus Column B Total $ _____
Present Acc't's Rec. Balance $ _____

Daily Cash

Opening Cash on Hand
at Beginning of Day $ _____   -0-
Cash Received During Day $ _____
Total $ _____

DAILY JOURNAL #103

DATE ___10/18/20- -___   SHEET NO. ___103___

	RECEIPT NUMBER	DATE	DESCRIPTION CODE	CHARGE	PAYMENT	ADJUSTMENTS	BALANCE	PREVIOUS BALANCE	NAME
1	1095	10/18	OV (WC)	44 00	—	—	44 00	—	Sun, Cheng
2	1096	10/18	OV	44 00	—	—	44 00	—	Jonathan, Charles
3	1097	10/18	CPE/LAB	278 00	—	—	278 00	—	Babcock, Sara
4									
5									
6									
7									
32									
33									
34									
				Column A	Column B	Column C	Column D	Column E	TOTALS

◄ ALL RECEIPTS MUST BE
IN NUMERICAL ORDER

Proof of Posting

Column E Total $	_____
Plus Column A Total $	_____
Subtotal $	_____
Minus Column B Total $	_____
Equals Column D Total $	_____

Accounts Receivable Control

Previous Balance $	_____
Plus Column A $	_____
Subtotal $	_____
Minus Column B Total $	_____
Present Acc'ts Rec. Balance $	_____

Daily Cash

Opening Cash on Hand at Beginning of Day $	_____
Cash Received During Day $	_____
Total $	_____

BLANK DAILY JOURNAL

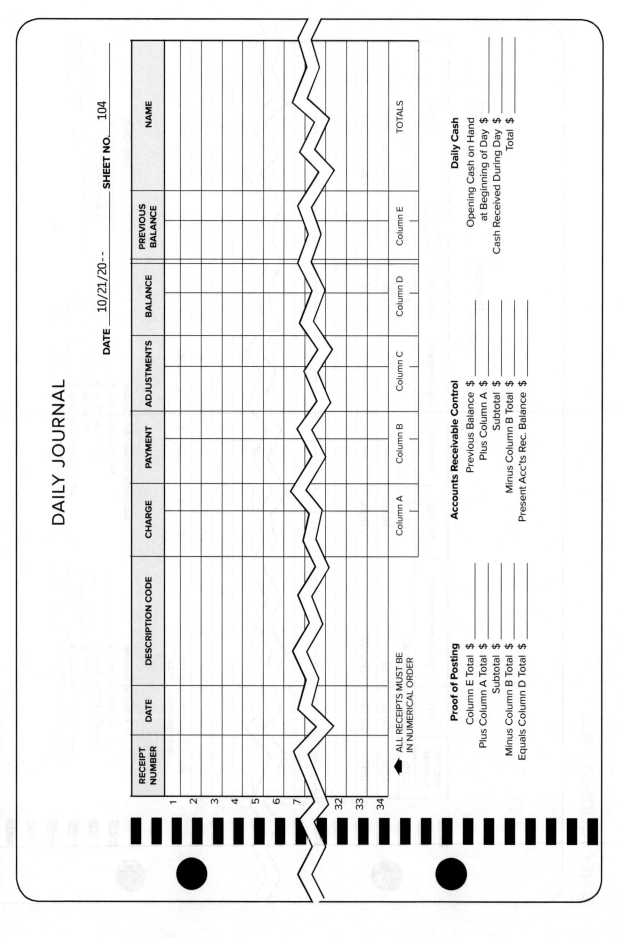

DAILY JOURNAL

DATE ___10/21/20- -___   SHEET NO. ___104___

RECEIPT NUMBER	DATE	DESCRIPTION CODE	CHARGE	PAYMENT	ADJUSTMENTS	BALANCE	PREVIOUS BALANCE	NAME
1								
2								
3								
4								
5								
6								
7								
32								
33								
34								
		TOTALS	Column A	Column B	Column C	Column D	Column E	

◀ ALL RECEIPTS MUST BE IN NUMERICAL ORDER

Proof of Posting

Column E Total $ _____
Plus Column A Total $ _____
Subtotal $ _____
Minus Column B Total $ _____
Equals Column D Total $ _____

Accounts Receivable Control

Previous Balance $ _____
Plus Column A $ _____
Subtotal $ _____
Minus Column B Total $ _____
Present Acc'ts Rec. Balance $ _____

Daily Cash

Opening Cash on Hand
at Beginning of Day $ _____
Cash Received During Day $ _____
Total $ _____

DEPOSIT SLIPS

DEPOSITED IN

FIRST NATIONAL BANK
CHICAGO, IL 60623-2791

THIS DEPOSIT ACCEPTED UNDER AND SUBJECT TO THE PROVISIONS
OF THE UNIFORM COMMERCIAL CODE

DATE _____

Karen Larsen, MD
2235 South Ridgeway Avenue
Chicago, IL 60623-2240

⑈07015550 ⑈2242027720 ⑈

	DOLLARS	CENTS
Cash		
Checks List Separately		
Total from Other Side		
Subtotal		
Less Cash Received		
TOTAL		

DEPOSITED IN

FIRST NATIONAL BANK
CHICAGO, IL 60623-2791

THIS DEPOSIT ACCEPTED UNDER AND SUBJECT TO THE PROVISIONS
OF THE UNIFORM COMMERCIAL CODE

DATE _____

Karen Larsen, MD
2235 South Ridgeway Avenue
Chicago, IL 60623-2240

⑈07015550 ⑈2242027720 ⑈

	DOLLARS	CENTS
Cash		
Checks List Separately		
Total from Other Side		
Subtotal		
Less Cash Received		
TOTAL		

DEPOSITED IN

FIRST NATIONAL BANK
CHICAGO, IL 60623-2791

THIS DEPOSIT ACCEPTED UNDER AND SUBJECT TO THE PROVISIONS
OF THE UNIFORM COMMERCIAL CODE

DATE _____

Karen Larsen, MD
2235 South Ridgeway Avenue
Chicago, IL 60623-2240

⑈07015550 ⑈2242027720 ⑈

	DOLLARS	CENTS
Cash		
Checks List Separately		
Total from Other Side		
Subtotal		
Less Cash Received		
TOTAL		

DEPOSITED IN

FIRST NATIONAL BANK
CHICAGO, IL 60623-2791

THIS DEPOSIT ACCEPTED UNDER AND SUBJECT TO THE PROVISIONS
OF THE UNIFORM COMMERCIAL CODE

DATE _____

Karen Larsen, MD
2235 South Ridgeway Avenue
Chicago, IL 60623-2240

⑈07015550 ⑈2242027720 ⑈

	DOLLARS	CENTS
Cash		
Checks List Separately		
Total from Other Side		
Subtotal		
Less Cash Received		
TOTAL		

TELEPHONE LOG

TIME	CALLER	TELEPHONE NUMBER	REASON	DONE

TELEPHONE LOG

Date _____

TIME	CALLER	TELEPHONE NUMBER	REASON	DONE

TO-DO LIST

Date _____

RUSH	ITEMS TO DO	DONE

TAI CLINIC, INC.
Grace Tai, MD
100 Sun Valley Road, Lisle, IL 60532
312-555-9300

October 19, 20--

Karen Larsen, MD
2235 South Ridgeway Avenue
Chicago, IL 60623-2240

Dear Dr. Larsen:

RE: David Kramer   DOB: 4/28/20--

David is up to date on his immunizations. His immunization record is as follows:

DTP: 3 months (7/26/20--)   Oral polio: 3 months (7/26/20--)
      6 months (10/22/20--)   6 months (10/22/20--)
      9 months (1/29/20--)   9 months (1/29/20--)

MMR: 2 years (5/2/20--)

David is due for a booster DTP before starting kindergarten.

If you have any questions, please contact our office.

Sincerely,

Grace Tai, MD

Grace Tai, MD

jz

KL
Please file.

RECEIPTS

No. _1214_

To _____

Date _____

For _____

Amount _____

_____

No. _1214_ _____ _20_____

Received from _____

_____ Dollars

For _____

_____

$ _____

No. _____

To _____

Date _____

For _____

Amount _____

_____

No. _____ _20_____

Received from _____

_____ Dollars

For _____

_____

$ _____

No. _____

To _____

Date _____

For _____

Amount _____

_____

No. _____ _20_____

Received from _____

_____ Dollars

For _____

_____

$ _____

No. _____

To _____

Date _____

For _____

Amount _____

_____

No. _____ _20_____

Received from _____

_____ Dollars

For _____

_____

$ _____

LAURA LUND'S PATIENT ENCOUNTER FORM

No.	Date	Description	Charge	Credit		Current Balance
				Payment	**Adjustment**	

Patient Information	Patient	Laura Lund

Patient Information

13419 S. Buffalo Avenue
Address

Chicago, IL 60633-2010
City, State, ZIP

312-555-4100
Home phone

father
312-555-8840
Work phone

Lawrence Lund
Responsible person

father
Relationship

Employee Benefit Plan
Insurance

525267A
Patient Insurance ID

Patient _____ Laura Lund _____

Date: 10/19/20--   **Chart #AA020**

Karen Larsen, MD
2235 S. Ridgeway Avenue
Chicago, IL 60623-2240

312-555-6022

Fax: 312-555-0025

Diagnoses:

1. _____ S13.8XXA _____

2. _____

3. _____

4. _____

OFFICE VISITS

New Patient	Established Patient

Preventive Medicine

	_____ 99381	under 1 year	_____ 99391	
	_____ 99382	1–4	_____ 99392	_____ 99211
_____ 99202	_____ 99383	5–11	_____ 99393	(99212)
_____ 99203	_____ 99384	12–17	_____ 99394	_____ 99213
_____ 99204	_____ 99385	18–39	_____ 99395	_____ 99214
_____ 99205	_____ 99386	40–64	_____ 99396	_____ 99215
	_____ 99387	65+	_____ 99397	

Hospital Visits
Initial:
_____ 99221
_____ 99222
_____ 99223
Subsequent:
_____ 99231
_____ 99232
_____ 99233
Discharge:
_____ 99238
_____ 99239
Nursing Facility
Initial:
_____ 99304
_____ 99305
_____ 99306

Other
_____
_____

Lab:
_____ 80048 Basic metabolic panel
_____ 87110 Chlamydia culture
_____ 85651 ESR; nonautomated
_____ 83001 FSH
_____ 82947 Glucose, blood
_____ 85025 Hemogram (CBC) with differential
_____ 80076 Hepatic function panel
_____ 85018 HGB
_____ 86701 HIV-1
_____ 83002 LH
_____ 80061 Lipid panel
_____ 86617 Lyme antibody

_____ 86308 Monospot test
_____ 88150 Pap
_____ 85610 Prothrombin time
_____ 84152 PSA
_____ 86430 Rheumatoid factor
_____ 82270 Stool hemoccult x 3
_____ 87430 Strep screen
_____ 84478 Triglycerides
_____ 84443 TSH
_____ 81001 UA with microscopy
_____ 87088 UC
_____ 84550 Uric acid, blood
_____ 81025 Urine pregnancy test
_____
_____

Injections:
_____ 90471 admin 1 vac
_____ 90472 each add'l vac
_____ 90716 Chickenpox
_____ 90702 DT
_____ 90700 DTaP
_____ 90657 Influenza 0.25mL
_____ 90658 Influenza 0.5mL
_____ 90710 MMRV, subcutaneous
_____ 90707 MMR
_____ 90649 4vHPV
_____ 90713 Polio vac inactivated (IPV)
_____ 90714 Td
ECG:
_____ 93000 ECG

Other
_____
_____

2021 Edition

ANA MENDEZ'S PATIENT ENCOUNTER FORM

No.	Date	Description	Charge	Credit		Current Balance
				Payment	Adjustment	

Patient Information	
3457 W. 63d Place	
Address	
Chicago, IL 60629-4270	
City, State, ZIP	
312-555-3606	
Home phone	**Work phone**
self	
Responsible person	**Relationship**
Blue Cross & Blue Shield	874669
Insurance	**Patient Insurance ID**

Patient _____ Ana Mendez _____

Date: 10/19/20-- | Chart #AA024

Karen Larsen, MD
2235 S. Ridgeway Avenue
Chicago, IL 60623-2240

312-555-6022

Fax: 312-555-0025

Diagnoses:

1. J03.90

2. I88.9

3. _____

4. _____

OFFICE VISITS

New Patient		Established Patient	

Preventive Medicine

	_____ 99381 under 1 year	_____ 99391	
	_____ 99382 1–4	_____ 99392	_____ 99211
_____ 99202	_____ 99383 5–11	_____ 99393	(99212)
_____ 99203	_____ 99384 12–17	_____ 99394	_____ 99213
_____ 99204	_____ 99385 18–39	_____ 99395	_____ 99214
_____ 99205	_____ 99386 40–64	_____ 99396	_____ 99215
	_____ 99387 65+	_____ 99397	

Hospital Visits
Initial:
_____ 99221
_____ 99222
_____ 99223
Subsequent:
_____ 99231
_____ 99232
_____ 99233
Discharge:
_____ 99238
_____ 99239
Nursing Facility
Initial:
_____ 99304
_____ 99305
_____ 99306

Other

_____
_____

Lab:
_____ 80048 Basic metabolic panel
_____ 87110 Chlamydia culture
_____ 85651 ESR; nonautomated
_____ 83001 FSH
_____ 82947 Glucose, blood
_____ 85025 Hemogram (CBC) with differential
_____ 80076 Hepatic function panel
_____ 85018 HGB
_____ 86701 HIV-1
_____ 83002 LH
_____ 80061 Lipid panel
_____ 86617 Lyme antibody

_____ 86308 Monospot test
_____ 88150 Pap
_____ 85610 Prothrombin time
_____ 84152 PSA
_____ 86430 Rheumatoid factor
_____ 82270 Stool hemoccult x 3
_____ 87430 Strep screen
_____ 84478 Triglycerides
_____ 84443 TSH
_____ 81001 UA with microscopy
_____ 87088 UC
_____ 84550 Uric acid, blood
_____ 81025 Urine pregnancy test

_____
_____

Injections:
_____ 90471 admin 1 vac
_____ 90472 each add'l vac
_____ 90716 Chickenpox
_____ 90702 DT
_____ 90700 DTaP
_____ 90657 Influenza 0.25mL
_____ 90658 Influenza 0.5mL
_____ 90710 MMRV, subcutaneous
_____ 90707 MMR
_____ 90649 4vHPV
_____ 90713 Polio vac inactivated (IPV)
_____ 90714 Td

ECG:
_____ 93000 ECG

Other

_____
_____

DONALD MITCHELL'S PATIENT ENCOUNTER FORM

| No. | Date | Description | Charge | Credit | | Current Balance |
				Payment	Adjustment	

Patient Information

Address
5231 W. School Street

City, State, ZIP
Chicago, IL 60651-2248

Home phone
312-555-8153

father
Work phone
312-555-6141

Responsible person
Alan Mitchell

father
Relationship

Insurance
New York Mutual

Patient Insurance ID
304253D

Patient Donald Mitchell

Date: 10/19/20--   **Chart #AA026**

Karen Larsen, MD
2235 S. Ridgeway Avenue
Chicago, IL 60623-2240

312-555-6022

Fax: 312-555-0025

Diagnoses:
1. Z00.129
2. _____
3. _____
4. _____

OFFICE VISITS

New Patient		Established Patient

Preventive Medicine

		under 1 year		99391		
_____ (99381)			_____ 99391			
_____ 99382	1–4	_____ 99392		
_____ 99202	_____ 99383	5–11	_____ 99393	_____ 99211
_____ 99203	_____ 99384	12–17	_____ 99394	_____ 99212
_____ 99204	_____ 99385	18–39	_____ 99395	_____ 99213
_____ 99205	_____ 99386	40–64	_____ 99396	_____ 99214
	_____ 99387	65+	_____ 99397	_____ 99215

Hospital Visits
Initial:
_____ 99221
_____ 99222
_____ 99223
Subsequent:
_____ 99231
_____ 99232
_____ 99233
Discharge:
_____ 99238
_____ 99239
Nursing Facility
Initial:
_____ 99304
_____ 99305
_____ 99306

Other
_____
_____

Lab:
_____ 80048 Basic metabolic panel
_____ 87110 Chlamydia culture
_____ 85651 ESR; nonautomated
_____ 83001 FSH
_____ 82947 Glucose, blood
_____ 85025 Hemogram (CBC) with differential
_____ 80076 Hepatic function panel
_____ 85018 HGB
_____ 86701 HIV-1
_____ 83002 LH
_____ 80061 Lipid panel
_____ 86617 Lyme antibody

_____ 86308 Monospot test
_____ 88150 Pap
_____ 85610 Prothrombin time
_____ 84152 PSA
_____ 86430 Rheumatoid factor
_____ 82270 Stool hemoccult x 3
_____ 87430 Strep screen
_____ 84478 Triglycerides
_____ 84443 TSH
_____ (81001) UA with microscopy
_____ 87088 UC
_____ 84550 Uric acid, blood
_____ 81025 Urine pregnancy test
_____
_____

Injections:
_____ 90471 admin 1 vac
_____ 90472 each add'l vac
_____ 90716 Chickenpox
_____ 90702 DT
_____ 90700 DTaP
_____ 90657 Influenza 0.25mL
_____ 90658 Influenza 0.5mL
_____ 90710 MMRV, subcutaneous
_____ 90707 MMR
_____ 90649 4vHPV
_____ 90713 Polio vac inactivated (IPV)
_____ 90714 Td

ECG:
_____ 93000 ECG

Other
_____
_____

2021 Edition

THERESA DAYTON'S PATIENT ENCOUNTER FORM

No.	Date	Description	Charge	Credit		Current Balance
				Payment	Adjustment	

Patient Information

Address
105 W. Chestnut Street

City, State, ZIP
Chicago, IL 60610-2816

Home phone
312-555-2231

Work phone
312-555-2583

Responsible person
self

Relationship

Insurance
Blue Cross/Blue Shield

Patient Insurance ID
DAY512374

Patient Theresa Dayton

Date: 10/19/20--

Chart #AA012

Karen Larsen, MD
2235 S. Ridgeway Avenue
Chicago, IL 60623-2240

312-555-6022

Fax: 312-555-0025

Diagnoses:

1. N60.01
2. Z30.9
3. _____
4. _____

OFFICE VISITS

New Patient	Established Patient

Preventive Medicine

	_____ 99381	under 1 year	_____ 99391	_____ 99211
	_____ 99382	1–4	_____ 99392	(99212)
_____ 99202	_____ 99383	5–11	_____ 99393	_____ 99213
_____ 99203	_____ 99384	12–17	_____ 99394	_____ 99214
_____ 99204	_____ 99385	18–39	_____ 99395	_____ 99215
_____ 99205	_____ 99386	40–64	_____ 99396	
	_____ 99387	65+	_____ 99397	

Hospital Visits
Initial:
_____ 99221
_____ 99222
_____ 99223
Subsequent:
_____ 99231
_____ 99232
_____ 99233
Discharge:
_____ 99238
_____ 99239
Nursing Facility
Initial:
_____ 99304
_____ 99305
_____ 99306

Other
_____
_____

Lab:
_____ 80048 Basic metabolic panel
_____ 87110 Chlamydia culture
_____ 85651 ESR; nonautomated
_____ 83001 FSH
_____ 82947 Glucose, blood
_____ 85025 Hemogram (CBC) with differential
_____ 80076 Hepatic function panel
_____ 85018 HGB
_____ 86701 HIV-1
_____ 83002 LH
_____ 80061 Lipid panel
_____ 86617 Lyme antibody

_____ 86308 Monospot test
_____ 88150 Pap
_____ 85610 Prothrombin time
_____ 84152 PSA
_____ 86430 Rheumatoid factor
_____ 82270 Stool hemoccult x 3
_____ 87430 Strep screen
_____ 84478 Triglycerides
_____ 84443 TSH
_____ 81001 UA with microscopy
_____ 87088 UC
_____ 84550 Uric acid, blood
_____ 81025 Urine pregnancy test
_____
_____

Injections:
_____ 90471 admin 1 vac
_____ 90472 each add'l vac
_____ 90716 Chickenpox
_____ 90702 DT
_____ 90700 DTaP
_____ 90657 Influenza 0.25mL
_____ 90658 Influenza 0.5mL
_____ 90710 MMRV, subcutaneous
_____ 90707 MMR
_____ 90649 4vHPV
_____ 90713 Polio vac inactivated (IPV)
_____ 90714 Td
ECG:
_____ 93000 ECG

Other
_____
_____

RAYMOND MURRARY'S PATIENT ENCOUNTER FORM

No.	Date	Description	Charge	Credit		Current Balance
				Payment	**Adjustment**	

Patient Information	Patient	Raymond Murrary

Patient Information

3908 N. Central Avenue
Address

Chicago, IL 60634-3276
City, State, ZIP

312-555-6343
Home phone   Work phone

self
Responsible person   Relationship

Medicare   1GE4-ET5-KM73
Insurance   Patient Insurance ID

Patient _____ Raymond Murrary _____

Date: 10/19/20--   **Chart #**AA030

Karen Larsen, MD
2235 S. Ridgeway Avenue
Chicago, IL 60623-2240

312-555-6022

Fax: 312-555-0025

Diagnoses:

1. _____ J44.1 _____

2. _____ J40 _____

3. _____

4. _____

OFFICE VISITS

New Patient	Established Patient

Preventive Medicine

	_____ 99381	under 1 year	_____ 99391
	_____ 99382	1–4	_____ 99392 _____ 99211
_____ 99202	_____ 99383	5–11	_____ 99393 _____ 99212
_____ 99203	_____ 99384	12–17	_____ 99394 _____ 99213
_____ 99204	_____ 99385	18–39	_____ 99395 _____ 99214
_____ 99205	_____ 99386	40–64	_____ 99396 _____ 99215
	_____ 99387	65+	_____ 99397

Hospital Visits
Initial:
_____ 99221
_____ 99222
_____ 99223
Subsequent:
_____ 99231
_____ 99232
_____ 99233
Discharge:
_____ 99238
_____ 99239
Nursing Facility
Initial:
_____ (99304)
_____ 99305
_____ 99306

Other
_____
_____

Lab:
_____ 80048 Basic metabolic panel
_____ 87110 Chlamydia culture
_____ 85651 ESR; nonautomated
_____ 83001 FSH
_____ 82947 Glucose, blood
_____ 85025 Hemogram (CBC) with differential
_____ 80076 Hepatic function panel
_____ 85018 HGB
_____ 86701 HIV-1
_____ 83002 LH
_____ 80061 Lipid panel
_____ 00017 Lyme antibody

_____ 86308 Monospot test
_____ 88150 Pap
_____ 85610 Prothrombin time
_____ 84152 PSA
_____ 86430 Rheumatoid factor
_____ 82270 Stool hemoccult x 3
_____ 87430 Strep screen
_____ 84478 Triglycerides
_____ 84443 TSH
_____ 81001 UA with microscopy
_____ 87088 UC
_____ 84550 Uric acid, blood
_____ 81025 Urine pregnancy test
_____
_____

Injections:
_____ 90471 admin 1 vac
_____ 90472 each add'l vac
_____ 90716 Chickenpox
_____ 90702 DT
_____ 90700 DTaP
_____ 90657 Influenza 0.25mL
_____ 90658 Influenza 0.5mL
_____ 90710 MMRV, subcutaneous
_____ 90707 MMR
_____ 90649 4vHPV
_____ 90713 Polio vac inactivated (IPV)
_____ 90714 Td
ECG:
_____ 93000 ECG

Other
_____
_____

DAILY JOURNAL #105

DAILY JOURNAL

DATE ___10/19/20-- ___   SHEET NO. ___105___

	RECEIPT NUMBER	DATE	DESCRIPTION CODE	CHARGE	PAYMENT	ADJUSTMENTS	BALANCE	PREVIOUS BALANCE	NAME
1	1098		VOID		—	—			
2	1099	10/19	OV	44 00	—	—			Lund, Laura
3	1100	10/19	OV	44 00	8 80	—			Mendez, Ana
4	1101	10/19	CPE/UA	163 00	—	—			Mitchell, Donald
5	1102	10/19	OV	44 00	—	—			Dayton, Theresa
6	1103	10/19	Nursing home visit	53 00	—	—			Murrary, Raymond
7									
32									
33									
34				Column A	Column B	Column C	Column D	Column E	TOTALS

◀ ALL RECEIPTS MUST BE
IN NUMERICAL ORDER

Proof of Posting

Column E Total $ _____
Plus Column A Total $ _____
Subtotal $ _____
Minus Column B Total $ _____
Equals Column D Total $ _____

Accounts Receivable Control

Previous Balance $ _____
Plus Column A $ _____
Subtotal $ _____
Minus Column B Total $ _____
Present Acc'ts Rec. Balance $ _____

Daily Cash

Opening Cash on Hand
at Beginning of Day $ _____
Cash Received During Day $ _____
Total $ _____

TELEPHONE LOG

TELEPHONE LOG

Date _____

TIME	CALLER	TELEPHONE NUMBER	REASON	DONE

TO-DO LIST

TO-DO LIST

Date _____

RUSH	ITEMS TO DO	DONE

MARC PHAN'S PATIENT ENCOUNTER FORM

No.	Date	Description	Charge	Credit		Current Balance
				Payment	Adjustment	

Patient Information	Patient	Marc Phan

Patient Information

9340 S. Green Street
Address

Chicago, IL 60620-8129
City, State, ZIP

312-555-3344   father 312-555-2577
Home phone   **Work phone**

Tam Phan   father
Responsible person   **Relationship**

University Health Plan,   626033-3
Insurance   **Patient Insurance ID**

Patient _____ Marc Phan _____

Date: 10/24/20--   **Chart #AA031**

Karen Larsen, MD
2235 S. Ridgeway Avenue
Chicago, IL 60623-2240

312-555-6022

Fax: 312-555-0025

Diagnoses:

1. ___ J40 ___

2. ___ L22 ___

3. _____

4. _____

OFFICE VISITS

New Patient	Established Patient

Preventive Medicine

	_____ 99381	under 1 year	_____ 99391	
	_____ 99382	1–4	_____ 99392	_____ 99211
_____ 99202	_____ 99383	5–11	_____ 99393	(99212)
_____ 99203	_____ 99384	12–17	_____ 99394	_____ 99213
_____ 99204	_____ 99385	18–39	_____ 99395	_____ 99214
_____ 99205	_____ 99386	40–64	_____ 99396	_____ 99215
	_____ 99387	65+	_____ 99397	

Hospital Visits
Initial:
_____ 99221
_____ 99222
_____ 99223
Subsequent:
_____ 99231
_____ 99232
_____ 99233
Discharge:
_____ 99238
_____ 99239
Nursing Facility
Initial:
_____ 99304
_____ 99305
_____ 99306

Other
_____
_____

Lab:
_____ 80048 Basic metabolic panel
_____ 87110 Chlamydia culture
_____ 85651 ESR; nonautomated
_____ 83001 FSH
_____ 82947 Glucose, blood
_____ 85025 Hemogram (CBC) with differential
_____ 80076 Hepatic function panel
_____ 85018 HGB
_____ 86701 HIV-1
_____ 83002 LH
_____ 80061 Lipid panel
_____ 86617 Lyme antibody

_____ 86308 Monospot test
_____ 88150 Pap
_____ 85610 Prothrombin time
_____ 84152 PSA
_____ 86430 Rheumatoid factor
_____ 82270 Stool hemoccult x 3
_____ 87430 Strep screen
_____ 84478 Triglycerides
_____ 84443 TSH
_____ 81001 UA with microscopy
_____ 87088 UC
_____ 84550 Uric acid, blood
_____ 81025 Urine pregnancy test
_____
_____

Injections:
_____ 90471 admin 1 vac
_____ 90472 each add'l vac
_____ 90716 Chickenpox
_____ 90702 DT
_____ 90700 DTaP
_____ 90657 Influenza 0.25mL
_____ 90658 Influenza 0.5mL
_____ 90710 MMRV, subcutaneous
_____ 90707 MMR
_____ 90649 4vHPV
_____ 90713 Polio vac inactivated (IPV)
_____ 90714 Td

ECG:
_____ 93000 ECG

Other
_____
_____

2021 Edition

SARAH MORTON'S PATIENT ENCOUNTER FORM

No.	Date	Description	Charge	Credit		Current Balance
				Payment	Adjustment	

Patient Information	
723 W. Sixth Place	
Address	
Chicago, IL 60621-2314	
City, State, ZIP	mother
312-555-2324	312-555-8876
Home phone	**Work phone**
Esther Morton	mother
Responsible person	**Relationship**
Northstar Insurance	7193584C
Insurance	**Patient Insurance ID**

Patient _____ Sarah Morton _____

Date: 10/24/20--   **Chart #**AA028

Karen Larsen, MD
2235 S. Ridgeway Avenue
Chicago, IL 60623-2240

312-555-6022

Fax: 312-555-0025

Diagnoses:

1. M41.20 _____
2. M21.769 _____
3. _____
4. _____

OFFICE VISITS

New Patient	Established Patient

Preventive Medicine

	_____ 99381	under 1 year	_____ 99391
	_____ 99382	1–4	_____ 99392 _____ 99211
_____ 99202	_____ 99383	5–11	_____ 99393 (99212)
_____ 99203	_____ 99384	12–17	_____ 99394 _____ 99213
_____ 99204	_____ 99385	18–39	_____ 99395 _____ 99214
_____ 99205	_____ 99386	40–64	_____ 99396 _____ 99215
	_____ 99387	65+	_____ 99397

Hospital Visits
Initial:
_____ 99221
_____ 99222
_____ 99223
Subsequent:
_____ 99231
_____ 99232
_____ 99233
Discharge:
_____ 99238
_____ 99239
Nursing Facility
Initial:
_____ 99304
_____ 99305
_____ 99306

Other
_____
_____

Lab:
_____ 80048 Basic metabolic panel
_____ 87110 Chlamydia culture
_____ 85651 ESR; nonautomated
_____ 83001 FSH
_____ 82947 Glucose, blood
_____ 85025 Hemogram (CBC) with differential
_____ 80076 Hepatic function panel
_____ 85018 HGB
_____ 86701 HIV-1
_____ 83002 LH
_____ 80061 Lipid panel
_____ 86617 Lyme antibody

_____ 86308 Monospot test
_____ 88150 Pap
_____ 85610 Prothrombin time
_____ 84152 PSA
_____ 86430 Rheumatoid factor
_____ 82270 Stool hemoccult x 3
_____ 87430 Strep screen
_____ 84478 Triglycerides
_____ 84443 TSH
_____ 81001 UA with microscopy
_____ 87088 UC
_____ 84550 Uric acid, blood
_____ 81025 Urine pregnancy test
_____
_____

Injections:
_____ 90471 admin 1 vac
_____ 90472 each add'l vac
_____ 90716 Chickenpox
_____ 90702 DT
_____ 90700 DTaP
_____ 90657 Influenza 0.25mL
_____ 90658 Influenza 0.5mL
_____ 90710 MMRV, subcutaneous
_____ 90707 MMR
_____ 90649 4vHPV
_____ 90713 Polio vac inactivated (IPV)
_____ 90714 Td

ECG:
_____ 93000 ECG

Other
_____
_____

2021 Edition

DORIS CASAGRANDA'S PATIENT ENCOUNTER FORM

No.	Date	Description	Charge	Credit		Current Balance
				Payment	**Adjustment**	

Patient Information	Patient	Doris Casagranda	

3132 W. 42d Street
Address

Chicago, IL 60632-1406
City, State, ZIP

312-555-1200
Home phone

George Casagranda
Responsible person

National Insurance
Insurance

father

312-555-1245
Work phone

father
Relationship

81813B
Patient Insurance ID

Date: 10/24/20--

Karen Larsen, MD
2235 S. Ridgeway Avenue
Chicago, IL 60623-2240

312-555-6022

Fax: 312-555-0025

Chart #AA008

Diagnoses:

1. L73.2

2. _____

3. _____

4. _____

OFFICE VISITS

New Patient	Established Patient

Preventive Medicine

	_____ 99381	under 1 year	_____ 99391	
	_____ 99382	1–4	_____ 99392	_____ 99211
_____ 99202	_____ 99383	5–11	_____ 99393	(99212)
_____ 99203	_____ 99384	12–17	_____ 99394	_____ 99213
_____ 99204	_____ 99385	18–39	_____ 99395	_____ 99214
_____ 99205	_____ 99386	40–64	_____ 99396	_____ 99215
	_____ 99387	65+	_____ 99397	

Hospital Visits
Initial:
_____ 99221
_____ 99222
_____ 99223
Subsequent:
_____ 99231
_____ 99232
_____ 99233
Discharge:
_____ 99238
_____ 99239
Nursing Facility
Initial:
_____ 99304
_____ 99305
_____ 99306

Other

_____
_____

Lab:
_____ 80048 Basic metabolic panel
_____ 87110 Chlamydia culture
_____ 85651 ESR; nonautomated
_____ 83001 FSH
_____ 82947 Glucose, blood
_____ 85025 Hemogram (CBC) with differential
_____ 80076 Hepatic function panel
_____ 85018 HGB
_____ 86701 HIV-1
_____ 83002 LH
_____ 80061 Lipid panel
_____ 86617 Lyme antibody

_____ 86308 Monospot test
_____ 88150 Pap
_____ 85610 Prothrombin time
_____ 84152 PSA
_____ 86430 Rheumatoid factor
_____ 82270 Stool hemoccult x 3
_____ 87430 Strep screen
_____ 84478 Triglycerides
_____ 84443 TSH
_____ 81001 UA with microscopy
_____ 87088 UC
_____ 84550 Uric acid, blood
_____ 81025 Urine pregnancy test

_____
_____

Injections:
_____ 90471 admin 1 vac
_____ 90472 each add'l vac
_____ 90716 Chickenpox
_____ 90702 DT
_____ 90700 DTaP
_____ 90657 Influenza 0.25mL
_____ 90658 Influenza 0.5mL
_____ 90710 MMRV, subcutaneous
_____ 90707 MMR
_____ 90649 4vHPV
_____ 90713 Polio vac inactivated (IPV)
_____ 90714 Td

ECG:
_____ 93000 ECG

Other

_____
_____

2021 Edition

RANDY BURTON'S PATIENT ENCOUNTER FORM

No.	Date	Description	Charge	Credit		Current Balance
				Payment	Adjustment	

Patient Information	Patient	Randy Burton

Patient Information

4345 W. Grace Street
Address

Chicago, IL 60641-6730
City, State, ZIP

312-555-7292
Home phone   **Work phone**

Paul Burton   father
Responsible person   **Relationship**

No insurance
Insurance   **Patient Insurance ID**

Patient _____ Randy Burton _____

Date: 10/24/20--   **Chart #**AA007

Karen Larsen, MD
2235 S. Ridgeway Avenue
Chicago, IL 60623-2240

312-555-6022

Fax: 312-555-0025

Diagnoses:

1. ___ZØØ.129___

2. _____

3. _____

4. _____

OFFICE VISITS

New Patient		Established Patient	

Preventive Medicine

	___ 99381	under 1 year	___ 99391	
	___ 99382	1–4	___ (99392)	___ 99211
___ 99202	___ 99383	5–11	___ 99393	___ 99212
___ 99203	___ 99384	12–17	___ 99394	___ 99213
___ 99204	___ 99385	18–39	___ 99395	___ 99214
___ 99205	___ 99386	40–64	___ 99396	___ 99215
	___ 99387	65+	___ 99397	

Hospital Visits
Initial:
___ 99221
___ 99222
___ 99223
Subsequent:
___ 99231
___ 99232
___ 99233
Discharge:
___ 99238
___ 99239
Nursing Facility
Initial:
___ 99304
___ 99305
___ 99306

Other
_____
_____

Lab:
___ 80048 Basic
    metabolic panel
___ 87110 Chlamydia
    culture
___ 85651 ESR;
    nonautomated
___ 83001 FSH
___ 82947 Glucose,
    blood
___ 85025 Hemogram
    (CBC) with
    differential
___ 80076 Hepatic
    function panel
___ 85018 HGB
___ 86701 HIV-1
___ 83002 LH
___ 80061 Lipid panel
___ 86617 Lyme
    antibody

___ 86308 Monospot
    test
___ 88150 Pap
___ 85610 Prothrombin
    time
___ 84152 PSA
___ 86430 Rheumatoid
    factor
___ 82270 Stool
    hemoccult x 3
___ 87430 Strep screen
___ 84478 Triglycerides
___ 84443 TSH
___ 81001 UA with
    microscopy
___ 87088 UC
___ 84550 Uric acid,
    blood
___ 81025 Urine
    pregnancy test
_____
_____

Injections:
___ (90471) admin 1 vac
___ (90472) each add'l
    vac
___ 90716 Chickenpox
___ 90702 DT
___ (90700) DTaP
___ 90657 Influenza
    0.25mL
___ 90658 Influenza
    0.5mL
___ 90710 MMRV,
    subcutaneous
___ 90707 MMR
___ 90649 4vHPV
___ (90713) Polio vac
    inactivated (IPV)
___ 90714 Td

ECG:
___ 93000 ECG

Other
_____
_____
_____

2021 Edition

GARY ROBERTSON'S PATIENT ENCOUNTER FORM

No.	Date	Description	Charge	Credit Payment	Credit Adjustment	Current Balance

Patient Information

3449 W. Foster Avenue
Address

Chicago, IL 60625-2377
City, State, ZIP

312-555-3360   312-555-8857
Home phone   **Work phone**

self
Responsible person   **Relationship**

Prudential Group Health   ROB512374
Insurance   **Patient Insurance ID**

Patient _____ Gary Robertson _____

Date: 10/24/20--   **Chart #AA038**

Karen Larsen, MD
2235 S. Ridgeway Avenue
Chicago, IL 60623-2240

312-555-6022

Fax: 312-555-0025

Diagnoses:

1. _N10_____
2. _____
3. _____
4. _____

OFFICE VISITS

New Patient	Established Patient

Preventive Medicine

New Patient	Preventive Medicine	Age	Established Patient	
	_____ 99381	under 1 year	_____ 99391	
	_____ 99382	1–4	_____ 99392	
_____ 99202	_____ 99383	5–11	_____ 99393	_____ 99211
_____ 99203	_____ 99384	12–17	_____ 99394	_____ 99212
_____ 99204	_____ 99385	18–39	_____ 99395	_____ 99213
_____ 99205	_____ 99386	40–64	_____ 99396	_____ 99214
	_____ 99387	65+	_____ 99397	_____ 99215

Hospital Visits

Initial:
_____ 99221
_____ 99222
_____ 99223

Subsequent:
x 3 (99231)
_____ 99232
_____ 99233

Discharge:
_____ 99238
_____ 99239

Nursing Facility

Initial:
_____ 99304
_____ 99305
_____ 99306

Other

_____
_____

Visits:
10/18
10/20
10/22

Lab:
_____ 80048 Basic metabolic panel
_____ 87110 Chlamydia culture
_____ 85651 ESR; nonautomated
_____ 83001 FSH
_____ 82947 Glucose, blood
_____ 85025 Hemogram (CBC) with differential
_____ 80076 Hepatic function panel
_____ 85018 HGB
_____ 86701 HIV-1
_____ 83002 LH
_____ 80061 Lipid panel
_____ 86617 Lyme antibody

_____ 86308 Monospot test
_____ 88150 Pap
_____ 85610 Prothrombin time
_____ 84152 PSA
_____ 86430 Rheumatoid factor
_____ 82270 Stool hemoccult x 3
_____ 87430 Strep screen
_____ 84478 Triglycerides
_____ 84443 TSH
_____ 81001 UA with microscopy
_____ 87088 UC
_____ 84550 Uric acid, blood
_____ 81025 Urine pregnancy test

_____
_____

Injections:
_____ 90471 admin 1 vac
_____ 90472 each add'l vac
_____ 90716 Chickenpox
_____ 90702 DT
_____ 90700 DTaP
_____ 90657 Influenza 0.25mL
_____ 90658 Influenza 0.5mL
_____ 90710 MMRV, subcutaneous
_____ 90707 MMR
_____ 90649 4vHPV
_____ 90713 Polio vac inactivated (IPV)
_____ 90714 Td

ECG:
_____ 93000 ECG

Other

_____
_____

CHECKS RECEIVED: DAILY JOURNAL #106

NO. 5321

20 – 62
710

October 24 20 --

PAY
TO THE
ORDER OF Karen Larsen, MD $ 44 00/100

Forty-four and no/100 _____ DOLLARS

First National Bank
Chicago, IL 60623-2791

FOR _____   Charles Jonathan

I:0710 III 0062 242 III 046580 II'

NO. 10082

20 – 62
710

October 24 20 --

PAY
TO THE
ORDER OF Karen Larsen, MD $ 44 and no/100

Forty-four and no/100 _____ DOLLARS

First National Bank
Chicago, IL 60623-2791

FOR Cheng Sun Worker's Comp   Billings, Inc.

I:0710 III 0062 202 III 056232 II'

NO. 152462

20 – 62
710

October 24 20 --

PAY
TO THE
ORDER OF Karen Larsen, MD $ 143 and 20/100

One hundred forty-three and 20/100 _____ DOLLARS

Chicago Bank
Chicago, IL 60621

FOR David Kramer   New York Mutual

I:0710 III 0155 262 III 025592 II'

NO. 152463

20 – 62
710

October 24 20 --

PAY
TO THE
ORDER OF Karen Larsen, MD $ 90 and 40/100

Ninety and 40/100 _____ DOLLARS

Chicago Bank
Chicago, IL 60621

FOR Erin Mitchell   New York Mutual

I:0710 III 0155 262 III 025592 II'

DAILY JOURNAL #106

DAILY JOURNAL

DATE ___October 24, 20-- ___ SHEET NO. ___106___

RECEIPT NUMBER	DATE	DESCRIPTION CODE	CHARGE	PAYMENT	ADJUSTMENTS	BALANCE	PREVIOUS BALANCE	NAME
1								
2								
3								
4								
5								
6								
7								
32								
33								
34								
TOTALS			Column A	Column B	Column C	Column D	Column E	

◄ ALL RECEIPTS MUST BE IN NUMERICAL ORDER

Proof of Posting

Column E Total $ ___
Plus Column A Total $ ___
Subtotal $ ___
Minus Column B Total $ ___
Equals Column D Total $ ___

Accounts Receivable Control

Previous Balance $ ___
Plus Column A $ ___
Subtotal $ ___
Minus Column B Total $ ___
Present Acc'ts Rec. Balance $ ___

Daily Cash

Opening Cash on Hand
at Beginning of Day $ ___
Cash Received During Day $ ___
Total $ ___

MONICA ARMSTRONG'S PATIENT ENCOUNTER FORM

No.	Date	Description	Charge	Credit		Current Balance
				Payment	**Adjustment**	

Patient Information

5518 Monroe Street
Address

Chicago, IL 60644-5519
City, State, ZIP

312-555-4413   312-555-8825
Home phone   **Work phone**

self
Responsible person   **Relationship**

Blue Cross/Blue Shield,   38521
Insurance   **Patient Insurance ID**

Patient _____ Monica Armstrong _____

Date: 10/25/20--   **Chart #AA001**

Karen Larsen, MD
2235 S. Ridgeway Avenue
Chicago, IL 60623-2240

312-555-6022

Fax: 312-555-0025

Diagnoses:

1. ZØ1.419
2. N92.Ø
3. N84.1
4. RØ1.1

OFFICE VISITS

New Patient		**Established Patient**	

Preventive Medicine

New Patient		age	Established Patient	
	_____ 99381	under 1 year	_____ 99391	
	_____ 99382	1–4	_____ 99392	_____ 99211
_____ 99202	_____ 99383	5–11	_____ 99393	_____ 99212
_____ 99203	_____ 99384	12–17	_____ 99394	_____ 99213
_____ 99204	_____ 99385	18–39	_____ 99395	_____ 99214
_____ 99205	_____ 99386	40–64	(99396)	_____ 99215
	_____ 99387	65+	_____ 99397	

Hospital Visits
Initial:
_____ 99221
_____ 99222
_____ 99223
Subsequent:
_____ 99231
_____ 99232
_____ 99233
Discharge:
_____ 99238
_____ 99239
Nursing Facility
Initial:
_____ 99304
_____ 99305
_____ 99306

Other
_____
_____

Lab:
_____ 80048 Basic metabolic panel
_____ 87110 Chlamydia culture
_____ 85651 ESR; nonautomated
_____ 83001 FSH
_____ 82947 Glucose, blood
_____ 85025 Hemogram (CBC) with differential
_____ 80076 Hepatic function panel
_____ 85018 HGB
_____ 86701 HIV-1
_____ 83002 LH
_____ 80061 Lipid panel
_____ 86617 Lyme antibody

_____ 86308 Monospot test
(88150 Pap)
_____ 85610 Prothrombin time
_____ 84152 PSA
_____ 86430 Rheumatoid factor
_____ 82270 Stool hemoccult x 3
_____ 87430 Strep screen
_____ 84478 Triglycerides
_____ 84443 TSH
_____ 81001 UA with microscopy
_____ 87088 UC
_____ 84550 Uric acid, blood
_____ 81025 Urine pregnancy test
_____
_____

Injections:
_____ 90471 admin 1 vac
_____ 90472 each add'l vac
_____ 90716 Chickenpox
_____ 90702 DT
_____ 90700 DTaP
_____ 90657 Influenza 0.25mL
_____ 90658 Influenza 0.5mL
_____ 90710 MMRV, subcutaneous
_____ 90707 MMR
_____ 90649 4vHPV
_____ 90713 Polio vac inactivated (IPV)
_____ 90714 Td
ECG:
_____ 93000 ECG

Other
_____
_____

2021 Edition

JEFFREY KRAMER'S PATIENT ENCOUNTER FORM

No.	Date	Description	Charge	Credit		Current Balance
				Payment	**Adjustment**	

<table>
<tr><th colspan="2">Patient Information</th></tr>
</table>

Patient Information	

510 N. Marine Drive
Address

Chicago, IL 60640-5607
City, State, ZIP

	father
312-555-1913	312-555-8820
Home phone	**Work phone**

Andrew Kramer	father
Responsible person	**Relationship**

Northstar Premium Insurance,	
	KRA9162D
Insurance	**Patient Insurance ID**

Patient _____ Jeffrey Kramer _____

Date: 10/25/20--	**Chart #AA017**

Karen Larsen, MD	**Diagnoses:**
2235 S. Ridgeway Avenue	
Chicago, IL 60623-2240	1. _H66.009_
312-555-6022	2. _H60.399_
Fax: 312-555-0025	3. _____
	4. _____

OFFICE VISITS

New Patient	Established Patient

Preventive Medicine

	_____ 99381	under 1 year	_____ 99391	
	_____ 99382	1–4	_____ 99392	_____ 99211
_____ 99202	_____ 99383	5–11	_____ 99393	(99212)
_____ 99203	_____ 99384	12–17	_____ 99394	_____ 99213
_____ 99204	_____ 99385	18–39	_____ 99395	_____ 99214
_____ 99205	_____ 99386	40–64	_____ 99396	_____ 99215
	_____ 99387	65+	_____ 99397	

Hospital Visits

Initial:
_____ 99221
_____ 99222
_____ 99223

Subsequent:
_____ 99231
_____ 99232
_____ 99233

Discharge:
_____ 99238
_____ 99239

Nursing Facility

Initial:
_____ 99304
_____ 99305
_____ 99306

Other
_____
_____

Lab:
_____ 80048 Basic metabolic panel
_____ 87110 Chlamydia culture
_____ 85651 ESR; nonautomated
_____ 83001 FSH
_____ 82947 Glucose, blood
_____ 85025 Hemogram (CBC) with differential
_____ 80076 Hepatic function panel
_____ 85018 HGB
_____ 86701 HIV-1
_____ 83002 LH
_____ 80061 Lipid panel
_____ 86617 Lyme antibody

_____ 86308 Monospot test
_____ 88150 Pap
_____ 85610 Prothrombin time
_____ 84152 PSA
_____ 86430 Rheumatoid factor
_____ 82270 Stool hemoccult x 3
_____ 87430 Strep screen
_____ 84478 Triglycerides
_____ 84443 TSH
_____ 81001 UA with microscopy
_____ 87088 UC
_____ 84550 Uric acid, blood
_____ 81025 Urine pregnancy test
_____
_____

Injections:
_____ 90471 admin 1 vac
_____ 90472 each add'l vac
_____ 90716 Chickenpox
_____ 90702 DT
_____ 90700 DTaP
_____ 90657 Influenza 0.25mL
_____ 90658 Influenza 0.5mL
_____ 90710 MMRV, subcutaneous
_____ 90707 MMR
_____ 90649 4vHPV
_____ 90713 Polio vac inactivated (IPV)
_____ 90714 Td

ECG:
_____ 93000 ECG

Other
_____
_____

2021 Edition

CHENG SUN'S PATIENT ENCOUNTER FORM

No.	Date	Description	Charge	Credit		Current Balance
				Payment	**Adjustment**	

Patient Information		Patient	Cheng Sun	

Patient Information

2235 W. School Street
Address

Chicago, IL 60618-5785
City, State, ZIP

312-555-3750   312-555-8149
Home phone   Work phone

self
Responsible person   Relationship

Metro State Plan,   CHE5679
Insurance   Patient Insurance ID

Patient _____ Cheng Sun _____

Date: 10/25/20--   **Chart #**AA042

Karen Larsen, MD
2235 S. Ridgeway Avenue
Chicago, IL 60623-2240

312-555-6022

Fax: 312-555-0025

Diagnoses:

1. _Z00.00_

2. _____

3. _____

4. _____

OFFICE VISITS

New Patient	Established Patient

Preventive Medicine

	____ 99381	under 1 year	____ 99391
	____ 99382	1–4	____ 99392	____ 99211
____ 99202	____ 99383	5–11	____ 99393	____ 99212
____ 99203	____ 99384	12–17	____ 99394	____ 99213
____ 99204	____ 99385	18–39	____ 99395	____ 99214
____ 99205	____ 99386	40–64	____ (99396)	____ 99215
	____ 99387	65+	____ 99397	

Hospital Visits

Initial:
____ 99221
____ 99222
____ 99223
Subsequent:
____ 99231
____ 99232
____ 99233
Discharge:
____ 99238
____ 99239

Nursing Facility
Initial:
____ 99304
____ 99305
____ 99306

Other
_____
_____

Lab:
____ (80048) Basic metabolic panel
____ 87110 Chlamydia culture
____ 85651 ESR; nonautomated
____ 83001 FSH
____ 82947 Glucose, blood
____ 85025 Hemogram (CBC) with differential
____ 80076 Hepatic function panel
____ 85018 HGB
____ 86701 HIV-1
____ 83002 LH
____ (80061) Lipid panel
____ 86617 Lyme antibody

____ 86308 Monospot test
____ 88150 Pap
____ 85610 Prothrombin time
____ (84152) PSA
____ 86430 Rheumatoid factor
____ (82270) Stool hemoccult x 3
____ 87430 Strep screen
____ 84478 Triglycerides
____ 84443 TSH
____ (81001) UA with microscopy
____ 87088 UC
____ 84550 Uric acid, blood
____ 81025 Urine pregnancy test
_____
_____

Injections:
____ 90471 admin 1 vac
____ 90472 each add'l vac
____ 90716 Chickenpox
____ 90702 DT
____ 90700 DTaP
____ 90657 Influenza 0.25mL
____ 90658 Influenza 0.5mL
____ 90710 MMRV, subcutaneous
____ 90707 MMR
____ 90649 4vHPV
____ 90713 Polio vac inactivated (IPV)
____ 90714 Td

ECG:
____ 93000 ECG

Other
_____
_____

2021 Edition

CHECKS RECEIVED: DAILY JOURNAL #107

NO. 1532106   20 – 62
710

October 25   20 --

PAY
TO THE
ORDER OF   Karen Larsen, MD $ 192 and 80/100

One hundred ninety-two and 80/100 _____ DOLLARS

First National Bank
Chicago, IL 60623-2791

FOR   Monica Armstrong   BC/BS

⑈0710 ⑈⑈0062 242 ⑈046580 ⑈⑈

NO. 1909242   20 – 62
710

October 25   20 --

PAY
TO THE
ORDER OF   Karen Larsen, MD $ 93 and no/100

Ninety-three and no/100 _____ DOLLARS

First National Bank
Chicago, IL 60623-2791

FOR   Laura Lund   Employee Benefit

⑈0710 ⑈⑈0062 202 ⑈056232 ⑈⑈

NO. 19646482   20 – 62
710

October 25   20 --

PAY
TO THE
ORDER OF   Karen Larsen, MD $ 222 and 40/100

Two hundred twenty-two and 40/100 _____ DOLLARS

Chicago Bank
Chicago, IL 60621

FOR   Sara Babcock   Kaiser Insurance

⑈0710 ⑈⑈0155 262 ⑈025592 ⑈⑈

NO. 1227847   20 – 62
710

October 25   20 --

PAY
TO THE
ORDER OF   Karen Larsen, MD $ 147 and 00/100

One hundred forty-seven and 00/100 _____ DOLLARS

First National Bank
Chicago, IL 60623-2791

FOR   Gary Robertson   Prudential Group Health

⑈0710 ⑈⑈0062 081 ⑈502249 ⑈⑈

DAILY JOURNAL #107

DAILY JOURNAL

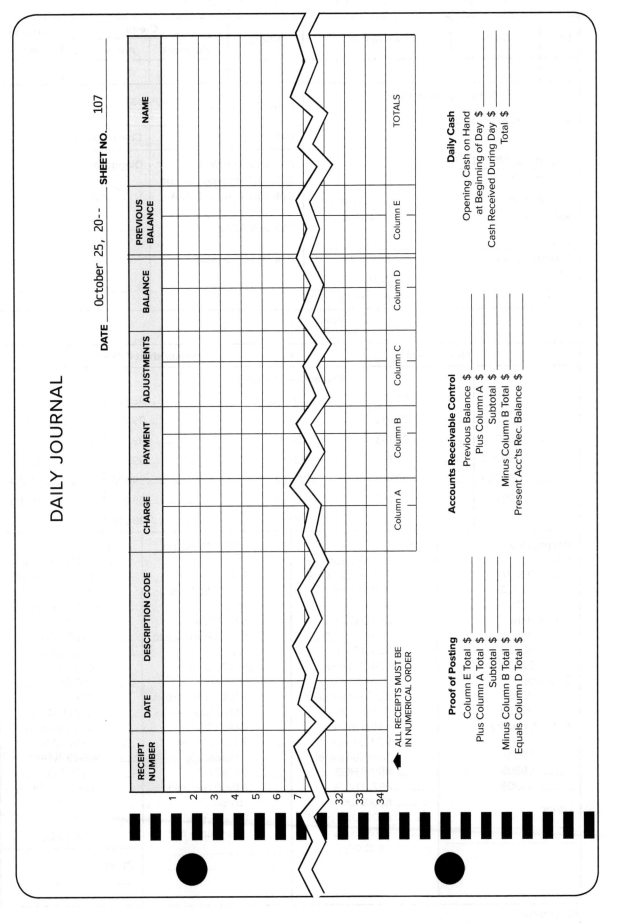

DATE __October 25, 20--__ SHEET NO. __107__

RECEIPT NUMBER	DATE	DESCRIPTION CODE	CHARGE	PAYMENT	ADJUSTMENTS	BALANCE	PREVIOUS BALANCE	NAME
1								
2								
3								
4								
5								
6								
7								
32								
33								
34								
		TOTALS	Column A	Column B	Column C	Column D	Column E	

◄ ALL RECEIPTS MUST BE IN NUMERICAL ORDER

Proof of Posting

Column E Total $ _____
Plus Column A Total $ _____
Subtotal $ _____
Minus Column B Total $ _____
Equals Column D Total $ _____

Accounts Receivable Control

Previous Balance $ _____
Plus Column A $ _____
Subtotal $ _____
Minus Column B Total $ _____
Present Acc'ts Rec. Balance $ _____

Daily Cash

Opening Cash on Hand
at Beginning of Day $ _____
Cash Received During Day $ _____
Total $ _____

THOMAS BAAB'S PATIENT ENCOUNTER FORM

No.	Date	Description	Charge	Credit		Current Balance
				Payment	**Adjustment**	

Patient Information	Patient	Thomas Baab	

Patient Information

5015 N. Ridgeway Avenue
Address

Chicago, IL 60625-1220
City, State, ZIP

312-555-3478   312-555-8830
Home phone   **Work phone**

self

Responsible person   **Relationship**
Blue Cross/Blue Shield
                           21659
Insurance   **Patient Insurance ID**

Patient _____ Thomas Baab _____

Date: 10/26/20-- | **Chart #AA002**

Karen Larsen, MD
2235 S. Ridgeway Avenue
Chicago, IL 60623-2240

312-555-6022

Fax: 312-555-0025

Diagnoses:

1. ___ E78.5 ___

2. _____

3. _____

4. _____

OFFICE VISITS

New Patient	Established Patient

Preventive Medicine

	_____ 99381	under 1 year	_____ 99391	
	_____ 99382	1–4	_____ 99392	_____ 99211
_____ 99202	_____ 99383	5–11	_____ 99393	(99212)
_____ 99203	_____ 99384	12–17	_____ 99394	_____ 99213
_____ 99204	_____ 99385	18–39	_____ 99395	_____ 99214
_____ 99205	_____ 99386	40–64	_____ 99396	_____ 99215
	_____ 99387	65+	_____ 99397	

Hospital Visits
Initial:
_____ 99221
_____ 99222
_____ 99223
Subsequent:
_____ 99231
_____ 99232
_____ 99233
Discharge:
_____ 99238
_____ 99239
Nursing Facility
Initial:
_____ 99304
_____ 99305
_____ 99306

Other
_____
_____

Lab:
_____ 80048 Basic
          metabolic panel
_____ 87110 Chlamydia
          culture
_____ 85651 ESR;
          nonautomated
_____ 83001 FSH
_____ 82947 Glucose,
          blood
_____ 85025 Hemogram
          (CBC) with
          differential
_____ 80076 Hepatic
          function panel
_____ 85018 HGB
_____ 86701 HIV-1
_____ 83002 LH
_____ 80061 Lipid panel
_____ 86617 Lyme
          antibody

_____ 86308 Monospot
          test
_____ 88150 Pap
_____ 85610 Prothrombin
          time
_____ 84152 PSA
_____ 86430 Rheumatoid
          factor
_____ 82270 Stool
          hemoccult x 3
_____ 87430 Strep screen
_____ 84478 Triglycerides
_____ 84443 TSH
_____ 81001 UA with
          microscopy
_____ 87088 UC
_____ 84550 Uric acid,
          blood
_____ 81025 Urine
          pregnancy test
_____
_____

Injections:
_____ 90471 admin 1 vac
_____ 90472 each add'l
          vac
_____ 90716 Chickenpox
_____ 90702 DT
_____ 90700 DTaP
_____ 90657 Influenza
          0.25mL
_____ 90658 Influenza
          0.5mL
_____ 90710 MMRV,
          subcutaneous
_____ 90707 MMR
_____ 90649 4vHPV
_____ 90713 Polio vac
          inactivated (IPV)
_____ 90714 Td

ECG:
_____ 93000 ECG

Other
_____
_____

2021 Edition

Working Papers

THERESA DAYTON'S PATIENT ENCOUNTER FORM

No.	Date	Description	Charge	Credit		Current Balance
				Payment	**Adjustment**	

Patient Information	Patient _____ Theresa Dayton _____

Patient Information

105 W. Chestnut Street
Address

Chicago, IL 60610-2816
City, State, ZIP

312-555-2231   312-555-2583
Home phone   Work phone

self

Responsible person   Relationship
Blue Cross/Blue Shield
                             DAY512374
Insurance   Patient Insurance ID

Patient _____ Theresa Dayton _____

Date: 10/26/20--   **Chart #AA012**

Karen Larsen, MD   **Diagnoses:**
2235 S. Ridgeway Avenue
Chicago, IL 60623-2240   1. __G44.209__

312-555-6022   2. _____

Fax: 312-555-0025   3. _____

                              4. _____

OFFICE VISITS

New Patient	Established Patient

Preventive Medicine

	_____ 99381	under 1 year	_____ 99391
	_____ 99382	1–4	_____ 99392	_____ 99211
_____ 99202	_____ 99383	5–11	_____ 99393	(99212)
_____ 99203	_____ 99384	12–17	_____ 99394	_____ 99213
_____ 99204	_____ 99385	18–39	_____ 99395	_____ 99214
_____ 99205	_____ 99386	40–64	_____ 99396	_____ 99215
	_____ 99387	65+	_____ 99397	

Hospital Visits
Initial:
_____ 99221
_____ 99222
_____ 99223
Subsequent:
_____ 99231
_____ 99232
_____ 99233
Discharge:
_____ 99238
_____ 99239
Nursing Facility
Initial:
_____ 99304
_____ 99305
_____ 99306

Other

_____
_____

Lab:
_____ 80048 Basic
   metabolic panel
_____ 87110 Chlamydia
   culture
_____ 85651 ESR;
   nonautomated
_____ 83001 FSH
_____ 82947 Glucose,
   blood
_____ 85025 Hemogram
   (CBC) with
   differential
_____ 80076 Hepatic
   function panel
_____ 85018 HGB
_____ 86701 HIV-1
_____ 83002 LH
_____ 80061 Lipid panel
_____ 86617 Lyme
   antibody

_____ 86308 Monospot
   test
_____ 88150 Pap
_____ 85610 Prothrombin
   time
_____ 84152 PSA
_____ 86430 Rheumatoid
   factor
_____ 82270 Stool
   hemoccult x 3
_____ 87430 Strep screen
_____ 84478 Triglycerides
_____ 84443 TSH
_____ 81001 UA with
   microscopy
_____ 87088 UC
_____ 84550 Uric acid,
   blood
_____ 81025 Urine
   pregnancy test

_____
_____

Injections:
_____ 90471 admin 1 vac
_____ 90472 each add'l
   vac
_____ 90716 Chickenpox
_____ 90702 DT
_____ 90700 DTaP
_____ 90657 Influenza
   0.25mL
_____ 90658 Influenza
   0.5mL
_____ 90710 MMRV,
   subcutaneous
_____ 90707 MMR
_____ 90649 4vHPV
_____ 90713 Polio vac
   inactivated (IPV)
_____ 90714 Td
ECG:
_____ 93000 ECG

Other

_____
_____

2021 Edition

ARDIS MATTHEWS' PATIENT ENCOUNTER FORM

No.	Date	Description	Charge	Credit		Current Balance
				Payment	**Adjustment**	

Patient Information

2000 North Lincoln Park West
Address

Chicago, IL 60614-1411
City, State, ZIP

312-555-3178   312-555-8848
Home phone   **Work phone**

Earl Matthews   husband
Responsible person   **Relationship**

Arling Employee Plan,   1037942-01
Insurance   **Patient Insurance ID**

Patient _____ Ardis Matthews _____

Date: 10/26/20-- | **Chart #**AA022

Karen Larsen, MD
2235 S. Ridgeway Avenue
Chicago, IL 60623-2240

312-555-6022

Fax: 312-555-0025

Diagnoses:

1. _____ R51.9 _____

2. _____

3. _____

4. _____

OFFICE VISITS

New Patient	Established Patient

Preventive Medicine

	_____ 99381	under 1 year	_____ 99391	
	_____ 99382	1–4	_____ 99392	_____ 99211
_____ 99202	_____ 99383	5–11	_____ 99393	(99212)
_____ 99203	_____ 99384	12–17	_____ 99394	_____ 99213
_____ 99204	_____ 99385	18–39	_____ 99395	_____ 99214
_____ 99205	_____ 99386	40–64	_____ 99396	_____ 99215
	_____ 99387	65+	_____ 99397	

Hospital Visits
Initial:
_____ 99221
_____ 99222
_____ 99223
Subsequent:
_____ 99231
_____ 99232
_____ 99233
Discharge:
_____ 99238
_____ 99239
Nursing Facility
Initial:
_____ 99304
_____ 99305
_____ 99306

Other
_____
_____

Lab:
_____ 80048 Basic
  metabolic panel
_____ 87110 Chlamydia
  culture
_____ 85651 ESR;
  nonautomated
_____ 83001 FSH
_____ 82947 Glucose,
  blood
_____ 85025 Hemogram
  (CBC) with
  differential
_____ 80076 Hepatic
  function panel
_____ 85018 HGB
_____ 86701 HIV-1
_____ 83002 LH
_____ 80061 Lipid panel
_____ 86617 Lyme
  antibody

_____ 86308 Monospot
  test
_____ 88150 Pap
_____ 85610 Prothrombin
  time
_____ 84152 PSA
_____ 86430 Rheumatoid
  factor
_____ 82270 Stool
  hemoccult x 3
_____ 87430 Strep screen
_____ 84478 Triglycerides
_____ 84443 TSH
_____ 81001 UA with
  microscopy
_____ 87088 UC
_____ 84550 Uric acid,
  blood
_____ 81025 Urine
  pregnancy test
_____
_____

Injections:
_____ 90471 admin 1 vac
_____ 90472 each add'l
  vac
_____ 90716 Chickenpox
_____ 90702 DT
_____ 90700 DTaP
_____ 90657 Influenza
  0.25mL
_____ 90658 Influenza
  0.5mL
_____ 90710 MMRV,
  subcutaneous
_____ 90707 MMR
_____ 90649 4vHPV
_____ 90713 Polio vac
  inactivated (IPV)
_____ 90714 Td

ECG:
_____ 93000 ECG

Other
_____
_____

2021 Edition

ANA MENDEZ'S PATIENT ENCOUNTER FORM

No.	Date	Description	Charge	Credit		Current Balance
				Payment	**Adjustment**	

Patient Information		Patient	Ana Mendez	

Patient Information

3457 W. 63d Place
_____
Address

Chicago, IL 60629-4270
_____
City, State, ZIP

312-555-3606
_____
Home phone   Work phone

self
_____
Responsible person   Relationship

Blue Cross & Blue Shield,   874669
_____
Insurance   Patient Insurance ID

Patient _____ Ana Mendez _____

Date: 10/26/20--   **Chart #AA024**

Karen Larsen, MD
2235 S. Ridgeway Avenue
Chicago, IL 60623-2240

312-555-6022

Fax: 312-555-0025

Diagnoses:

1. ___ JØ1.9Ø ___

2. _____

3. _____

4. _____

OFFICE VISITS

New Patient	Established Patient

Preventive Medicine

New Patient				Established Patient	
	_____ 99381	under 1 year	_____ 99391		
	_____ 99382	1–4	_____ 99392	_____ 99211	
_____ 99202	_____ 99383	5–11	_____ 99393	(99212)	
_____ 99203	_____ 99384	12–17	_____ 99394	_____ 99213	
_____ 99204	_____ 99385	18–39	_____ 99395	_____ 99214	
_____ 99205	_____ 99386	40–64	_____ 99396	_____ 99215	
	_____ 99387	65+	_____ 99397		

Hospital Visits

Initial:
_____ 99221
_____ 99222
_____ 99223

Subsequent:
_____ 99231
_____ 99232
_____ 99233

Discharge:
_____ 99238
_____ 99239

Nursing Facility

Initial:
_____ 99304
_____ 99305
_____ 99306

Other

_____
_____

Lab:

_____ 80048 Basic metabolic panel
_____ 87110 Chlamydia culture
_____ 85651 ESR; nonautomated
_____ 83001 FSH
_____ 82947 Glucose, blood
_____ 85025 Hemogram (CBC) with differential
_____ 80076 Hepatic function panel
_____ 85018 HGB
_____ 86701 HIV-1
_____ 83002 LH
_____ 80061 Lipid panel
_____ 86617 Lyme antibody

_____ 86308 Monospot test
_____ 88150 Pap
_____ 85610 Prothrombin time
_____ 84152 PSA
_____ 86430 Rheumatoid factor
_____ 82270 Stool hemoccult x 3
_____ 87430 Strep screen
_____ 84478 Triglycerides
_____ 84443 TSH
_____ 81001 UA with microscopy
_____ 87088 UC
_____ 84550 Uric acid, blood
_____ 81025 Urine pregnancy test

_____
_____

Injections:

_____ 90471 admin 1 vac
_____ 90472 each add'l vac
_____ 90716 Chickenpox
_____ 90702 DT
_____ 90700 DTaP
_____ 90657 Influenza 0.25mL
_____ 90658 Influenza 0.5mL
_____ 90710 MMRV, subcutaneous
_____ 90707 MMR
_____ 90649 4vHPV
_____ 90713 Polio vac inactivated (IPV)
_____ 90714 Td

ECG:
_____ 93000 ECG

Other

_____
_____

2021 Edition

GARY ROBERTSON'S PATIENT ENCOUNTER FORM

No.	Date	Description	Charge	Credit		Current Balance
				Payment	**Adjustment**	

Patient Information	**Patient** _____ Gary Robertson

Patient Information

3449 W. Foster Avenue
_____
Address

Chicago, IL 60625-2377
_____
City, State, ZIP

312-555-3360   312-555-8857
Home phone   **Work phone**

self
_____
Responsible person   **Relationship**

Prudential Group Health   ROB512374
Insurance   **Patient Insurance ID**

Patient _____ Gary Robertson

Date: 10/26/20--   **Chart #**AA038

Karen Larsen, MD
2235 S. Ridgeway Avenue
Chicago, IL 60623-2240

312-555-6022

Fax: 312-555-0025

Diagnoses:

1. __N10__

2. _____

3. _____

4. _____

OFFICE VISITS

New Patient		**Established Patient**	

Preventive Medicine

New Patient				Established Patient	
	_____ 99381	under 1 year	_____ 99391		
	_____ 99382	1–4	_____ 99392	_____ 99211	
_____ 99202	_____ 99383	5–11	_____ 99393	(99212)	
_____ 99203	_____ 99384	12–17	_____ 99394	_____ 99213	
_____ 99204	_____ 99385	18–39	_____ 99395	_____ 99214	
_____ 99205	_____ 99386	40–64	_____ 99396	_____ 99215	
	_____ 99387	65+	_____ 99397		

Hospital Visits
Initial:
_____ 99221
_____ 99222
_____ 99223
Subsequent:
_____ 99231
_____ 99232
_____ 99233
Discharge:
_____ 99238
_____ 99239
Nursing Facility
Initial:
_____ 99304
_____ 99305
_____ 99306

Other
_____
_____

Lab:
_____ 80048 Basic metabolic panel
_____ 87110 Chlamydia culture
_____ 85651 ESR; nonautomated
_____ 83001 FSH
_____ 82947 Glucose, blood
_____ 85025 Hemogram (CBC) with differential
_____ 80076 Hepatic function panel
_____ 85018 HGB
_____ 86701 HIV-1
_____ 83002 LH
_____ 80061 Lipid panel
_____ 86617 Lyme antibody

_____ 86308 Monospot test
_____ 88150 Pap
_____ 85610 Prothrombin time
_____ 84152 PSA
_____ 86430 Rheumatoid factor
_____ 82270 Stool hemoccult x 3
_____ 87430 Strep screen
_____ 84478 Triglycerides
_____ 84443 TSH
_____ 81001 UA with microscopy
_____ 87088 UC
_____ 84550 Uric acid, blood
_____ 81025 Urine pregnancy test
_____
_____

Injections:
_____ 90471 admin 1 vac
_____ 90472 each add'l vac
_____ 90716 Chickenpox
_____ 90702 DT
_____ 90700 DTaP
_____ 90657 Influenza 0.25mL
_____ 90658 Influenza 0.5mL
_____ 90710 MMRV, subcutaneous
_____ 90707 MMR
_____ 90649 4vHPV
_____ 90713 Polio vac inactivated (IPV)
_____ 90714 Td

ECG:
_____ 93000 ECG

Other
_____
_____

FLORENCE SHERMAN'S PATIENT ENCOUNTER FORM

No.	Date	Description	Charge	Credit		Current Balance
				Payment	Adjustment	

Patient Information

6111 N. Lincoln Avenue
Address

Chicago, IL 60608-3173
City, State, ZIP

312-555-1217
Home phone   **Work phone**

self
Responsible person   **Relationship**

Medicare   4GM3-PT6-XR91
Insurance   **Patient Insurance ID**

Patient _____ Florence Sherman _____

Date: 10/26/20--   **Chart #AA040**

Karen Larsen, MD
2235 S. Ridgeway Avenue
Chicago, IL 60623-2240

312-555-6022

Fax: 312-555-0025

Diagnoses:

1. ___ S00.93XA ___
2. ___ S40.029A ___
3. _____
4. _____

OFFICE VISITS

New Patient	Established Patient

Preventive Medicine

	_____ 99381	under 1 year	_____ 99391	
	_____ 99382	1–4	_____ 99392	_____ 99211
_____ 99202	_____ 99383	5–11	_____ 99393	(99212)
_____ 99203	_____ 99384	12–17	_____ 99394	_____ 99213
_____ 99204	_____ 99385	18–39	_____ 99395	_____ 99214
_____ 99205	_____ 99386	40–64	_____ 99396	_____ 99215
	_____ 99387	65+	_____ 99397	

Hospital Visits
Initial:
_____ 99221
_____ 99222
_____ 99223
Subsequent:
_____ 99231
_____ 99232
_____ 99233
Discharge:
_____ 99238
_____ 99239
Nursing Facility
Initial:
_____ 99304
_____ 99305
_____ 99306

Other
_____
_____

Lab:
_____ 80048 Basic metabolic panel
_____ 87110 Chlamydia culture
_____ 85651 ESR; nonautomated
_____ 83001 FSH
_____ 82947 Glucose, blood
_____ 85025 Hemogram (CBC) with differential
_____ 80076 Hepatic function panel
_____ 85018 HGB
_____ 86701 HIV-1
_____ 83002 LH
_____ 80061 Lipid panel
_____ 86617 Lyme antibody

_____ 86308 Monospot test
_____ 88150 Pap
_____ 85610 Prothrombin time
_____ 84152 PSA
_____ 86430 Rheumatoid factor
_____ 82270 Stool hemoccult x 3
_____ 87430 Strep screen
_____ 84478 Triglycerides
_____ 84443 TSH
_____ 81001 UA with microscopy
_____ 87088 UC
_____ 84550 Uric acid, blood
_____ 81025 Urine pregnancy test
_____
_____

Injections:
_____ 90471 admin 1 vac
_____ 90472 each add'l vac
_____ 90716 Chickenpox
_____ 90702 DT
_____ 90700 DTaP
_____ 90657 Influenza 0.25mL
_____ 90658 Influenza 0.5mL
_____ 90710 MMRV, subcutaneous
_____ 90707 MMR
_____ 90649 4vHPV
_____ 90713 Polio vac inactivated (IPV)
_____ 90714 Td
ECG:
_____ 93000 ECG

Other
_____
_____

2021 Edition

CHECKS RECEIVED: DAILY JOURNAL #108

NO. 439205   20 – 62
710

October 26   20 --

PAY
TO THE
ORDER OF   Karen Larsen, MD $ 114 and ⁿᵒ/100

One hundred fourteen and ⁰⁰/100 _____ — DOLLARS

First National Bank
Chicago, IL 60623-2791

FOR   Todd Grant   Prudential Plan

⑈0710 ⑊0062 081 ⑊502249 ⑈

NO. 1983425   20 – 62
710

October 26   20 --

PAY
TO THE
ORDER OF   Karen Larsen, MD $ 42 and ⁴⁰/100

Forty-two and ⁴⁰/100 _____ — DOLLARS

First National Bank
Chicago, IL 60623-2791

FOR   Raymond Murrary   Medicare

⑈0710 ⑊0062 242 ⑊046580 ⑈

NO. 475   20 – 62
710

October 26   20 --

PAY
TO THE
ORDER OF   Karen Larsen, MD $ 86 and ²⁰/100

Eighty-six and ²⁰/100 _____ — DOLLARS

First National Bank
Chicago, IL 60623-2791

FOR _____   Clarence Rogers

⑈0710 ⑊0062 202 ⑊056232 ⑈

NO. 704382   20 – 62
710

October 26   20 --

PAY
TO THE
ORDER OF   Karen Larsen, MD $ 66 and ⁴⁰/100

Sixty-six and ⁴⁰/100 _____ — DOLLARS

Chicago Bank
Chicago, IL 60621

FOR   Stephen Villano   Employee Benefit Plan

⑈0710 ⑊0155 262 ⑊025592 ⑈

DAILY JOURNAL #108

DAILY JOURNAL

DATE ___October 26, 20- -___   SHEET NO. ___108___

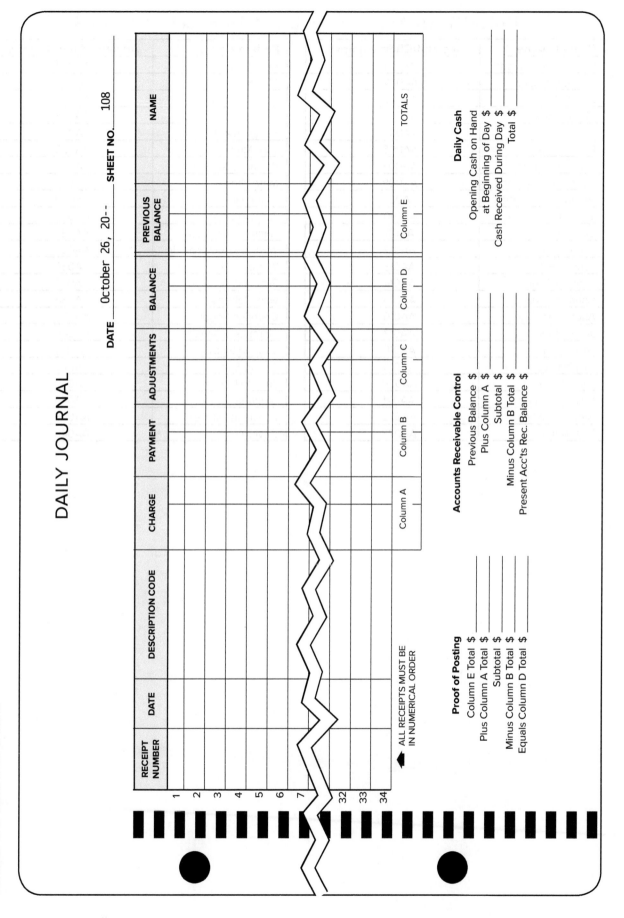

RECEIPT NUMBER	DATE	DESCRIPTION CODE	CHARGE	PAYMENT	ADJUSTMENTS	BALANCE	PREVIOUS BALANCE	NAME
1								
2								
3								
4								
5								
6								
7								
32								
33								
34								
			Column A	Column B	Column C	Column D	Column E	TOTALS

◄ ALL RECEIPTS MUST BE IN NUMERICAL ORDER

Proof of Posting

Column E Total $ _____
Plus Column A Total $ _____
Subtotal $ _____
Minus Column B Total $ _____
Equals Column D Total $ _____

Accounts Receivable Control

Previous Balance $ _____
Plus Column A $ _____
Subtotal $ _____
Minus Column B Total $ _____
Present Acc'ts Rec. Balance $ _____

Daily Cash

Opening Cash on Hand
at Beginning of Day $ _____
Cash Received During Day $ _____
Total $ _____

WP 86

PATIENT NAMES AND ACCOUNT/CHART NUMBERS

Patient Name	Account/Chart Number	Patient Name	Account/Chart Number
Monica T. Armstrong	AA001	Ana Mendez	AA024
Thomas R. Baab	AA002	Alan Mitchell	AA025
Sara Babcock	AA003	Donald Mitchell	AA026
Allison Becker	AA004	Esther Morton	AA027
Michael Becker	AA005	Sarah Morton	AA028
Paul Burton	AA006	Clair Munson	AA029
Randy T. Burton	AA007	Raymond Murrary	AA030
Doris L. Casagranda	AA008	Marc Phan	AA031
George Casagranda	AA009	Tam Phan	AA032
Joseph W. Castro	AA010	Janet Provost	AA033
Lena Crac	AA011	Nancy J. Richards	AA034
Theresa Dayton	AA012	Warren L. Richards, Jr.	AA035
Todd Grant	AA013	Warren Richards	AA036
Alma Jackson	AA014	Suzanne Roberts	AA037
Charles Jonathan III	AA015	Gary Robertson	AA038
Andrew Kramer	AA016	Clarence Rogers	AA039
Jeffrey Kramer	AA017	Florence Sherman	AA040
Jack Kyser	AA018	Eugene Sinclair	AA041
Cynthia Kyser	AA019	Cheng Sun	AA042
Laura Lund	AA020	Juan Villano	AA043
Lawrence Lund	AA021	Stephen Villano	AA044
Ardis Matthews	AA022	Erin Jean Mitchell	AA045
Earl Matthews	AA023	David Kramer	AA046